PAIN

ACUTE AND CHRONIC

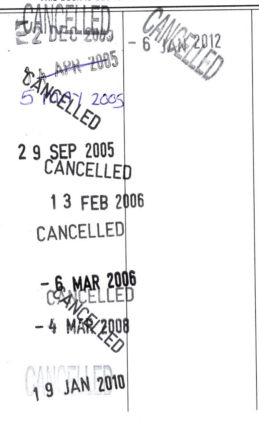
Don Gresswell Ltd., London, N21 Cat. No. 1207   DG 02242/71

PAIN
ACUTE AND CHRONIC

Edward A Shipton
MBChB, DA, FFA, FRCA (Hon), M MED, D MED

Full Professor and Academic Head
Department of Anaesthesia
University of Otago
Christchurch
New Zealand

A member of the Hodder Headline Group
LONDON
Co-published in the United States of America by Oxford University Press Inc., New York

First published in South Africa in 1993 by
Witwatersrand University Press, Johannesburg

Second edition published in Great Britain in 1999 by
Arnold, a member of the Hodder Headline Group,
338 Euston Road, London NW1 3BH

http://www.arnoldpublishers.com

Co-published in the United States of America by
Oxford University Press Inc.,
198 Madison Avenue, New York, NY 10016
Oxford is a registered trademark of Oxford University Press

Whilst the advice and information in this book are believed to be true and
accurate at the date of going to press, neither the author not the publisher can
accept any legal responsibility or liability for any errors or omissions that may
be made. In particular (but without limiting the generality of the preceding
disclaimer) every effort has been made to check drug dosages; however, it is
still possible that errors have been missed. Furthermore, dosage schedules are
constantly being revised and new side-effects recognized. For these reasons the
reader is strongly urged to consult the drug companies' printed instructions
before administering any of the drugs recommended in this book.

British Library Cataloguing in Publication Data
A catalogue record for this book is available from the British Library

Library of Congress Cataloging-in-Publication Data
A catalog record for this book is available from the Library of Congress

ISBN 0 340 64612 8

2 3 4 5 6 7 8 9 10

Publisher: Jo Koster
Project Editor: Melissa Morton
Production Editor: Rada Radojicic
Production Controller: Sarah Kett
Cover Design: Richard Kwan

Typeset in 9/11pt Palatino by Saxon Graphics Ltd, Derby
Printed and bound in Great Britain by The Bath Press, Bath

What do you think about this book? Or any other Arnold title?
Please send your comments to feedback.arnold@hodder.co.uk

CONTENTS

To my family, who have filled my life with so much love, joy, and purpose –
my wife, Elspeth, and my children, Catherine, David and Ashleigh.

FOREWORD

The field of pain management was launched by the publication of the first edition of John J Bonica's *Management of Pain* in 1953. His experiences in World War II had made it clear to him that pain was more than a by-product of illness or disease. He first recognized that the complexities of pain diagnosis and management were beyond the knowledge and skills of any one health care provider. He called for research, both basic and clinical, better education of health care providers, increased scientific and medical interchange of information and the recognition of pain management as a bona fide medical treatment specialty.

It is now 46 years since his clarion call. If he were still alive to review the status of pain as this millenium comes to a close, he would be very pleased. Not that we have eliminated the scourge of pain, as that is not true, especially in the less developed regions of the world. What has been accomplished is reflected in the contents of this comprehensive textbook about pain management. There are now pain clinics located in every developed country in addition to which there are many that are still in the process of development. Regional, national and international societies devoted to pain research and pain management have evolved and are very healthy. Clinicians and scientists can attend meetings focused upon pain to hear the latest research and clinical observations. Journals, web pages, books and multimedia shows about pain are now readily available. The scientific basis of pain management has been dramatically broadened. Animal models for human clinical pain states have permitted the study of chronic pain phenomena. New technologies such as MRI and PET scanning have offered windows on the nervous system and its functioning. Finally, the public has become aware of and interested in many of the issues in pain research and management, as reflected by the articles in news media, popular journals and books.

The shift to outcomes-based medicine will effect pain management, as many of the things that we do for patients in pain lack good data on efficacy. Fortunately, leaders of the pain world have initiated the development of proper clinical trials to validate our patients' care strategies, and we will not be left behind in this new development in health care. Better epidemiological studies will demonstrate the need for pain management services in every society. Professorial pronouncements are no longer the standard of care; instead we look for properly conducted clinical trials. This means that we are measuring relevant outcomes, which is not an easy issue in pain patients. Patient self-reported pain levels are only one of the many measures of adequate treatment. Others include functional status, health care consumption and work status. It is, after all, the disability ascribed to pain that is the major cost of pain to any industrialized society.

However, we must not lose sight of the primary reasons for the existence of the profession of medicine: to provide information, guidance, prognosis, sympathy and caring for those who are ill. Such tasks are hard to quantify and do not find much favour with those who pay the bills for health care. They do not lend themselves to a numerical code for services rendered. It is hard to determine their efficacy. The needs of different patients may vary widely. The addition of technology to the physician's armamentarium is relatively new in our history. Pills, injections, operations, behavioural engineering and physical therapies are important, but they are not sufficient for the pain clinician. A broad, biopsychosocial perspective on the pain patient is required to confront adequately all of the issues that impair normal functioning.

There is no agreement upon the proper training and strategies for the pain management specialist. We have little data on the outcomes of alternative management strategies. Vast sums are spent on high technology interventions with little data on efficacy. The biomedical model still reigns supreme in health care and in pain management. The roles of cognitive, affective and environmental factors are often not considered by physicians who assess and treat those who complain of pain. Increasing evidence from clinical studies suggests that past pain experiences and anticipated consequences play a large role in the interpretation of stimuli from within and outside the body. We must learn how to integrate this information into our practices.

This comprehensive text covers all the contemporary bases of the sciences basic to pain and the management of patients with acute and chronic pain.

Professor Shipton has read widely and distilled the essence of each of the facets of pain treatment. He has put great efforts into the development of this text. Books of this quality will advance our field by providing enhanced education for our colleagues, our students and trainees. Our patients also owe him a great deal of gratitude.

John D Loeser, MD
University of Washington School of Medicine,
Seattle, USA
Immediate Past President:
International Association for
the Study of Pain

PREFACE

Pain medicine is rapidly approaching recognition as a speciality in its own right. However, if pain management specialists and pain relief units are to survive, their efficacy and relative value compared with other forms of health care will have to demonstrated. There has been a shift from inpatient to outpatient care, as well as a shift towards outcome-based medical practice and research of pain management.

The scientific study of pain has flourished over the past two decades. New concepts in the management of pain have come about from strengthening the alliance between basic science and clinical practice. There has been an explosion of knowledge in the basic sciences in addition to enormous advances in the development of basic research in the study of pain, with clinical application relevant to acute and chronic (including cancer) pain. A revolution in molecular biology has allowed, for the first time, the study of pain at the level of the gene. Advances in neurotransmitter and receptor pharmacology have allowed the development of neurotransmitter antagonists, the modulation of ionic channels and the use of enzyme inhibitors.

In acute pain, it is becoming increasingly clear that one remedy for poor pain management lies not so much in the development of new techniques as in the development of acute pain services to exploit existing expertise. Currently, the majority of clinical data focusing on outcome with respect to the type of post-traumatic or postoperative pain management are inconclusive. Only the availability of high-quality evidence will provide a firm foundation for building better post-traumatic and perioperative care

It was thus decided to write a handbook on pain with a style that is simple and practical, based on clinical practice instead of only experimental data – to appeal to undergraduates and postgraduates alike from a variety of medical disciplines when faced with a patient 'in pain'.

Introduced in this book are the types of pain encountered, pain assessment and the pain services available. Advances in pharmacological formulations with the synthesis of different classes of active drugs, new routes of drug administration and the increasing sophistication of technical systems for drug delivery are all discussed. The problem of the patient with a complex regional pain syndrome is highlighted. Research seeking to clarify the psychological processes affecting the pain experience, as well as the necessity of psychological intervention in dealing with chronic as well as acute pain, is presented. Also included is the role of diagnostic and therapeutic interventions in pain management (including in children, patients with fibromyalgia and those suffering from AIDS).

Unfortunately, in a handbook, it is not possible to describe every painful condition (e.g. headaches back pain, sickle cell disease, rheumatology and pain in the elderly) or every diagnostic technique in depth, but only to provide the basic principles on which to build an approach. The importance of rehabilitation with patient self-help is emphasized. An holistic, yet scientific, approach is desirable. Finally, the book reviews the latest progress made and concludes with a vision of 'The future' to bring the reader to the cutting edge of recent advances in the management of pain.

It is hoped that this handbook will stimulate much greater attention to this most important subject, especially in our medical postgraduate and undergraduate training, which will result in the acceptance by all health care professionals that pain care and prevention should enjoy the highest priority.

E A Shipton

ACKNOWLEDGEMENTS

I wish to acknowledge the help given by friends and colleagues in the second edition of this book. I am most grateful to the following people:

- Mr Terry Borain for the medical illustrations.
- Professor John Loeser, Past-President of the International Association for the Study of Pain, Director of the Multidisciplinary Pain Center, and Professor in the Departments of Neurological Surgery and Anesthesiology at the University of Washington School of Medicine, Seattle, USA, for kindly writing the Foreword.
- Annalisa Page, Melissa Morton and Rada Radojicic of Arnold Publishers for interacting with me so positively and patiently in the publication of this book.
- Mr Hugh Lane, my close friend, who assisted me so generously with his valuable legal advice.
- Professor Selma Browde and Mr Hannes Botha, For their support and vision.
- Dr Keith Budd, Council member of The Royal College of Anaesthetists and recently retired Director of the Pain Relief Unit, Royal Infirmary, Bradford, UK, for always being available for advice, direction and encouragement.
- My physiotherapist colleagues, Phyllis Berger, Manfred Zipfel and Didi Stenerson, who taught me so much about the physiotherapist's input in pain management.
- Dr Partrick Dessein, a rheumatologist ahead of his time, for teaching and guiding me through the rheumatological aspects of pain.
- Professor Michael Cousins, Past-President of the International Association for the Study of Pain, and Head of the Department of Anaesthesia and Pain Management, University of Sydney, Royal North Shore Hospital, St Leonards, Australia, and Professor Winston Parris, former Director of the Vanderbilt Pain Center, Nashville, USA, for their encouragement and friendship.
- Professor David Bevan, Head of the Department of Anaesthesia at the University of British Columbia, and Editor-in-Chief of the *Canadian Journal of Anaesthesia* for placing his faith in me and for giving me the opportunity to develop further in the area of pain management.
- My colleagues, Drs John Lloyd, Chris Glynn and Henry McQuay of the Oxford Regional Pain Relief Unit, University of Oxford, UK, for providing me in the first place with the opportunity of studying pain management.
- Finally, my dear wife, Elspeth, who has in the past 3 years once again been so willing to bear the brunt of having to cope with the extra load of parenting out young children while her husband spent a great deal of his extra time rewriting this book, and without whose constant encouragement and support this book would not have been written.

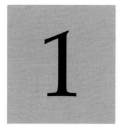

1 INTRODUCING PAIN:
The physiology, biochemistry, classification and assessment of pain

DEFINITION

Pain is a multidimensional phenomenon involving sensory, affective, motivational, environmental and cognitive components. The International Association for the Study of Pain has defined pain as: 'An unpleasant sensory or emotional experience associated with actual or potential tissue damage, or described in terms of such damage'.[1] This does not apply to living people capable of self-report.[2] Thus, non-verbal behavioural information is often needed and used for pain assessment.[2]

Pain is always subjective. Each individual learns the application of the word through experiences related to injury in early life.[1] It is unquestionably a sensation in a part of the body, but it is also unpleasant and therefore also an emotional experience. Many people report pain in the absence of tissue damage or any likely pathophysiological cause; this usually happens for psychological reasons. If we accept this subjective report, there is no way to distinguish their experience from that resulting from tissue damage.[1]

There are four components of the clinical phenomenon of pain.[3] These are nociception, pain, suffering and pain behaviour. Their roles need to be determined before effective treatments can be planned and carried out. Nociception is the detection of tissue damage caused by thermal, mechanical or chemical energy (transmitted to the central nervous system [CNS] by A delta and C fibres).[3] Pain is the perception of a noxious stimulus that occurs when nociceptive information reaches the CNS or when injury to the CNS leads to altered afferent input or central processing, when there is

pain without nociception.[3] Suffering is a negative affective response generated in higher nervous centres (e.g. the limbic lobe) by pain or by other affective states (depression, isolation, fear and anxiety).[3] Pain behaviours (closely linked to suffering) are the things that a patient says, or does or does not do, that suggest that tissue damage has occurred (e.g. talking about pain, moaning, grimacing, limping, taking pain medicine, going to doctors, or collecting compensation payments).[3]

Afferent pathways first synapse in the dorsal horn, the second-order neurones transmitting activity to the supraspinal areas, mostly via pathways in the ventrolateral white matter of the spinal cord, which are named according to their projecting areas.[4] The spinothalamic tract projects directly to the ventro-posterior lateral nucleus in the thalamus for the perception of well-localized pain.[4] The spinothalamic tract terminates in the somatosensory area of the cerebral cortex. The spinoreticular tract contacts limbic areas involved with emotional functioning. The spinomesencephalic tract projects to areas responsible for sensori-discriminative functions, emotional responses and descending inhibitory pathways.[4] Dorsal horn, thalamic and somatosensory cortex neurones are classified as nociceptive specific or multireceptive wide-dynamic range (WDR) neurones and are somatotopically organized.[4]

Some brain stem areas make an important contribution to pain modulation in the descending inhibitory pathways.[4] The peri-aqueductal grey matter, the raphi nuclei and the locus coeruleus are key sites for pain inhibition and are activated by pathways in the cortical or thalamic areas, or from ascending tracts via collaterals.[4] Activating nociceptive activity reaching the brain stem results in increased descending activity to the dorsal horn, decreasing nociception.[4] The axons descend mainly in the dorsolateral funiculus, terminating in the dorsal horn at different spinal levels, where they may directly inhibit nociceptive neurones or activate inhibitory interneurones.[4] The transmitters involved in the descending inhibitory pathways at spinal cord level are mainly 5-hydroxytryptamine (5-HT) and noradrenaline (NA). The action of local interneurones in the dorsal horn is generally mediated via endogenous opioid peptides or NA.[4] With intact spinal cord and brain stem connections, diffuse noxious inhibitory controls can occur, whereby nociceptive activity can inhibit spinal cord neurones other than those directly activated by the afferents.[4]

Major landmarks concerning the physiopathology of pain are: the liberation of substance P and other neuropeptides at both spinal and peripheral endings; the anatomical and functional analysis of the nociceptive pathways; and the characterization of endomorphin ligands and receptors.[2] Models of neuropathic pain have advanced the understanding of its specific pathophysiology. Sensori-discriminative aspects of pain involve lateral thalamic nuclei and corresponding somaesthetic cortices, whereas medial thalamic nuclei encode nociceptive stimuli during attention-directed tasks.[2] Their cortical connections, namely the anterior cingular cortex and insular cortex, support their role in the affective-motivational dimensions of pain.[2] The sympathetic nervous system plays an important role in modulating sensory processing in animal models of neuropathic pain and clinical observations in certain chronic pain states.[5] However, in postoperative pain and in inflammation, the interaction of the sympathetic nervous system and the somatic nervous system needs further investigation.

An impressive increase in the number and quality of randomized clinical trials has been observed since 1950.[2] The use of primary and secondary analgesics, new interventional techniques and drug delivery routes, physical and psychological interventions are discussed, ending with a glimpse into future developments in the field of pain.

Acute pain

Acute pain (e.g. surgical procedures, injury and childbirth) often announces the presence of a disease process or injury, which needs to be treated, while the pain is relieved. It is a signal of ongoing or impending tissue damage that provokes the organism to escape from the injurious circumstances and

seek treatment.[6] Acute pain typically results from soft tissue injury or inflammation (typically seen postoperatively).[7] It is rarely difficult to follow the pain to the injured part of the body.[3] It has a reparative function by enabling healing and repair to occur undisturbed. This is achieved by making the injured/inflamed area and the surrounding tissue hypersensitive to all stimuli so that contact with any external stimulus is avoided.[7] It may bring about immobility to promote healing. Since acute pain is reparative, it may be sufficient to reduce it to a level where it is no longer distressing but can still fulfil a protective function.[4] The patient's culture, gender, age and past experience, and the anticipated consequences, may modify the expression of acute pain[3]. The physician focuses on the injury and the reduction of nociceptive information coming from the injury to the CNS as the primary treatment activity (pharmacological, physical and/or psychological).[3] Acute pain is a symptom that must be treated or its cause eliminated.[3] Nature (not the physician) heals the acute injury.

However, if acute pain is not soon relieved, the segmental, suprasegmental and neuroendocrine reflex responses that occur may produce serious pathophysiological responses.[8] Very brief acute pain is transmitted in a simple way and rarely produces difficulties in treatment. The situation within the spinal cord changes if the stimulus continues.[9] After only seconds of C fibre stimulation, additional peptides are released from the C fibres, and spinal N-methyl-D-aspartate (NMDA) receptor activation and nitric oxide (NO) production occur.[9] Soon after, genes are induced in central neurones, and increases and decreases in diverse pharmacological systems involved in pain transmission and modulation occur over periods of only a few hours.[9] This rapid plasticity has important implications for the pharmacological treatment of acute pain as both the level of the pain transmission and the pain modulation will be changing over time.

These might later progress to a chronic pain state. How does this occur? It has been found that patients who develop chronic pain report a higher pain intensity, higher anxiety and distress, less certainty that their pain will resolve, longer hospitalization, less dependence on ambulation, a diagnosis of trauma and less need for surgery.[10] Recognition of these factors may lead to early identification of those with acute pain who are at risk of developing chronic pain.[10] Neuropathic pain in the postoperative period may be associated with unnecessary suffering, if the diagnosis is not made and treatment modalities are ineffective.[11] It is likely that the inadequate management of acute pain may set the scene for progression to a chronic pain state.[11] The possibility arises that acute, intensive intervention may avoid or reduce mechanisms whereby short-term stimuli may lead to long-term plasticity and structural changes in the nociceptive pathways, and subsequent chronic pain.[11] There is a need for further research in this area to determine whether or not such a theoretical potential can be turned into a therapeutic advantage.

Chronic pain

How and when acute pain becomes chronic is the most important dichotomy in the pain world. This is controversial and lacks clear definition. If pain persists beyond the usual course of an acute injury or disease, or recurs every few months or years, it is regarded as chronic.[8] Although the labels suggest an obligate temporal difference, there is more than the remoteness of onset of the pain problem that distinguishes these two types of pain.[3] It is now apparent that acute pain can lead to CNS changes (e.g. in the dorsal horn) that far outlast the nociceptive generation from the periphery.[3] Injuries in the nervous system can generate chronic pain in the absence of pathology in the part that hurts (e.g. phantom limb pain and trigeminal neuralgia).[3] Some laboratory rats appear particularly pain prone, and the hunt is on for the gene(s) predisposing individuals (estimated at 10 per cent of the general population) to chronic pain resulting from noxious stimuli, to which normal individuals would produce only short-lived pain.[12] This may be result in differing CNS responses to both bodily and nervous system injury, and thereby perpetuate painful states.[3] The affective responses to a perceived noxious stimulus may be related to the individual's genetics, past experience, mood or interpretations of the meaning of the pain to generate and perpetuate chronic pain. Regardless of the originating factors of a chronic pain, environmental forces will play a larger or smaller role, depending on the relationships between the individual and their family, friends or workplace, and can perpetuate pain behaviours without any measurable internal generators of nociception or pain (e.g. low back pain duration representing the fraction of the pre-injury wage paid by the compensation system).[3] It is therefore essential that the issues of the return to normal behaviour patterns as well as the relief of symptoms are addressed.[3]

Pain perception begins with the activation of peripheral nociceptors and conduction through A delta and unmyelinated C fibres to the dorsal root ganglion.[13] From here, signals travel via the spinothalamic tract to the thalamus and somatosensory cortex. The modulation of sensory input (that is, pain) occurs at many levels. Nociceptors are also neuro-effectors, and transmission can be modulated by their cell bodies, which secrete inflammatory mediators, neuropeptides or other pain-producing substances.[13] Descending pathways from the hypothalamus, which has opioid-sensitive receptors and is stimulated by arousal and emotional stress, can transmit signals to the dorsal horn that modulate ascending nociceptive transmissions.[13] The relative balance between the activity of the inhibitory gamma-aminobutyric acid (GABA) and the excitatory amino acids (glutamate) appears to determine the level of pain transmission.[14] The NMDA receptor for glutamate has been implicated in the generation and maintenance of central (spinal) states of hypersensitivity.[14] It has been shown that the activation of this receptor underlies wind-up, whereby the transmission of noxious messages is potentiated. This is why and how a painful response is not always matched to the stimulus.[14] Antagonists at this receptor–channel complex prevent or block enhanced (hyperalgesic) pain states induced by tissue damage, inflammation, nerve damage and ischaemia.[14] Amplification systems within the spinal cord have parallels with other plastic events, such as long-term potentiation in the hippocampus. The roles of inhibitory transmitter systems can also change, and opioid, adenosine and GABA transmission can vary in different pain states.[14] Hyperalgesia would appear to be balanced by inhibitions during inflammatory but not in neuropathic states.[14] In the latter case, events reminiscent of long-term potentiation may predominate. Modulation to alter pain perception can also occur at higher centres (e.g. frontal cortex, midbrain and medulla) by opioids and anti-inflammatory agents, as well as antagonists and agonists of neurotransmitters.[13] It is apparent that some types of chronic pain have both a peripheral and supraspinal component.[15]

Peripheral noxious stimuli or tissue injury induces the release of excitatory amino acids and other transmitters from primary afferent terminals in the spinal dorsal horn, which may lead to the expression of immediate early genes in dorsal horn neurones via the activation of intracellular messengers including calcium ions and various protein kinases.[16] Various immediate early genes of the fos, jun and zinc finger families are differentially expressed in dorsal horn neurones in a time-dependent manner.

Protein products of these genes function as transcription factors and trigger long-lasting plastic changes in CNS neurones.[16] Simultaneously, excitatory amino acids may activate the synthesis of prostanoids and NO, which may affect the sensitivity of dorsal horn neurones.[16] In addition, peripheral chemical mediators such as 5-HT contribute to peripheral hyperalgesia.[16] These events may contribute to the establishment of persistent pain and hyperalgesia in a concerted way. It has been shown that pre-treatment, but not post-treatment, with local anaesthetics or analgesics reduces the expression of c-fos in the spinal cord neurones and pain responses in animals, suggesting that the inhibition of intracellular events by pre-treatment with local anaesthetics and analgesics is effective for the reduction of persistent pain following tissue injury.[16] C-fos has been found to be necessary for prodynorphin transactivation.[17] The induction of dynorphin peptide leads to a reduction of thermal hyperalgesia and mechanical allodynia during chronic pathological pain.[17] Recently, a partial nerve ligation model for chronic pain has been used to investigate whether there are changes in the expression of mRNA for several immediate early genes that correlate in time with the initial adaptive behavioural changes and with the development of allodynia in this model.[18] Except for c-jun mRNA, all changes were transient despite behavioural evidence of continuing allodynia.[18] Also, specific mutations leading to an increased risk of rare forms of migraine have been identified in both mitochondrial DNA and a calcium channel gene.[19] Thus, gene therapy by insertion of DNA into a patient's cells (with gene expression or gene transfer) is now a possibility for the treatment of pain.[20] Several routes of administration – intraparenchymal, intrathecal and intrathecal with pial-glial membrane disruption – are possible.[20]

Therefore, when pain persists in spite of therapy, it becomes chronic, loses its distinct signal function and includes aspects of physical, emotional and psychosocial disarray, as well as neural imprinting, that markedly influence that pain's perceived severity and its consequences.[6] Chronic pain can be a sustained sensory abnormality occurring as a result of ongoing peripheral pathology (such as chronic inflammation), or it can be autonomous, independent of the trigger that initiated it.[7] In the latter case, it is changes in the nervous system that have become the pathology, and the pain is maladaptive, offering no survival advantage.[7] Spontaneous chronic pain occurs in most chronic pain conditions, especially the denervation syndromes,

where the sensory channel from the periphery to the CNS is disrupted (anaesthesia dolorosa, phantom limb pains and brachial plexus avulsion injuries).[7] Provoked pain is elicited by a peripheral stimulus, but the response is exaggerated in amplitude and duration[7]. The pain may be generated by stimuli quite unlike those which would normally be required to elicit pain (e.g. post-herpetic or trigeminal neuralgia, and complex regional pain syndrome [CRPS] type 2).[7] A distinctive feature of clinical pain is then sensory hypersensitivity, comprising both an exaggerated and increased response to suprathreshold stimuli, and pain production by low-intensity or formerly subthreshold stimuli.[7] In both cases, the responsiveness of the pain system is altered, with pain increase in the former and a reduction in pain threshold in the latter.[7] Chronic pain can linger even when the original source is gone because physical deconditioning, behavioural consequences and/or neurophysiological changes persist.[6] The chronic bombardment of the CNS with nociceptive input thus changes the neurophysiological response based on alterations in the neural threshold, chemistry and modulation.[6] Chronic pain rarely has any biological function and results in tremendous emotional, physical, economic and social suffering for patients and their families. The protocol for patient evaluation must be systematic and thorough, encompassing the physical and behavioural components, and respecting the neurophysiological mechanisms that are operative.[6] Outcomes-based treatment strategies according to outcome measures (e.g. self-assessment of pain levels and pain relief, health care and medication consumption, functional abilities and work status) are needed in both acute and chronic pain[3].

Clinical pain is present when ongoing discomfort and abnormal sensitivity are features of the patient's symptomatology.[7] The usual three features of clinical pain are: spontaneous pain, which may be dull, burning or stabbing, exaggerated pain in response to noxious stimuli (hyperalgesia), and pain produced by stimuli that would never normally do so (allodynia). It is useful to analyse clinical pain from the perspective of the injured tissue;[7] in terms of inflammatory pain (which is associated with tissue damage), inflammation or both; and neuropathic pain, the pain that results from a lesion of the peripheral or central nervous system; and from a temporal perspective, considering acute and chronic pain[7].

Another heuristically useful way to divide chronic pain syndromes to facilitate diagnosis and treatment, is as follows:[3]

■ Chronic pain caused by cancer is best thought of as acute pain persisting over time. The management principles are basically the same as for acute pain, although added neuropathic pain and mood disturbances need to be addressed.

■ Chronic pain as a result of peripheral or central nervous system injury may be from a malignant disease, or follow trauma or any other pathological process that affects the nerves, spinal cord or brain, and is more likely to respond to antidepressants and anticonvulsants.

■ Chronic pain can be associated with a chronic disease, such as diabetic neuropathy or arthritis. Different therapies are needed at different times to treat the underlying disease and chronic pain state, as well as the acute flare-ups.

■ The largest group, forming the bulk of the epidemic of chronic pain in developed countries, comprises the chronic pain syndromes of unknown aetiology (e.g. only 20 per cent of patients with low back pain can be accurately diagnosed). Physicians inadvertently contribute to the medicalization of all complaints and may act as gatekeepers for disability systems.

INCIDENCE

Epidemiological studies have shown that chronic pain represents a major public health problem.[21] The prevalence of chronic pain obtained from epidemiological studies ranges from 7 to 40 per cent, due in part to the definitions of pain that were used.[21] One careful survey showed that while 37 per cent of people reported recurrent pain, only 8 per cent had severe and persistent pain, and fewer than 3 per cent had severe and persistent pain lasting more than 6 days.[21] Several population surveys (in Canada, Sweden and the UK) found chronic and unrelieved pain to be widespread.[22–25] A recent survey found that 7 per cent of the adult population in UK households were in pain.[22] In the USA, it is estimated that 3.3 per cent of the population are permanently disabled as a result of pain.[26] In New Zealand, most (of the 1498) adults interviewed reported more than one life-disrupting experience of pain.[27] The epidemiology of pain in children and adolescents is still relatively undocumented.[28] Pain is thus a common health care problem that carries severe personal and economic consequences.

Even in the acute postoperative situation, about 75 per cent of patients report insufficient pain relief, which is often poorly relieved by traditional analgesic practices.[29] Patients have been found to have low expectations of pain relief and to display a reluctance to request analgesia, although 'customer demand' from patients for improved comfort after surgery is becoming apparent in some countries.[29,30] The immediate postoperative course as well as the long-term outcome may be influenced by the quality of pain relief after surgery.[30]

What is needed is detailed information on the nature of pain problems in a community, the adequacy of their current management and the types of health care facility that would be required for optimal care.[21] Strategies for the prevention of pain are firstly, primary prevention, which is the rationale behind pre-emptive analgesia (to prevent phantom pain in amputees, post-thoracotomy and post-mastectomy chronic pain syndromes, and post-herpetic neuralgia).[21] Secondary protection involves early detection of the disease (e.g. in neuropathic pain and low back pain) so that prompt and effective measures can be undertaken to minimize ill-health.[21] Tertiary prevention aims to minimize suffering from irremediable conditions.[21] This area may be the most fruitful in chronic pain in preventing the development of pain-related behaviour and psychological morbidity (as seen in the association between chronic pain and depression).[21] The challenge of epidemiological studies of pain is to identify the patient groups for which particular preventative strategies are appropriate.[21] To do this, standard definitions of pain need to be developed and used in studies that focus on specific syndromes rather than aggregating diverse conditions.

Chronic pain differs from acute pain in that it serves no useful function, causes suffering, limits activities of daily living and increases health care payments, disability and litigation fees.[13] Based on data from the USA, chronic pain costs society more than heart disease and cancer combined.[12] The amount of money expended on research and therapy does not begin to reflect this fact.[12]

TYPES OF PAIN

Nociceptive pain

Normally, pain is felt when impulses reach a conscious brain along fine, myelinated (A delta) and/or unmyelinated (C) nociceptive nerve fibres (Figure 1.1).[31] The sensory endings of these afferent fibres

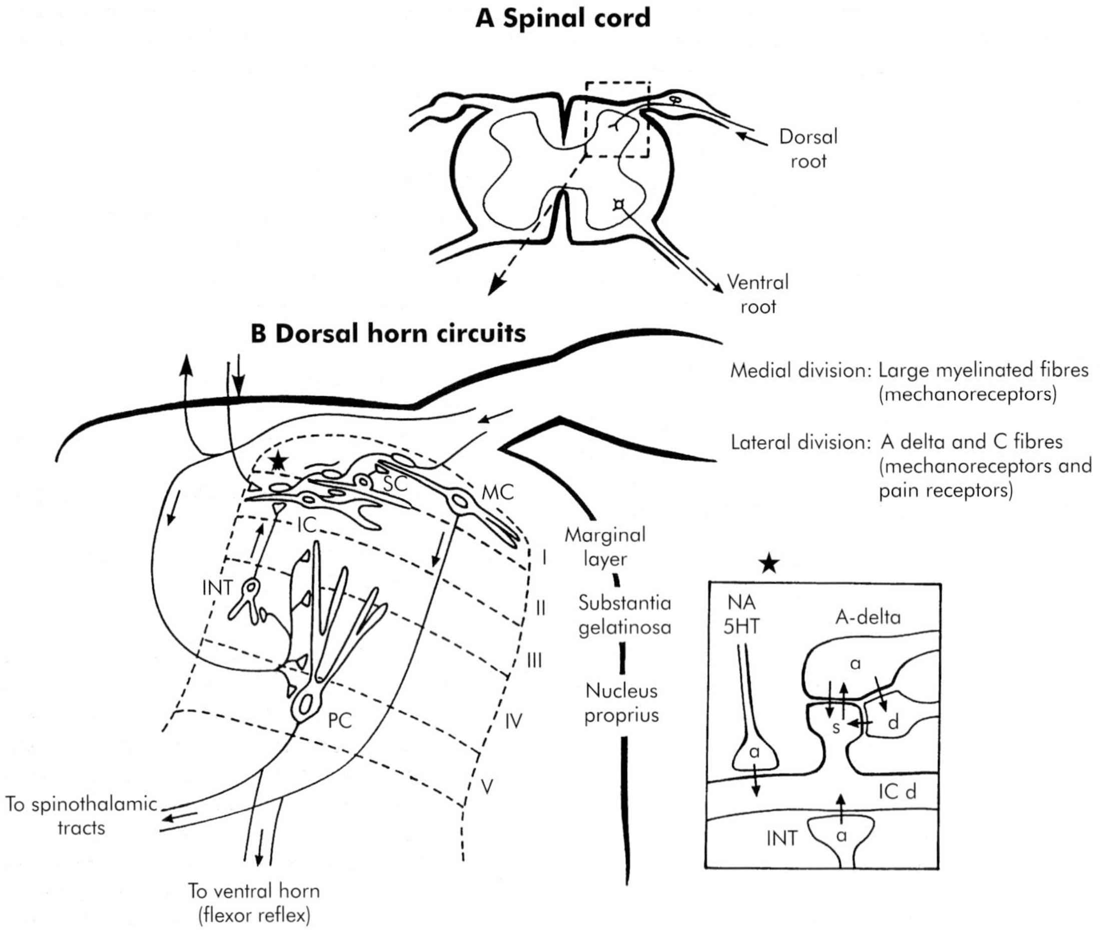

A Spinal cord

B Dorsal horn circuits

Medial division: Large myelinated fibres (mechanoreceptors)

Lateral division: A delta and C fibres (mechanoreceptors and pain receptors)

Marginal layer

Substantia gelatinosa

Nucleus proprius

To spinothalamic tracts

To ventral horn (flexor reflex)

Figure 1.1 Somatosensory circuits in the mammalian spinal cord. (A) Diagram of cross-section of spinal cord. (B) Some of the main neurone types and synaptic connections that have been identified in the dorsal horn. I–V, laminae of the dorsal horn; MC, marginal cell; SC, stalked cell; IC, islet cell; INT, interneurone; PC, projection cell. The large myelinated fibres are believed to be glutamanergic; pain fibres contain substance P, somatostatin, vasoactive intentinal peptide or cholecystokinin; descending fibres contain noradrenaline or serotonin. Inset: Synaptic organization of microcircuits in the marginal layer (site marked by an asterisk in B). a, axon; d, dendrite; s, spine; INT, interneurone; IC, islet cell; NA, noradrenaline; 5HT, serotonin.

are normally activated only by strong, noxious stimuli, and the brain interprets input arriving along them as being painful. It is this matching between the high threshold of the afferent endings in the periphery and their corresponding central connections that makes the pain system an effective sensory signalling apparatus.[31] Pain is 'normal' ('nociceptive') when it results from the activity of healthy nociceptive afferents aroused by intense stimuli.[31] Nociceptors are not a homogeneous population of sensory receptors with high thresholds but are extremely diverse in nature.[32] A nociceptor is a dynamic entity, shifting its properties under the influence, and according to the necessities, of its environment.[32] Cutaneous nociceptors consist of high-threshold mechanoreceptors (thinly myelinated, mainly A delta fibres with free nerve endings, the A mechano-heat fibres) and polymodal nociceptors (unmyelinated C fibres with free nerve endings).[33,34] The latter respond to intense mechanical or thermal stimuli, and to a variety of chemical irritants. The majority of thermal and mechanical pain arises from the activation of these polymodal nociceptors, which are innervated by C fibres.[35] Nociceptors occur in other somatic structures (such as muscle, fascia, tendons, joints, cornea and tooth pulp). Signals are carried by the A delta and C fibres.[36]

Physiological pain from high-intensity noxious stimuli (mechanical, thermal and chemical) that activate nociceptive receptors is highly localized and transient.[33] Flexion and autonomic reflexes are activated, and pain is produced. Pathological pain arises after tissue damage.[33] This may result in various types of injury, including ischaemia, inflammation and gross tissue destruction (trauma or surgery).[36] These nociceptors respond to local chemical stimulation and also become sensitized to chemical, mechanical and thermal stimuli.[35] Blood vessels become leaky as the result of some of these chemical mediators so that other mediators gain access to the damaged site from the vasculature.[35] Tissue damage generates the synthesis of arachidonic acid metabolites from adjacent membranes, the cleavage of the precursor of bradykinin to release the active peptide from the circulation, and the release of peptides such as substance P and calcitonin gene-related peptide (CGRP) from the C fibres via the afferent reflex.[35] This inflammatory soup, also containing serotonin, and potassium and hydrogen ions, activates and sensitizes the peripheral endings and causes vasodilatation and plasma extravasation, thereby eliciting the swelling, pain and tenderness of inflammation.[35] Pain is enhanced by their actions on the terminals of nociceptive peripheral sensory fibres, creating peripheral hyperalgesia.[35] In addition, there are the effects of other mediators (cytokinins, nerve growth factors, catecholamines and prostanoids) from the sympathetic nervous system.[35] This leads to a peripheral sensitization of nociceptors and silent afferents. Nociceptor-mediated pain generated by low-intensity stimuli ensues.

The blocking or reduction of the generation of nociceptive messages at the first stage in the periphery is expected to prevent some of the central alterations that induce central hypersensitivity.[35] Injury- or disease-triggered sensitization of primary afferent neurones, results in an increase in the responsiveness of 'normal' sensory endings in peripheral tissues as a result of inflammatory mediators, and perhaps also of the upregulation of certain channel and receptor molecules in the sensory cell body, and the generation of ectopic firing at sites of nerve injury and in the dorsal root ganglion.[31] Thus, even in the peripheral nervous system, the responses of neurones are not fixed, being dependent on previous stimulation and the chemical environment of the receptor.[37] There is sensory specialization in the peripheral nervous system associated with nociception. Specialized neurones encode the sensory features associated with tissue damage.[37] The activation

of nociceptors is a significant factor in chronic pain states such as chronic degenerative joint disease, cancer and myofascial syndromes.[38] Nociceptive pain and neuropathic pain often co-exist.

Neuropathic pain

Neuropathic pain arises because of malfunction in the peripheral or central nervous system, in comparison with pain caused by inflammatory aetiologies or evoked by the controlled injury of surgery.[6,39] Probable causes of neuropathic pain include:[6]

- mechanical factors (nerve compression/scarring after trauma, surgery or entrapment);
- toxicity (from lead, arsenic and chemotherapeutic drugs);
- metabolic disease (such as diabetes, alcoholism or malnutrition);
- post-inflammatory changes (after herpes zoster infection or in Guillain–Barré disease);
- idiopathic causes.

Terms used to describe some (but not all) forms of neuropathic pain include 'neurogenic pain', 'deafferentation pain' and 'central pain'. Its mechanism is entirely different from that of normal physiological (nociceptive) types of pain, which depend on a labelled line system.[40] Neuropathic pain affects at least 25 per cent of patients attending most pain clinics.[39]

Because the delicate balance of facilitation and inhibition within the nervous system is disrupted after injury to and subsequent scarring within the nervous system, patients with neuropathic pain often present with symptoms that are variously described.[6] The psychological devastation is augmented by the patient's failure to obtain a satisfactory response for the severity and duration of the pain, the poor response to the innumerable treatments prescribed and the perception gained over time that the physician no longer understands or truly cares.[6] Neuropathic pain symptoms and signs are described below.[39,40]

Spontaneous, continuous and paroxysmal pain

In the same patient, a combination of spontaneous and abnormal evoked (e.g. cold or touch allodynia) pain can be seen at the same time.[40] Deep tissue pain (polyradiculitis and brachial neuropathy) is a cramping, aching or squeezing pain.[40] Superficial skin pain has a burning, smarting or pricking character.[40] Episodic paroxysmal pain (trigeminal neuralgia, entrapment neuropathies and luetic diseases) has a shooting, shock-like or stabbing character.[40]

Sensory deficit and pain

A feature of neuropathic pain is a partial or complete loss of afferent sensory function and the paradoxical presence of certain hyperphenomena in the painful area.[40] In some patients, the sensory deficit may be gross, while it is subtle in others. It may involve a loss of all sensory abnormalities, but a loss of spinothalamic functions (cold, warmth and pinprick) appears crucial.[40]

Allodynia and hyperalgesia

A classical feature is the presence of abnormal evoked pain (allodynia) or unpleasant sensations (dyaesthesias) arising from non-noxious stimuli.[40] Mechanical allodynia is either A beta mediated or dynamic (evoked by gentle brush stimuli), or high threshold or static (evoked by high-threshold non-noxious stimuli).[40] Examples include pain caused by light stroking in trigeminal and diabetic neuralgias.[40] Recent findings in post-stroke pain suggest that allodynia may also manifest from deep tissues.[40] Allodynia and hyperalgesia can be quantified by measuring intensity, threshold for elicitation, duration and area of allodynia. Following complete injury, abnormal sensations may occasionally develop from the apparently de-afferentated body part as a result of changes in peripheral territory innervation areas, or because of the expansion of peripheral receptive fields, having lost their normal innervation.[40] Hyperalgesia can be provoked in normal subjects after large-diameter afferent blockade. Pinprick or cold is perceived as burning or squeezing, suggesting that afferent fibres normally exert an inhibitory input on dorsal horn neuronal activity, which can be disrupted in neuropathic pain.[40]

Hyperpathia

Hyperpathia is the prototypical disorder seen in neuropathic pain whenever there is loss of fibres. It is a variant of allodynia and hyperalgesia in which an explosive pain response is suddenly evoked from cutaneous areas with an increased sensory detection threshold when the stimulus intensity exceeds the sensory threshold.[40] It is a reflection of the peripheral or central deafferentation elevating the threshold and a central hyperexcitability as a result of lost or abnormal afferent input from peripheral afferents and their cells.[40]

Referred pain and abnormal pain radiation

The pain duration may be increased with abnormal spread (e.g. myelopathies and capsaicin-induced hyperalgesia). There is a direct link between pain intensity, duration and referral.[40] In post-traumatic pain, the presence of large areas with abnormal sensations and pain may be partly related to pathological dorsal horn changes encoding noxious information.[40] WDR neurones are characterized by small receptive zones activated by non-noxious stimuli (touch and gentle pressure) surrounded by a larger zone from which noxious stimuli (pinch, firm pressure and a temperature over 45°C) can evoke neuronal discharges.[40] A noxious stimulus will activate several WDR neurones. Increasing stimulus intensity activates more WDR neurones rostrocaudally, reflecting the degree of radiation and referral.[40]

Wind-up like pain and after-sensations

Wind-up pain or abnormal temporal summation corresponds clinically to the increasing neuronal activity following repetitive C fibre stimulation of over 3 Hz evoked by repetitive noxious or non-noxious stimulation from normal or hyperalgesic cutaneous areas respectively.[40] When repetitive, low-threshold stimuli (activating the A beta fibres) elicit pain, this means that access has been obtained to central wind-up mechanisms normally reserved for C fibre input.[40] Wind-up pain can be produced by mechanical, electrical or thermal stimuli. After-sensations (pain persisting after the termination of the painful stimulus) are another feature of neuropathic pain, the WDR neurones showing persistent discharges following noxious recruitment.[40]

NEURONAL AND MOLECULAR MECHANISMS IN NEUROPATHIC PAIN

Peripheral mechanisms

Peripheral neuropathic pain is defined as pain initiated or caused by a primary lesion or dysfunction in the peripheral nervous system.[41] This includes neuralgia and painful neuropathy. Neuralgia is pain in the distribution of a nerve or nerves.[41] Painful polyneuropathies are usually symmetrical and distal (affecting the feet and sometimes the hands). These conditions may present with or without paraesthesia, hypoaesthesia, hyperalgesia and allodynia.[41] The difference between peripheral neuropathic pain and the complex regional pain syndrome type 2, is that diagnosis of the latter requires evidence of oedema, cutaneous blood flow changes or abnormal sudomotor activity.[41] Peripheral neuropathic pains can be divided into those presenting with shooting pain or allodynia with no sensory deficit (e.g. trigeminal

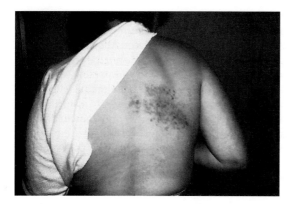

Figure 1.2   An example of a peripheral neuropathic pain – a patient with intercostal post-herpetic neuralgia.

neuralgia and metatarsalgia) and those presenting with a sensory deficit with other (usually burning) pains (e.g. diabetic mellitus neuropathy, post-herpetic neuralgia and causalgia)[39] (Figure 1.2). 'Sympathetic pain' will be discussed in Chapter 10. Studies on peripheral neuropathic pain accounted for only 0.2 per cent of the controlled pain studies published from 1950 to 1990.[41] Following experimental nerve injury, peripheral mechanisms that may contribute to neuropathic pain can be summarized as follows:[40]

- Afferent nerve fibre
  - post-injury nerve discharges;
  - nerve sprouting;
  - release of local factors (interleukins and nerve growth factors);
  - increased sensitivity of sprouts to mechanical and chemical stimuli.
- Dorsal root ganglion cell
  - spontaneous activity, increased evoked activity;
  - increased innervation of A cells by sympathetic terminals.
- Spinal cord
  - sprouting of large afferent terminals into 'nociceptive laminae';
  - central sensitization;
  - loss of inhibitory (GABA-ergic/?glycine-ergic) neurones;
  - dorsal horn reorganization.

Several abnormalities may contribute to peripheral neuropathic pain, namely:[40] nociceptor sensitization; an increased activity of damaged axons and their sprouts; nociceptor sensitization by the sympathetic nervous system; discharges in dorsal root ganglion cells; and collateral sprouting from neighbouring undamaged nerves to invade deafferented

territory. Regenerating sprouts are hypersensitive to mechanical stimuli, noradrenaline, potassium channel blockers, prostanoids and cytokines.[40] In injured axons and regenerating nerve fibres, there is an accumulation of sodium channels.[40] The spontaneous discharges in the dorsal root ganglia can be detected within a few hours. All this abnormal neuronal activity generates an abnormal barrage to the dorsal horn.[40] A role of the sympathetic nervous system is indicated, as a sympathectomy and phentolamine may relieve some types of neuropathic pain.[40]

Following axotomy/nerve constriction, there is a loss of substance P and CGRP, while cells not normally synthesizing peptides begin to release neuropeptide Y, galanin and vasoactive intestinal polypeptide.[40] Following an afferent barrage, released glutamate and aspartate cause excitation of postsynaptic neurones by acting at ionotropic (amino-methyl propionic acid [AMPA], NMDA and kainate) and metabotropic receptors.[40] At higher activity rates, the substance P released causes excitation of neurokinin$_1$ (NK$_1$) receptors on postsynaptic inter- or projection neurones, and further increases calcium ion entry through voltage-gated channels.[40] The activation of the metabotropic glutamate receptors results in an increase of phospholipase C and facilitates the formation of the second messengers (inositol triphosphate and diacylglycerol).[40] The increase of intracellular calcium ion concentration from several sources (voltage-gated, ligand-gated channels, NMDA-operated channels and intracellular stores) gives rise to a new cascade of events (the translocation of protein kinases, the formation of nitric oxide (NO) and the expression of proto-oncogenes such as *c-fos, c-jun, krox-24, jun-D, fos-b* and others).[40] Products from these immediate early genes facilitate the production of enzymes and neuropeptides, and may thereby induce long-term changes in the postsynaptic cells.[40] This phenomenon, known as long-term potentiation and primarily described in the hippocampus, is similar to the temporal facilitation of WDR neurones in the dorsal horn.[40] The facilitation of WDR neurones gives rise to the hyperalgesia and ongoing pain of neuropathic pain.[40] Spinal projection neurones of the WDR type are also influenced by enkephalinergic interneurones from descending bulbospinal fibres and by large-diameter afferent fibres.[40] The latter may be under the control of GABA- and glycine-containing interneurones.[40] A loss or reduced activity of these inhibitory interneurones may result in the production of allodynia following large-fibre input.[40]

Central mechanisms

Neuropathic pain can also be seen after damage to central somatosensory structures. Much less is known about the underlying mechanisms, although damage to the spinothalamic pathways is a necessary condition for the development of a central neuropathic pain syndrome.[40] Included are central post-stroke pain (with associated hyperalgesia or allodynia in the painful body part) as well as those resulting from cerebral vascular accidents, post-cordotomy pain dysaesthesias and pain arising in multiple sclerosis and in syringomyelia.[39,40] Sensitization of neuronal populations in the CNS which is directly or indirectly related to a loss of input, is an essential element in central neuropathic pain syndromes.[40] Neurones showing a sensitization in central neuropathic pain syndromes may be multiple and originate from many sources (spinal, brain stem, cortical and subcortical structures).[40] Particular interest has been directed at the thalamus, which receives input from internal and external sites, with a convergence of noxious and non-noxious information.[40]

BRAIN IMAGING IN NEUROPATHIC PAIN

Pain imaging is described later in this chapter. Only a few studies have analysed cerebral blood flow in chronic neuropathic pain patients. Two positron emission tomography (PET) studies showed decreased contralateral thalamic blood flow and, recently, activation of the right gyrus cinguli in eight patients with chronic neuropathic pain.[40] With single photon emission computed tomography (SPECT), decreased activity has been found in one patient with central pain, and increased contralateral thalamic activity in two patients with post-stroke pain.[40] Resolution refinement or technique combination (e.g. functional magnetic resonance imaging [fMRI], magnetoencephalography [MEG] and, ligand studies) will help to clarify the underlying pathology of neuropathic pain.[40]

NEUROBIOLOGY OF NEUROPATHIC PAIN

Understanding the neurobiological basis of neuropathic pain is facilitated by using animal models of nerve injury produced by the peripheral manipulation of rat nerves.[42] Recent animal models involve constriction of the sciatic nerve distal to the spinal cord, with a tight ligation of a portion, the loose ligation of the entire nerve (chronic constriction injury model) or the tight ligation of the two out of the three spinal nerves that form the sciatic nerve (spinal nerve ligation model).[42] Allodynia, hyperalgesia, spontaneous pain, sensory deficits and, in some cases, a sympathetic component are not a replicated ensemble seen in acute models.[42] Despite an inherent variability consistently injuring the same ratio of myelinated and unmyelinated fibres and in the differing degeneration of fibre types, similar behavioural results have been reported, suggesting that common consequences can result from variable peripheral changes.[42] Aberrations in somatosensory processing following partial nerve injury are the culmination of changes in the peripheral nervous system.[42] After nerve section, ectopic discharges within the neuroma and dorsal root ganglia contribute to these changes.[42] Following partial denervation (chronic constriction injury model), high-frequency spontaneous activity originating in the dorsal root ganglion targets the spinal neurones via injured A fibres.[42] Both fibres and dorsal root ganglia contribute to the behavioural responses (including allodynia) associated with the spinal nerve ligation model.[42] In this same model, a modified, rapidly adapting mechanoreceptor has been reported as innervating the partially deafferented foot, suggesting changes in transduction processes.[42] A structural reorganization of large (A beta) fibre terminations at the spinal cord level has been reported, so it is possible that low-threshold inputs can now gain access to spinal nociceptive transmission circuits.[42]

Few electrophysiological studies of spinal neurones in nerve injury models have been reported, and there have been no studies on the effects of spinal nerve ligation on neuronal responses.[42] In the chronic constriction injury model, a high percentage of spinal neurones showed abnormal levels of spontaneous activity, although many neurones had unexpectedly absent somatic fields.[42] Spinal neurones showed increased after-discharges and were sensitive to tapping of the nerve injury site.[42] The number of neurones sensitive to low-intensity mechanical stimuli and the magnitude of the neuronal evoked mechanical responses were reduced.[42] After partial ligation, only subtle, late changes in spinal neuronal responses, with a temporal profile different from that of the associated allodynia, have been reported.[42] Also reported were neurones with absent or enlarged mechanical receptive fields.[42] It remains unclear how changed peripheral and central neuronal responses contribute to the resultant pain states.

PHARMACOLOGY OF NEUROPATHIC PAIN

The pharmacology of both pain transmission and analgesia exhibits considerable plasticity, which can provide a rational basis for neuropathic pain treatment, where the pathology leads to alterations in both peripheral and central pain systems.[42] NMDA-mediated events are relevant to nerve injury-evoked pain – in the induction and maintenance of spinal nociceptive events, leading to hyperalgesia following tissue damage, nerve dysfunction and surgery.[42] Noxious stimuli enhance spinal excitatory events. High-frequency, constant intensity C fibre stimulation results in a marked, prolonged increase in the flexion withdrawal reflex, central hypersensitivity and wind-up, whereby the responses of dorsal horn nociceptive neurones suddenly increase in magnitude and duration despite the constant input into the spinal cord (NMDA receptor mediated).[42] Other causal factors (including phenotype and anatomical changes) will, by decreasing neuronal thresholds, allow the access of different afferent inputs to central nociceptive transmission.[42] Behavioural studies in the loose sciatic nerve ligation model show NMDA activation to be required for the induction and maintenance of pain-related behaviours.[42] In the spinal nerve ligation model, NMDA antagonism can relieve behavioural symptoms (mechanical and cold allodynia, hyperalgesia and spontaneous pain), although little difference exists between the receptor and channel blockers (ketamine, dextrorphan, MK-801 and memantine).[42] Aberrant peripheral activity is thus amplified by NMDA receptor-mediated spinal mechanisms in neuropathic pain.

In allodynia, central inhibitory neurones set the transmission level, as blocking the glycine or $GABA_A$ receptors in normal animals produces NMDA-mediated allodynia, against which morphine is ineffective, since low-threshold pathways are minimally controlled by opioid receptors.[42] GABA levels are reduced in neuropathic states (although enhanced after inflammation).[42] Neuropathic pain has a reduced opioid sensitivity, indicating a loss of inhibitory function.[42] After nerve damage, the rise in cholecystokinin (CCK) level and the presynaptic opioid receptor loss add to the diminishing opioid efficacy.[42] However, poorly opioid-responsive pains (as well as those in which the NMDA receptor is operative) may be overcome by opioid (morphine) dose escalation, although side-effects may confound this tactic.[42] Another (unproven) approach may be to use high-efficacy opioids such as alfentanil or sufentanil. The ability of morphine to control neuropathic pain, and its relative effectiveness by the neuraxial or systemic route, remains unclear.[42] There is a strong association between the NMDA receptor for glutamate and hyperalgesia/allodynia, and reduced opioid sensitivity.[42] There are many experimental drugs that effectively block the NMDA receptor, the channel or associated sites. The NMDA antagonists would be effective only in reducing hyperalgesia, rather than in abolishing the pain. However, NMDA antagonists have proved useful in treating allodynia/hyperalgesia sensitive to NMDA antagonists but not to opioids, by co-administering morphine with low doses of an NMDA antagonist (ketamine, memantine, dextrorphan or dextromethorphan), which may restore or potentiate the opioid effects.[42] Both dextrorphan and dextromethorphan also reduce wind-up. In human pain states with clear evidence for central change, it has been shown that these are entirely dependent on peripheral inputs for maintenance.[42] Consequently, there is a place for the use of peripheral local anaesthetics, although the symptoms may reappear once the block has worn off.[42] Spinal local anaesthetics do reduce NMDA-mediated activity and wind-up.[42] Systemic local anaesthetics also have selective effects on ectopic foci in damaged peripheral nerves, at doses that do not alter nerve conduction.[42] In peripheral nerve pathology, α_2-adrenergic agonists (clonidine) may persist and provide a target at postsynaptic sites, where presynaptic opioid receptors are reduced. They also potentiate opioid analgesia and, systemically and neuraxially, have sympathetic blocking effects in sympathetically maintained pain.[42]

Treatment requires decreasing the frequency and/or pain intensity. Thereafter, additional treatment will be required to help the patient both cope with pain that cannot be relieved, or is slower to change, and access physical and psychosocial rehabilitation.[6] The drugs available for the treatment of neuropathic pain need full assessment in controlled studies and against individual symptoms of the pain state. The current mainstay treatment for neuropathic pain remains anticonvulsants (carbamazepine and gabapentin), excitability blockers (lignocaine and mexiletine) and tricyclic antidepressants (amitriptyline, desipramine and dothiepin).[42] Carbamazepine is effective in about 50 per cent of patients with neuropathic pain, with minor side-effects.[42] Although it is a sodium channel blocker, the relative contribution of peripheral and central actions to its therapeutic effects is unclear. It is effective against neuronal responses in the spinal nerve ligation model.[42] In the chronic constriction injury model, gabapentin (systemic and neuraxial) partially reverses cold allodynia, mechanical allodynia and heat hyperalgesia, as well as mechanical allodynia in the spinal nerve ligation model.[42] In a limited number of cases, gabapentin has analgesic activity in neuropathic pain patients, and there is an expectation that the newer anticonvulsants will have therapeutic effects in neuropathic pain states.[42] The actions of the excitability blockers may be central and peripheral as well, and the relative contribution of the two sites remains unclear.[42] The basis for the role of antidepressants and other adrenergic agents in neuropathic pain treatment is also unclear as both central and peripheral actions, including sympathetic effects, are possible.[42] Anticonvulsants that increase inhibition, such as felbamate, have actions on the GABA-ergic inhibitory system.[42] Recent behavioural and electrophysiological studies have shown that anticonvulsants and sodium channel blockers (mexiletine) are effective in both neuropathic and inflammatory pain states.[42] Also, carbamazepine and gabapentin have been found to be effective in both conditions, providing evidence for a similar spinal processing of both neuropathic and inflammatory pain states, which appear to share a range of common physiological and pharmacological substrates.[42] Other antidepressants used include trazadone and some of the selective serotonin uptake inhibitors (sertraline), while other anticonvulsants include valproate and clonazepam[6]. Additional drugs tried include baclofen and the topical preparations of capsaicin, clonidine and EMLA (the eutectic mixture of lignocaine and prilocaine) cream.[6] Alternative methods encompass local anaesthetic infiltration or lignocaine infusion, sympathetic nervous system blockade, stimulation analgesia (transcutaneous or post-epidural trial spinal column stimulation) and further interventional approaches (cryotherapy and radiofrequency lesioning) following diagnostic local anaesthetic blocks.[6]

Analysis of controlled clinical trial data for peripheral neuropathic pain give consistent support to the analgesic effectiveness of tricyclic antidepressants, intravenous and topical lignocaine, intravenous ketamine, carbamazepine and topical aspirin.[41] There is limited support for the analgesic effectiveness of oral, topical and epidural clonidine, or for subcutaneous ketamine.[41] Trial method analysis has indicated that mexiletine and intravenous morphine are probably effective analgesics for peripheral neuropathic pain, while non-steroidal anti-inflammatory drugs (NSAIDs) are probably ineffective[41].

The description of a novel TTX (tetrodotoxin-resistant) sodium channel in C fibres may lead to possible therapeutic intervention.[42] Certain calcium channels also make important contributions to the genesis of neuropathic pain.[42] Opioids should never be discounted in neuropathic pain treatment. New drugs acting on other aspects of the central excitation cascade, such as GMI gangliosides and calcium channel blockers may prove effective in neuropathic pain.[40] Phorbol esters that stimulate protein kinase C formation increase the excitability of dorsal horn neurones projecting to the thalamus.[40] Electrophysiological and human scanning studies are essential if the relationship between peripheral damage and neuropathic pain is to be clarified.[42] Unanswered questions include the fact that, despite severe pain, human studies have reported deficits in thalamic activity.[42] In future, gene therapy may allow the patient's nervous system to overcome the injury by the restoration of neural function.[6]

VISCERAL PAIN

The sensibility of some visceral tissue differs profoundly.[43] The lung, liver and kidney parenchyma appear not to give rise to pain at all, while the mesenteries are sensitive to tension/clamping.[43] The gastrointestinal tract from the oesophagus to the rectum, the urinary tract from the kidney pelvis to the bladder, and the gallbladder, all yield pain upon distension.[43] Visceral ischaemia (e.g. angina) is also another stimulus for visceral pain.[43] Algogenic chemicals (e.g. bradykinin) produce pain when applied to visceral tissues.[43] Inflammatory states may trigger visceral pain, such as in the urinary and gastrointestinal tracts.[43] Spatial summation of the visceral inputs may explain the failure of localized mechanical stimuli (even damaging ones) to produce pain.[43]

To explain the encoding of visceral receptors, it has been found that both specific and intensity-coding receptors exist together, and their afferent fibres are found to travel in sympathetic and vagal afferent nerves.[44] Thus, both specific and intensity-encoding receptors are operating in the same organ and within the same afferent pathway. Silent nociceptors (sleeping unmyelinated afferent neurones) are an important subcategory of receptors that may contribute to pain sensation when the visceral organ is inflamed.[44] Organ distension (e.g. the bladder or joints) does not commonly produce pain sensation until the disease process causes inflammation of the organ. Visceral afferent fibres from visceral organs conduct information to cell bodies in the dorsal root ganglia.[44] Most visceral fibres are unmyelinated C fibre axons, but a few are myelinated A delta axons. Most of the afferent fibres forming the cardiopulmonary nerves enter the spinal cord at segments T2 and T3.[44] Renal, lumbar, colonic and hypogastric afferents are found primarily in the second, third and fourth lumbar dorsal root ganglia, respectively. The pelvic nerve contains visceral afferent fibres that enter the second sacral segment. Spinal visceral afferent fibres extend rostrally and caudally for several segments, periodically giving off collaterals that end primarily in the ipsilateral spinal grey matter, some penetrating the contralateral grey matter.[44] (Somatic afferents are more limited and focused.) The extensive distribution of visceral afferent fibres in the grey matter explains the diffuse and poorly localized nature of visceral sensations. Visceral afferent fibres terminate primarily on cells in laminae I, II, V and VI.[44] The spinothalamic tract transmits visceral information to the lateral (ventroposterolateral and ventroposteromedial) and medial thalamus. The cells of the lateral thalamus then project to the primary, and possibly the secondary, somatosensory, cortex. Information processed in these regions may be important for the sensori-discriminative nature of the pain, which refers to the capacity to analyse the location, intensity and duration of the nociceptive stimulus.[44] The association cortex may be responsible for the motivational-affective components of pain, including autonomic adjustments. Activity-dependent plasticity of the nociceptive systems may occur in the pathways, particularly in the nuclei that process nociceptive information from visceral organs. Little information exists about the reorganization or plasticity of the thalamic structures regarding visceral pain.[44] Other pathways carrying visceral information include the spinomesencephalic, the spinosolitary, the spinohypothalamic and the spinoreticular, which transmits visceral information to the reticular formation, where it mediates motor responses as well as escape and alerting behaviour.[44] The parabrachial nuclei of the pons function as an important region for processing viscerosomatic nociceptive information, which it transmits to the amygdala and hypothalamus, and is involved with emotional-affective, behavioural and autonomic reactions to noxious events.[44] The dorsal columns may process noxious visceral information.[44] The dorsal column medial lemniscal system and the spinal cord ventrolateral quadrant pathways are involved in processing information interpreted supraspinally as pain sensation. It is possible that the ventrolateral pathway transmits

information about diffuse, poorly localized pain, and the dorsal-column nuclei and pathways are important for changes associated with the cutaneous sensation associated with visceral pain.[44] Supraspinal nuclei are known to inhibit the activity of the spinothalamic tract cells in the spinal cord that receive visceral input, and the neuronal mechanisms in the C1 and C2 segments of the spinal cord participate in intraspinal inhibition.[44] Visceral pain is thus driven by both somatic and visceral input.[45] Its final perception depends on the interaction between visceral excitation, segmental and supraspinal inhibitory systems and descending excitatory systems.[45,46]

Unlike pain from skin stimulation, much visceral pain might be localized or referred to distant structures. The area of referral is generally segmental and superficial (e.g. to muscle and skin), innervated by the same spinal nerves as the affected viscus, or may be deep within the body, as visceral and somatic primary sensory neurones converge onto discrete populations of dorsal horn projection neurones.[43] The referral site may additionally show primary hyperalgesia (from sensitization of the primary sensory nociceptors) and secondary hyperalgesia (from central sensitization after strong visceral stimulation).[43,44] The change in the somatic referral of visceral pain often outlasts the duration of the noxious visceral stimulus.[44] Referred pain from two viscera close to each other may have overlapping somatic receptive fields of referral because their afferent input may converge to a common pool of spinothalamic tract cells (as seen in gallbladder disease mimicking angina pectoris).[44] The altered sensitivity of visceral tissue (e.g. with chemical bladder irritants or in cystitis) in inflammation suggests that new neural mechanisms of pain signalling may emerge.[43] After experimental inflammation of the bladder, the slope of the stimulus–response functions of the mechanosensitive afferents increases in the periphery, additionally leading to the recruitment of previously mechanically insensitive afferents.[43] The stimulus–response functions of the dorsal horn cells also show increase in excitability, both to bladder and to convergent somatic nociceptors.[43] Recent observations suggest that visceral afferents encode information according to an intensity rather than a specificity theory, implying that the pain threshold might be variable and set by the CNS rather than being determined principally by the recruitment of a particular high-threshold population of afferents.[43] There is thus evidence for a slowly developing and maintained increase in the excitability of central neurones following bladder inflammation.[43] It is still unclear whether central sensitization selectively affects sensory discriminative components of pain or other forms of sensory processing, such as the afferent control of bladder motility, and generalized autonomic responses.[43] There is evidence the nerve growth factor (NGF) is a mediator of persistent visceral pain and that it is upregulated in inflamed tissues (from macrophages, T- and B-lymphocytes, mast cells and Schwann cells).[43] NGF binds selectively to tyrosine kinase A (trkA), which is selectively expressed on nociceptive afferents.[43] Systemic synthetic trkA–IgG prevents exaggerated bladder reflexes after experimental inflammation of the bladder, offering new therapeutic possibilities for treating inflammatory pain.[43] There is evidence that the availability of NGF may contribute indirectly to central sensitization.[43] This is apparent in recordings from dorsal horn neurones, which exhibit increased responsiveness after the chronic application of exogenous NGF.[43]

In chronic pelvic pain, 25–80 per cent of patients have no visible pathology on laparoscopy, and a substantial proportion may have peripheral pain sources outside the pelvis and not associated with obvious tissue distortion.[47] They also have a high incidence of concurrent psychopathology.[47] Endometriosis can be shown in 15–40 per cent of these patients, and the pain is strongly associated with deep infiltrating lesions.[47] Pelvic congestion syndrome is also associated with chronic pelvic pain, and patients with dysmenorrhoea have been treated successfully by anaesthetizing the site of referred pain in the abdominal wall.[47] The hyperalgesia and persistent changes in autonomic reflex activity seen in many patients with chronic pelvic pain could be related to alterations in excitatory or inhibitory phenomena.[47] The stimulus for these changes or the effect of cyclical hormonal changes in these chronic pelvic pain patients remains unknown.

'Psychogenic' pain

Psychological factors contribute to the genesis and maintenance of many chronic pain syndromes. Chronic pain *per se* is also associated with psychological disorders (depression, anxiety and excessive dependence).[36] In somatoform pain disorders, patients believe they have pain but there is scant organic basis for their pain.[36] Pain that is inconsistent with the extent of tissue injury or co-existing neurological disease may be 'psychogenic' pain.[36] A precipitating nociceptive event for some patients may produce a persistent pain behaviour.[38] Pain-

associated psychological/psychiatric illness is, however, discussed further in Chapter 14.

Cancer pain management

The World Health Organisation (WHO) estimates that at least 4 million out of about 14 million people living with cancer experience chronic pain.[48] It occurs in at least 30 per cent of patients with metastatic disease, and about 75 per cent with advanced disease.[48] The pain sites vary, and there are different pathophysiological aspects and responses to treatment, which compound measurement difficulties. Pain changes over time in cancer (because of the concurrent involvement of different anatomical structures and because it is always evolving as a result of local tumour progression and metastatic spread) and breakthrough pains are common.[48] In assessment, quality of life and multiple symptom evaluation must also be considered.[48] Assessment instruments used include the McGill Pain Questionnaire, the Memorial Pain Assessment Card and the Brief Pain Inventory. Physical, psychological, social and spiritual factors, as well as the pain (mainly peripheral somatic nociceptive from the tumour but also neuropathic from nerve or CNS damage), all contribute to patient suffering.[48] Pain assessment includes physical (including neurological) and psychosocial evaluation. Peripheral nerve lesions (from the tumour, surgery and chemotherapy) give rise to neuropathic pain, in which secondary analgesics play a major therapeutic role (although this should not exclude a therapeutic opioid trial).[48]

One must have a clear understanding of the nature of a particular cancer and its pathogenesis in order to treat it effectively.[49] Because pain is a commonly associated feature of cancer, and because many of the therapeutic strategies for cancer may produce pain, it is important to understand the specific pain syndromes associated with the cancer *per se*.[49] Aggressive pain therapy and a continued reassessment of pain and of the patient's general condition represent the best approach to treating cancer-related pain syndromes.[49] It is customary to classify cancer pain into that caused by the cancer itself, that resulting from cancer treatment and that unrelated to the disease and its treatment.[48] No classification of cancer pain has been clinically validated, but staging systems are being used to describe patient groups within areas of cancer pain treatment.[48] Twenty per cent of pain syndromes are due to surgery, radiation and chemotherapy. These include:[48]

- post-surgical neuropathic pain syndromes (after a mastectomy, thoracotomy, nephrectomy, limb or rectal amputation or inguinal and axillary dissection, and also include stump pain);
- a non-healing incision;
- post-radiation pain syndromes (enteritis, dermatitis, muscle fibrosis, osteonecrosis, plexus fibrosis, myelopathy and radiation-induced peripheral nerve tumours);
- post-chemotherapy pain syndromes (as in aseptic bony necrosis, diffuse polyneuropathy and steroid pseudorheumatism).

An analytical classification by direct tumour involvement includes:[48]

- tumour infiltration of the bones and joints (base of skull syndromes, vertebral syndromes and diffuse and focal bone pain);
- visceral tumour infiltration (oesophageal mediastinal pain of the diaphragm with shoulder pain, an upper abdominal/pancreatic tumour with epigastric pain, splenomegaly with left upper quadrant pain, intestinal/peritoneal disease with diffuse abdominal pain, pleural pain, gastrointestinal perforation, biliary or ureteric obstruction, bladder tumour with suprapubic pain, and perirectal/rectal tumour with perineal pain);
- soft tissue tumour infiltration (skin/subcutaneous tissue, trunk and neck muscle/fascia mucous membrane and retroperitoneal tissue infiltration);
- neural tumour compression (peripheral nerve syndromes, radiculopathy, polyneuropathy, plexopathy, cranial nerve lesions and epidural spinal cord compression);
- tumour-related headache (skull lesion and intracranial tumour with or without raised intracranial pressure).

The pain specialist interacts with other specialists in diagnosing and planning the treatment of specific pain syndromes. Radiation therapy can be effective in reducing cancer-induced bone and visceral pain.[50] Surgery may be needed to stabilize pathological fractures, decompress entrapped nerves or bypass obstructed viscera.[50]

Informing patients of the reasons for their pain helps them to deal better with that pain and reduces their overall suffering.[50] The WHO has urged that resources begin shifting from biologically focused antitumour treatment to analgesia and palliative care relatively early in each patient's course.[51] The WHO analgesic ladder (in which

analgesic drugs are selected in a step-wise fashion based on the overall severity of the pain), if properly administered, can control pain in 70–90 per cent of patients with chronic cancer pain, although about 20 per cent of patients need other interventions.[48] There are also no true validation studies on the WHO ladder.[48] As the first step, NSAIDs are given for mild to moderate pain. Patients with moderate to severe pain, and those who fail an NSAID trial, should receive an opioid conventionally used for moderate pain, usually combined with an NSAID.[48] Severe pain or inadequate pain relief with the second step indicates the use of an opioid conventionally used for severe pain, possibly combined with an NSAID.[48] Adjuvant drugs can be added at any step to treat side-effects or other symptoms, or secondary analgesics may be used.[48] Opioid therapy strategy is:[48]

- to establish an initial dose;
- to prescribe fixed around-the-clock therapy, with other doses available as needed;
- to titrate the dose to the effect;
- to treat side-effects.

The right dose for any one patient is the dose that causes analgesia without toxicity.[50] Opioid tolerance and addiction are common concerns for patients, families and clinicians.[50] None of these is a clinically significant reality in the opioid analgesic therapy of terminally ill cancer patients.[50]

The agonist–antagonist opioids have a limited role in treating chronic cancer pain due to their ceiling effect for analgesia, their psychotomimetic effects and the possible precipitation of an abstinence syndrome (in patients physically dependent on pure opioid agonists).[48] Because of the CNS excitatory effects of the metabolite norpethidine, pethidine should not be used for chronic pain management. The so-called 'weak opioids' include codeine, hydrocodone, dihydrocodeine, oxycodone and propoxyphene (which has a toxic metabolite that does not usually pose a clinical problem).[48] They have no ceiling analgesic effect but have a limited available dose range because of the combination with aspirin or paracetamol with their maximum safe dose.[48] On their own, their doses can be titrated to effect. Tramadol is used as a step 2 drug.[48] In renal failure, metabolite accumulation can occur with morphine and propoxyphene.[48] For severe pain, a physician should have at least three strong opioids available (such as morphine, hydromorphone, fentanyl, oxymorphone, methadone or levorphanol) to rotate them, thus reducing the emergence of side-effects and minimizing the number of patients unresponsive to opioids when one opioid is not producing sufficient analgesia.[48] Patients may be started on immediate-release, short-acting morphine liquids (or tablets).[50] Once a patient's 24-hour morphine requirement has been established, optimal pain prevention may be achieved with 12-hourly controlled-release morphine tablets.[50] Immediate-release morphine should still be available for intermittent acute pains and dose titration. When switching opioids, equi-analgesic doses should generally be reduced by 25–50 per cent to account for incomplete cross-tolerance between different opioids.[48] Pain severity, age, metabolic abnormalities and concurrent treatments need to be taken into account in assessing the size of the dose reduction. For rapid dose titration, opioids with short half-lives are used.[48] The oral dose equivalency of tramadol to morphine is 4:1, with less nausea and constipation with tramadol.[48] Methadone (with a half-life of 12–100 hours) should not be used in the elderly or in severe metabolic dysfunction.[48] When changing to an opioid, an equivalent dose reduction of at least 75 per cent is preferable. For changing patients from oral hydromorphone to oral methadone, the clinically effective ratio is 1.2 ± 1.3 for methadone/hydromorphone oral doses.[48]

The oral route is preferred for its efficacy and simplicity.[48] For rapid onset, rapid dose titration, gastrointestinal dysfunction or because of side-effects, alternative routes can be used. Continuous opioid infusions (intravenous and subcutaneous) reduce plasma concentration fluctuations and are used in dysphagia, gastrointestinal obstruction, nausea and vomiting with oral opioids and excessive side-effects with parenteral bolus therapy.[48] When continuous intravenous or subcutaneous infusions are used to treat advanced cancer with other symptoms at home, the opioid (morphine or hydromorphone) can be combined with other drugs (metoclopramide, dexamethasone, haloperidol, scopolamine or midazolam) in the same infusion.[48] Because of its greater bioavailability, subcutaneous morphine should be given at one third of the dose of oral morphine.[50] Subcutaneous infusions are considered equi-analgesic to intravenous infusions, and volumes up to 3 ml per hour can be given for about a week via butterfly needles (25–27 gauge) or longer by using Teflon cannulae. More frequent infusion site rotation overcomes local skin reactions. Neuraxial routes are used for patients with opioid-responsive pain with excessive side-effects from systemic therapy. Transdermal fentanyl patches (25, 50, 75 or 100 μg per hour) are used for indications similar to those for intravenous/subcutaneous infusions.[48] The peak plasma concentrations are seen between 24 and 48 hours, the elimination half-life is about 24 hours, and the dosing interval is 48–72 hours.[48] Individual dose titration is essential. A simple rule of dose equivalency is to prescribe a fentanyl patch every 3 days in the same number of micrograms per hour as the patient was using orally in milligrams per 12 hours of long-acting morphine.[50] Rectal formulations (oxymorphone, morphine and hydromorphone) have a bio-availability similar to those given via the oral route and are useful in treating breakthrough pain in patients on parenteral opioids who lack the oral route.[48] Controlled-release formulations are now available. The oral transmucosal fentanyl lollipop might prove practical in treating breakthrough pain.[48] Sublingual buprenorphine is used for mild to moderate cancer pain.

Treatment is given prophylactically (with a stool softener and a cathartic titrated to effect) to prevent opioid constipation and ensure a bowel movement every 1–2 days.[48,50] Oral naloxone (0.8 mg twice daily, titrated to effect) is effective in patients with refractory constipation (in advanced cancer and poor hydration).[48] Unrelieved constipation is a common reason for opioid-associated nausea.[50] With dose titration, tolerance to nausea and vomiting usually develops, but opioid- and route-switching may be helpful. Drug treatment includes using metoclopramide, prochlorperazine, haloperidol, scopolamine, ondansetron and tropisetron. Similarly, tolerance to sedation develops rapidly but can be treated with methylphenidate or pemoline, or by selectively switching to the neuraxial route.[48] Opioid-induced delirium (dose-dependent) can be treated by haloperidol, by switching opioid or by switching to the neuraxial route.[48] Opioid-induced myoclonus (dose-dependent) can be treated by clonazepam or by switching opioid or route. Tolerance often develops to opioid-induced urinary retention (especially with neuraxial opioids), but if not, an opioid switch or a non-pharmacological approach can be tried.[48] Opioid-induced respiratory depression is always associated with decreased consciousness, and opioid tapering rather than naloxone administration (0.4 mg in 10 ml saline, titrated to effect) is used for oversedation without clinically significant respiratory depression, as tolerance usually develops rapidly.[48]

Although they are extensively used, it has never been formally proved that secondary analgesics employed to treat chronic benign pain improve analgesia in cancer pain.[48] Antidepressants used include, among others, amitriptyline (50–150 mg daily), desipramine and nortriptyline (less sedation and fewer anticholinergic effects), paroxetine, venlefaxine.[48] For lancinating neuropathic cancer pain, carbamazepine (400–1600 mg per day, although marrow toxicity limits its use), valproate and clonazepam can be used. The $GABA_B$ agonist baclofen can similarly be used. The α_2-adrenergic agonist clonidine can be used epidurally for sympathetically maintained pain, and transdermally in polyneuropathies.[48] Oral clonidine needs to be tested in cancer pain. Corticosteroids have an efficacy in improving the quality of life by relieving pain and improving appetite, nausea and mood.[48] Dexamethasone (10–100 mg) can result in marked analgesia in raised intracranial pressure, spinal cord compression, superior vena cava syndrome, metastatic bone pain, nerve plexus or peripheral nerve compression, symptomatic lymphoedema and hepatic capsular distension.[48] NSAIDs are indicated for mild to moderate pain related to bone and soft tissue invasion.[48] Their mechanism of action and side-effect profile is discussed in Chapter 4. Unlike opioids, NSAIDs have a ceiling effect for analgesia but do not produce tolerance or physical dependence. The risk of gastroduodenal toxicity is low with ibuprofen and diclofenac.[48] Low initial doses with dose titration are recommended with NSAIDs, although the use of the strong opioids should not be delayed if they are thought necessary. Bisphosphonates (clodronate, etidronate and pamidronate) inhibit osteoclastic activity and are useful in the treatment of cancer-associated hypercalcaemia or bone pain (reducing metastatic bone pain by 30–60 per cent).[48] In bone pain, the best analgesic effects are obtained with pamidronate.[48] In multiple myeloma, the bisphosphonates may also slow tumour growth and should be used early on.[48] Other potent bisphosphonates (aminohexane, risedronate and alendronate) and other bone resorption inhibitors (gallium nitrate and paclitaxel) offer better symptom control and survival.[48] For neuropathic pain, oral tocainamide, mexiletine and subcutaneous lignocaine infusions can be used, and there is a potential role here for the new NMDA receptor antagonists.[48]

Local and regional pain-blocking procedures can be invaluable in the 10–15 per cent of cancer pain patients whose systemic analgesic and secondary analgesic therapy has not provided pain relief or has been associated with intolerable toxicity.[50] The neuraxial opioid route is used in patients on systemic opioids experiencing unacceptable and untreatable side-effects (e.g. nausea, vomiting and drowsiness) or whose pain is uncontrolled.[48] Epidurally, the increase of low-dose bupivacaine (0.125–0.25 per cent) can increase the analgesic effect without increasing the toxicity. The common side-effects are usually self-limiting and manageable with dose titration.[48] Respiratory depression is rare. Systemic opioids may need tapering as withdrawal symptoms can occur if systemic opioids are suddenly stopped. Most hospice programmes should be willing to cover the maintenance and refilling of external or internal spinal opioid pumps.[50] Neurolytic blocks (with phenol in glycerine, and alcohol, and primarily for nociceptive pain) are indicated for patients with a short life expectancy with well-localized pain resistant to other pain control methods.[48]

The intrathecal and epidural (e.g. sacral phenol injection) as well as the subdural routes have been used.[48,50] For neoplastic infiltration of the upper abdominal viscera (pancreas, upper retroperitoneum, liver, gallbladder and proximal small bowel), a neurolytic coeliac plexus block can be performed, obtaining good analgesia in 80–90 per cent of patients for 2–4 weeks or longer.[48] With neuroablative procedures (e.g. percutaneous radiofrequency cordotomy), careful opioid dose titration is needed to avoid sedation, respiratory depression and withdrawal symptoms.[48] The indications, contraindications and complications of neuraxial and neurolytic interventions and neuroablative procedures are extensively discussed in later chapters. Cognitive behavioural therapies (autogenic relaxation, music therapy, visual imagery and distraction) have their own opioid-sparing effect.[50] Quality-improvement action plans must continuously be applied for an evidence-based, patient-centred, outcome-driven cancer pain health care system to become a reality.[51]

To summarize, uncontrolled pain is agony to the cancer patient and represents a true emergency[52] (Figure 1.3). The optimal control of pain and related symptoms in the cancer patient improves functioning and enhances quality of life.[53] This enables patients to focus on those things which give meaning to their life. Cancer patients are often undergoing treatment with surgery, radiation therapy and chemotherapy. Types of cancer pain include nociceptive, visceral and neuropathic pain. In general, cancer pain responds in a predictable way to orally administered primary and secondary analgesics.[54] Drug therapy (with opioids) is the mainstay of cancer pain treatment. Two major problem areas are pain associated with nerve damage and bone pain (both of which can be opioid non-responsive).

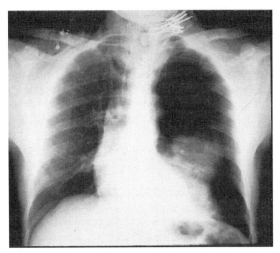

Figure 1.3   Cancer pain – an x-ray of a patient with carcinoma of the left bronchus.

It is so important to realize that the same management principles apply in cancer pain as in other acute and chronic pain problems. Thus, drug therapy for cancer pain can be found in the Chapters 3–6. Diagnostic and therapeutic nerve blocks and other interventional therapy used in these patients are covered in the remaining relevant chapters. The cancer patient's emotional response, and important aspects of therapy such as communication and support, are dealt with in Chapter 14.

THE ASSESSMENT OF PAIN

Pain is a highly complex phenomenon precluding objective assessment. The sensation of pain is not directly measurable because pain is a unique personal experience. There are no reliable and usable physiological indices of pain (e.g. increased blood pressure, hyperventilation and withdrawal movements). The only criterion possible for the scientific investigation of pain is that based on voluntary responses. Methods are, however, available to reliably and validly assess a patient's pain experience.

The prevention and control of acute pain can be enhanced if the severity and duration of patient discomfort in a clinical setting can be monitored.[55] In chronic pain, appraisals of pain are important for determining a patient's diagnosis, for evaluating a patient's cognitive perspective and for establishing a treatment plan.[56] Although the same technology can be applied to measuring acute and chronic pain, the goals of assessment and interpretation of the measures usually differ. In chronic pain, patterns over time (traits) are more useful measures than are day-to-day changes (states) in pain intensity.[55] It is also important to measure the impact of pain on patterns of physical and psychosocial functioning.

Experimentally induced pain

Pain can be experimentally induced by electrical, mechanical, chemical and thermal stimuli. Pain stimuli are chosen based on controllability, measurability, range of intensity, convenience and safety.[57] Conflicting results are obtained on the influence of chronic pain experiences on the thresholds of experimental pain stimuli. From a psychological point of view, the hypervigilance and adaptive level theories predict opposite reactivity for chronic pain patients exposed to experimental stimuli. A recent study found that chronic clinical pain did not significantly modify experimental pain measures.[57]

Two levels for patient response can be seen.[58] The first, known as the pain perception threshold, is the point at which the stimulus is perceived by the patient as painful. The second, known as the tolerance, is the maximum intensity of painful stimulus that can be endured.

Two types of stimulation occur, namely phasic and tonic.[59] In phasic stimulation, the sensation ceases when the stimulus does. Examples include thermal (radiant heat) stimulation and electrical stimulation.[59] Thermal stimulation is precise and simple, allowing rapid repetition without injury to the skin. With electrical stimulation, a clearly detectable pain sensation is produced. The stimulus intensity may be exactly determined. In tonic stimulation, the sensation does not cease with cessation of the stimulus. Examples include the cold pressor technique, in which the patient's hand is emerged in ice for a period of time, and the tourniquet pain technique.[59]

MEASUREMENT TECHNIQUES[59]

Submaximal effort tourniquet technique[58]

First, a pain estimate is obtained by asking the patient to rate his or her pain on a numerical scale ranging from 0 to 100 (see below). In this method, blood is first drained from the arm using a rubber bandage, and the limb ischaemia is maintained by use of a pressure cuff set well above systolic blood pressure. A hand exerciser is then squeezed 20 times. Following this, a stop watch is started and two times are recorded: the first when the pain reaches a level similar to that of the patient's usual pain, and the second, the time taken to reach the maximum pain bearable. Then:

Tourniquet pain ratio (TPR)

$$= \frac{\text{Time to reach clinical pain}}{\text{Time to reach maximum pain tolerated}} \times 100$$

If the pain estimates are markedly higher than the TPR, psychological factors are thought to play a significant part.[58]

Signal detection – sensory decision theory

In this, a version of signal detection is applied to the measurement of experimental pain.[60] By analysing responses to a series of stimuli, two determinants of threshold performance are identified, namely the ability to discriminate between stimuli and a willingness to call a stimulus painful. Sensory decision theory has been found to predict the status of chronic pain patients 6 months after its measurement.[61]

Experimental pain production measurement paradigm

An experimental pain production measurement paradigm has been produced using electrical stimuli that permit the separation of sensory from motivational factors in pain thresholds.[62] Electrical shock stimuli are rated against a standard stimulus with numerical estimates. Affective rating of shock intensity occurs at the same time.

Functional measurement scaling

This measurement requires that aspects of two stimuli be converted into a single response that relates the two stimuli.[63]

Descriptor differential scale

Here, 12 description items are used for each pain dimension assessed.[64] Subjects rate their pain as equal to, greater than or less than the anchoring description on a 10-point graphic scale.

MEASUREMENT APPARATUS

Algometers

Algometers have been used for the quantitative determination of pain parameters such as pain threshold and pain tolerance. Stimuli (e.g. pressure) are applied to various parts of the body (especially to the trigger points).

There are several types of algometer.

Mechanical algometer. This consists of a plunger mounted on a calibrated spring. The plunger of a force gauge is connected to a circular dial, calibrated in kg/cm^2, in accordance with the area of the tip.

Electrical algometer. The advantage of an electrical algometer over a mechanical one is its ability to record the force signal. A recently described pressure algometer uses a force–displacement transducer with two modifications:[65] a tip made of teflon (with a tip area of $0.25\ cm^2$) that covers one of the two beam shafts, and a handle mounted fully on the transducer to facilitate the maintenance of continuous pressure on a selected point. The transducer is connected to a carrier amplifier and plugged into a two-channel recorder. The patient is instructed to activate the marker of the recorder, by pressing a hand-held button, when the pain is first perceived and again when the pain becomes unacceptable. The marks, along with the simultaneous force tracing, allow for a quantitative and precise determination of the subject's response to these two pain pressure stimuli.[65]

Lithotripter. The power and nociceptive intensity of shock waves generated by the Dornier HM3 extracorporeal shockwave lithotripter are voltage dependent.[66] They have been used for precise and quantitative measurements of induced truncal pain.

Surface electromyography

Non-invasive quantitative surface electromyography has been found to be effective in quantifying severe acute pain.[67] The efficacy of surface electromyography in the pharmacological analgesic management of patients unable to verbalize pain intensity is currently being studied. Electromyography (with needles) is used to assess muscle tension in painful muscles in fibromyalgia.[68]

Pain imaging techniques

A number of relatively non-invasive methods of producing images of functional brain activity, such as single photon emission computed tomography (SPECT), positron emission tomography (PET) and functional magnetic resonance imaging (fMRI), are available.[69] They can all produce images of changes in regional cerebral blood flow during neural activity and have been applied to localizing brain areas associated with a variety of experimental and clinical pain conditions.[69] The major problem with PET and SPECT techniques is that it is not easy to determine whether decreased or increased metabolic activity reflects synaptic excitation or inhibition.[40] With the available resolution, it is also not possible to analyse activity within specific nuclei. Although the other imaging methods provide a more detailed temporal resolution (evoked potentials, magnetoencephalography) and spatial localization (fMRI), PET has the advantage of combining statistical quantification with the simultaneous detection of patterns of regional activity through the forebrain and brain stem.[70] It uses radioactive isotopes attached to metabolically active molecules to provide markers for the amount of neurological activity in various parts of the brain. Using PET to map changes in regional cerebral blood flow in response to nociceptive input, allows an increased understanding of the underlying neurophysiological mechanisms related to pain perception.[71] Several studies have described structures within the human forebrain that show increased blood flow during painful stimulation.[71] A close relationship between cerebral blood flow changes and electrical neuronal activity occurs.[71] In PET studies of experimentally phasic or tonic pain (giving differences in the activation pattern), increases in regional cerebral blood flow take place in the anterior cingulate cortex (most consistently), the somatosensory cortex, the insula of the contralateral thalamus, the prefrontal cortex, the lentiform nucleus and the cerebellum.[40]

Quantitative stimulus–response relationships within and between pain-activated regions need to be identified.[70] The potential impact of pain imaging is the development of new pharmacotherapies based on a knowledge of the specific biochemistry and pharmacology of functionally identified critical components of the pain network, and the identification of pain-specific reorganizations that take place in the CNS following disease or trauma affecting the peripheral or central nervous system.[70] This should result in the development of physical and pharmacological methods to prevent and to treat neuropathic pains.

Microneurography

Microneurography recording has provided information about the somatosensory system, although the data provided for tactile sensation are clearer than those for nociception.[72] A microelectrode is inserted percutaneously and is manually or electrically guided into a peripheral nerve fascicle.[72] Optimal recording conditions (a high signal-to-noise ratio) are then obtained for a particular axon.[72] Nociceptor fibres are not easy to study with

microneurography, this mostly being limited to the C polymodal nociceptors.[72] The nature of somatic nociceptors and nociception has been elucidated considerably using microneurography.[72] A few studies have investigated the pathophysiology of chronic pain and the mechanisms of action of some analgesic strategies, and the technique has also been used to study efferent autonomic activity.[72]

Analgesic drug monitoring

Although analgesics are generally perceived to be safe agents, serious toxicity may occur in the setting of acute overdose, chronic abuse or overuse.[73] The indications for drug monitoring in patients using these medications appropriately are as yet not well defined.[73] Colorimetric, enzymatic and immunoassays are used for the routine monitoring of paracetamol and salicylates. Recent advances include achiral and chiral chromatographic assays, restricted access media and automated chromatographic systems for the analysis of ibuprofen, naproxen and tramadol.[73]

ANIMAL PAIN – RAT PAW FORMALIN TEST

Localized inflammation of the rat hind paw caused by the subcutaneous injection of formalin has been used as a model for tonic pain.[74] A biphasic firing pattern of lumbar dorsal horn neurones from the receptive field of the ipsilateral hind paw occurs. An initial (0–10 minutes) high-frequency increase in firing is followed after a quiescent period by a more persistent (20–65 minutes) low-frequency discharge.[74] This model can be used to test pre-emptive analgesia.[75]

Another animal model, making use of the development of autotomy after peripheral nerve sectioning, is discussed in Chapter 10.

Clinical pain

Clinical pain assessment must rely on subjective or behavioural variables since available measurements of the peripheral and central generators are lacking.[57] It is standard to refer to the three dimensions of pain: the sensory and physiological, the behavioural, and the cognitive and affective.[76] Measurement across the various areas is not routine. Since all measurement is context dependent, no single score can ever represent pain.[76] To demonstrate efficacy, patient ratings of pain and activity, preferably retrospective for pretreatment levels, and therapists' ratings of global benefit are probably of most use.[76] Rehabilitation aims to increase activity levels and decrease use of health care resources. However, the use of reliable, valid and appropriate measures is no more difficult than the use of uninterpretable or unsuitable measures.

MEASURES OF PHYSICAL PERFORMANCE

There is a lack of available physical measures with well-demonstrated reliability and validity.[76] Measures used include mechanically derived measures (spinal mobility, trunk strength, endurance, positional tolerance and the approximation of repetitive daily activities/exercises) and speed and distance on an exercise bicycle.[76] Follow-up patient counts can be requested by mail, electronic mail or by telephone. For good-quality data, a simple physical measure (one that can be administered by a trained lay-person) consists of a 5-minute walk distance test, a 1-minute stair-climbing test and 1 minute of repeated standing and sitting from a chair.[76] Measures of activity include patient activity (plus parallel measurements by the partner) counts, a specific activities report and a checklist of painful pain-limited or no longer painful activities.[76] Trivial (tying shoelaces) or major (holding a full-time job) goals can be weighted according to their importance. An 'up-time' recorder can be used to record time spent reclining.[76]

MEASURES OF FUNCTION/QUALITY OF LIFE

Tools used consist of the Sickness Impact Profile (with 136 weighted questions), the Oswestry Low Back Pain Disability Questionnaire (consisting of a single question with six possible response levels on pain intensity, personal care, lifting, walking, sitting, standing, sleeping, sexual activity, social life and travelling, with the score as a percentage), the Arthritis Impact Measurement Scales (covering mobility, physical activity, dexterity, household activities, activities of daily living, social activity, pain, depression and anxiety).[76] Quality of life measures are popular among the managerial strata of health services.

PHYSIOLOGICAL MEASURES

Electromyograph (EMG) measures have proved more useful than cardiovascular function for measuring the impact of pain.[76] Dynamic EMG recordings have been used in low back pain.[76] Studies of sleep problems in pain patients are rare.[76] Results obtained using patient ratings (difficulty in falling asleep, and feeling rested on wakening) give as satisfactory results as when using expensive polysomnography.[76] An automated device for recording the time to fall asleep is available for home use.[76]

PAIN QUANTITY AND QUALITY

The visual analogue scale (VAS) has been validated against estimates by the treating surgeon, the observation of activity level and analgesic use.[76] Pain ratings (verbal, numerical and spatial) are widely used but with insufficient data on the effects of context.[76] Another poorly addressed area is the differentiation between statistical and clinical significance. So few studies clearly state that the pain is not expected to change that it is not possible to test the association of expectation with findings.[76] It may be better to anchor pain estimates by taking an average of 12 ratings over 4 days.[76] Pain intensity measurement has been compared by VASs, numerical rating scales (NRSs) (0–100, and an 11-point box scale) and four- and five-item verbal scales for ease of scoring, ease of patient understanding, sensitivity in the number of response categories, statistical power sensitivity and relationships with other pain indices.[76] The 0–100 NRSs were the simplest to administer, were not subject to scoring error and presented fewer problems than the VASs for older subjects. While verbal scales had the lowest error rate, few response options can make for less sensitivity to change.[76] Most respond to 0–100 scales in multiples of five. A mechanical VAS minimizes measurement error.[76]

Self-report measurement procedures: single-dimensional self-reporting

Single-dimensional scaling is simple, rapid to administer and can be used in a variety of different

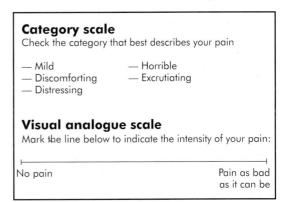

Category scale
Check the category that best describes your pain

— Mild   — Horrible
— Discomforting   — Excruciating
— Distressing

Visual analogue scale
Mark the line below to indicate the intensity of your pain:

|————————————————————————————|
No pain   Pain as bad
                                     as it can be

Figure 1.4 Category and visual analogue scales.

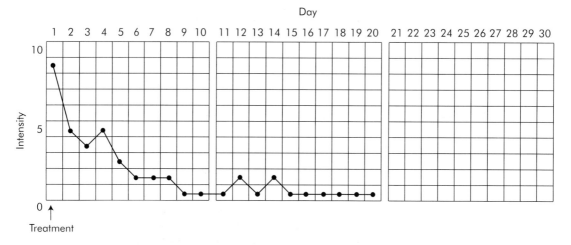

Figure 1.5   Daily visual analogue pain scale in the treatment of a patient suffering from post-herpetic neuralgia.

settings (even in children).[77] However, it tends to oversimplify the assessment of the pain problem.

Verbal descriptor (category) scales. In this verbal rating scale, the best word descriptor (e.g. mild, distressing or excruciating) is chosen by the patient to fit the pain[77] (Figure 1.4). Such scales are easy to use, but equal interval adjectives should be assigned to pain from 0–5, or 5–10, to appreciate the divergence from the ideal.[76] A facial expression picture scale can be used in the same way. This, unfortunately, produces simple category data with a limited range.[77]

Numerical rating scales. Patients are asked to choose a number from 0 to 101 to describe the intensity of their pain, 0 being 'No pain' and 101 'Worst pain imaginable'[77] (Figures 1.4 and 1.5). This can be easily administered in the oral or written form.

Visual analogue scale. The VAS has been shown to be one of the best paper and pencil instruments for assessing clinical pain intensity.[59] Its estimates are reliable over time and are sensitive to changes over time.[59] Although there are many variables, it typically consists of a 10 cm horizontal line bounded by 'No pain' at the left end and 'Worst pain imagin-

able' at the right. Patients indicate their pain intensity on either a 1–10 or a 1–100 scale.

Graphic rating scale. Here, descriptive words such as 'mild', 'moderate' and 'severe' are placed along the VAS at specified intervals, and patients are asked to indicate the degree of their pain[59] (Figure 1.6).

Self-report measurement procedures: multiple dimensional self-reporting

Cross-modal validation. With this technique, pain is quantified by matching it to the experience of a precisely controlled stimulus in another sensory modality (e.g. auditory). It offers potentially more reliable and valid data than the simpler VASs.[55] Using a cross-modality approach, a Pain Perception Profile has been developed to assess pain through the use of psychophysically scaled verbal descriptors. Advancement in this field is required before scores from pain patients can be confidently interpreted.[77]

McGill Pain Questionnaire. This is the best known and most extensively tested multidimensional pain questionnaire designed to provide quantification of pain on more than an intensity dimension, which can be treated statistically[59,77] (Figure 1.7). It takes 5–15 minutes to complete. Pain is scaled in four categories: sensory, affective, evaluative and miscellaneous. Sensory descriptors include words such as 'throbbing', 'pinching', 'aching', 'dull', 'splitting' and 'piercing'.[78] Evaluative descriptors include 'bearable', 'mild', 'violent', 'agonizing' and 'intense'. Affective descriptors include 'exhausting', 'wicked', 'frightful', 'vicious' and 'punishing'.[78]

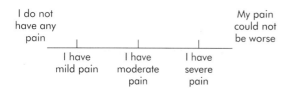

Figure 1.6   Graphic rating scale.

McGill Pain Questionnaire

(MODIFIED).

Name: . . . . Date: . . . .

PRI: S ____ A _____ E___ M(S)_____ M(AE)____ M(T)_____ PRI(T)___ PPI ___
(1–10)   (11–15)   (16)   (17–19)   (20)   (17–20)   (1–20)

PART 1: What does your pain feel like?

> Some of the words below describe your *present* pain.
> Tick *only* those words that best describe it. *Leave out* any
> category that is *not* suitable. Use only a *single word* in
> each appropriate category (the one that applies best).

1 Flickering . . . . Quivering . . . . Pulsing . . . . Throbbing . . . . Beating . . . . Pounding	**8** Tingling . . . . Itchy . . . . Smarting . . . . Stinging	**16** Annoying . . . . Troublesome Miserable Intense . . . . Unbearable . . . .
2 Jumping . . . . Flashing . . . . Shooting	**9** Dull . . . . Sore . . . . Hurting . . . . Aching . . . . Heavy	**17** Spreading . . . . Radiating Penetrating . . . . Piercing . . . .
3 Pricking . . . . Boring . . . . Drilling Stabbing . . . . Lancinating	**10** Tender . . . . Taut . . . . Rasping Splitting	**18** Tight . . . . Numb . . . . Drawing Squeezing . . . . Tearing . . . .
4 Sharp . . . . Cutting . . . . Lacerating	**11** Tiring . . . . Exhausting	**19** Cool . . . . Cold . . . . Freezing . . . .
5 Pinching . . . . Pressing . . . . Gnawing . . . . Cramping . . . . Crushing	**12** Sickening . . . . Suffocating	**20** Nagging . . . . Nauseating . . . . Agonizing . . . . Dreadful Torturing . . . .
	13 Fearful . . . . Frightful . . . . Terrifying	**PPI**
6 Tugging . . . . Pulling . . . . Wrenching	**14** Punishing . . . . Cruel . . . . Vicious . . . . Killing	**0** No pain . . . . **1** Mild . . . . **2** Discomforting . . . . **3** Distressing . . . .
7 Hot . . . . Burning . . . . Scalding . . . . Searing	**15** Retching . . . . Blinding	**4** Horrible . . . . **5** Excruciating . . . .

Figure 1.7 McGill pain questionnaire (*continued overleaf*)

PART 2: How does your pain change with time?

> Which word or words would
> you use to describe the
> *pattern* of pain?

Brief   . . . . .
Momentary . . . . .
Transient . . . . .

Rhythmic   . . . . .
Periodic   . . . . .
Intermittent . . . . .

Continuous . . . . .
Steady   . . . . .
Constant   . . . . .

PART 3: Where is your pain?

> Please mark on the drawing below, the areas where you
> feel pain. Put an **E** if external, or an **I**, near the area
> which you mark. Put **EI** if both external and internal.

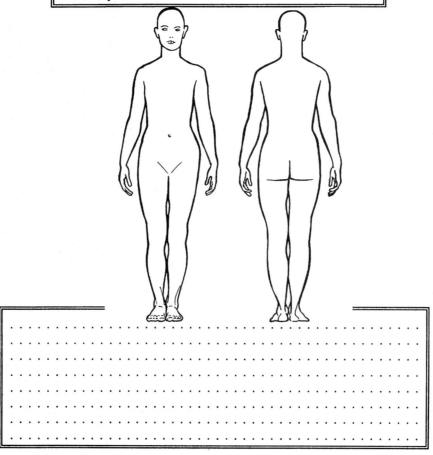

Figure 1.7 McGill pain questionnaire – continued.

Patients are presented with 20 sets of words that describe pain and are asked to select those sets which seem relevant to their pain, circling the words that best describe their pain within each selected set.[55] The total of the four sections is known as the Pain Rating Index. Each set has 2–6 words listed in order of increasing discomfort.[59] The score in each section is the sum of the ranks of words chosen in each set. An adjective is chosen from each set that best describes the patient's current pain experience. The Present Pain Intensity is then rated on a verbal rating scale from 0 (no pain) to 5 (maximum pain). The total number of adjectives chosen is also noted.[59] In sick patients, it is possible to administer the scale orally. A shortened form that relates well to the standard questionnaire has also been developed.[59]

Several studies have evaluated the structure of the McGill Pain Questionnaire responses in patients with clinical pain conditions.[69,80] It is reported to possess strong concurrent validity, internal consistency, and test and retest reliability, especially of the affective distress of pain patients.[59] The evidence of its diagnostic value for pain description is more questionable.[81] The theoretical nature of the McGill Pain Questionnaire has been confirmed in acute clinical pain.[82] The standard psychological indices of discriminant validity may not, however, apply to multidimensional pain measures.[79] Studies using factor analytic techniques to determine whether the McGill Pain Questionnaire assesses the dimension of pain it was postulated to assess have yielded conflicting results.[80] More work needs to be done on the multidimensional evaluation of factors that evoke or modulate pain responses. Since its attractions are to provide separate sensory and affective scores, the inconsistencies between factor analytical solutions are of some concern.[76] A Pain Discomfort Scale, consisting of 10 items (each rated on a 5-point scale), covers fear, helplessness and interference by pain with daily life.[76] The use of pain drawings (two dimensions) is rather unstandardized.[76]

Dartmouth Pain Questionnaire. The Dartmouth Pain Questionnaire allows the assessment (with acceptable levels of validity and reliability) of additional factors such as a general affective dimension, the time course and intensity of the pain, and behaviours affected by pain.[77] An advantage is its consideration of the remaining aspects of positive functioning.[55]

West Haven–Yale Multidimensional Pain Inventory. This 52-item inventory was designed to assess overall dimensions specific to chronic pain problems.[55] It consists of three parts composed of 12 scales that examine the impact of pain on the patients' lives, the responses of others to the patients' communications of pain and the extent to which patients participate in common daily activities.[83,84] Scales covering pain severity, interference by pain with daily life, control, distress, spouse support, frequency of three types of spouse response (solicitous, distracting and punishing) and four types of activity (household, outdoor, away from home and social) are combined into a general activity score.[76]

Pain Disability Index. The Pain Disability Index is a self-report instrument to assess the degree to which chronic pain interferes with various daily activities.[85] It has test–retest reliability and validity. The Pain Disability Index also seems to be associated with levels of pain behaviour shown by patients.

Illness Behaviour Questionnaire. Another self-report instrument is the 52-item Illness Behaviour Questionnaire.[86] It attempts to identify illness behaviour syndromes associated with chronic pain. Patients are divided into three groups: those with a reality-orientated attitude towards illness, those with abnormal illness behaviour and those with hysteria or hypochondriasis. Unfortunately, its construction is unsatisfactory, and it does not appear to predict treatment response.[76]

Cognitive and coping measures. Three measures of the patient's coping response to pain are the Vanderbilt Management Inventory, the Coping Strategies Questionnaire, and the Ways of Coping Checklist.[87] The purpose of a coping strategy may be more important than the activity itself.[76] Attitudes, or statements of belief, are not related in any simple way to behaviour. Important points have been made about separating the dimensions of beliefs, adjustment and coping, and about the problem of mixing cognitive and behavioural measures within a single questionnaire scale.[76] Pain-specific scales to relate patient's behaviour to their sense of control include both the 13- and 20-item Locus of Control. Less well tested but currently used pain-related cognitive scales include the Pain Beliefs and Perceptions Inventory, the Pain Cognition List, the Cognitive Errors Questionnaire, the Pain Cognitions Questionnaire, the Pain-Related Self-Statements Scale and the Pain-Related Control Scale.[76] The Pain Anxiety and Symptoms Scale, and the Fear Avoidance Beliefs Questionnaire focus on the fear of pain related to disability.[76] The Distress Risk

Assessment Measure identifies stress associated with a poorer medical treatment outcome.[76]

■ *Vanderbilt Management Inventory.* The Vanderbilt Management Inventory studies the frequency with which active or passive coping mechanisms are used when faced with increased pain levels. Active coping includes such responses as exercise, activity and ignoring pain sensations.[88] Passive coping includes withdrawal or giving responsibility for pain management to an outside source. Applying statistical techniques rather than intuitive grouping means that questionable labels such as 'active or 'passive' tend to be used, which are not adequately validated but are instead influenced by the level of activity or inactivity, the time well spent and independence.[76]

■ *Coping Strategies Questionnaire.* This contains 42 items assessing seven pain coping strategies (such as diverting attention and ignoring pain sensations). Two additional items ask patients to rate their ability to control and decrease their pain.[89] The questionnaire has shown its usefulness across a range of questions, especially the catastrophizing subscale.[76]

■ *Ways of Coping Checklist.* The checklist was designed to assess categories of coping posited by a transactional model of stress.[87] It is not pain specific and can present options that are not open to pain patients.[76]

Brief Pain Inventory. This is a quick pain measure (5–15 minutes), covering analgesics and their effects, and the cause, type, location and level (on a 0–10 scale) of pain. It has shown reliability and validity in both cancer and arthritis pain.[79]

Memorial Pain Assessment Card. This measure scales pain, pain relief and mood on a VAS and adds a set of adjectives reflecting pain intensity.[55]

QDSA. This is a French adjective list questionnaire to discriminate neuropathic pain from non-neuropathic pain[84].

Behavioural scaling

Here, pain is defined as a pattern of observable behaviours. Measurement consists of identifying behaviours and scoring them according to frequency, speed, rate and accuracy.[77] Many pain programmes observe and measure the frequency of pain behaviours (facial, vocal and bodily pain complaints), sleep and appetite disturbances, medication intake, activity level and socialization.[59] These

behavioural patterns can be quantified by trained observers either directly (e.g. measuring frequency) or using videotapes, which requires patient observation over a range of activities. Specific pain behaviours, such as guarding, grimacing, groaning and verbal pain complaint, are, surprisingly, rarely measured in chronic pain treatment.[76] Several behaviours, if sustained, are likely to contribute to further disability.[76] Behavioural approaches also try to determine the operants that reinforce and maintain pain behaviours. Patients' attitudes towards and beliefs about their pain influence their behaviour.[90] A major disadvantage of behavioural observation is that pain behaviours are highly specific for each pain syndrome.[55] More recently developed scales used include the Keefe and Block System, the Richard's Pain Behaviour Scale and the Millon Behavioural Pain Inventory.[76] Facial expressions have been extensively studied, but coding and interpretation require considerable training.[76]

Pain diary. Pain diaries used for behavioural self-support typically consist of a log of daily activities (sitting, walking and reclining) allocated to small intervals of time (usually three times daily for half-hour blocks of time). Hourly pain levels (on a 0–10 scale), medication use and the effect of other pain-relieving devices may also be recorded and validated against an up-time monitor, partner sampling and pill counts (Figure 1.8).[76] One limitation is that the reliability is unknown and varies from patient to patient.[77]

UAB Pain Behaviour Scale. This scale quantifies 10 target behaviours: verbal and non-verbal vocal complaints, down-time, facial grimaces, standing position, mobility, body language, use of supportive equipment, stationary movement and medication.[91]

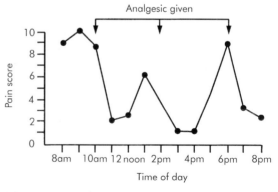

Figure 1.8 Hourly pain levels (0–10 scale) as part of a pain diary.

Checklist for Interpersonal Pain Behaviours. This assesses pain behaviour in terms of the interaction between patients and their direct environment.[92]

Prognostic scoring system

A prognostic scoring system for analgesic procedures has recently been described.[93] A one-page questionnaire comprising eight sections is filled in by an observer to assess pain frequency, pain intensity, pain depth, pain duration, previous procedures, analgesics used, specific analgesics and the use of psychotropic agents. It has a high correlative value in predicting outcome in various pain syndromes (other than trigeminal neuralgia).

Psychometric assessment measures

The emotional response to the state of pain is mostly depression as well as anger and frustration.[94,95] Psychometric assessment measures include the Minnesota Multiphasic Personality Inventory, the Beck Depression Inventory, the modified Zung Depression Scale, the Hamilton Rating Scale for depression, the Hospital Anxiety and Depression Scale, the Profile of Mood States, the Spielberger State Trait Inventory and the Eysenck Personality Inventory. The Minnesota Multiphasic Personality Inventory is designed as a personality test, although, with respect to pain, the subscales of depression, hypochondriasis and hysteria are most often used.[76] The lack of evidence for personality characteristics of chronic pain patients has not discouraged users of this inventory. Psychometric assessment will be further discussed in Chapter 14.[96]

Social support and the significant other

Patients frequently cite social (especially partner and familial) support, or the lack of it, as an important factor in sustaining change.[76] Spouse behaviour is rarely measured as part of pain management (although it appears, for example, in the Dyadic Adjustment Scale).[76] Other family members, employers or workmates may all have considerable influence over various areas of the patient's function. A Significant Others' Scale provides 10 items covering emotional support.[76]

Cultural influences and patient expectations

Although ethnic identity has been found to have an important influence on experimental and acute pain intensity and response, little work has been directed towards understanding how ethnicity affects the chronic pain experience.[97]

Using the McGill Pain Questionnaire in several languages and questions about lifestyle, chronic pain expression was found to vary across six ethnic groups as a function of affiliation to the ethnic group.[76] Broad patient satisfaction with treatment has only been assessed in a minority of studies.[76] Treatment programmes for multi-ethnic populations should include a thorough cultural assessment, and providers need to be aware of the potential effect of ethnic background on chronic pain patients' communications, concerns and coping styles related to the chronic pain experience.[97]

Drug use and use of other health care resources

Drug intake is a major focus of treatment and an important outcome measure that can be quantified and costed.[76] The classification and measurement of drug effects is unstandardized and poorly addressed.[76] Drug use can contribute significantly to associated problems: inactivity can be related to oversedation, and cognitive function can be adversely affected by opioids and benzodiazepines, as may sexual function, which can also be affected by antidepressants.[76] Antidepressant plasma levels can vary considerably, and urinary screening may be used to check patient information.[76] Among measures used in pain management studies (by self-reporting from 3 months to over 2 years) are hospital admissions and visits, physician visits and the receipt and expense of further treatment.[76]

Work and compensation

Most studies of pain management have relied on the self-reporting of a return to work or failure to do so at a certain point.[76] Measures used include work-related function (using the Sickness Impact Profile [SIP], Life Impact Checklist, Oswestry Low Back Pain Questionnaire or Maruta Index), interference with work, compliance with ergonomic techniques, termination of compensation claims and receipt of pain-related benefits.[76] During the long time it can take to resolve insurance remunerations, patients adapt to the sick role, becoming increasingly difficult to rehabilitate to a productive, active life.[76] Few studies have used an external information source, such as disability payments, or contact with employers/compensation-payers during follow-up.[76] The use of methods to monitor treatment adherence after discharge (such as the use of relaxation tapes) is rare.[76]

PAEDIATRIC PAIN ASSESSMENT AND MANAGEMENT

Neonates

Paediatric pain management has rapidly developed into a speciality in its own right.[98] Considerable improvements have been made by acknowledging that children's pain is different from that of adults and by consideration of their special needs. Evidence has accumulated that pain perception in infants is not dependent on the degree of myelinization and that pain pathways are formed before birth.[99] Premature neonates have the neuroanatomical substrate and functional neurophysiological and neurochemical processes responsible for mediating pain/nociception.[100] Multiple lines of evidence indicate that preterm neonates have a greater sensitivity to pain than term neonates or any older age group, and that they also maintain a prolonged hypersensitivity following exposure to a painful stimulus or experience.[100] Neonates and infants can remember pain, resulting in altered pain thresholds and pain-related behaviours being documented during early childhood.[99,100] Newborns circumcized without anaesthesia, when compared to those circumcized with a eutectic mixture of local anaesthetics (EMLA), showed more intense and prolonged behavioural responses to the pain of immunization at 4 and 6 months of age. Acute painful stimuli in neonates elicit motor withdrawal reflexes and arousal, with increases in heart rate, respiratory rate, blood pressure and intracranial pressure, decreases in systemic oxygen saturation, and changes in hormonal, metabolic and immune functions dependent on the degree of pain and tissue injury.[100] Significant responses occur to venepuncture, endotracheal suctioning, nursing procedures and mechanical ventilation.[100] The use of judicious analgesia during the intensive care of newborns demonstrates the beneficial effects of stress reduction (e.g. decreased hypoxic episodes, increased haemodynamic stability, a decreased incidence of intraventricular haemorrhage and improved neurobehavioural outcomes).[100] Retrospective surveys have reported a lack of standard practices and the use of a wide variety of drugs, with significant differences in the use of analgesics in neonates (and older children).[100] Routine analgesia for neonates was most commonly provided with opioids (fentanyl, morphine and pethidine), and sedation was most often given in the form of benzodiazepines (lorazepam, midazolam and diazepam).[100] Phenobarbitone, paracetamol and chloral hydrate were less commonly used analgesics/sedatives.[100] Most of these medications were prescribed infrequently, in inadequate doses or 'as needed' treatment.[100] A large proportion of neonates exposed to mechanical ventilation and other invasive therapies did not receive any analgesia or sedation.[100]

For newborn intubation and ventilation, low-dose morphine (10 μg/kg per hour) or fentanyl (1.5 μg/kg per hour) infusions are generally safe and may blunt some but not all of the hormonal and metabolic stress responses (e.g. giving rise to a lower plasma cortisol).[101] Further studies of the risk-benefit ratios of different analgesic infusions in neonates is necessary. Recognizing that the pain system is highly developed in neonates, and considering the substantial evidence for clinical, physiological and psychological sequelae of inadequately treated pain, mandate therapeutic approaches to analgesia and sedation be investigated and optimized.[100]

Assessment and measurement of pain

The measurement of pain in the paediatric population is a major challenge,[102] yet the accurate and reliable measurement of pain is necessary for diagnostic purposes and for evaluating pain management programmes.[103] Even premature newborns respond to noxious stimulation with behavioural and physiological signs of stress and distress.[104] The measurement of pain denotes the assessment of one dimension of the pain experience (such as intensity), whereas assessment involves all facets of pain experiences (such as intensity, frequency, duration and quality).[99] The measurement and assessment of pain in infants and children remain a challenge. Children's verbal and cognitive limitations hamper communication, their overt pain behaviours do not always provide an accurate pain measurement, and the 'meaning' attached to a certain type of behaviour may vary.[103] Paradoxically, there are better behavioural pain measures for use with newborns than with 2–4-year-olds as measures are confounded by fear and anxiety in the latter group.[101] Multicomponent behavioural measures have been used in prematures and neonates.[101] Intensity scales are best suited to assessing acute, short-duration pain.[99] Behavioural and physiological measures used together, can provide a more accurate picture of pain in neonates and very young infants.[99] Multidimensional methods are most appropriate for assessing chronic and recurrent pain in children.[99] Of the numerous methods now available, none has been universally accepted, and none is truly applicable to all age groups.[98] However, the tools most commonly used and most vigorously validated include those described below.[99]

SELF-REPORT MEASURES

Unidimensional methods (for children 3 years and older) include VASs and their variations, poker chips, photographs, graphic and numerical rating scales and thermometer-like derivatives, verbal rating scales, projected measures where pain is inferred from drawings, the selection of colours, pain maps with colours to indicate intensity, the interpretation of cartoon pictures, and faces scales.[99,102] The addition of happy and sad faces is the most common modification of the VAS.[98] Face interval scales measuring pain affect are considered preferable for younger children and have been validated for children as young as 3 years old.[55] Several face scales have been developed (Figure 1.9). A faces pain scale using derivatives from children's drawings of facial expressions of pain has been shown to be a reliable index over time of self-reported pain.[102] All, however, fall short in terms of validity, reliability, sensibility and practical applicability.[102]

Multidimensional methods (for those 6 years and older) require more developed communication skills and abstract thinking; they include the Abu-Saad Paediatric Pain Assessment Tool and the children's form of the McGill Pain Questionnaire.[99] The Abu-Saad Paediatric Pain Assessment Tool can be used in children as young as 7 years of age.[105] It consists of 30 word descriptors in the sensory affective and evaluative domains, as well as a 10 cm scale that measures the present and worst pain experienced by the child.[105] On analysis of self-report scales using a range of facial expressions, it was concluded that there were limitations to each and no reason to pick one as the 'best' of this type of scale.[101]

BEHAVIOURAL METHODS

Behavioural observation methods are unobtrusive, are independent of verbal skills, reflect the social environment and may be more objective.[106] These methods are used when children are unable to speak (e.g. neonates, infants and intubated children), are too ill or are sedated.[99] Indicators using crying, body movement and facial expressions are employed.[99] Based on these indicators, a number of observational tools have been developed and tested.[99] The coding of facial actions has been found to be more accurate with tissue-injuring procedures than with factors that increase arousal *per se*. It has also been shown that these measures change appropriately with analgesic treatments and that they correlate with physiological variables in restricted settings.[101] The utility of both the neonatal facial action coding and the neonatal infant pain scale have been independently supported.[101] Toddler pain behaviour may include rocking, kicking, rubbing, hitting, biting, trying to run away and opening the eyes wide.[55] Behavioural observation methods include the Procedural Behavioural Rating Scale, the Procedure Behaviour Checklist, the Childrens' Hospital of Eastern Ontario Pain Scale, the Infant Pain Behaviour Rating Scale and the Observation Scale of Behavioural Distress. Categories are weighted according to intensity. They include crying, screaming, physical restraint, verbal resistance, requests for emotional support, rigidity, verbal expressions of fear, nervous behaviour and information-seeking.[55] In pain ratings, it has been found that those made by the child, nurse and parent reflect different perspectives.[103] An assessment of parental anxiety may also be valuable.[55] The measurement of longer lasting pain by non-verbal means, as well as an understanding of the interrelationships between self-report, behaviours and biological measures, is lacking.[107]

PHYSIOLOGICAL METHODS

Physiological pain measures in the neonate continue to be studied but with little evidence of

5   4   3   2   1

Figure 1.9 Faces pain scale (visual analogue scale as a sequence of faces).

specificity across a range of physiological circumstances.[101] These include variability of heart rate, respiratory rate, blood pressure, intracranial pressure, oxygen saturation and stress hormone levels.[99]

Postoperative pain management

Children need to be psychologically prepared by informing them how much pain they are likely to experience and how this pain will be controlled.[98] It should also be remembered that pain is better prevented than treated. The presence of a parent will help most children experiencing pain.[98] Children settle more quickly in the recovery room if loading doses of analgesics have been given in theatre.[98] For a rapid onset of effect, opioids can be titrated intravenously. Recently, very good efficacy and safety have been reported with tramadol infusions in infants and toddlers undergoing major surgery.[101] Intrapleural analgesia remains problematic in children because of the high bupivacaine dosing used.[101] The intravenous use of the NSAID ketorolac provides a marked (over 50 per cent) reduction in morphine use and a lowering of pain scores.[101] In a double-blinded patient-controlled analgesia (PCA) comparison, morphine and hydromorphone were equal in terms of efficacy and side-effects.[101] Low doses of clonidine have shown promise as a supplement to local anaesthetics, either for single-shot caudal use or for epidural infusions in children, because of a favourable analgesia-to-side-effect profile.[101] Repeated doses of paracetamol 20 mg/kg per rectum every 6 hours have produced safe plasma concentrations in neonates.[101] With the amino-amide local anaesthetics, there is a narrower margin between the effective and toxic doses in infants.[101] An epidural bupivacaine bolus of 1.8 mg/kg followed by an infusion of 0.2 mg/kg per hour showed safe plasma concentrations for 48 hours, but many neonates had steadily rising plasma concentrations at 48 hours.[101] Infusion rates should be reduced in patients at risk of seizures.

Epidural infusions remain labour intensive, and the side-effects, technical problems (catheter dislodgement) and dose limitations can result in inadequate analgesia in a significant percentage of cases.[98] Yet epidural techniques are gaining general acceptance for children.[98] The most common are the single-shot caudal block for circumcisions, hypospadias and epispadias repair, and continuous caudal catheter infusions (via 18 gauge or 19 gauge Tuohy or Crawford needles) following more major repairs.[98] Continuous epidural catheter techniques via the lumbar approach or via catheters fed up to the lumbar/thoracic levels from the caudal canal can be used for abdominal surgery (e.g. ureteric re-implantation, pyeloplasty and bladder operations). An analgesic epidural mixture of bupivacaine 0.1 per cent (1 mg/ml) and fentanyl 2 μg/ml can be infused at 0.2 ml/kg per hour for abdominal/thoracic surgery, and at 0.1 ml/kg per hour for continuous sacral analgesia.[98] A loss of resistance to saline technique safeguards against air embolism.[98] A single dose of epidural morphine 0.05–0.10 mg/kg provides analgesia lasting 10–12 hours.[98] Delayed respiratory depression is uncommon in children.[98] Methods need to be found to improve the success rates of systemic and epidural analgesic infusions, and to diminish factors that delay adequate analgesic provision.

Children undergoing outpatient surgery commonly experience inadequate pain relief because pain scores are high, perioperative analgesia and neural blockade are inadequate, and parents under-recognize pain so are reluctant to give analgesics.[101]

Pharmacology of analgesic drugs

Paracetamol (acetaminophen) is effective, well tolerated in a number of formulations and (unlike aspirin) is not associated with bleeding, asthma or Reye's syndrome.[98] Children are more resistant to its hepatotoxicity than are adults.[98] It is used for minor procedures, for day case surgery and to supplement regional blockade. Children can be premedicated with paracetamol 20 mg/kg 30–60 minutes before surgery and given paracetamol 15–20 mg/kg 4-hourly postoperatively[98]. Alternatively, rectal paracetamol 25–30 mg/kg can be given after induction.[98] The benefit of using NSAIDs is to provide analgesia at least equal to that with paracetamol, without sedation and the high incidence of nausea and vomiting associated with opioids.[98] The use of NSAIDs, however, remains controversial, mainly because of problems with platelet dysfunction, although NSAIDs such as ibuprofen, diclofenac and naproxen are used in paediatric formulations.[98] Ketorolac has been shown to be an effective analgesic in children, although intravenous ketorolac is not approved for paediatric use.[98]

When pain is inadequately covered by simple analgesics or local anaesthetics, opioids become the agents of choice. Side-effects (nausea, vomiting, sedation and pruritus) limit the degree of analgesia achievable. Caution (decreased infusion rates and increased respiratory monitoring) is needed with opioid use in premature and term newborns because of increased susceptibility to the respiratory depressant effects as a result of reduced clearance, possibly increased blood–brain permeability and immature responses to hypoxia and hypercarbia.[100] When postoperative pain is not severe, codeine is commonly used as it is well tolerated in syrup or tablet form and, in doses of 0.5–1.0 mg/kg, appears to work synergistically with paracetamol.[98] Morphine is the opioid of choice for severe postoperative pain, although pethidine, fentanyl and sufentanil are commonly used alternatives.[98] Pethidine, becaue of the agitation and seizures caused by its metabolite (norpethidine), is not used for long-term analgesia, especially in patients with impaired renal function.[98] Fentanyl and sufentanil, with their rapid redistribution and short duration of action are best given as infusions or in PCA.[98]

Methods of paediatric drug administration

The administration method is more important than the choice of drug. Administration routes include oral, rectal, intravenous, subcutaneous, oral and nasal transmucosal, transdermal and inhalational.[98] Most children fear intramuscular injections (which have a variable effect), so that the oral and intravenous routes are most often employed. Intermittent injections of morphine (0.05 mg/kg) or pethidine (0.5 mg/kg) infused over 5–20 minutes are rapid acting and painless but time-consuming (needing frequent doses).[98] Continuous opioid infusions (used in preschool children or those unsuitable for PCA) provide smooth uninterrupted analgesia by maintaining a constant blood level of the drug.[98] Using a 50 ml syringe pump, morphine 0.5 mg/kg or pethidine 5 mg/kg diluted to 50 ml with normal saline or 5 per cent dextrose solution can be run at 0–4 ml/hour.[98] For infants less than 3 months of age, the infusion rate is halved, while apnoea monitoring, pulse oximetry and a high level of nursing care are desirable.[98] Subcutaneous morphine infusions have been successfully used for postoperative analgesia in patients ranging from 7 months to 20 years of age.[98] However, the vast majority of children (unlike adults), following postoperative opioid administration, do not experience multiple episodes of clinically significant oxygen desaturation.[98]

PCA allows for individual variability, is generally safe and results in high patient satisfaction. It can be offered to all children who can understand the concept of pressing the button when they hurt. Common settings for morphine are a bolus dose of 15–25 μg/kg, and a lockout time of 5 minutes.[98] The use of a background infusion remains controversial.[98] Long-term PCA usage in children with prolonged acute pain episodes (as in burns, cancer and sickle cell disease) promises to be a valuable technique.[98] PCA is extensively discussed in Chapter 7.

Peripheral nerve blocks in infants and children

Regional blockade techniques have been developed for children of all ages, including newborns, the benefits being complete analgesia without sedation or opioid side-effects, and a quicker recovery. They are most often used to provide perioperative analgesia in association with general anaesthesia.[98] Neonates may be at greater risk of local anaesthetic toxicity because of reduced albumen and alpha-1-acid glycoprotein levels, giving higher levels of free drug in the plasma.[98] Their greater volume of distribution (similar to to that of children) may, however, confer some protection against cardiovascular and CNS local anaesthetic toxicity (especially highly protein bound bupivacaine).[98] Children (6 months and over) eliminate local anaesthetics faster than adults.[98] Arm blocks can provide relaxation and analgesia/anaesthesia for fracture reductions and laceration repairs.[108] For brachial plexus block, the axillary approach is the safest and most successful. More peripheral blocks, such as those of the median, radial and ulnar nerves, may be performed at the wrist, while the digital nerves may be blocked using a metacarpal approach. Femoral nerve blocks are used in children presenting with femoral shaft fractures.[98] With a fascia lata block, patients with femur fractures or femur osteotomies experience excellent analgesia with full urinary function and motor and sensory function in the contralateral leg.[109] Combined femoral nerve and lateral cutaneous nerve of the thigh blocks provide analgesia for skin graft donor sites.[98] The inguinal paravascular block can be used for lower limb surgery or for diagnostic muscle biopsy. Sciatic nerve blockade (anterior, posterior and lateral approaches) is used for surgery on the foot[98]. Ankle nerve blocks and metatarsal nerve blocks are also used. Intercostal nerve blocks will provide analgesia in both the chest wall (upper six nerves) and abdomen (lower six nerves) after surgery or trauma. Continuous interpleural local anaesthetic infusions have been used for analgesia after coarctation repair or anterior spinal fusions. Ilio-inguinal and ilio-hypogastric nerve blocks relieve pain after herniotomy or orchidopexy.[108,110] Blockade of the dorsal nerve of the penis provides analgesia following circumcision; topical lignocaine will do the same. Wound infiltration with plain bupivacaine 0.25 per cent (up to 3 mg/kg) or lignocaine aerosol sprayed into the wound can be a successful way of providing post-operative analgesia, especially after inguinal herniotomy or pyloromyotomy.[110] Continuous peripheral blocks can extend the block duration of the blockade. In infants undergoing coarctation repairs and ductus arteriosus ligations, continuous intercostal blockade reduces analgesic requirements and accelerate tracheal extubation.[109] Sympathetic blockade (stellate and lumbar) may be indicated in children with peripheral ischaemia, in accidental intra-arterial injections or for the treatment of sympathetically maintained pain.[98] Continuous administration of bupivacaine via a catheter can be used for lumbar sympathetic blockade.

Procedural pain in children

Procedures such as changing dressings, suturing, intravenous cannulation, blood-taking and lumbar punctures strike fear into many children.[98] The advantages of the satisfactory analgesia (in about 80 per cent of patients) from 50 per cent nitrous oxide in oxygen include rapid onset and offset, a lack of need for intravenous access and good acceptance of a face mask, nasal mask or self-activated inhalation device by most, although not all, children.[101] Recommended repeated administrations are for an hour a day only with folinic acid supplements.[98] EMLA (the eutectic mixture of prilocaine and lignocaine) is applied under an occlusive dressing for at least an hour before intravenous cannulation, lumbar puncture needle insertion and accessing infusaports, and for superficial skin procedures.[98] In an infant below 3 months of age, the prilocaine may give rise to methaemoglobinaemia. For broken skin and wound suturing in children, topical tetracaine 0.5 per cent, adrenaline 1:2000 and cocaine 11.8 per cent are instilled onto gauze in the wound (not supplied by end-arteries) for 10–20 minutes[98]. Transmucosal midazolam has been given via orally (described above), intranasally (0.3 mg/kg), and sublingually.[98] The induction agent propofol (in small doses) is effective for procedural pain, either alone or supplemented with fentanyl.[101]

Children (especially related to oncology and burns) have been shown to respond well to hypnotherapy and other behavioural methods (distraction, relaxation, therapeutic plays, music and art therapy).[98] Audiovisual distraction before venepuncture reduces fear and distress scores.[101] Sucrose pacifiers, the prone position and automated lancets have been found to reduce heelstick pain in neonates.[101]

Pain in the burns patient is caused by the initial injury, dressing changes and debridement and grafting. Following oral premedication with midazolam (0.5 mg/kg), inhalational 50 per cent nitrous oxide in oxygen, intravenous midazolam or fentanyl titration, or PCA (IV or SC for difficult venous access), together with behavioural therapy, can be used.[98] Oral sustained-release morphine or methadone can be used as a baseline for longer-term analgesia.

Cancer pain and palliative care

Aggressive therapy with chemotherapy, radiotherapy and surgery results in many pain management problems.[98] Almost 50 per cent of cases of childhood cancers are haematological malignancies (leukaemias and lymphomas), requiring bone marrow aspiration, lumbar puncture, intravenous therapy and surgery. Procedural pain is treated as described above. For mild pain, intermittent paracetamol and codeine in syrup, tablet or rectal formulations, are used, but are individualized. For bony pain, the use of NSAIDs (e.g. tablet, syrup or rectal formulations of naproxen) can be given twice daily, the benefits often outweighing the problems of platelet dysfunction in the terminally ill patient.[98] Sustained-release morphine tablets, methadone syrup and oxycodone suppositories are commonly used in combination with NSAIDs.[98] In the terminal phase, with effort directed to home care, analgesic treatments, including tramadol, NSAIDs and corticosteroids, oral or subcutaneous morphine and transdermal fentanyl, result in 80 per cent of children feeling comfortable.[101] Antidepressants and anticonvulsants can be added for stubborn neuropathic pain, and midazolam (orally, rectally or intravenously) for relieving distress. PCA (with patient, nurse or parental control) has been successfully used, especially in patients undergoing total body irradiation and bone marrow transplantation.[101] For oral mucositis, systemic opioids (often with PCA), topical local anaesthetics and mouth washes are used.[98]

Chronic non-cancer pain in children

Headache is common in about 75 per cent of children.[98] Serious causes are first ruled out, but tension headaches and migraines remain the most common causes.[98] If mild, they are treated with rest, simple analgesics, massage, relaxation, biofeedback and 'help yourself' training.[98,101] In migraine, both ibuprofen and paracetamol have shown impressive efficacy.[101] Sumatriptan is not as effective as in adults, and dihydroergotamine is associated with a recurrence of headaches.[101] Recurring abdominal pain without a clear-cut cause is found in about 15 per cent of schoolchildren.[98] Sympathetically maintained pain is found in female adolescents (a female-to-male ratio of about 6:1) and is treated by a combination of interventional therapy (sympathetic blockade and pharmacotherapy), physical therapy and psychological therapy.[98] Adenosine infusions may help, and higher neuropeptide Y and CGRP levels have been found in the affected limbs.[101] The episodic pain caused by small vessel occlusion in sickle cell crises should, if severe, be treated with aggressive opioid dosing (including PCA) in day treatment programmes.[98,101] There is a need for further study of therapeutic efficacy in both acute and chronic pancreatitis, and better clarification of the risks and benefits of long-term opioids.[101]

Conclusion

Advances in paediatric pain management are found from the neonate to the adolescent, in acute, chronic and recurrent pain, in pain pathways and pain perception, in tools to access and measure pain, and in testing the effectiveness of specific pain intervention strategies to relieve and prevent pain.[99] Despite these, however, problems remain. The doses prescribed are often too small and the frequency of administration too low. There is a great discrepancy between what nurses know and what they apply in pain interventions.[99] This is because of the time needed to apply the intervention, motivation, work load and ward policy.[99] The establishment of an acute pain service within a hospital will provide the following benefits:[98]

- the development of a clear pain policy for the institution;
- the facilitation and co-ordination of pain management methods;
- the provision of prescription guidelines and protocols, and a guarantee of their implementation (e.g. the avoidance of 'as needed' medications as much as possible, and never in the first few days postoperatively);
- the development of clear lines of responsibility and accountability;
- the provision of continuing training and education;
- the introduction of standard pain assessment tools appropriate for age and the clinical population;
- the appropriate charting and reporting of pain;
- the facilitation of non-pharmacological techniques such as adjuvants;
- the maintenance of pain management equipment.

REFERENCES

1. **International Association for the Study of Pain.** 1979: Pain terms: a list with definitions and notes on usage. *Pain* **6**, 249–52.
2. **Cesaro, P, and Ollat, H.** 1997: Pain and its treatments. *European Neurology* **38**(N3), 209–15.
3. **Loeser, J.D.** 1996: *Pain: concepts and management. 150 years on – a selection of papers presented at the 11th World Congress of Anaesthesiologists.* Rosebery, NSW: Bridge Printery, 67–72.
4. **Ekblom, A. and Rydh-Rinder, M.** 1998: Pain mechanisms: anatomy and physiology. In Rawal, N. (ed.) *Management of acute and chronic pain.* London: BMJ Books, 1–22.
5. **Raja, S.N.** 1995: Role of the sympathetic nervous system in acute pain and inflammation. *Annals of Medicine* **27**(2), 241–6.
6. **Rowlingson, J.C.** 1996: Neuropathic pain. *International Symposium of Regional Anaesthesia,* 120–6.
7. **Woolf, C.J.** 1995: Somatic pain – pathogenesis and prevention. *British Journal of Anaesthesia* **75**, 169–76.
8. **Bonica, J.J.** 1992: Importance of the problem. In Aronoff, G.M. (ed.) *Evaluation and treatment of chronic pain,* 2nd edn. Baltimore: Williams & Wilkins, xx-xxviii.
9. **Dickenson, A.H.** 1995: Central acute pain mechanisms. *Annals of Medicine* **27**(2), 223–7.
10. **White, C.L., Le Fort, S.M., Amsel, R. and Jeans M.E.** 1997: Predictors of the development of chronic pain. *Research Nurse Health* **20**(4), 309–18.
11. **Hayes, C. and Molloy, A.R.** 1997: Neuropathic pain in the perioperative period. *International Anesthesiology Clinics* **35**(2), 67–81.
12. **Thompson, E.N.** 1997: Chronic pain. *Canadian Journal of Anaesthesia* **44**(3), 243–6.

13. **Markenson, J.A.** 1996: Mechanisms of chronic pain. *American Journal of Medicine* **101**(1A), 6S-18S.

14. **Dickenson, A.H., Chapman, V. and Green, G.M.** 1997: The pharmacology of excitatory and inhibitory amino-mediated events in the transmission and modulation of pain in the spinal cord. *General Pharmacology* **28**(5), 633–8.

15. **Pleuvry, B.J. and Lauretti, G.R.** 1996: Biochemical aspects of chronic pain and its relationship to treatment. *Pharmacology and Therapeutics* **76**(3), 313–24.

16. **Tokunage, A. and Senba, E.** 1996: Molecular mechanisms of chronic pain. *Masui* **45**(5), 547–57.

17. **Taylor, J.S., Morcuende, S. and Naranjo, J.R.** 1997: Molecular pathways of pain: knockdown of the prodyorphin gene reveals an involvement in antinociception. In Borsook, D. (ed.) *Molecular neurobiology of pain, progress in pain research and management*, vol. 9. Seattle: IASP Press, 201–218.

18. **Delander, G.E., Schott, E., Brodin, E. and Fredholm, B.B.** 1997: Spinal expression of mRNA for immediate early genes in a model of chronic pain. *Acta Physiologica Scandinavica* **161**(4), 517–25.

19. **Peroutka, S.J.** 1998: Genetic basis of migraine. *Clinical Neuroscience* **5**(1), 34–7.

20. **Iadarola, M.J., Lee, S. and Mannes, A.J.** 1997: Gene transfer approaches to pain control. In Borsook, D. (ed.) *Molecular neurobiology of pain, progress in pain research and management*. Seattle: IASP Press, **9**, 337–59.

21. **Crombie, I.K., Davies, H.T.O. and Macrae, W.A.** 1994: The epidemiology of chronic pain: time for new directions. *Pain* **57**, 1–3.

22. **Bowsher, D., Rigge, M. and Sopp, L.** 1991: Prevalence of chronic pain in the British population: a telephone survey of 1037 households. *Pain Clinic* **4**(4), 223–30.

23. **Crook, J., Rideout, E. and Browne, G.** 1984: The prevalence of pain complaints in a general population. *Pain* **18**, 299–314.

24. **Brattberg, G., Thorslund, M. and Wikman, A.** 1989: The prevalence of pain in a general population: the results of a postal survey in a country of Sweden. *Pain* **37**, 215–22.

25. **Chan, A.W., MacFarlane, I.A., Bowscher, D., Wells, J.C., Bessex, C. and Griffith, K.** 1990: Chronic pain in patients with diabetes mellitus: comparison with a non-diabetic population. *Pain Clinic* **3**, 147–59.

26. **Lipton, S.** 1991: Introduction. *British Medical Bulletin* **47**(3), i-iv.

27. **James, F.R., Large, R.G., Bushnell, J.A. and Wells, J.E.** 1991: Epidemiology of pain in New Zealand. *Pain* **44**, 279–83.

28. **Goodman, J.E. and McGrath, P.J.** 1991: The epidemiology of pain in children and adolescents: a review. *Pain* **46**, 247–64.

29. **Lavies, N., Hart, L., Rounsefell, B. and Runciman, W.** 1992: Identification of patient, medical and nursing staff attitudes to postoperative opioid analgesia: stage I of a longitudinal study of postoperative analgesia. *Pain* **48**, 313–19.

30. **Breivik, H.** 1995: Cost effectiveness of postoperative pain management. *European Society of Anaesthesiologists Refresher Course Lectures*, vol. 1, 183–88.

31. **Devor, M.** 1996: Pain mechanisms and pain syndromes. In Campbell, J.N. (ed.) *Pain 1996 – an updated review*. Seattle: IASP Press, 103–13.

32. **Schmidt, R.F., Schaible, H.G., Meblinger, K., Heppelmann, B., Hanesch, U. and Pawlak, M.** 1994: Silent and active nociceptors: structure, functions, and clinical implications. In Gebhardt, G.F., Hammond, D.L. and Jensen, T.S. (eds) *Progress in pain research and management – Proceedings of the 7th World congress on pain*, vol. 2. Seattle: IASP Press, 213–50.

33. **Woolf, C.J.** 1991: Generation of acute pain: central mechanisms. *British Medical Bulletin* **47**(3), 523–33.

34. **Rang, H.P., Bevan, S. and Dray, A.** 1991: Chemical activation of nociceptive peripheral neurones. *British Medical Bulletin* **47**(3), 534–48.

35. **Dickenson, A.H.** 1996: Pharmacology of pain transmission and control. In Campbell, J.N. (ed.) *Pain 1996 – an updated review*. Seattle: IASP Press, 113–21.

36. **Cimino, C.** 1992: Painful neurological syndromes. In Aronoff, G.M. (ed.) *Evaluation and treatment of chronic pain*, 2nd edn. Baltimore: Williams & Wilkins, 56–66.

37. **Dubner, R.** 1997: Neural basis of persistent pain: sensory specialization, sensory modulation and neuronal plasticity. In *Current concepts in acute, chronic, and cancer pain management*. New York: World Foundation for Pain Relief and Research, 1–8.

38. **Murphy, T.H.** 1990: Chronic pain. In Miller, R.D. (ed.) *Anesthesia*, 3rd edn. New York: Churchill Livingstone, 1927–50.

39. **Bowsher, D.** 1991: Neurogenic pain syndromes and their management. *British Medical Bulletin* **47**(3), 644–66.

40. **Jensen, T.S.** 1996: Mechanisms of neuropathic pain. In Campbell, J.N. (ed.) *Pain 1996 – an updated review*. Seattle: IASP Press, 77–86.

41. **Kingery, W.S.** 1997: A critical review of controlled clinical trials for peripheral neuropathic pain and complex regional pain syndromes. *Pain* **73**, 123–39.

42. **Dickenson, A.** 1997: Current strategies and pharmacological basis for the treatment of neuropathic pain. In *Current concepts in acute, chronic, and cancer pain management*. New York: World Foundation for Pain Relief and Research, 25–32.

43. **McMahon, S.B., Dmitrieva, N. and Koltzenburg, M.** 1995: Visceral pain. *British Journal of Anaesthesia* **75**, 132–44.

44. **Foreman, R.D.** 1996: Mechanisms of visceral pain: visceral sensory processing. In Campbell, J.N. (ed.) *Pain 1996 – an updated review*. Seattle: IASP Press, 339–49.

45. **Ness, T.J. and Gebhart, G.F.** 1990: Visceral pain: a review of experimental studies. *Pain* **41**, 167–234.

46. **Cervero, F.** 1991: Mechanisms of acute visceral pain. *British Medical Bulletin* **47**(3), 549–60.

47. **Rapkin, A.J.** 1995: Pelvic visceral pain in women. *IASP Newsletter* (Sep/Oct) 4–6.

48. **Ventafridda, V., Caraceni, A. and Sbanotto, A.** 1996: Cancer pain management. *Pain Reviews* **3**, 153–79.

49. **Parris, W.C.V.** 1997: Cancer pain syndromes and their management. In Parris, W.C.V. (ed.) *Cancer pain management: principles and practice.* Boston: Butterworth-Heinemann, 279–92.

50. **Levy, M.H.** 1997: Current concepts in the management of cancer pain in a hospice environment. In *Current concepts in acute, chronic, and cancer pain management.* New York: World Foundation for Pain Relief and Research, 167–71.

51. **Miaskowski, C.** 1994: Effective cancer pain management: from guidelines to quality improvement. *Pain – clinical updates* II(2) 1–4.

52. **Burchmann, S.C.** 1990: Introduction to cancer pain management. In Abram, S.E. (ed.) *The pain clinic manual.* Philadelphia: J.B. Lippincott, 238–41.

53. **Patt, R.B.** 1992: Control of pain associated with advanced malignancy. In Aronoff, G.M. (ed.) *Evaluation and treatment of chronic pain*, 2nd edn. Baltimore: Williams & Wilkins, 313–39.

54. **Hanks, G.W.** 1991: Opioid-responsive and opioid non-responsive pain in cancer. *British Medical Bulletin* **47**(3), 718–31.

55. **Chapman, C.R. and Syrjala, K.L.** 1990: Measurement of pain. In Bonica, J.J. (ed.) *The management of pain*, 2nd edn. Philadelphia: Lea & Febiger, 580–94.

56. **Jamison, R.N. and Brown, G.K.** 1991: Validation of hourly pain intensity profiles with chronic pain patients. *Pain* **45**, 123–8.

57. **Boureau, F., Luu, M. and Doubrere, J.F.** 1991: Study of experimental pain measures and nociceptive reflex in chronic pain patients and normal subjects. *Pain* **44**, 131–8.

58. **Bond, M.R.** 1984: *The measurement of pain – its nature, analysis, and treatment*, 2nd edn. Edinburgh: Churchill Livingstone, 34–9.

59. **Hebben, N.** 1992: Toward the assessment of clinical pain in adults. In Aronoff, G.M. (ed.) *Evaluation and treatment of chronic pain*, 2nd edn. Baltimore: Williams & Wilkins, 384–93.

60. **Clark, W.C.** 1974: Pain sensitivity and the report of pain: an introduction to the sensory decision theory. *Anesthesiology* **40**, 272–87.

61. **Young, J.C., Clark, W.C. and Janal, M.N.** 1991: Sensory decision theory and visual analogue score indices predict status of chronic pain patients six months later. *Journal of Pain and Symptom Management* **6**, 58–64.

62. **Tursky, B.** 1976: The pain perception profile: a psychological approach. In Weisenberg, M. and Tursky, B. (eds) *Pain: new perspectives in therapy and research.* New York: Plenum Press.

63. **Gracely, R.H. and Wolskee, P.J.** 1983: Semantic functional measurement of pain: integrating perception and language. *Pain* **15**, 389–98.

64. **Gracely, R.H. and Kwilosz, D.M.** 1988: The descriptor differential scale: applying psychological principles to clinical pain assessment. *Pain* **35**, 279–88.

65. **Adler, D., Magora, F., Shapira, S.C., Veler, A. and Mahler, Y.** 1991: A new recording pressure algometer. *Pain Clinic* **4**(3), 183–6.

66. **Bromage, P.R., Husain, I., El-Faqih, S., Bonsu, A.K., Kadiwal, G.H. and Seraj, P.** 1990: Critique of the Dornier HM3 lithotripter as a clinical algesimeter. *Pain* **40**, 255–65.

67. **Ackerman, W., Edmonds, H., Cases Cristobal, V.** *et al.* 1992: Quantitative assessment of severe pain using non-invasive surface electromyography. *Anesthesia and Analgesia* **74**, S1.

68. **Zidar, J., Backman, E., Bengtsson, A. and Henriksson, K.G.** 1990: Quantitative EMG and muscle tension in painful muscles in fibromyalgia. *Pain* **40**, 249–54.

69. **Berman. J.** 1995: Imaging pain in humans. *British Journal of Anaesthesia* **75**, 209–16.

70. **Casey, K.L. and Minoshima, S.** 1997: Can pain be imaged? In Jensen, T.S. Turner, J.A. and Wiesenfeld-Halin, Z. (eds) *Progress in pain research and management – Proceedings of the 8th World Congress on Pain*, vol. 8. Seattle: IASP Press, 855–66.

71. **Svensson, P., Johannsen, P., Troels, S.J.** *et al.* 1997: Cerebral representation of graded painful phasic and tonic heat in humans: a positron emission tomography study. In Jensen, T.S. Turner, J.A. and Wiesenfeld-Halin, Z. (eds) *Progress in pain research and management – Proceedings of the 8th World Congress on Pain*, vol. 8. Seattle: IASP Press, 867–78.

72. **Rice, A.S.C. and Casale, R.** 1994: Microneurography and the investigation of pain mechanisms. *Pain Reviews* **1**, 121–37.

73. **White, S., and Wong, S.H.** 1998: Standards of laboratory practice: analgesic drug monitoring. *Clinical Chemistry* **44**(5), 1110–23.

74. **Wheeler-Aceto, H., Porreca, F. and Cowan, A.** 1990: The rat paw formalin test: comparison of noxious agents. *Pain* **40**, 229–38.

75. **McQuay, H.J.** 1992: Pre-emptive analgesia. *British Journal of Anaesthesia* **69**(1), 1–3.

76. **Williams, A. C.deC.** 1995: Pain measurement in chronic pain management. *Pain Reviews* **2**, 39–63.

77. **Chapman, C.R.** 1989: Assessment of pain. In Nimmo, W.S. and Smith, G. (eds) *Anaesthesia.* Oxford: Blackwell Scientific Publications, 1149–65.

78. **Thompson, G.E.** 1990: Regional anesthesia and central mechanisms of pain. In Barash, P.G. (ed.) *American Society of Anesthesiologists Annual Refresher Course Lectures*, vol. 41, 287–98.

79. **Gracely, R.H.** 1992: Evaluation of multidimensional pain scales. *Pain* **48**, 297–300.

80. **Holroyd, K.A., Holm, J.E., Keefe, F.J.** *et al.* 1992: A multicentre evaluation of the McGill Pain Questionnaire: results from more than 1700 chronic pain patients. *Pain* **48**, 301–12.

81. **Boureau, F., Doubrere, J.F. and Luu, M.** 1990: Study of verbal description in neuropathic pain. *Pain* **42**, 145–52.

82. **Lowe, N.K., Walker, S.N. and MacCullum, R.C.** 1991:

Confirming the theoretical structure of the McGill Pain Questionnaire in acute clinical pain. *Pain* **46**, 53–60.

83. **Kerns, R.D., Turk, D.C. and Rudy, T.E.** 1985: The West Haven-Yale Multidimensional Pain Inventory (WHYMPI). *Pain* **23**, 345–56.

84. **Pilowsky, I.** 1994: Pain and illness behaviour: assessment and management. In Wall, P.D. and Melzack, R.M. (eds) *Textbook of pain*, 3rd edn. Edinburgh: Churchill Livingstone, 1309–20.

85. **Tait, R.C., Chiball, J.T. and Krause, S.** 1990: The Pain Disability Index: psychometric properties. *Pain* **40**, 171–82.

86. **Pilowsky, I. and Spence, N.D.** 1976: Illness behaviour syndromes associated with intractable pain. *Pain* **2**, 161–71.

87. **Turner, J.A.** 1990: Coping strategies of patients with chronic pain. *Pain* supplement 5, S251.

88. **Jensen, M.P., Turner, J.A., Romano, J.M. and Kardy, P.** 1991: Coping with chronic pain: a critical review of the literature. *Pain* **47**, 249–83.

89. **Katz, J. and Melzack, R.** 1990: Pain memories in phantom limbs: review and clinical observation. *Pain* **43**, 319–36.

90. **Strong, J., Ashton, R. and Chant, D.** 1992: The measurement of attitudes towards and beliefs about pain. *Pain* **48**, 227–36.

91. **Richards, J.S., Neopomuceno, C., Riles, M. and Suer, Z.** 1982: Assessing pain behaviour: the UAB Pain Behaviour Scale. *Pain* **14**, 393–8.

92. **Vlaeyen, J.W., Pernot, D.F., Kole, S.A., Schuerman, J.A., Van, E.H. and Groenman, N.H.** 1990: Assessment of the components of observed chronic pain behaviour: the Checklist for Interpersonal Pain Behaviours. *Pain* **43**, 337–47.

93. **Brydon, H.L. and Hitchcock, E.** 1992: A prognostic scoring system for analgesic procedures. *Pain Clinic* **5**(2), 91–9.

94. **Haythornthwaith, J.A., Sieber, W.J. and Kerns, R.D.** 1991: Depression and the chronic pain experience. *Pain* **46**, 177–84.

95. **Wade, J.B., Price, D.P., Hamer, R.M., Schwartz, S.M. and Hart, R.P.** 1990: An emotional component analysis of chronic pain. *Pain* **40**, 303–10.

96. **Mendelson, G.** 1990: Psychological and social factors predicting responses to pain treatment. *Pain* supplement 5, S252.

97. **Bates, M.S. and Edwards, W.T.** 1992: Ethnic variations in the chronic pain experience. *Ethnic Disease* **2**(1), 63–83.

98. **Gaukroger, P.B. and Van Der Walt, J.** 1995: The clinical aspect of pain control in neonates and children. *Pain Reviews* **2**, 92–110.

99. **Abu-Saad, H.H.** 1996: Pain assessment and management in children. In Campbell, J.N. (ed.) *Pain 1996 – an updated review.* Seattle: IASP Press, 3–8.

100. **Anand, K.J.S.** 1995: Pain in the neonatal intensive care unit. *IASP Newsletter* (Nov/Dec), 3–4.

101. **Berde, C.B.** 1997; Pediatric pain update: presentations at the fourth International Symposium on Pediatric Pain in Helsinki. *IASP Newsletter* (Sep/Oct), 3–6.

102. **Bieri, D., Reeve, R.A., Champion, G.D., Addicoat, L. and Ziegler, J.B.** 1990: The faces pain scale for the self assessment of the severity of pain experienced by children: development, initial validation and preliminary investigation for ratio scale properties. *Pain* **41**, 139–50.

103. **Manne, S.L., Jacobsen, P.B. and Redd, W.H.** 1992: Assessment of acute pediatric pain: do child self-report, parent ratings, and nurse ratings measure the same phenomenon? *Pain* **48**, 45–52.

104. **Berde, C.** 1992: Chronic pain in pediatrics. In Aronoff, G.M. (ed.) *Evaluation and treatment of chronic pain*, 2nd edn. Baltimore: Williams & Wilkins, 349–57.

105. **Abu-Saad, H.H., Kroonen, E. and Halfens, R.** 1990: On the development of a multidimensional Dutch pain assessment tool for children. *Pain* **43**, 249–56.

106. **Lloyd-Thomas, A.R.** 1990: Pain management in paediatric patients. *British Journal of Anaesthetia* **64**, 85–104.

107. **McGrath, P.J.** 1990: Paediatric pain: a good start. *Pain* **41**, 253–4.

108. **Broadman, L.** 1990: Regional anesthesia for pediatric patients. *American Society of Anesthesiologists Annual Refresher Course Lectures*, vol. 41, 1–7.

109. **Berde, C.** 1996: Regional anesthesia in children: what have we learned? *Anesthesia and Analgesia* **83**, 897–900.

110. **Lloyd-Thomas, A.R.** 1990: Pain management in paediatric patients. *British Journal of Anaesthesia* **64**, 85–104.

2

INTRODUCING PAIN:
Pain management services

ACUTE PAIN MANAGEMENT SERVICES

A synopsis of the management of acute pain is described, which is expanded upon throughout the book.

Introduction

Perioperative and post-traumatic pain problems persist despite the availability of very efficient drugs and adequate techniques. One editorial stated it as follows: 'A visit to most postoperative wards will show you the time-honoured ritual of inadequate postoperative pain management. Patients expect ineffective pain relief, and their carers ensure that they are not disappointed.'[1] About 50 per cent of anaesthesiologists and surgeons still do not inform their patients about perioperative analgesia.[2] The rational approach to the relief of acute pain is to use the highest-quality evidence available from systematic reviews of valid randomized trials.[3] The parenteral administration of fixed doses of systemic opioids at fixed intervals for the treatment of postoperative pain is the most widespread technique currently used.[4] Many studies over the past decades have demonstrated the inadequacy of such an approach, about 75 per cent of patients reporting insufficient pain relief and 80 per cent of these experiencing moderate to extreme pain.[4,5] In the USA, 57 per cent of those patients who had surgery cited concern about pain after surgery as their primary fear experienced before surgery.[5] In 1989, the National Health and Medical Research Council, in its publication on *Severe pain*, described the situation in Australia as 'areas of enlightenment in a sea of misery'.[6] The

first official guidelines were established in the early 1990s by the Royal College of Surgeons of England, and by the US Department of Health and Human Services.[7] A recent 17-nation survey was undertaken to study the availability of acute pain services and the use of newer analgesic techniques.[8] It showed that over 50 per cent of the anaesthesiologists were dissatisfied with postoperative pain management, that very few hospitals used quality assurance measures (such as frequent pain assessments and documentation) and that only 34 per cent of hospitals had an organized acute pain service (APS).[8] Also, a recent study showed that nurses as well as physicians overestimated low and underestimated high levels of pain indicated by patients.[9]

The American Society of Anesthesiologists' Task Force on Pain Management recommends:[7]

- proactive individualized planning for patient care;
- staff training for the effective, safe use of the available options;
- information for and the education of patients;
- the assessment and documentation of therapeutic efficacy and side-effects;
- protocols (for drug ordering, administration and discontinuation, and for the transfer of responsibility);
- the availability of appropriate therapeutic techniques (PCA, patient-controlled epidural analgesia [PCEA], regional anaesthesia or a multimodal approach);
- the 24-hour availability of a responsible anaesthesiologist, who should also be familiar with paediatric, geriatric and ambulatory surgery pain management.

Physiology

Surgery produces a barrage of nociceptive input into the CNS, via afferent C and A delta fibres, which is caused by direct nerve trauma, local tissue damage and the subsequent release of sensitizing algogenic compounds and algesic mediators.[4] Their effects may well outlast the acute perioperative period by days and evoke exaggerated changes in neuroplasticity, such as primary and secondary hyperalgesia, and allodynia.[4] Segmental and suprasegmental reflex responses, as well as cortical activation, initiate positive feedback loops via sympathetic and motor efferents, leading to continuing pain. This may trigger the impairment of pulmonary, cardiovascular, gastrointestinal, neuroendocrine, immunological and metabolic functions. Pain impairs breathing and coughing. Gastrointestinal motility is impaired, and mobility is restricted, making thromboembolism more likely.[10] Poor pain control may result in a longer hospital stay.

Psychology

Four principal categories of preparatory procedure have been identified: the provision of information (e.g. regarding the procedure), behavioural instructions (e.g. training the patient to relax and instructing him to cough), cognitive methods (e.g. positive thinking) and psychotherapeutic approaches (e.g. exploring emotional responses).[10]

Pain charts

The fact that there is a chart (e.g. the Burford chart) is more important than its form.[3] Pain measurements are recorded at the same time as sedation, respiratory rate, frequency and nausea.[3] There are special charts for children.

Acute pain services

It is becoming increasingly clear that one remedy for poor pain management lies not so much in the development of new techniques as in the development of acute pain services (APS) to exploit existing expertise.[3,11] Training and education should be the main aims of an APS. During recent years, APSs have been established in many countries, including the USA (in 42 per cent of hospitals, with an additional 13 per cent planning an APS) and Canada, the countries of Western Europe (about 37 per cent of hospitals), the UK (about 43 per cent of hospitals) and New Zealand and Australia.[5,7] In 1991, the first acute pain relief service in Southern Africa was established at Hillbrow Hospital, Johannesburg, under the auspices of the Department of Anaesthe-

siology.[10] The proposed steps for introducing an APS are as follows:[7]

- form a multidisciplinary steering group (which includes surgeons and nurses) to survey current practice;
- train medical and nursing staff and dedicated APS nurses;
- monitor pain and sedation;
- introduce new techniques in a phased and controlled manner;
- develop guidelines (especially to manage side-effects and breakthrough pain);
- offer patient information leaflets;
- audit the efficacy.

Up to 80 per cent of APSs in the USA, but only about 50 per cent of the APSs in Western Europe, were headed by anaesthesiologists.[7,11] In the USA, fewer than 30 per cent of the surgical patient population have access to an APS, as only patients selected by anaesthesiologists or surgeons receive the benefits of these services.[2]

PATIENT SELECTION

Any patient requiring analgesia for the relief of postoperative pain or any acutely painful condition (e.g. pancreatitis, fractured ribs, burns or sickle cell crises) should receive attention from the APS.

METHODS USED

New routes of drug administration, technical advances in delivery systems, the concept of pre-emptive analgesia, and multimodal (or balanced) analgesia have enhanced the standard acute pain care. Advances include the use of patient-controlled analgesic pumps (via the subcutaneous, intravenous, epidural and nasal routes), intrathecal opioid analgesia and the constant epidural infusion of multimodal drug mixtures (local anaesthetics, opioids, α_2-adrenergic agonists, etc.), combined spinal-epidurals and the use of constant infusion regional local anaesthetic (plus opioids or α_2-adrenergic agonists) techniques[12] (see also Chapter 7).

ORGANIZATION

The establishment of an APS requires the cooperation of the hospital administrative, nursing and medical staff. Close communication is essential between the theatre anaesthetists and the APS, which assumes responsibility for analgesia when surgery has been completed. Initial equipment (e.g.

PCA pumps) needs to be purchased. The hospital pharmacy must develop reliable stocking and dispensing procedures for opioids self-administered via PCA pumps.[12] It may also become involved with special preparations of opioids/local anaesthetics for epidural injection or infusion. Comprehensive pain management teams usually consist of anaesthetists (both consultant and junior medical staff), specially trained nurses, pharmacists and physiotherapists, who regularly visit and assess patients under their care.[2] The APS must be available to provide needed analgesic techniques 24 hours a day and to provide monitoring of ventilatory, cardiovascular and CNS functions. The team is responsible for the maintenance and filling of the PCA pumps and catheters, and for carrying out clinical ward rounds on all patients. The preoperative planning of patients' postoperative analgesic care is carried out. Various pain scoring methods (e.g. VASs) are used to assess pain on at least a daily basis. Some expertise in psychological methods should be available within the team to create well-informed, prepared and participating patients.[13] In cooperation with the surgeons, appropriate protocols, pain management guidelines, standard orders and monitoring routines are developed. The economic costs of such a service can be high (US$200–$300 per patient).[2]

Thus, the employment of a dedicated APS nurse is probably more effective than sophisticated technical equipment, and low-cost, nurse-based, anaesthesiologist-supervised models (as in about 13 per cent of Swedish hospitals) can be used as only 10–25 per cent of surgical patients require PCA or PCEA.[7,10,11] With attentive nursing, greater administration flexibility, better understanding of the pharmacokinetics of prescribed analgesics and regular pain scoring, intramuscular or intravenous opioids and/or non-opioids can provide excellent analgesia.[11] At the time of preoperative evaluation, patients are informed about pain assessment by 3-hourly VAS recordings, the pain management techniques available and the importance of requesting pain medication before the pain becomes too severe.[2] Routine pain scoring is as important as recording the temperature, heart rate and blood pressure. With PCA or epidural pain therapy, the VAS is recorded hourly. A specially trained APS nurse makes daily rounds of all surgical departments to check VAS recordings on charts, help with technical problems (PCA or epidural route) and refer problem patients to the anaesthetist specializing in pain management.[2] The cost of nurse-based, anaesthesiologist-supervised models is less than

US $4 per patient.[2] Ward nurses are given the flexibility to administer analgesics when necessary (based on standard orders and protocols). The pain anaesthetist selects the patients for special pain therapies (PCA, epidurals and peripheral neural blockade), and is available for consultation or for any emergencies.[2] The pain anaesthetist is also responsible for all monitoring routines and staff teaching programmes. All epidural catheters should be placed in the operating room holding area, while PCA is initiated in the post-anaesthesia care unit or in the operating room and continued on the wards.

SAFETY ISSUES

Ongoing nurse and physician education (the relevant anatomy, physiology, pharmacology and goals and risks of therapy) are crucial for successful implementation of an APS.[2,14] The development of nursing protocols and appropriate nurse training should precede the expansion of PCA and epidural infusions of local anaesthetics to all post-surgical wards (as well as the burns unit).[12] Hospital printed protocols and standard orders permit opioid use via the intramuscular, intravenous, subcutaneous PCA and epidural routes.[2] This helps to standardize clinical practice. The monitoring of patients, order-writing and epidural catheter identification should be covered by the same issue of 'standing orders'. Nurses are delegated to administer epidural opioids and local anaesthetics, and to set up PCA pumps.[2]

STANDING ORDERS

An example for analgesic use on surgical wards is as follows:[2]

- 3-hourly VAS recordings to be terminated only if a score of 3 or less is obtained without treatment on three consecutive occasions;
- as a base analgesic, every adult patient to be given rectal paracetamol 1 g 4–6 times daily (children 15–20 mg/kg) unless contraindicated, until VAS is terminated;
- intramuscular morphine 7.5–10 mg to be given when the VAS score is over 3 (doses being reduced by 50 per cent in the elderly and the very sick), the VAS being rechecked about 45 minutes later. If the VAS is still over 3, 50 per cent of the initial morphine dose is given; if the VAS remains greater than 3 after the second dose, the pain anaesthetist should be contacted.

For PCA (intravenous or subcutaneous) on the ward, a standing order may be as follows:[2]

- As a base analgesic, every adult patient is given rectal paracetamol 1 g 4–6 times daily (children 15–20 mg/kg) unless contraindicated, until the VAS is terminated.
- In the operating theatre or post-anaesthesia care unit, the loading dose of morphine is titrated to clinical effect (a VAS of less than 3).
- A bolus dose of morphine 1.0–1.5 mg (depending on surgery type and patient clinical status) is given with a lockout time of 6 minutes.
- Respiratory rate, sedation level and VAS scores are recorded hourly.
- After PCA has been stopped, 3 hourly VAS recordings are continued until the VAS is 3 or less without treatment on three consecutive occasions.
- For inadequate analgesia or PCA problems, the APS nurse should be contacted.

For epidural morphine administration on the ward, an example of standing orders is given below:[2]

- As a base analgesic, every adult patient is given rectal paracetamol 1 g 4–6 times daily (children 15–20 mg/kg) unless contraindicated, until the VAS is terminated.
- 4 mg of morphine via a titration of 0.4 mg/mL are given when the VAS is over 3 (doses being reduced by 50 per cent in the elderly and the very sick).
- After every injection, the respiratory rate and sedation level are recorded every 30 minutes for 2 hours, and then hourly for 10 hours.
- If no urine has been passed within 6 hours after surgery, the bladder is catheterized (in and out).
- Intravenous naloxone 0.4 mg is given with a respiratory rate of less than 10 or with deep sedation without response, and the pain anaesthetist is called.
- Intravenous access is maintained for at least 12 hours after the last dose of epidural morphine.
- 3-hourly VAS recordings are continued until the VAS score is 3 or less without treatment on three consecutive occasions.
- For inadequate analgesia or PCA problems, the APS nurse is contacted.

CONCLUSION

Innovations resulting from an APS may include routine local anaesthetic infiltration of the wound at surgery – subcutaneous or intramuscular morphine injections via an indwelling catheter, intravenous morphine titrated to effect instead of repeated intramuscular injections, alternative pain assessment tools and the frequent recording of pain on movement and/or deep inspiration.[2] Patients can only benefit enormously from the more effective analgesia provided by an APS. The benefits of effective analgesia include earlier ambulation and decreased postoperative morbidity.[15] Research is being conducted into the cost–benefit ratio of such a service, especially in relationship to a decrease in patient hospital stay.[15]

Oral analgesics

Analgesia is improved by offering analgesics to patients on a regular basis around the clock, especially for the first 24–48 hours post-trauma or surgery.[10] Analgesic orders should allow for the great variation in individual opioid requirements, including a regularly scheduled dose and 'rescue' doses for instances in which the usual regimen is insufficient.[10] As most perioperative pain relief is managed solely with oral medication and much takes place in the home, when patients can swallow (even after major surgery), the oral route is preferred for pain relief. In order to know which oral medications to recommend to patients, the treatment-specific number-needed-to-treat (NNT) needs to be calculated.[3] This is the number of patients with moderate or severe perioperative pain who need to receive the active drug for one patient to achieve at least 50 per cent pain relief compared with placebo over a 6-hour treatment period.[3] Using the NNT, the strongest oral analgesic regimen would be oral NSAIDs, provided that no contraindications exist, supplemented as necessary with paracetamol and opioid.[3] As the pain wanes, paracetamol, supplemented by NSAIDs if necessary, is given.[3] In day case surgery, this regimen results in high-quality pain relief.[3] There is no evidence that NSAIDs given rectally or by injection perform better than the same drugs at the same dose given by mouth.[3]

Other opioid routes

For severe, acute pain, opioids are the first-line treatment.[3] The classical nurse-administered intramuscular opioids have disadvantages, summarized as 'too little, too late', because of staffing shortages, ward distractions, the fear of side-effects, and controlled drug regulations.[3,7] Making intramuscular opioids more patient controlled by the nurse immediately reacting to a patient's request may improve intramuscular analgesia.[7] When comparing the relative efficacy of injected opioids and NSAIDs, the following has been found:

- Injecting morphine 10 mg provides analgesia similar to that of oral NSAIDs.
- Injecting morphine 10–20 mg provides analgesia similar to that of injected NSAIDs.
- Injecting NSAIDs provides analgesia similar to that of oral NSAIDs.
- Injecting morphine 20 mg gives greater analgesia than injecting morphine 10 mg and greater analgesia than the best performers on the oral league table.

Continuous intravenous infusions avoid the peaks and troughs of intermittent administration and allow smoother pain control.[10] Careful respiratory monitoring is essential. If intravenous application is deemed inappropriate, subcutaneous rather than intramuscular opioids should be the next choice.[10]

Inhalational route

Fentanyl (100–300 μg) can provide postoperative analgesia when administered as a nebulized aerosol via an oxygen-driven nebulizer.[16] A liposomal-encapsulated formulation of fentanyl as a nebulized aerosol delivery system providing a controlled, sustained release has been used to increase absorption and prolong duration.[16]

Transmucosal route

With the sublingual route, opioids with a high lipid solubility (buprenorphine, fentanyl and methadone) have better bio-availability than those with low lipid solubility (morphine).[17] Oral transmucosal fentanyl has been used for postoperative analgesia in adults undergoing hip or knee arthroplasty.[16] A variety of drugs (fentanyl, sufentanil, butorphanol, ketamine, calcitonin and midazolam) have been administered intranasally.[18,19]

Transdermal route

EMLA cream (lignocaine and prilocaine) provides local anaesthesia for venepuncture.[20] Transdermal fentanyl patches (25, 50, 75 and 100 cm²) provide sustained infusion rates of about 25, 50, 75 and 100 μg per hour for 48–72 hours. Transdermal fentanyl should not replace intravenous PCA for postoperative pain management because of its delayed onset and prolonged residual effects.[21] The transdermal drug delivery of ionized drugs can be enhanced by electromotive drug administration. The electromotive administration of morphine hydrochloride has been used to reduce postopera-tive intravenous opioid requirements.[17] Plasma morphine levels were related to the iontophoresis current. With the electromotive administration of fentanyl, analgesic concentrations are rapidly reached (like morphine within 15–30 minutes).[16] A PCA delivery system for the electromotive administration of fentanyl is currently being investigated.[16] With opioids, switching off the current stops drug delivery and avoids a depot effect. The electromotive administration of lignocaine has been used for superficial surgical procedures.[22]

Intra-articular route

A systematic review of valid trials of intra-articular morphine in knee surgery has shown that morphine can indeed provide analgesia for up to 24 hours.[3]

Encapsulation matrices

The action of rapidly cleared drugs (such as local anaesthetics and opioids) can be prolonged by incorporating them into a variety of encapsulation matrices. Local anaesthetics have been encapsulated into liposomes for topical application, around nerve structures (peripheral nerves and the spinal cord) or intra-articularly to prolong their analgesic effects.[23,24] The epidural and brachial plexus administration of liposome-encapsulated bupivacaine leads to a prolongation of human postsurgical pain relief with minimal or absent motor blockade.[23] Encapsulating bupivacaine in poly(D,L)-lactide-coglycolide microspheres prolongs analgesia and diminishes systemic toxicity.[25]

Stimulation-induced analgesia

Transcutaneous electrical nerve stimulation (TENS) is not effective for post-traumatic and perioperative pain relief, and is of limited value for labour pain.[3]

Pre-emptive analgesia

To prevent persistent pain, should prophylactic measures be undertaken or should physicians wait until it happens?[3] Also, why do some patients end up with chronic pain after surgery? Is this a result of traumatic or surgical nerve damage, or of uncontrolled severe postoperative pain, implying that if the acute pain were better controlled, chronic pain would not develop?[3] Pre-emptive analgesia implies that analgesia given before the painful stimulus prevents or reduces subsequent pain. Its purpose is to prevent or reduce functional changes in the CNS (central sensitization).[10] The evidence for the clinical advantage of intervening before pain occurs as opposed to giving the same intervention after the pain has developed is still unconvincing, most probably because of a number of confounding factors and the use of study designs that have made it difficult to find any reliable answers.[3] The evidence from randomized controlled trials has been reviewed.[26] In the four studies with opioids, there was weak evidence of a pre-emptive effect in three. It may be that any pre-emptive effect of opioids is counteracted by the induction of acute tolerance. The evidence that long-term pain syndromes (e.g. phantom pain) can be pre-empted by pre-pain manoeuvres remains tentative, because of the small patient numbers involved, inadequate randomization and unclear methods.[3] This underscores some of the current controversies surrounding pre-emptive analgesia: how intensely and how long must the pre-emptive intervention be sustained in the post-traumatic or postoperative period to guarantee a prolonged benefit?

Multimodal analgesia

The plasticity in opioid controls illustrates the advantage of combining opioids with local anaesthetics, α_2-agonists, and NMDA antagonists where reducing excitability or enhancing inhibition improves opioid efficacy.[27] The rationale is that each drug exerts its analgesic effect via a different mechanism. Thus, a low-dose combination might offer the best therapeutic effect while minimizing the risks of the unwanted side-effects seen with high doses of each of these drugs. This is known as multimodal (or balanced) analgesia. There is clinical evidence that the neuraxial combination of local anaesthetics and opioids produces optimal analgesia and patient satisfaction in a variety of acute pain states, with fewer side-effects when compared to neuraxial opioids alone.[7] Evidence shows that perioperative epidural anaesthesia/analgesia:[7]

- reduces thromboembolic complications;
- allows a faster recovery of gastrointestinal function, inhibits the endocrine metabolic stress response to surgery and reduces cardiovascular complications;
- helps to shorten the rehabilitation time, hospital stay and return to work time;
- reduces incidence/severity of chronic pain syndromes.

Recent data suggest that these effects are beneficial in patients at high risk of cardiac, pulmonary and infectious morbidity, especially after major surgery.[4]

Multimodal approach to postoperative rehabilitation

The key pathogenic factor in postoperative morbidity is the surgical stress response, with increased demands on organ function.[28] The development of pain-alleviating regimens that allow early ambulation, techniques to reduce nausea, vomiting and ileus, a realization that early enteral nutrition is important for recovery and the reduction of infective complications, and the use of well-established antithrombotic and antimicrobial regimens, represent a global approach to perioperative care.[28]

Patient-controlled analgesia

With its proven efficacy, PCA is now used in paediatric surgery, obstetrics, trauma, burns, patients receiving immunotherapy and a variety of medical conditions.[29,30] PCA has been successfully used for patient-controlled sedation in patients undergoing surgical procedures under local anaesthesia.[31] It has also been used as patient-controlled neuroleptanalgesia in patients undergoing minor surgical procedures.[31] Although most PCA is administered via the intravenous route, this has in some areas been replaced by sublingual, intramuscular, subcutaneous, neuraxial and intraventricular PCA, and most recently by the oral and intranasal routes (PCINA).[3,31,32] PCA equipment ranges from simple disposable pumps (from Baxter Health Care, Go-Medical and Vygon) to very sophisticated microprocessor systems (from CADD-Pharmacia Deltic, Graseby-PCA and Abbott Pain Manager).[31] PCINA devices (Go Medical Lockout Nasal Spray) consist of a specially designed spray bottle with a bolus spray of 0.2 mL and filling (lockout) times of 3 or 4 minutes. The maximum volumes that can be delivered per hour are 4 and 3 mL, respectively. A study using sufentanil in these devices has recently been completed for perioperative paediatric pain (Roelofse and Shipton, 1999, unpublished data). Informed prescribing is based on a maximum knowledge (of pharmacokinetic and pharmacodynamic factors) of the drugs involved. It seems that the success of this method is independent of the opioid used.[31] Fentanyl produces no known pharmacologically active metabolites and appears to be the least complex and most efficacious of the agents commonly used in the PCA setting.[33] The point at which the patient becomes uncomfortable enough to make a demand has become known as the minimum effective (blood drug) concentration (MEC). There are no reliable MECs for individual drugs during PCA, and intra-individual variability (of up to 30 per cent) can occur.[31] While most patients seem to demand some pattern whereby they load and then maintain pain relief at a relatively stable level, the end-point that they are demanding is influenced by factors other than their state of pain at that time. The PCA drug demand decision is determined by the pain felt, which, will in turn, be dependent on any interaction of factors that influence the hierarchy of states (anatomical, physiological, biochemical, pharmacological and psychological) pertaining to the pain and its treatment.[31] There is strong evidence that PCA should be used without continuous (background) infusion, because of the increased risk of respiratory depression.[7] There is very little difference in outcome between efficient intermittent injection and PCA.[3] However, PCA patients are almost always more satisfied with their pain control.[31] New research concepts on PCA technique include changing the lockout interval, the use of variable-dose PCA and patient-maintained, target-controlled infusions, and iontophorectic non-invasive PCA systems.[31,34,35]

Neuraxial opioids

The unique feature of neuraxial opioid analgesia is the lack of sympathetic, or motor, block, which allows patients to ambulate without the risk of orthostatic hypotension or motor incoordination usually associated with neuraxial local anaesthetics or with opioids administered parenterally.[36] The advantages of neuraxial opioids are particularly beneficial in high-risk patients undergoing major surgery, those with compromised pulmonary or cardiovascular function, and grossly obese or elderly patients.[36] Preservative-free morphine, with its hydrophilicity, remains the prototypical agent. This characteristic allows morphine to travel cephalad by passive cerebrospinal fluid (CSF) flow to provide analgesia at sites distant to its placement. The intrathecal route offers a certain availability of the drug in the CSF. Studies with intrathecal injections tend to show a ceiling effect above which only the side-effects increase with increasing dose.[36] Better spinal localization of opioid ensures the resulting segmental analgesia with smaller doses. Compar-

isons of epidural versus intravenous lipid-soluble opioids (alfentanil, sufentanil, fentanyl and butorphanol) have uniformly shown no significant difference in analgesic power or side-effects between the two routes of administration.[36] Highly lipid-soluble opioids have a rapid onset of action (5–15 minutes).[36] They have a relatively short duration of action (2–4 hours). Thus, in general, highly lipid-soluble opioids should preferably not be given epidurally as the sole agent for postoperative analgesia.[36] Epidural PCA (or PCEA) using fentanyl or hydromorphone has been successfully given as an alternative to intravenous PCA for post-surgical pain (e.g. caesarean section – with fentanyl; post-thoracotomy – with fentanyl; upper abdominal surgery – with hydromorphone; and vascular surgery – with morphine).[37–40] Much less opioid is consumed, with similar or even improved analgesia, emphasizing the spinal action of opioids. The majority of PCEA studies have concentrated on bupivacaine/opioid (fentanyl, diamorphine and pethidine) combinations in which the addition of the local anaesthetic was shown to lead to some improvement of efficacy and less opioid-induced pruritus, but usually also to minor cardiovascular depressions.[41] If the MECs of opioids are used, PCEA is a safe technique, incurring a low risk of dose-dependent side-effects.[42] Patients given PCEA with morphine or fentanyl seem to recover more quickly, as judged by shorter mechanical ventilatory times, higher satisfaction with analgesia and fewer postoperative complications, than patients given intravenous PCA.[42] Thus, the length of stay in hospital and intensive care units, and subsequently hospital costs, may be reduced.[42]

Neuraxial local anaesthetic/other drug combinations

Human studies evaluating labour pain and postoperative pain have demonstrated synergistic effects between local anaesthetics (bupivacaine and lignocaine) and opioids (morphine and fentanyl).[43,44] Combinations result in a reduction in the dose of agents needed, the maintenance or enhancement of the degree of pain relief, and the minimization of the risk of unwanted side-effects.[43] Insertion of the epidural catheter should be at the mid-dermatomal level of the incision when local anaesthetics/lipid soluble opioids are used. Dose-ranging studies will be necessary to determine the ideal concentrations of opioids and local anaesthetics to obtain optimal analgesia with a minimal incidence of side-effects. For postoperative analgesia in children, a caudal bupivacaine–morphine mixture has been successfully used.[45] Dosing of morphine should be reduced by at least 50 per cent for infants less than 6 months of age.[46] The addition of the α_2-adrenergic agonist clonidine to epidural combination regimens of local anaesthetic and opioid will increase analgesic power, but the infusion rates studied so far (19–25 μg per hour) have resulted in hypotension, which is exaggerated in hypertensive patients and thoracic neuraxial administration.[46,47] Epidural clonidine in the dose range 3–10 μg/kg may prolong postoperative analgesia by 4–7 hours when added to local anaesthetics.[47] Epidural ketamine 4–30 mg has been used for lower abdominal surgery, with an onset of 20 minutes and a duration of 3–4 hours.[47] The addition of caudal ketamine 0.5 mg/kg to bupivacaine for postoperative analgesia in children significantly improves both quality and duration of analgesia.[47] Human studies to show the efficacy of neuraxial NSAIDs in reducing neuraxial opioid doses still need to be undertaken.[48] In labour, interest has focused on the ideal dose and combination of drugs to produce excellent analgesia without motor block (the walking epidural). In labour, the pain of most patients is successfully relieved with a loading dose of 10–15 mL bupivacaine 0.04–0.25 per cent and fentanyl 50 μg or sufentanil 5 mg followed by an infusion of bupivacaine 0.04–0.0625 per cent and fentanyl 1.5–2.5 μg/mL or sufentanil 0.10–0.25 μg/mL at a rate of 10–15 mL per hour.[49–51] This provides excellent analgesia in the first two stages of labour, with minimal maternal motor weakness, no detrimental effects on uterine or umbilical arterial flow, and no loss of beat-to-beat heart rate variability.[52]

Combined spinal-epidurals (CSEA)

CSEA provides flexibility of technique and drug choice with the ability to 'kick-start' analgesia with a variety of local anaesthetics/opioids and to continue analgesia via the epidural catheter.[53] The needle-through-needle technique is the most popular variety of CSEA. Although the dominant use of CSEA has been in obstetrics and gynaecology, it is increasingly being used in orthopaedic, urological and vascular surgery.[54] For example, with CSEA techniques for walking epidurals in labour, patients can receive an intrathecal dose of bupivacaine 2.5 mg plus fentanyl 25 μg, with epidural boluses of bupivacaine 0.1 per cent plus fentanyl 2 μg/mL to maintain analgesia.[53]

Regional analgesia

Wound infiltration with local anaesthetics is safe and cost-effective.[55] The implantation of polyethylene catheters into the surgical wound followed by an infusion of local anaesthetics can also provide effective analgesia and have an opioid-sparing effect following major surgery.[56] Lignocaine aerosol has been used to provide effective postoperative analgesia when sprayed into herniorrhaphy and tonsillectomy wounds.[56] Lignocaine self-adhesive tape relieves needle insertion pain (for stellate ganglion blockade) after an application time of 7 minutes or more.[57] Any peripheral nerve blocks performed with long-acting local anaesthetics provide analgesia for about 12 hours.[56] Wrist, ankle and elbow blocks are easy to perform. Ilio-inguinal and ilio-hypogastric blocks can give quite effective analgesia after herniorrhaphy.[56] Infraorbital blocks can give effective analgesia after cleft lip repair.[58] Intercostal nerve blocks can be used to provide pain relief after upper abdominal and thoracic surgery. A suprascapular nerve block has recently been shown to be effective for pain relief in arthroscopic shoulder surgery.[59] Paravertebral somatic nerve blocks can be used for the relief of perioperative thoraco-abdominal pain. Interpleural analgesia with local anaesthetics (bupivacaine) has been used for postoperative analgesia, as well as for the treatment of post-traumatic pain.[60] Catheters can be introduced into the brachial plexus, femoral nerve lumbar plexus and paravertebral and intercostal spaces. Continuous regional anaesthetic techniques using an indwelling catheter inserted into the vicinity of the neural structures involved are most effective in providing post-traumatic or perioperative pain relief.[4] With the correct local anaesthetic dose (even down to 0.625 per cent bupivacaine and ropivacaine), selective nociceptive transmission with intact motor function can be obtained for up to several days.[4] This is especially beneficial for those with a prior history of chronic pain, an affected compromised limb circulation or the need for immediate postoperative physiotherapy to maintain joint integrity, and those who have undergone revascularization or re-implantation surgery.[4] All major plexuses (cervical, brachial, lumbar and sacral) can be blocked by a single injection of local anaesthetic.[61] For prolonged local anaesthesia, regional clonidine can be added.[4]

Intraperitoneal analgesia

Intraperitoneal analgesia is obtained by instilling local anaesthetic into the peritoneal cavity to reduce perioperative abdominal and pelvic pain.[62] Pelvic local anaesthetic instillation during laparoscopic sterilization results in no pain during clip application, a marked reduction in postoperative pain and a fall in the incidence and severity of postoperative shoulder pain.[62] Recommended lignocaine dosages (diluted to 80 mL before peritoneal instillation) are 500 mg for postpartum patients and 1000 mg for non-pregnant patients.[62] In laparoscopic cholecystectomy, 30 mL 0.5 per cent bupivacaine has led to a marked reduction in postoperative pain for 8 hours post-surgery.[62] Future trials will undoubtedly clarify the desirability and safety of this practice.

Conclusion

The majority of clinical data focusing on outcome with respect to the type of post-traumatic or post-operative pain management are currently inconclusive.[4] Only the availability of high-quality evidence will provide a firm foundation for building better post-traumatic and perioperative care.[3]

CHRONIC PAIN MANAGEMENT SERVICE

As these patients are usually in the sixth or seventh decade of life, the burden of chronic pain has increased substantially in the past decade.[63] A detailed study of the costs incurred by users of speciality pain clinic services has shown that users of the services incur less direct health care expenditure than do non-users with similar conditions.[63,64] In the UK, such information as is available indicates that pain clinics result in direct health care savings of over £1000 per patient per year and that the total savings may be twice the cost of the chronic pain service.[63] Multicentre trials (with a common protocol and central randomization) with about 500 patients per group will be necessary to determine the 'true' NNT (plus or minus 0.5 units) in order to demonstrate the 'true' clinical relevance of an intervention.[63]

Pain treatment centres have been categorized as multidisciplinary comprehensive, modality orientated and syndrome orientated.[65] An estimated 2000 pain management centres/pain clinics exist in the USA today, whose treatment approaches are often biased by the background of the centres medical

director.[65] However well intended, it is now clear that no single discipline or mode of therapy will suffice. Only a multidisciplinary approach will prevail.

Multidisciplinary pain centre

The primary objective of a multidisciplinary pain centre (MPC) is to return the patient to full functioning.[65] Other objectives include the relief or decrease of pain with the abolition of pain medication, the elimination of assistive devices, a low or zero disability rating, job satisfaction with return to work, leisure activities without limitations, independence from the health care system, the prevention of re-injury and optimum wellness.[65]

An MPC is one that offers multidisciplinary evaluation, treatment and rehabilitation, and a cohesive pain team approach.[66] The organizational structure will depend on available resources (facilities and staff) and the needs of the surrounding patient population. The exact composition will depend on the emphasis and philosophy of the clinic.[67]

Ideally, staffing should include physicians (from a variety of disciplines) and other health-care professionals, as well as secretarial and reception personnel.[68] The director should be a physician with a wide knowledge and experience of chronic pain management. He or she must also have the maturity and wisdom to direct and coordinate the work of the entire team.[69] An MPC should have an expert in the behavioural sciences (psychiatrist or psychologist) on the team,[67] who can be assigned as a counsellor to each patient and can administer psychopharmacology, biofeedback and behavioural modifications.[65] Access to physicians from anaesthetics (to provide nerve blocks, spinal stimulators and opioid pumps), oncotherapy, orthopaedics, neurosurgery, neurology and rheumatology is preferable. Available services should include physiotherapy, occupational therapy, pharmacy, social services, diagnostic radiology and laboratory services.[67] Nurses trained in rehabilitation and pain behaviour can monitor patient progress and serve as case managers.[65] A vocational rehabilitation division can evaluate and direct job placement, and an ergonomics division can undertake job simulation and adapt the patients and/or work site, while computing daily achievement goals.[65] Most therapy can be undertaken on an outpatient basis. Therapeutic facilities offered usually include pharmacological, cognitive, physical and interventional modalities. Inpatient status is preferred for difficult, complicated cases.

Ideally, all patients (with adequate history, physical examinations and laboratory work-up) should be referred by a physician. At the initial (screening) visit, a patient's history is taken and a thorough clinical examination (including neurological investigation, the six motions of the back and a soft tissue examination) is carried out (Figure 2.1).[65] A psychological interview and testing are usually performed at the same visit. Patients with major psychiatric disorders are not precluded as long as they have compensated for them.[65] Patients must have the ability to understand and carry out instructions, must be compliant and cooperative, and must not display aggressive behaviour. A baseline measurement of the patient's pain may be carried out, and a pain diary may be given to the patient to fill in. The patient should be assigned to a particular physician who will be primarily responsible for coordinating that patient's care.[67] The need for further evaluation is also determined. Other assessments should include physiotherapy evaluation and family and vocational assessments.[66] Ideally, all patients should undergo an evaluation in which a problem-solving group attempts to identify the medical, behavioural, vocational, financial, social and other significant patient problems.[65]

Once the assessment has been completed, a decision is then made regarding the most likely diagnosis, and a treatment plan is formulated. This is discussed with the patient, his or her family and significant others (lawyers, employers and insurers), and specific goals are decided upon. Inpatient treatment is required for patients with major behavioural problems or those needing detoxification. Specific therapy, such as nerve blocks or trigger point injections, may be undertaken as an outpatient.

An intense multidisciplinary programme involves a full-time multidisciplinary staff, complete patient involvement, weight control, physical restoration and conditioning, home programme maintenance, pacing, body mechanics, energy-saving techniques, re-injury prevention education, pain control and elimination, drug detoxification, behavioural modification, biofeedback, relaxation, imagery, individual and group therapy, family therapy, assertiveness training, stress management, coping skills, vocational counselling, job planning and simulation, achievement of maximal function, immediate return to work at discharge (ideally) and follow-up care.[65]

Patients who have not benefitted from conventional pain treatments, whose lives are severely disrupted by pain, and those with psychological problems are best treated at an MPC.[66] Interaction with fellow patients helps many to focus less on their pain. Follow-up studies have shown that MPCs reduce suffering and pain behaviour in patients and improve their functional ability and quality of life.[66,67,70] A recent meta-analytic study review has confirmed that the MPC approach (using chronic back pain patients) is superior to unimodal treatments.[71] Both in- and outpatient MPC management programmes have been found to produce improvements in illness-related behaviour and psychological distress.[72] Most patients treated in this way are able to resume many of their formerly abandoned activities and regain a sense of purpose and worth.[66] Following a comprehensive MPC pain management programme lasting 4 weeks, the vast majority of these patients return to work, although they have some residual pain, which should eventually remit.[65] Failures are usually hard-core patients with major behavioural problems. In the USA, if only a 1 per cent reversal of social security disability occurred as a result of the pain programme, $900 000 000 would be saved over a 5-year period.[65]

A systematic review of outpatient services for chronic pain control has recently been conducted, and an evidence-based resource for pain relief established.[63,73] Effective interventions included the following.[63,73]

- minor analgesics, with NNTs ranging from 17 for codeine 60 mg to 2.5 (good) for ibuprofen 400 mg;[73]

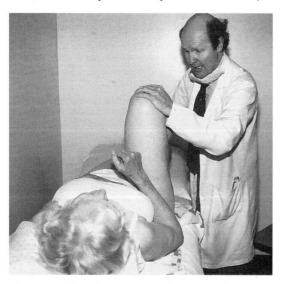

Figure 2.1   Clinical examination of a pain patient in a multidisciplinary clinic.

- antidepressants and anticonvulsants with NNTs in the order of 2.5;
- systemic local anaesthetic-like drugs for nerve damage pain;
- topical NSAIDs in rheumatological conditions;
- topical capsaicin in diabetic neuropathy;
- epidural corticosteroids for back pain and sciatica.

Interventions for which evidence for effectivity is lacking include:[63,73]

- transcutaneous electrical nerve stimulation (TENS) in chronic pain (TENS was shown not to be effective in postoperative and labour pain);
- relaxation;
- spinal cord stimulators.

Ineffective interventions were found to be intravenous regional sympathetic blockade and injections of corticosteroids in or around shoulder joints for pain.[63,73]

Modality-orientated clinic

Such clinics offer a single or limited treatment options, for example nerve blocks applied by anaesthetists and behavioural and cognitive management protocols used by psychologists.[68] The physician in charge should be aware of the clinic's limitations and not treat patients who are unlikely to respond.

Syndrome-orientated clinic

Here, a specific type of pain problem is managed. Examples include clinics for arthritis, headache and facial pain.[68]

Hospice

Hospices, 'resting places for travellers or pilgrims', have been established to provide terminal care 'that incorporates the skills of a hospital with the more leisurely hospitality and warmth of a home'.[74] Care shifts from the disease to the patient. Strictly speaking, hospice is primarily a concept of care rather than a specific place of care.[75] Hospice affirms life and regards dying as a normal process.[75] Hospice neither hastens nor postpones death. It provides personalized services and a caring community so that patients and their families can attain the necessary preparation for a death that is satisfactory to them.[75] The focus of care is to alleviate the physical, emotional, social and spiritual pain related to death and dying. Hospice nursing care focuses on helping hospice patients to live each day as fully and

autonomously as possible until their death in an environment that is familiar and comfortable.

From the humble beginnings of many hospices in back rooms and church basements, hospice programmes are now also being run by large home-care organizations and hospital systems.[75] The British and Canadian hospice movements began within their health care delivery systems and provided services primarily in free-standing hospice buildings in Britain and inpatient palliative care units in Canada.[76] In the USA, the National Hospice Organization (representing over 1900 hospice programmes) provides palliative care to terminally ill patients, and supportive services to patients, their families and significant others, 24 hours a day, 7 days a week, in both home- and facility-based settings.[76] In 1992, this organization provided palliative care for 246 000 patients, of whom 78 per cent had cancer, 10 per cent had heart-related diagnoses and 4 per cent had AIDS.[75,76] In 1995, the total figure had grown to 390 000 patients.[75] By June 1996, there were more than 2700 hospices in the USA.[75] Other terminal non-neoplastic diseases include amyotrophic lateral sclerosis, end-stage respiratory disease and end-stage Alzheimer's disease.[75]

Physical, social, spiritual and emotional care is provided during the last stages of illness, during the dying process and during bereavement by a medically directed interdisciplinary team consisting of patients/families, professionals (one or more physicians, nurses, a psychologist, a social worker, a minister of religion), home health aides (to provide assistance with the personal care of the patient) and volunteers. A fully fledged hospice will offer inpatient, outpatient and day care, as well as community nursing, home and bereavement care.[74] To be eligible for hospice care, a patient must have a disease for which disease-orientated, life-prolonging therapies are no longer effective, appropriate or desired, and have a predicted survival of about 6 months or less.[76]

The major goals of terminal care are to relieve pain and other distressing symptoms (e.g. opioid side-effects), to provide psychological care (for the patient and family) and to help patients to live as actively and as comfortably as possible. Moderate to severe pain is usually controlled effectively with oral opioids and secondary analgesics. Every intervention considered for the hospice patient must be carefully evaluated to assure that it causes more benefit than harm.[76] Effective physical pain relief in hospice patients is essential for the relief of their social, psychological, and spiritual pains.[76] Inadequate analgesia or excessive analgesic toxicity can interfere with successful therapy of this total pain. Assuring a comfortable death also reduces the pain of the patient's loved ones. The hospice nurse keeps the patient's physician informed of the patient's changing condition.[75] Care is available on an on-call basis 24 hours a day, 7 days a week, and is provided regardless of the ability to pay or the source of reimbursement.[75] Social workers provide emotional support and counselling to hospice patients and their families, as well as bereavement services (from support groups to individual counselling) for up to a year after the patient's death.[75] The goal of the hospice chaplain is to meet with patients wherever they are in their spiritual path and to walk with them to the end of their life.[75] The hospice volunteer maintains communication with patients and family members on a weekly basis and is often the most sensitive to the individual's unique needs. Volunteers are more like friends during a time of need and provide respite, companionship, emotional support, errands and transportation.[75] Volunteerism is the major personnel resource of a hospice.[75] Comprehensive pain management and hospice support require interdisciplinary collaboration and commitment.[76]

Home care

An extension of an MPC or the hospital palliative care team can provide home care for terminal patients. Some countries operate a national oncology palliative care service. Hospice care has developed primarily as a home-based service.[77] Ideally, the hospice establishment serves as an extension of the home-care service and functions as a unit with it.[69] It is the operating base for the home-care team. Factors influencing the decision to treat patients at home include the patient's and family's acceptance of the appropriateness of palliative care and their desire for death to occur in familiar surroundings.[77] The concept of palliative care has achieved legitimacy in mainstream medical education, patient care and health policy throughout the world.[78] In terminal patients, the main aim is quality of life, including functional and psychosocial well-being.[78] Home pain management offers many advantages, such as cost savings and patient and family satisfaction. The goals are to provide optimal pain control, preserve autonomy at home and secure continuity of care.[78]

The foundations of a successful home programme to manage cancer and HIV/AIDS include the collaboration of involved health care providers (general practitioners, hospital physicians and home care nurses), communication based on valid pain assessment tools, professional competence and a definition of the role of each health care provider within the team.[78] Health care providers can obtain a global pain score by using the following method:[78]

- The patient's new VAS pain rating is compared with the previous one, and a value of 0, 1, or 2 assigned if the score has decreased, remained unchanged or increased respectively.
- Using a verbal rating scale, patient-rated pain intensity is rated on a scale of 0–4 (from 'none' to 'excruciating').
- The percentage patient-rated pain relief during the current treatment is rated on a scale of 0–4.
- Adding the scores from these three scales calculates a global pain score ranging from 0 (no pain at all) to 10 (maximum, increasing pain).

The simplest route (often the oral) for analgesic administration is usually the best. Some patients require multiple routes of administration to provide the best pain control with minimal side-effects. Patients are treated with oral opioids, intravenous opioids or subcutaneous opioid infusions.[78] PCA is helpful to treat unstable pain (e.g. breakthrough pain and incident pain), whereas transdermal fentanyl is more suitable for chronic, stable and prolonged pain.[78] Both options increase the autonomy of home-care patients. Opioid side-effects should be approached aggressively through ongoing monitoring, assessment, the use of adapted tools and pre-emptive therapy such as a 'bowel regime' at the start of opioid therapy.[78] Relaxation, distraction, guided imagery, biofeedback, massage, rest, cold and heat applications, exercise and stretching can reinforce drug therapies.[78]

While initial assessments are made by a hospice (or hospital) physician, continuing review is carried out by the nursing team, with adjustment to medication as required. Ideally, the family general practitioner should be actively involved. The services of a psychologist and a social worker should be available to the nursing team. Education and involvement of the family are also important. They must understand the regimen in detail, the function of each drug and its timing, and any particular problems.[69] The home-care nurse then begins daily home visits to assess pain and other symptoms. The nurse adjusts the drug dosage and provides adjuvants according to a predetermined protocol until pain control and symptoms are satisfactory. Side-effects are also assessed and treated with previously agreed therapies. Social services, physiotherapy, housekeeping and psychological support are also provided in the patient's home. In a recent study of patients in the palliative (67 per cent) and the terminal (33 per cent) phases of their illness, the mean duration of home care before death was 88.7 days and the mean length of inpatient hospitalization only 3.5 days.[78] If care breaks down (e.g. because of the development of a neuropathic pain syndrome or a difficult home situation), the patient can be admitted. Very rarely, the pain clinic may have to be consulted for the insertion of a spinal drug delivery system, neuroablative procedures, radiotherapy or fracture stabilization.[69] Symptom control with oral medication, emotional support and physical care will enable most terminal patients to remain at home until death or very near it.[69] Adopting an organized, aggressive and anticipatory approach to pain and symptom control will enhance the quality of life for both the patient and family.

Caring for pain in the patient with AIDS[79]

A variety of pain syndromes have been identified with HIV disease and AIDS, and their prompt recognition helps to ensure effective treatment.[80] When possible, treatment is directed towards the underlying source of pain, in combination with carefully individualized pharmacotherapy and attention to psychosocial factors. Pain in AIDS impairs most aspects of quality of life and worsens its psychological and functional morbidity.[80] Estimates of the prevalence of pain in HIV-infected individuals range from 30 to 80 per cent, the prevalence of pain increasing as the disease progresses.[81] Up to 85 per cent of patients with AIDS pain are undertreated, a situation more widespread than with cancer pain.[80] Women with HIV and pain are twice as likely to be undertreated than are their male counterparts.[80] Lack of education and a history of drug abuse are other predictors of the undertreatment of AIDS pain.[80] Like cancer pain, AIDS pain tends to be more than one type, to involve more than one location and to increase as the disease progresses.[80] The same broad pharmacological principles (such as the titration of opioids and secondary analgesics, and scheduled 'by-the-clock' administration combined with 'as needed' doses) that apply for treating cancer pain have been successfully applied to AIDS pain.[80] Sixty per cent of patients have pain resulting from viral burden or immunological suppression, 30 per cent have pain arising from treatment, and 10 per cent have pain due to chronic non-HIV-related conditions.[80]

Neuropathic pain syndromes occur in up to 40 per cent of AIDS patients with pain.[81] About 30 per cent develop symmetrical predominantly sensory neuropathy, which characteristically presents as symmetrical distal burning, numbness and a pins and needles sensation.[80] The predominant symptom in about 60 per cent of patients is pain in the soles of the feet.[81] Another 10 per cent may develop myelopathy from viral infection of the spinal cord.[80] Other causes of neuropathic pain include:

- immune-mediated neuropathy (acute Guillain–Barré syndrome and inflammatory demyelinating polyneuropathies);
- toxic neuropathies (alcohol);
- nutritional neuropathies (folate and vitamins B_6 and B_{12});
- antiretroviral therapy (didanosine and zalcitabine);
- antiviral agents (foscarnet);
- antibacterial agents (dapsone and metronidazole);
- antimycobacterial preparations (isoniazid, rifampicin and ethionamide);
- antineoplastic drugs (vincristine and vinblastine);
- infectious polyradiculopathies associated with cytomegalovirus (CMV) infection;
- radiotherapy;
- surgery;
- treatment with phenytoin.[80,81]

The type of neuropathy varies with the infection stage, such as the seroconversion stage (mononeuritides, brachial plexopathy and acute demyelinating polyneuropathy), the latent phase (demyelinating polyneuropathies), the transition phase (shingles and mononeuritis multiplex) and the late phase (predominantly sensory neuropathy).[81] Other common pain in AIDS includes that arising from the abdomen, mouth, skin and joints.[80]

The abdomen is the primary site of pain in 12–25 per cent of patients.[81] Abdominal pain may arise from infections that can lead to organomegaly and obstruction, such as cryptosporidiosis (Shigella, Salmonella and Campylobacter enteritis (giving repeated small intestinal intussusception), CMV ileitis (leading to bowel perforation) and mycobacterial (MIA) infection.[81] Lymphoma and Kaposi's sarcoma can present with bowel obstruction. Other causes of abdominal pain include ileus, aseptic peritonitis, toxic shock herpes zoster and the Fitzhugh–Curtis syndrome.[81] Cholecystitis (from CMV or cryptosporidiosis) and extrahepatic biliary obstruction (from Kaposi's sarcoma and MAI infection) may occur.[81] Hepatitis may be caused by opportunistic liver infections (CMV, MAI and fungi) or drugs (didanosine and pentamidine), while pancreatitis may be due to drugs (didanosine, dideoxycytidine and pentamidine) or infections (CMV, MAI and Cryptococcus).[81] Infectious causes of anorectal pain include periectal abscesses, CMV proctitis, fissure-in-ano and herpes simplex virus.[81]

Headache is reported in up to 40 per cent of patients in the later stages of disease.[81] It is mostly of the tension, zidovudine-induced (AZT, in 15–30 per cent) or vascular/migrainous type.[80] When the T-cell count falls below 200, ominous causes such as HIV encephalitis and atypical meningitis, opportunistic CNS infections (toxoplasmosis, cryptococcal meningitis, CMV, herpes simplex and herpes zoster infection, tuberculosis and candidiasis), and CNS lymphoma arise.[80,81]

A variety of rheumatological conditions (associated with up to 40 per cent of pain syndromes) have been reported in AIDS, ranging from various forms of arthritis, arthropathy, arthralgia and myopathy to myositis and myalgias.[81] These include Reiter's syndrome, psoriatic arthritis, septic arthritis, HIV-associated arthritis, non-specific arthralgias, HIV-associated painful articular syndrome (large joints), vasculitis, Sjögren's syndrome, polymyositis, AZT myopathy and dermatomyositis.[80,81]

Oropharyngeal and oesophageal pain from ulcers is common, causing dysphagia and odynophagia.[80] Oropharyngeal and oesophageal candidiasis occurs in up to 75 per cent of HIV-positive individuals. Oral and oesophageal ulcerations can be caused by herpes simplex virus, CMV, Epstein–Barr virus, myobacteria, Cryptococcus, histoplasmosis, or AZT.[81] Dental abscesses are common. Up to 75 per cent of patients with cutaneous Kaposi's sarcoma have intra-oral lesions.[81] Lymphomas and Kaposi's sarcoma can invade the oesophagus.

Chest pain occurs in about 10 per cent of AIDS pain syndromes.[81] Infectious causes include pneumocystis pneumonia, oesophagitis, pleuritis/pericarditis (viral, bacterial or tuberculosis) and post-herpetic neuralgia.[81] Lymphoma and Kaposi's sarcoma can invade the pericardium, chest wall, lung, oesophagus and pleura.[81]

HIV-related conditions that cause pain in children include meningitis, sinusitis, otitis media, herpes zoster infection, cellulitis, abscesses, candida dermatitis, dental caries, intestinal infections (MAI and cryptosporidiosis), hepatosplenomegaly, oral and oesophageal candidiasis, and encephalopathic spasticity.[80]

Not only is the symptom burden high in AIDS, but also the majority of symptoms are psychological in nature (depression, anxiety and hopelessness).[80] Both depression and negative thoughts related to pain were significantly correlated to the presence and intensity of pain,[81] emphasizing the need for interdisciplinary assessment and management. A multidimensional model of AIDS pain calls for access to pharmacological, psychotherapeutic, cognitive-behavioural, anaesthetic, neurosurgical and rehabilitative interventions.[80] The WHO has devised guidelines for the analgesic management of cancer pain (WHO ladder), which the US Agency for Health Care Policy and Research has endorsed for the management of HIV positive/AIDS pain.[81] Clinical reports describe the successful application of the WHO ladder principles in AIDS pain, with particular emphasis on the use of morphine.[80]

The initial step in pain management is a comprehensive assessment of pain symptoms. The pain is more commonly associated with treatable, underlying causes than is cancer pain.[80] Aggressive antiretroviral therapy and the treatment of opportunistic infections have dramatically increased survival in children with HIV/AIDS.[82] A careful history and clinical examination may disclose an identifiable syndrome (herpes zoster or bacterial infection, or neuropathy) that can be treated in a standard fashion.[81] Qualitative pain features, its time course and any manoeuvres that change its intensity should be elicited.[80] Pain intensity (current, average, at best and at worst) should be assessed to determine the analgesics needed for moderate to severe pain, and to evaluate treatment efficacy.[80] Pain descriptors (burning, shooting, dull, sharp, etc.) help to determine the pain mechanism (somatic nociceptive, visceral nociceptive, neuropathic or mixed) and the likelihood of response to secondary analgesics (antidepressants, anticonvulsants, oral local anaesthetics, corticosteroids, etc.).[80] Additionally, detailed medical, neurological, and psychosocial assessments (including a history of drug use or abuse) must be obtained.[80] Family members or partners should be interviewed. During the assessment phase, pain should be aggressively treated.[81] Fundamental aspects requiring ongoing evaluation include pain intensity and relief, pain-related functional interference (mood state and activities) and the monitoring of drug effects (side-effects and abuse behaviour).[80,81] Pain assessment tools include the Brief Pain Inventory and the Memorial Pain Assessment Card.[81] The latter is a helpful clinical tool consisting of VASs that measure pain intensity and relief, and mood, which a patient can complete in less than 30 seconds.[80]

The first step of the WHO ladder employs paracetamol (which can give interaction problems with azidothymidine, and hepatotoxicity with overdose) or NSAIDs (which may cause problems with bleeding, gastric ulceration and renal and hepatic morbidity).[82] The non-acetylated salicylates (salsalate, sodium salicylate and choline magnesium salicylate) theoretically have fewer gastrointestinal effects and less inhibition of platelet aggregation.[81] Opioids are the mainstay of pharmacotherapy of moderate to severe pain in the HIV patient.[81] The following principles apply:

- Choose an appropriate drug and route.
- Start with lowest possible dose and titrate.
- Use 'as needed' doses selectively.
- Be aware of equivalent analgesic doses.
- Use a combination of an opioid, a non-opioid and a secondary analgesic.
- Be aware of tolerance.
- Understand physical and psychological dependence.

In step 2 of the WHO ladder, oxycodone (in sustained-release form or in combination with paracetamol or a NSAID when not contraindicated), hydrocodone or codeine can be used.[81] Because opioid agonist–antagonist drugs (pentazocine, nalbuphine and butorphanol) can reverse opioid effects and precipitate opioid withdrawal syndromes, their use is limited in AIDS pain.[81] More severe pain is managed with morphine (or other stronger opioids such as hydromorphone, methadone, levorphanol and fentanyl).[81] The oral route is preferred (every 3–4 hours with morphine, or hydromorphone), but sustained-release oral morphine provides 8–12 hours of analgesia (with immediate-release, short-acting opioid rescue supplementation).[81] With the use of transdermal fentanyl patches, an alternate opioid must be provided until adequate fentanyl levels are obtained. In AIDS, the transdermal fentanyl absorption may be increased with fever, resulting in increased plasma levels and a shorter duration of analgesia.[81] Opioid sedation usually resolves after the patient has been maintained on a steady dosage.[81] Intravenous haloperidol (1–2 mg) can be used to treat opioid-induced delirium.

Individuals who inject drugs are among the AIDS exposure categories with the highest rate of increase of AIDS.[81] The dilemma of opioid administration to individuals who are suspected or actual abusers is a difficult one, raising treatment questions, including:[81,82] how to treat patients with a high opioid tolerance; how to distinguish between active abusers, those on methadone maintenance and those in recovery; and how to distinguish between tolerance, physical dependence and addiction (psychological dependence or drug abuse).[80] It is, however, possible to manage pain in substance abusers with AIDS safely and responsibly using the following approach:[81]

- Set clear goals and conditions for opioid therapy.
- Set limits.
- Recognize drug abuse behaviours.
- Make consequences clear.
- Use written contracts.
- Establish a single prescriber.
- Use pharmacological as well as non-pharmacological interventions.
- Pay attention to psychosocial issues.
- Use a team approach.

Commonly used secondary analgesics include antidepressants, anticonvulsants, neuroleptics, psychostimulants, corticosteroids and oral local anaesthetics.[81] Paroxitene (a serotonin selective uptake inhibitor) has proved a highly effective analgesic in neuropathy.[81] Newer antidepressants such as sertraline, venlafaxine and nefazodone may eventually prove useful as secondary analgesics.[81] Advantages of the psychostimulant pemoline include mild abuse potential, only mild sympathomimetic effects and the fact that it can be absorbed via the buccal mucosa as a chewable tablet.[81] There is an increased risk of extrapyramidal side-effects from neuroleptics in AIDS patients.[81] Non-pharmacological interventions include physical therapies (cutaneous stimulation with heat, cold and massage), psychological therapies (relaxation, imagery, biofeedback, distraction and reframing, hypnosis and patient education) and nerve blocks.[81] The climate of medical care is changing, and patients and their families are more willing to relinquish futile attempts at cure in favour of palliative care.[82]

REFERENCES

1. **Harmer, M.** 1991: Postoperative pain relief – time to take our heads out of the sand? *Anaesthesia* **46**, 167–8.
2. **Rawal, N. and Berggren, L.** 1994: Organization of acute pain services: a low-cost model. *Pain* **57**, 117–23.
3. **McQuay, H. and Moore**, A. 1997: The concept of postoperative care. *Current Opinion in Anaesthesiology* **10**, 369–73.

4. **Nierhaus, A. and Am Esch, J.C.** 1997: Postoperative pain management. *Pain Reviews* **4**, 149–57.

5. **Warfield, C.A. and Kahn, C.H.** 1995: Acute pain management. *Anesthesiology* **83**, 1090–4.

6. **Gouke, C.R. and Owen, H.** 1995: Acute pain management in Australia and New Zealand. *Anaesthesia and Intensive Care* **23**, 715–7.

7. **Wulf, H. and Neugebauer, E.** 1997: Guidelines for postoperative pain therapy. *Current Opinion in Anaesthesiology* **10**, 380–5.

8. **Rawal, N. and Allvin, R.** 1998: Acute pain services in Europe: a 17-nation survey of 105 hospitals – the EuroPain Acute Pain Working Party. *European Journal of Anaesthesiology* **15**(3), 354–63.

9. **Sjostrom, B., Haljamae, H., Dahlgren, L.O. and Lindstrom, B.** 1997: Assessment of postoperative pain: impact of clinical experience and professional role. *Acta Anaesthesiologica Scandinavica* **41**(3), 339–44.

10. **Shipton, E.A.** 1996: The relief of acute pain. *South African Journal of Surgery* **34**(1), 40–3.

11. **Rawal, R.** 1996: Organization models for acute pain services (APS). In Campbell, J.N. (ed.) *Pain 1996 – an updated review*. Seattle: IASP Press, 195–8.

12. **Ready, L.B.** 1990: Acute Pain Management Service. *International Anesthesia Research Society Review Course Lectures* 123–6.

13. **Shipton, E,A.** 1992: Postoperative pain – an update. *South African Journal of Surgery* **30**(1), 2–5.

14. **Rose, D.K., Cohen, M.M. and Yee, D.A.** 1997: Changing the practice of pain management. *Anesthesia and Analgesia* **84**, 764–2.

15. **Shipton, E.A., Beeton, A.G., Minkowitz, H.S.** 1993: An acute pain relief service – the first ten months. *South African Medical Journal* **83**, 501–5.

16. **Sandler, A.N.** 1997: New drug delivery systems for acute pain management. In Jain, S. Mauskop, A. and Vietsauskop, B. (eds) *Current concepts in acute, chronic, and cancer pain management*. New York: World Foundation for Pain Relief and Research, 77–81.

17. **Ashburn, M.A. and Stanley, T.H.** 1992: Drug delivery systems in the 1990's. *International Anesthetic Research Society Review Course Lectures,* 129–35.

18. **Biddle, C. and Gilliland, C.** 1992: Transdermal and transmucosal administration of pain-relieving and anxiolytic drugs: a primer for the critical care practitioner. *Heart and Lung* **21**(2), 115–24.

19. **Theroux, M., West, D., Corddry, D., Kettrick, R. and Bachrach, S.** 1992: Efficacy of midazolam administered nasally for suturing lacerations in emergency rooms. *Anesthesiology* **77**(3A), A1172.

20. **Kano, T., Nakamura, M., Hashiguchi, A.** *et al.* Skin pretreatments for shortening onset of dermal patch anesthesia with 35 GA MHPh 2Na-10% lidocaine gel mixture. *Anesthesia and Analgesia* **75**, 555–7.

21. **Sevarino, F.B., Naulty, J.S., Sinatra, R.** *et al.* Transdermal fentanyl for postoperative pain management in patients recovering from abdominal gynecologic surgery. *Anesthesiology* **77**, 463–6.

22. **Petelenz, T., Petelenz, A.I., Iwinski, T.J. and Dubel, S.** 1984: Mini set for iontophoresis for topical analgesia before injection. *International Journal of Clinical Pharmacology Therapy and Toxicology* **22**, 152–5.

23. **Malinovsky, J.M., Benhamou, D., Alafandy, M.** *et al.* Neurotoxicological assessment after intracisternal injection of liposomal bupivacaine in rabbits. *Anesthesia and Analgesia* **85**, 1331–6.

24. **Grant, G.J.** 1997: Effect of liposomal encapsulation of bupivacaine on plasma drug levels after intraarticular administration in rabbits. *Anesthesia and Analgesia* **84**, S296.

25. **Fletcher, D., Le Corre, P., Guilbaud, G. and Le Verge, R.** 1997: Antinociceptive effect of bupivacaine encapsulated in poly-(D,L)-lactide-co-glycolide microspheres in the acute inflammatory pain model of carrageenin-injected rats. *Anesthesia and Analgesia* **84**, 90–4.

26. **McQuay, H.J.** 1995: Pre-emptive analgesia: a systematic review of clinical studies. *Annals of Medicine* **27**, 249–56.

27. **Dickenson, A.H.** 1995: Spinal cord pharmacology of pain. *British Journal of Anaesthesia* **75**, 193–200.

28. **Shipton, E.A.** 1998: The relief of acute pain: moving the frontiers forward. *South African Journal of Anaesthesiology and Analgesia* **4**(3), 2–7.

29. **Kluger, M.T. and Owen, H.** 1991: Patient-controlled analgesia: can it be made safer? *Anaesthesia and Intensive Care* **19**(3), 412–20.

30. **Shipton, E.A, Minkowitz, H.S. and Becker, P.** 1993: Patient-controlled analgesia in burn injuries: the subcutaneous route. *Canadian Journal of Anaesthesia,* **40**, 898.

31. **Shipton, E.A.** 1998: Patient controlled analgesia – quo vadis? *Hospital Supplies* (Mar), 2.

32. **Dickenson, A.H., Sullivan, A.F and McQuay, H.J.** 1990: Intrathecal etorphine, fentanyl, and buprenorphine on spinal nociceptive neurones in the rat. *Pain* **42**, 227–34.

33. **Mather, L.E. and Woodhouse, A.** 1997: Pharmacokinetics of opioids in the context of patient controlled analgesia. *Pain Reviews* **4**, 20–32.

34. **Shipton, E.A.** 1996: Patient controlled analgesia (PCA) – an update. *Hospital Supplies* (Feb), 12–16.

35. **Love, D.R., Owen, H., Ilsley, A.H., Plummer, J.L, Hawkins, R.M. and Morrison, A.** 1996: A comparison of variable-dose patient-controlled analgesia with fixed-dose patient-controlled analgesia. *Anesthesia and Analgesia* **83**, 1060–4.

36. **Shipton, E.A.** 1996: Modern use of neuraxial opioids in acute pain. *South African Journal of Surgery* **34**(4), 180–5.

37. **Parker, R.K. and White, P.F.** 1992: Epidural patient-controlled analgesia: an alternative to intravenous patient-controlled analgesia for pain relief after cesarean delivery. *Anesthesia and Analgesia* **75**, 245–51.

38. **Grant, R.P., Dolman, J.F., Harper, J.A.** 1992: Patient-controlled lumbar epidural fentanyl compared with patient-controlled intravenous fentanyl for post-

thoracotomy pain. *Canadian Journal of Anaesthesia,* **39**(3), 214–19.

39. **Welchew, E.A. and Breen, D.P.** 1991: Patient-controlled on-demand epidural fentanyl: a comparison of patient-controlled on-demand fentanyl delivered epidurally or intravenously. *Anaesthesia* **46**, 438–41.

40. **Bustamante, J., Sawaki, Y. and White, P.F.** 1992: Comparison of IV-PCA vs Epidural-PCA following major vascular surgery. *Anesthesia and Analgesia* **74**, S39.

41. **Lehmann, K.A.** 1997: Update of patient-controlled analgesia. *Current Opinion in Anaesthesiology* **10**, 374–9.

42. **Chrubasik, S. and Chrubasik, J.** 1995: The use of patient-controlled epidural analgesia for acute and chronic pain. *Pain Reviews* **2**, 29–37.

43. **De Leon-Casasola, O.A. and Lema, M.J.** 1996: Postoperative epidural opioid analgesia: what are the choices? *Anesthesia and Analgesia* **83**, 867–75.

44. **Kehlet, H. and Dahl, J.B.** 1993: The value of multimodal or balanced analgesia in postoperative pain treatment. *Anesthesia and Analgesia* **77**, 1048–56.

45. **Berde, C.** 1993: Acute postoperative pain management in children. *American Society of Anesthesiologists' Annual Refresher Course Lectures,* **136**, 1–7.

46. **Abuzaid, H., Prys-Roberts, C., Wilkins, D.G. and Terry, D.M.S.** 1993: The influence of diamorphine on spinal anaesthesia induced with isobaric 0.5% bupivacaine. *Anaesthesia* **48**, 492–5.

47. **Rawal N.** 1996: Opioids and nonopioids – efficacy, safety and cost-benefit. *Pain Reviews* **3**, 31–62.

48. **Malmberg, A.B. and Yaksh, T.L.** 1993: Pharmacology of the spinal action of ketorolac, morphine, ST-91, U50488H, and L-PIA on the formalin test and an isobolographic analysis of the NSAID interaction. *Anesthesiology* **79**, 270–81.

49. **Russell, R. and Reynolds, F.** 1993: Epidural infusions for nulliparous women in labour. *Anaesthesia* **48**, 856–61.

50. **Yee, I., Carstoniu, J., Halpern, S. and Pittini, R.** 1993: A comparison of two doses of epidural fentanyl during caesarean section. *Canadian Journal of Anaesthesia* **40**(8), 722–5.

51. **Le Polain, B., De Kock, M., Scholtes, J.L. and Van Lierde, M.** 1993: Clonidine combined with sufentanil and bupivacaine with adrenaline for obstetric analgesia. *British Journal of Anaesthesia* **71**, 657–60.

52. **Wittels, B., Glosten, B., Faure, E.A.M.** *et al.* Opioid antagonist adjuncts to epidural morphine for postcesarean analgesia: maternal outcomes. *Anesthesia and Analgesia* **77**, 925–32.

53. **Carrie, L.E.S.** 1996: Combined spinal epidural anaesthesia (CSEA) in obstetric practice. In Carrie, L.E.S., Urmey, W.F. and Hanaoka, K. (eds) *New advances in combined spinal epidural anaesthesia – a global update.* Auckland: Customised Medical Communications, International Symposium of Regional Anaesthesia, 1–7.

54. **Hanaoka, K.** 1996: Combined spinal epidural anaesthesia: the Japanese experience. In Carrie, L.E.S.,

Urmey, W.F. and Hanaoka, K. (eds) *New advances in combined spinal epidural anaesthesia – a global update.* Auckland: Customised Medical Communications, International Symposium of Regional Anaesthesia, 13–16.

55. **Dahl, J.B., Frederiksen, H.J.** 1995: Wound infiltration for operative and postoperative analgesia. *Current Opinion in Anaesthesiology* **8**, 435–40.

56. **Raj, P.P.** 1991: Regional techniques for postoperative analgesia. *McGill University Annual Review Course in Anaesthesia,* (May), 311–21.

57. **Inada, T., Uesugi, F., Kawachi, S. and Inada, K.** 1997: Lidocaine tape relieves pain due to needle insertion during stellate ganglion block. *Canadian Journal of Anaesthesia* **44**(3), 259–62.

58. **Nicodemus, H.F., Ferrer, M.J.R., Cristobal, V.C. and De Castro, L.R.** 1991: Bilateral infraorbital blocks with 0.05% bupivacaine in children. *Anesthesiology* **75**(3A), A690.

59. **Ritchie, E.D., Tong, D., Chung, F., Norris, A.M., Miniaci, A. and Vairavanathan, S.D.** 1997: Suprascapular nerve block for postoperative pain relief in arthroscopic shoulder surgery: a new modality? *Anesthesia and Analgesia* **84**, 1306–12.

60. **Levine, C.B. and Levin, B.H.** 1992: Long-term interpleural analgesia using a subcutaneous implantable infusion system. *Canadian Journal of Anaesthesia* **39**(4), 408.

61. **Winnie A.P.** 1991: Regional anesthesia of the extremities. *American Society of Anesthesiologists Annual Refresher Course Lectures* **19**, 233–51.

62. **Starbuck, N.** 1999: Intraperitoneal analgesia. *South African Journal of Anaesthesiology and Analgesia* **5**(1), 30–1.

63. **McQuay, H.J. and Moore, R.A.** 1998: *An evidence-based resource for pain relief.* Oxford: Oxford University Press, 251–7.

64. **Weir, R., Browne, G.B., Tunks, E., Gafni, A. and Roberts, J.** 1992: A profile of users of speciality pain clinic services: predictors of use and cost estimates. *Journal of Clinical Epidemiology* **45**, 1399–415.

65. **Rosomoff, H.L.** 1996: Multidisciplinary approaches in pain treatment centers. In Campbell, J.N. (ed.) *Pain 1996 – an updated review.* Seattle: IASP Press, 279–85.

66. **Aronoff, G.M. and McAlary, P.W.** 1992: Pain centres: treatment of intractable suffering and disability from chronic pain. In Aronoff, G.M. (ed) *Evaluation and treatment of chronic pain,* 2nd edn. Baltimore: Williams & Wilkins, 416–29.

67. **Abram, S.E.** 1989: Pain – acute and chronic. In Barash, P.G., Cullen, B.F. and Stoelting, R.K. (eds). *Clinical anesthesia.* Philadelphia: J.B. Lippincott, 1427–54.

68. **Abram, S.E. and Lynch, N.T.** 1990: Pain clinic organization and staffing. In Abram, S.E. (ed.) *The pain clinic manual.* Philadelphia: J.B. Lippincott, 4–13.

69. **Raftery, H.** 1991: Integration of hospital and home care for patients dying with cancer pain. *Pain Clinic* **4**(2), 1–2.

70. **Maruta, T., Swanson, D.W. and McHardy, M.J.** 1990: Three-year follow-up of patients with chronic pain who were treated in a multidisciplinary pain management center. *Pain* **41**, 47–53.

71. **Flor, H., Fydrich, T. and Turk, D.C.** 1992: Efficacy of multidisciplinary pain treatment centres: a meta-analytic review. *Pain* **49**, 221–30.

72. **Peters, J.L. and Large, R.G.** 1990: A randomised control trial evaluating in- and outpatient pain management programmes. *Pain* **41**, 283–93.

73. **McQuay, H.J., Moore, R.A., Eccleston, C., Morley, S. and Williams, A.C.** 1997: Sytematic review of outpatient services for chronic pain control. *Health Technology Assessment* **1**(6), I-IV.

74. **Twycross, R.G.** 1990: Terminal care of cancer patients: hospice and home care. In Bonica, J.J. (ed.) *The management of pain*, 2nd edn. Philadelphia: Lea & Febiger, 445–60.

75. **Dunlap, D.L.** 1997: The hospice movement: a philosophical approach. In Parris, W.C.V. (ed.) *Cancer pain management: principles and practice.* Boston: Butterworth-Heinemann, 499–505.

76. **Levy, M.H.** 1997: Current concepts in the management of cancer pain in a hospice environment. In *Current concepts in acute, chronic, and cancer pain management.* New York: World Foundation for Pain Relief and Research, 167–71.

77. **Patt, R.B.** 1992: Control of pain associated with advanced malignancy. In Aronoff, G.M. (ed.) *Evaluation and treatment of chronic pain*, 2nd edn. Baltimore: Williams & Wilkins, 313–39.

78. **Poulain, P., Langlade, A. and Goldberg, J.** 1997: Cancer pain management in the home. *Pain – clinical updates* **V**(1), 1–4.

79. **Shipton, E.A.** 1998: Pain in AIDS. *South African Journal of Anaesthesiology and Analgesia* **4**(2), 4–7.

80. **Breitbart, W., Passik, S.T., Lefkowitz, M., Patt, R.B. and Reddy, K.S.** 1996: Pain in AIDS: a call to action. *Pain – clinical updates* **IV**(1), 1–4.

81. **Breitbart, W.** 1997: Pain in AIDS. In *Current concepts in acute, chronic, and cancer pain management.* New York: World Foundation for Pain Relief and Research, 315–36.

82. **Carr, D.B.** 1995: Pain in HIV/AIDS. *Current Opinion in Anaesthesiology* **8**, 441–4.

3 PRIMARY ANALGESICS:
The opioids

OPIOID RECEPTORS AND LIGANDS

Endogenous opioid peptides and opioid receptors constitute a physiological system widely distributed in the mammalian central and peripheral nervous systems, where it has a putative neurotransmitter/neuromodulator role.[1] In addition, endogenous opioid peptides participate in the modulation of the cardiovascular, endocrine, gastrointestinal and immune systems. To date, three genetically independent families of endogenous opioid peptides (enkephalins, dynorphins and beta-endorphins) have been found, derived from different precursors:

pro-enkephalin, prodynorphin and pro-opiomelanocortin) (Figure 3.1).[2] They include approximately 20 peptides with opioid-like activity (putative transmitters). The endogenous opioid peptides constitute the endogenous ligands for different types of opioid receptors (mu, delta and kappa), which are present in pre- and postsynaptic membranes. Both endogenous opioid peptides and opioid receptors are found in supraspinal, spinal and probably peripheral sites in close association with sensory pathways that convey nociceptive information.[1] The endogenous opioid peptides are probably activated by nociceptive stimuli and, as a consequence, an inhibitory modulation of sensory information occurs. Thus, at each anatomical site where sensory information is processed,

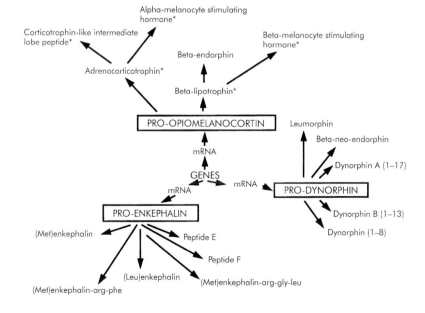

Figure 3.1 Opioid peptides and precursors. *No opioid receptor activity.

nociceptive transmission will occur as a result of the simultaneous activation of the endogenous excitatory and inhibitory systems.

The endogenous ligands for the opioid receptors are a family of peptides in the CNS that originate by proteolytic cleavage of three independent precursor proteins: pro-opiomelanocortin (POMC), pro-enkephalin (A) and prodynorphin (pro-enkephalin B). In humans, most peptides with opioid-like activity include one of the amino acid sequences tyr-gly-gly-phe-met (met-enkephalin) or tyr-gly-gly-phe-leu (leu-enkephalin).[1] POMC contains one copy of the met-enkephalin sequence, while it is also a common precursor of alpha, beta and gamma-melanocyte stimulating hormone, corticotrophin and beta-endorphin. Pro-enkephalin contains seven copies of met-enkephalin and originates four met-enkephalins, one leu-enkephalin, one met-enkephalin-arg6-phe7 and one met-enkephalin-arg6-gly7-leu8.[1] Pro-dynorphin contains four copies of leu-enkephalin and induces the formation of dynorphin A and B, and alpha- and beta-neoendorphin.[1] Precursor maturation into active neuropeptides involves cleavage at basic residues within these molecules. The physiological factors that trigger the activation of enzymes inducing the formation of biologically active peptides are not well established.

The anatomical distribution of the endogenous opioid peptides and their precursors has been elucidated with immunocytochemical and *in situ* hybridization techniques. The genes are expressed in tissues of different embryological origin, such as reproductive tissue, chromaffin cells, the immune system (leucocytes, macrophages T-helper cells, thymus and spleen) and neuronal tissues.[1] The hypophysis (anterior and intermediate lobes) is the major site of POMC synthesis, while in the brain, high levels are found in the arcuate nucleus of the hypothalamus and the medullary nucleus tractus solitarius. Pro-enkephalin A and pro-dynorphin are widely distributed in the CNS. Areas of pro-enkephalin A and prodynorphin synthesis include the hypothalamus, striatum, thalamus, lateral geniculate nucleus, peri-aqueductal grey matter, colliculi, substantia nigra, raphe magnus, nucleus reticularis paragigantocellularis, tractus solitarius, spinal trigeminal nucleus and dorsal horn of the spinal cord. In addition, prodynorphin is also found on the anterior lobe of the pituitary gland.[1] The widespread distribution of these peptides in the neuraxis suggests their involvement in multiple neuronal functions and 'co-operation' between the systems. Mu receptors are distributed widely in the brain and spinal cord, especially in areas associated with pain regulation and sensorimotor integration.[3] The existence of mu isoreceptors needs to be verified. Delta receptors are distributed less widely and are most densely located in areas involved with olfaction and motor integration.[2] Kappa receptors are located mainly in brain areas associated with pain perception (peri-aqueductal grey) and the regulation of water and food.[2] No epsilon receptors have been detected with any degree of certainty in any tissue except the rat vas deferens.[2]

The anatomical distribution of opioid receptors is being re-evaluated using molecular biological tools and immunohistochemical studies with antireceptor antibodies.[1] Opioid receptors are present in the peripheral terminals of primary afferent sensory fibres in the dorsal root ganglia and in the superficial layers of the dorsal horn of the spinal cord and in the brain.[1] Endogenous opioid peptides are released either tonically or following stimulus-evoked depolarization. They produce their physiological effects by binding to specific receptors close to the release site (enkephalins and dynorphins) and/or in remote locations (beta-endorphin).[1] They are inactivated in the extracelluar space by peptidases, which cleave biologically active peptides into inactive fragments. No endogenous opioid peptide-specific degrading enzymes have been described to date.[1] The better-characterized enzymes are those which participate in the inactivation of enkephalins, mainly metallopeptidases and aminopeptidase-N. Drugs that block these enzymes (e.g. RB101, a systemically active mixed peptidase inhibitor) have recently been developed. They would have important advantages over exogenously administered opioids, such as lack of tolerance and dependence.

The opioid receptors differ in their configuration, anatomical distribution and affinity for various opioid ligands. The different receptors do, however, differ in the type of pain they suppress as well as in several of their other functions.[1] Most of the ligands show a relative lack of specificity for an individual receptor type/subtype. The molecular characteristics of the opioid receptors (mu, delta and kappa) have been defined through cloning of their genes and DNA sequencing.[4] These receptors belong to the large family of seven transmembrane spanning receptors that signal through G proteins and apparently form an independent gene subfamily.[4] Studies of the relationships between the structures of the opioid receptors and their ligand binding properties will provide valuable information for the development of novel type-selective opioids agonists and antagonists with limited side-effects. Opioid receptor subtypes include mu$_1$ and mu$_2$, kappa$_1$, kappa$_2$ and kappa$_3$, and delta$_1$ and delta$_2$.[4] Future molecular biological studies will clarify whether these subtypes are attributable to different genes or different post-translational modifications. The molecular mechanism of desensitization will be elucidated by the use of cell lines established by transfection with the opioid receptor cDNA.[4] Receptor desensitization is considered to be a phenomenon involved in tolerance. The physiological significance of the opioid receptors will be studied by using 'knockout' mice, in which the opioid receptor gene is inactivated.[4]

Mechanisms of opioid action

There are three main mechanisms (Figure 3.2) thought to underlie opioid actions. First is a presynaptic action whereby opioid receptor activation reduces transmitter release from neurone terminals (tachykinins and excitatory amino acids).[5] This results from the opening of potassium channels (mu and delta receptors) or a closing of calcium channels (kappa), both of which lead to a reduction in calcium ion influx into C fibre terminals, thus diminishing transmitter release. The second mechanism is a postsynaptic hyperpolarization that affects the cell bodies of output neurones, interneu-

rones or dendrites and reduces the evoked activity in neuronal pathways (again via the opening of potassium channels or the closing of calcium channels). Third, there is a disinhibition in a circuit of two inhibitory neurones (via GABA$_A$-mediated disinhibition, or vice versa, of enkephalin neurones in the substantia gelatinosa), in which the second cell is held in check by the other inhibitory neurone. Inhibition of the first neurone by the opioid allows the second cell to become active, resulting in inhibition of activity.[5] Recent studies of cDNA expression systems using cultured cells and frogs' oocytes have shown that the activation of the mu receptor as well as the delta-receptor reduces neurotransmitter release by inhibition of the conotoxin-sensitive calcium channels.

Transmembrane signal transduction occurs by the sequential interaction of three membrane components: the recognition site (receptor), a pertussis-sensitive G protein and an effector system, which in the case of opioid receptors can be an enzyme (adenyl cyclase or phospholipase C) or an ion channel.[1] The agonist binds to the receptor and mobilizes the G protein.[4] The G protein incorporates an inorganic phosphate (GDP is transformed to GTP) and dissociates into subunits (alpha, beta and gamma). The alpha subunit activates the effector system, while the beta/gamma unit coordinates stimuli from different pathways.[1] The interaction of the G protein with the receptor determines the ligand affinity, while the duration of dissociation of the alpha from the beta/gamma subunits defines its efficacy. G proteins coupled to opioid receptors can alter the activity of enzymes that regulate the intracellular levels of cAMP and inositol 1,4,5-triphosphate (IP$_3$) and/or directly modify ion channel conductance.[1] Changes in intracellular levels of second messengers alter the phosphorylation of intracellular proteins, and short-term cellular responses occur. These modifications would explain the acute effects of opioids on membrane permeability. Altered protein phosphorylation also causes the induction of nuclear proteins (creb and fos-like transcription factors), which bind to specific DNA sequences in the promoter region of genes.[1] As a consequence, the rate of generation of these genes increases or decreases. Altered gene expression in target neurones could contribute to the addictive actions of opioids.[1]

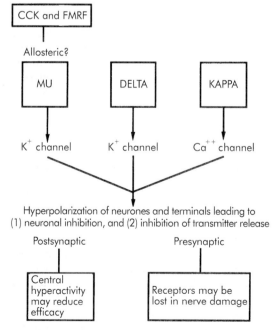

Figure 3.2 Opioid receptor subtypes and their effector mechanisms. CCK, cholecystokinin; FMRF, FMRFamide (Phe-Met-Arg-Phe-NH$_2$) – (a neuropeptide for opioid receptor subtypes); K$^+$, potassium ion; Ca^{++}, calcium ion.

Spinal analgesia

Recent studies on the spinal opioid systems have begun to address the extent of plasticity in opioid

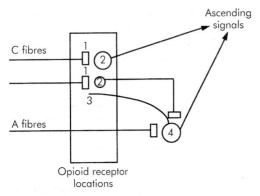

Opioid sites of action

1. Presynaptic block of transmitter release
2. Inhibition of neurones
3. Inhibition on dendrites
4. Postsynaptic inhibition – non-selective

Figure 3.3 Sites of opioid action in the spinal cord.

spinal function, with indications that opioid activity and function are not immutable even to the extent of activation of opioid peptide genes by particular stimuli.[5] Most opioid receptors are concentrated around the C fibre terminal zones in lamina 1 and the substantia gelatinosa (Figure 3.3).[3] Although species differences occur, opioid receptors in the rat spinal cord consist of 70 per cent mu, 24 per cent delta and 6 per cent kappa receptors.[3] The proportion of presynaptic sites in the spinal cord varies from 50 to 70 per cent for the subtypes based on drops in levels after rhizotomy.[5] More than 70 per cent of the total mu receptor sites are on the afferent terminal.[5] Mu and delta receptors appear to be coupled in that the activation of one receptor changes the affinity of the other.[2] Both mu and delta opioid receptors can modulate the input of nociceptive information in the dorsal horn. Delta receptors are less effective with visceral pain. Mu ligands include dermorphin and DAGOL (an enkephalin).[6,7] Opioids can, however, have facilitatory effects on C fibre transmission at low doses (which could explain the itching of the extremities following spinal morphine), while inhibition predominates at higher doses.[5]

Most mu and delta opioids have similar dose ranges after intrathecal application, but the most potent opioids are the mu ligands, presumably reflecting the many opioid sites in the spinal cord.[5] The intrathecal combination of a selective mu agonist (DAGOL) and a selective delta agonist (DPDPE) produces marked synergistic effects of the evoked activity of the WDR neurones.[8] The intrathecal application of a mu agonist (morphine) and the

delta agonist (DADLE) shows little evidence of cross-tolerance.[9] The spinal application of kelatorphan (a peptidase inhibitor) can be reversed by a selective delta antagonist. The inverse relationship between lipophilicity and potency is due to binding (in lipid-rich fibre tracts) or vascular redistribution.[3] Systemic potency ratios are thus poor predictors of spinal effectiveness.[10]

The antinociceptive effect of spinal kappa opioids is unclear. Dynorphin, the endogenous kappa agonist, has some effects that differ from those of typical opioid actions. It promotes the action of some neurones and inhibits other nociceptive neurones when applied spinally.[5] The analgesic activity of kappa agonists on kappa receptors may depend upon the intensity of the stimulus rather than its modality.[2,8] Certainly, all kappa agonists that have analgesic activity in man also have significant mu agonist activity. The facilitation of spinal opioid (morphine)-induced antinociception by local anaesthetics (bupivacaine) may be associated with a conformational change in the spinal opioid receptors induced by local anaesthetics.[11] All three subtypes of opioid receptor can interact to produce antinociceptive synergy.[12] However, the independent analgesic effects following the activation of non-mu receptors indicates that there is potential for opioid analgesics that are delta or kappa agonists.[5]

Non-opioid sigma receptors may be identical to the phenyl cyclohexylpiperidine (PCP) receptor. The PCP receptor appears to be coupled to the NMDA-L-glutamate receptor complex.[2,8] As discussed in Chapter 16, the NMDA receptor complex may be involved in sustaining or even magnifying pain transmission in the cord (wind-up).

Peripheral analgesia[13]

Human peripheral nerves have been found to contain endogenous opioid ligands (beta-endorphin and met-enkephalin) as well as opioid receptors.[14] Opioid receptors have been demonstrated on the peripheral terminals of thinly myelinated and unmyelinated sensory nerves in animals and humans. The opioid receptor messenger RNA has been detected in dorsal root ganglia.[15] These findings are in line with functional studies indicating that C fibre neurones mediate the peripheral antinociceptive effects of morphine.[15] Recent animal and human studies reveal that immune cells produce endogenous opioids during inflammation.[15] This production of opioids is matched by an increased expression of different opioid receptors on primary afferent nociceptors, where they can exert analgesic activity. Endogenous ligands of peripheral opioid receptors, opioid peptides (endorphin, enkephalin and dynorphin) and their respective mRNAs have been discovered in inflamed tissue.[15] These peptides can be produced by immune cells, including T- and B-lymphocytes, monocytes and macrophages. The injection of mu, delta and kappa selective agonists produces selective peripheral antinociceptive effects that can be blocked by the selective respective antagonists.[15] If the function of peptide-containing primary afferents is impaired with capsaicin, this enhancement of opioid responsiveness is lost.[16] Peripheral opioid mechanisms can also be activated by stress.[16] All three opioid receptor types can be functionally active in peripheral tissues.[5]

Following the agonistic occupation of neuronal opioid receptors, the excitability of the nociceptive input terminal or the propagation of action potentials is attenuated and the peripheral release of excitatory neuropeptides (e.g. substance P) is inhibited.[15] The increased efficacy of peripheral exogenous opioids administered during inflammation may be a result of perineural disruption, the activation of inactive neuronal opioid receptors and their upregulation.[15] The prolonged elevation of endogenous opioids may not lead to a downregulation of opioid receptors and tolerance.[15]

Opioids also act peripherally on sympathetic fibres.[15] These data suggest that both primary afferent nociceptors and sympathetic fibres could be targets for peripherally acting opioids, which would lack the central sedative and psychotropic effects (respiratory depression, nausea and dysphoria) of existing opioids, as well as avoiding the dependence problem.[15,16] Such drugs would affect neither the motor nor autonomic systems (unlike local anaesthetics), and they would not have NSAID-like effects (gastrointestinal irritation, bleeding, and kidney or liver damage).[15] Opioids (fentanyl) injected at very low doses into the rat brachial plexus sheath give rise to a localized, potent and prolonged antinociceptive effect, which is naloxone reversible.[17] Opioids (fentanyl and pethidine) can block peripheral conduction.[18,19] A growing number of controlled clinical studies examining the local analgesic effects of opioids is emerging, the majority of which support the efficacy of locally applied opioids.[15] A wide variety of regional analgesic techniques could be enhanced by using exogenous opioids to bind to endogenous peripheral nerve opioid receptors.[15] In humans, local injections of opioids have been tried to exploit their peripheral sites of action, for example treating pain after arthroscopic knee procedures by the intra-articular injection of morphine.[20] These studies have examined perineural, interpleural, regional intravenous or intra-articular opioid application (mostly using morphine in the postoperative setting).[21] They show prolonged regional analgesia after giving opioids (morphine, fentanyl or buprenorphine) combined with local anaesthetics.[22] It is also plausible that opioids will prove more effective when applied near peripheral terminals of nerves at sites of injury rather than along the nerve trunk at a distance from the central or proximal terminals.[23] Trials of better methodological quality are needed to provide stronger evidence for clinical utility.

Several laboratories have recently developed various opioid compounds that do not cross the blood–brain barrier; some of these are already showing promising results in preclinical testing.[15] For example, a kappa agonist, GR-94839, with limited brain penetration has been found to be antinociceptive in the rat model in the presence of inflammation only.[16] Clinically, peripheral opioid effects may prove advantageous in inflammatory pain (e.g. postoperative pain, cancer, arthritis, trauma and burns).[5,15] The local activation of these intrinsic antinociceptive substances will open new vistas in research.

Using a similar rationale, methylnaltrexone, a quaternized derivative of the opioid antagonist naltrexone, has been administered systemically to block opioid-induced ileus, urinary retention, pruritus and nausea.[23] Animal studies confirm that nausea and ileus are antagonized without a reduction in opioid analgesia.[23] Human studies are in progress.

Supraspinal analgesia

Supraspinal sites of opioid analgesia are now well established and have been localized to areas in the medial brain stem around the nucleus raphe magnus, extending rostrally to the peri-aqueductal and periventricular grey areas.[5] Particularly dense opioid receptor binding is observed in limbic structures, thalamic nuclei and neural areas that control visceral function.[1] Mu, kappa, and delta receptors elicit supraspinal analgesia.[3] The mechanisms of action of opioids at supraspinal levels, in particular how they interact with descending inhibitory controls, are still unclear.[5] It is thought that supraspinal opioids might alter the unpleasant nature of the pain, modulate nociception from the cord by activating descending control systems or interfere with descending controls (which are turned off by noxious stimuli), thus allowing nociception to occur.[3] Nociception might also be modulated by opioids at the thalamic and sensory cortical levels. The simplest situation is that supraspinal opioids increase descending inhibitory influences, these in turn blocking spinal transmission. This is demonstrated by intraventricular morphine reducing the spinal induction of C-fos (a marker of noxious evoked activity).[5] Other findings, however, do not show this direction of effect.[5] Diffuse noxious inhibitory controls are descending controls induced by heterosegmental noxious stimulation, involving both opioid and serotonergic mechanisms.[5] Morphine reduces these descending controls. The multiplicity of the descending controls (in terms of their locations, pharmacology and spinal projections) forms a framework within which the various directions of effect of opioids can be incorporated.[5] The direct spinal actions of opioids in blocking the spinal transmission of pain would prevent the initial activation of diffuse noxious inhibitory controls and reduce segmental excitations and descending controls.[5]

Supraspinal opioids produce behavioural analgesia. Opioids modulate transmitters involved in other non-nociceptive functions. Respiratory depression, nausea and vomiting may be mediated via opioid receptors in the area of the solitary tract.[3] Dependence may be related to receptor sites in the locus coeruleus and ventral tegmental areas.[3] Delta- and kappa-mediated analgesia is less associated with respiratory depression, dependence and tolerance than is mu-mediated analgesia.[8,10]

The molecular neurobiology of the endogenous opioid peptides could facilitate enzyme modification of the maturation/degradation of active peptides, the development of analgesic receptor-specific opioids, the characterization of receptor type/subtype physiological effects, the manipulation of transmembrane signalling and the study of the molecular basis of tolerance and addiction.[1]

CLINICAL PHARMACOLOGY

Opioids are often prescribed incorrectly because of the fear of respiratory depression and addiction. Pain acts as a physiological antagonist of the CNS depressant effects (e.g. respiratory depression) of opioids and may also antagonize other side-effects (e.g. nausea and vomiting).[24] In opioid-responsive pain, opioids need to be titrated (i.e. used in appropriate doses) against pain for minimal respiratory depression or tolerance.[25] If pain is relieved by some other means (e.g. nerve block), opioid dosage should be reduced (by 75 per cent) to avoid respiratory depression. It thus follows that opioid-induced respiratory depression (or tolerance) may occur if inappropriately high doses are used, if opioids are used for indications other than analgesia or if they are used for opioid-(relatively) non-responsive pain.[25,26] The use of neuraxial opioids is discussed in Chapter 9. Combinations of opioids with other drugs (e.g. local anaesthetics, α_2-adrenergic agonists, NMDA receptor antagonists and NSAIDs) are dealt with in Chapter 16.

General characteristics

With opioids, a kinetic and dynamic variability can occur which can be as great as five-fold for a seemingly similar group of patients.[27] Variability can even occur within the same patient in different conditions. The opioid concentration required to achieve a given degree of effect is influenced by a number of dynamic variables, for example opioid tolerance, drug interaction, ageing, disease states and probably a large number of other factors.[27] Also, opioid requirements vary for different types and intensities of noxious stimulation. It has been suggested that genetic factors may be an important determinant of opioid response.[28] The challenge is to titrate dose to the individual patient's needs and, in reality, 'to listen to those on the receiving end'.[29]

Opioids from the same pharmacological class (i.e. mu agonists) have quantitatively different effect profiles that can be explained by differences in their physicochemical properties and kinetics.[29] When opioids are compared at plasma concentrations producing equianalgesia, none causes significantly less respiratory depression or less intensive subjective side-effects.[29]

Opioids are still the most commonly used analgesics for postoperative pain. Intravenous opioids should be front-loaded to achieve the minimum effective analgesic concentration in a reasonable time period. In the acute intraoperative situation, opioids can be used intermittently, titrated manually (a loading dose plus a continuous infusion) or given by computer control of infusion pumps (programmed with average kinetic data for the patient population).[27] Alfentanil, fentanyl and sufentanil are the opioids most widely used to supplement general anaesthesia or be given as primary anaesthetic agents in very high doses (e.g. during cardiac surgery).[30]

In acute pain, opioids should be administered when required, titrating to an effective dose size and interval. In chronic pain, the effective dose size and interval are again first established. Doses are then given 'by the clock' to prevent the pain returning.[25] Generalizations about opioid-responsiveness should not be based on the effects of a single drug.[28]

Classification

The opioid analgesics are the major class of drugs used in the management of pain of moderate or greater severity. This remains true irrespective of the pathophysiological mechanism underlying the pain.[31] Structurally, opioids may be divided into the morphinans (e.g. morphine), the 4-phenylpiperidines (e.g. pethidine and fentanyl), and the 3,3-diphenylpropylamines (e.g. methadone and dextropropoxyphene), and opioids with ester linkages (e.g. remifentanil).[32]

Based on their interactions with the various receptor subtypes, the opioids can be divided into agonist and agonist–antagonist classes. The pure agonist drugs are most commonly used and recommended. Their major advantage is that they have no clinically relevant ceiling effect to their analgesia. As the dose is raised, their analgesic effects increase in a log-linear function until either analgesia is achieved or dose-limiting side-effects (e.g. confusion, sedation, nausea, vomiting or respiratory depression) supervene.[31] Codeine, dextropropoxyphene, hydromorphone and oxycodone are low-efficacy opioid agonists. High-efficacy opioid agonists include morphine, pethidine, papaveretum, methadone, fentanyl, alfentanil, sufentanil and remifentanil (see Chapter 16), phenazocine, dextramoramide, levorphanol and diamorphine.[33]

Partial agonists and mixed agonists–antagonists are classified according to their action on opioid receptor types. Partial agonists are less effective at a specific opioid receptor type than is a full agonist. Mixed agonist–antagonists have both agonistic activity (complete or incomplete) at different receptor type(s) and antagonistic activity at others. Pentazocine, butorphanol and nalbuphine (nalorphine-like) have an agonistic action on the kappa receptor.[34] Each of them has an affinity for, but not efficacy at, the mu receptor. Buprenorphine, dezocine and meptazinol have partial agonistic activity (morphine-like) at the mu receptor.[26] Buprenorphine has an extremely high affinity for and relatively low efficacy at mu receptors.[34]

Dezocine is slightly more potent than morphine when used for postoperative pain.[35] The subjective effects of mu partial agonists are morphine-like throughout their dose range.[34]

The mixed agonists–antagonists have a much higher incidence of psychotomimetic reactions such as dysphoria and hallucinations.[26] These are thought to be mediated by the non-opioid sigma receptors and can restrict the use of some of these agents in chronic pain. These drugs do, however, have a lower dependence liability and a lower abuse potential than pure agonists.[34] This may result in more relaxed inventory controls, an advantage in their use for patient-controlled analgesia (PCA). Tolerance and physical dependence can occur with mixed agonists–antagonists, but the withdrawal syndrome is usually brief.[34]

A ceiling effect occurs on their efficacy. However, this appears to be clinically restrictive only for nalbuphine as the ceiling effect for the others occurs outside the clinical dose range.[36] The ceiling effect for nalbuphine is equivalent to 30 mg morphine.[36] They have, however, been shown to be sufficient for the treatment of postoperative pain, labour pain and renal colic, and as part of a balanced anaesthetic technique.[34] They have been given intramuscularly, orally, sublingually, intranasally and intravenously (by bolus or continuous infusion), and used in PCA.[34] Several have been used successfully via the spinal route (e.g. epidural butorphanol for caesarean sections). Mixed agonists–antagonists have been shown to be useful adjuncts (both intravenously and epidurally) to lessen or eliminate undesirable side-effects (pruritus, nausea and respiratory depression) from the administration of pure mu agonists.[37]

A ceiling effect for respiratory depression (equivalent to 20–30 mg morphine) has also been demonstrated.[25] Respiratory depression after 2–4 mg butorphanol is equivalent to that produced by 10 mg morphine.[34] Respiratory depression reaches a maximum after approximately 30 mg nalbuphine.[36] This should (in theory) make these drugs safer in the overdose situation.

The mixed agonists–antagonists have been shown to produce less spasm of the gastrointestinal tract smooth muscle and less of a rise in intrabiliary pressure than the agonists, and there should (in theory) be a ceiling effect to constipation.[25,34]

Some of the mixed agonist–antagonists (pentazocine and butorphanol) can, in high doses, increase myocardial oxygen consumption by increasing heart rate, systolic and pulmonary arterial pressure and cardiac work.[38,39] The antagonistic effects of these drugs can be used to antagonize other pure mu agonists. This interaction has not been a problem in the acute clinical situation (where combinations may give additive analgesia) but only after chronic exposure or in opioid-dependent individuals.[25,34]

To summarize, the mixed agonist–antagonists have good safety profiles. Life-threatening respiratory depression is uncommon, and minor toxic effects such as nausea, constipation and urinary retention occur less frequently than with morphine.[34] The mixed agonist-antagonist opioids and the partial agonists have limited utility, however, because of a ceiling effect for analgesia, the precipitation of withdrawal in patients physically dependent on opioid agonists and a high prevalence of dose-dependent psychomimetic side-effects (pentazocine and butorphanol).[31] The use of the opioid antagonists (naloxone, naltrexone and nalmephene) is discussed in Chapter 6.

Morphine is the parent molecule of the morphinans, with an oral and rectal bio-availability of about 25 per cent.[32] Conjugate metabolism with glucuronic acid occurs in the liver, giving rise to the metabolites morphine-6-glucuronide and morphine-3-glucuronide, which are excreted in the urine and accumulate with renal damage.[32] If one is titrating dose to effect, this will not matter as less morphine will be needed.[40] Accumulation can be a problem with unconscious intensive care patients on fixed dose schedules with inadequate renal function.[40] Normorphine can be produced via demethylation. Morphine-6-gluceronide is an active metabolite (of morphine, codeine and diamorphine) with a greater potency than that of morphine.[32] Morphine-3-glucuronide may have an antagonistic-like effect.[32] Recently, intrathecal morphine-6 glucuronide has been found to have greater analgesic activity than intrathecal morphine in man.[41] It persists in the cerebral spinal fluid (CS), which may make it useful as an intrathecal analgesic where prolonged pain relief is required. Intrathecal morphine-6-glucuronide 100 µg and 150 µg have been shown to give excellent analgesia following total hip replacement.[42]

Codeine (3-methoxy morphine) undergoes hepatic metabolism by glucuronidation, N-demethylation (norcodeine) and O-demethylation (about 10 per cent to morphine via the CYP2D6 enzyme, absent in about 7 per cent of Caucasians).[32] It is often formulated in combinations with aspirin or paracetamol. Dihydrocodeine is a synthetic opioid with a structure and pharmacodynamics similar to those of codeine.[40] In postoperative pain, it is less

effective than other analgesics when administered as a single oral dose.[40] Multiple doses may improve its analgesic efficacy but increase the number of side-effects.[40] Controlled-release codeine has been shown to be an effective oral analgesic for the continuous suppression of pain in patients with chronic non-malignant pain.[43] The 12-hour analgesic duration provided patients with enhanced quality of life outcomes and increased control over their pain management.

Dextropropoxyphene is an opioid used alone or in combination with paracetamol. For a single dose of dextropropoxyphene 65 mg in postoperative pain, the NNT for at least 50 per cent pain relief is 7.7 when compared with placebo over 4–6 hours.[38] Pooled data show increased CNS effects of the combination with paracetamol compared with placebo.[44]

Diamorphine (3,6-diacetyl morphine) is rapidly cleared mainly in the liver to 6-monoacetyl morphine, a potent metabolite.[32] Hydromorphone is about six times more potent than morphine, with a greater bio-availability than but similar duration to that of morphine.[32] It is mainly excreted as the 3-glucuronide.[32] Controlled-release hydromorphone has a 12-hour analgesic duration and has been successfully used orally for the relief of severe pain.[45]

Pethidine (merperidine) has an oral bio-availability of about 50 per cent and is hydrolysed to inactive compounds and demethylated to norpethidine, which can accumulate in multiple doses (so multiple dosing is contraindicated), especially with compromised renal functions.[32,40] This can act as a CNS irritant and cause convulsions.[40] Its duration of action is 2–3 hours.[32] It has an anticholinergic effect yet is no better than other opioids at dealing with colicky pain.[40] It may be used neuraxially for its local anaesthetic (membrane-stabilizing) effects.

Methadone has a high oral bio-availability, albeit with a long elimination half-life (20–45 hours), a longer time to reach steady state (up to 10 days) and the potential for significant accumulation.[32] An initial therapy of 10 mg at 0, 6, 12 and 24 hours, followed by 10 mg on day 3 has been recommended.[32] It is used in drug rehabilitation and in cancer pain.[32]

The 4-phenylpiperidines, in order of increasing potency and lipid solubility, are fentanyl, alfentanil and sufentanil.[32] Fentanyl has a high hepatic clearance (so is not given orally) and is metabolized to inactive metabolites (via dealkylation to norfentanyl) that are excreted in the urine.[32] It is used intravenously (as intermittent boluses or a continuous infusion), in PCA (intravenously or subcutaneously) and in transdermal patches, where the amount released is proportional to the surface area.[46] Delayed-release preparations (transdermal or oral) should not be used in acute pain as delayed onset and offset are dangerous in this context.[40] In cancer pain, fentanyl patches may effectively substitute morphine-causing side-effects.[32] A new short-acting opioid in this group is remifentanil (see Chapter 16).

Tramadol hydrochloride is among the atypical opioids. It is a unique, centrally acting opioid analgesic with an analgesic efficacy and potency comparable to those of pentazocine or pethidine.[47,48] It can also be given orally. Tramadol has been used to treat postoperative pain. Although it is a weak agonist at all types of opioid receptors (with some selectivity for mu receptors), it causes the *in vitro* inhibition of noradrenaline uptake and the stimulation of serotonin release.[48,49] Its L-isomer is more active at the opioid receptors and its D-isomer at other sites.[48] Each component independently contributes to the overall analgesic activity, in concert thus resulting in a significant reduction in the side-effect profile typically associated with opioids.[47] Tramadol has not been associated with clinically significant side-effects such as respiratory depression, constipation or sedation. Tolerance and psychological dependence have not been a problem in the long term,[47] so it is not a controlled drug in most countries. The unique composition of this agent will promote further research in this area. Several formulations are available. The racemate seems to have superior efficacy and safety when compared with either enantiomer (L or D).[50]

The oral bio-availability is 70 per cent following single doses and 90 per cent in multiple dose studies.[51,52]Adverse effects can best be prevented by commencing therapy at 50 mg three times daily and gradually increasing the dose until analgesia is achieved. Oral administration is comparable to intramuscular injection both in the time taken to reach both onset of analgesia and peak plasma level. Given intravenously, tramadol will produce analgesia in doses ranging from 50 to 400 mg. With a loading dose of 200 mg and incremental doses of 20 mg, its use in PCA regimens has been effective in acute pain.[51,52] Its intravenous use has recently been compared with that of epidural morphine for immediate post thoracotomy pain.[53] In postoperative pain, tramadol 50, 100 and 150 mg had NNTs for at least 50 per cent total pain relief of 7.3, 4.8 and 2.4, respectively, comparable to aspirin 650 mg plus codeine 60 mg, and paracetamol 650 mg plus propoxyphene 100 mg.[54] Tramadol shows a dose–response for analgesia in both postoperative and dental pain patients.[54] Its advantages over traditional opioids are the lack of tolerance and addiction, and minimal respiratory depression.[32] It may cause vomiting, sedation, dry mouth and headache in a dose-related fashion.[32,54]

Kapanol is a pellitized sustained-release capsule with a profile that is superior to that of MST Continus® (slow-release morphine sulphate), resulting in a flat plasma morphine concentration–time profile, which allows it to be administered at 12-hourly intervals.[55,56] A new sustained-release morphine suppository has recently been tested, showing efficacy and safety profiles equivalent to those of the morphine sustained-release tablets.[57] It provided 12 hours of pain relief. A lipid-based, injectable drug delivery system has been developed for the epidural sustained-release of morphine (DTC401).[58] As a single epidural injection, it significantly prolonged the duration of analgesia when compared with epidural morphine.

Opioid tolerance

The development of tolerance to opioid analgesia is manifest as a shift to the right of the dose–response curve, or as a decrease in the intensity of the response when a constant dose is repetitively administered.[59] The possibility of rapid dose escalation for pain control is one of the major fears surrounding opioid prescription, regardless of the nature of the pain. At least three factors may be operating simultaneously to cause dose escalation. There may be an increase in the nociceptor stimulus, changes in the receptors or alterations in opioid pharmacokinetics by either self-induction or drug administration, resulting in enhanced elimination.[60] In cancer pain, dose escalation is predominantly the consequence of a continual increase in nociceptive stimulus. However, in chronic non-terminal pain states, a continual increase in the nociceptive focus is less probable. Changes in receptor association dynamics and pharmacokinetic considerations have a greater influence.[60]

Preclinical pharmacological studies show no opioid receptor reduction on the target neurones, or any change in their affinity, when tolerance occurs.[16] Cell surface receptors may become uncoupled from the intracellular mechanisms (responsible for the increase in potassium ion conductance, etc.).[16] The translocation and activation of protein kinase C may be a critical step in the development of tolerance.[61] Chronic exposure to opioids (like chronic exposure to noxious stimulation) results in long-term changes in the CNS.[62,63] Tolerance to morphine in rodents can be blocked by the NMDA receptor antagonists MK-801 and LY-274614, and the oral antitussive dextromethorphan, or by the inhibition of nitric oxide synthetase, as well as being attenuated by the use of cholecystokinin antagonists and dynorphin.[16,59,63] In hyperalgesia, similar excitatory amino acid receptor-mediated and intracellular mechanism changes have now been implicated, as for opioid tolerance.[64] In the rat model, there is now evidence to support the putative role of the morphine metabolite morphine-3-glucuronide in the development of tolerance to the antinociceptive effects of morphine.[65] Lack of opioid efficacy after chronic use may be caused not only by changes secondary to opioid use, but also by the fact that these changes are exacerbated by the inputs associated with the pain itself.[62]

Analgesic tolerance appears to be a rare limiting factor during opioid pharmacotherapy.[63] Tolerance to most adverse effects is anticipated and welcomed, increasing a favourable balance between analgesia and side-effects. Escalating pain in a patient previously receiving a stable opioid dose should never be attributed to tolerance but be evaluated for progressive disease.[63] Any patient on opioids must be provided with an ongoing titration designed to identify the optimal balance between analgesia and side-effects. Controlled clinical studies are needed to address opioid tolerance and responsiveness.

Opioid dependence

Psychological dependence is hardly ever seen after pain relief with opioids, although physical withdrawal may occur if the dose is suddenly reduced.[26] In mice, pretreatment with pertussis toxin will reduce the incidence of withdrawal signs in animals given chronic high-dose morphine, reinforcing the idea that the development of physical dependence may involve pertussis-sensitive G proteins.[16] It is thus important to withdraw patients from opioid medication of any considerable duration in a gradual manner. Withdrawal can be demonstrated in isolated tissues and even on single neurones.[16] Dependence, however, is a combination of the abortion of withdrawal, a psychological preference for the drug-induced state and circumstance.[16] Many individuals can take opioids for long periods of time without becoming clinically dependent, whereas others rapidly become so.[16] It may be possible to avoid some of the clinical dependence problems associated with the use of mu opioids by using selective ligands for the other receptor subtypes.[16]

Addiction is a behavioural pattern of drug use characterized by compulsive self-administration on a continuous or periodic basis in order to experience the drug's psychic effects or to avoid the discomfort associated with its absence.[32] Supplies are usually obtained by deceptive or illegal means. Addiction is extremely rare in cancer patients with no history of drug abuse,[32] and is not a problem with opioid use in acute pain.[40]

Opioids in non-malignant pain

Over 130 countries have enacted legislation consistent with the aims of the Single Convention, which requires controls on the production, distribution and illicit consumption of opioid drugs.[60] The Single Convention also established the International Narcotics Control Board, one of whose functions is to record statistics for the amount of opioids consumed for licit purposes.[60] The use of opioid analgesics can increase significantly without increases in opioid diversion and abuse if reasonable controls are exercised during drug distribution.[66] If diversion occurs, the answer is to stop those responsible for the diversion rather than to limit the necessary supply or opioid distribution to patients. Recently, the treatment of various non-malignant chronic pain syndromes with opioids has been proposed based on an accumulation of case reports and uncontrolled open studies.[67] The only consensus is that opioid tolerance, physical dependence or addiction seldom causes difficulties. These studies suggest that opioids may be effective in nociceptive pain and in some types of neuropathic pain, but not in idiopathic pain.[67] However, in all of these trials, opioids were given only over short periods of time, limiting the conclusions that may be drawn therefrom. There is only one placebo-controlled study investigating long-term opioid use in chronic non-malignant pain (that of soft tissue or musculoskeletal origin, using morphine).[68] The authors concluded that morphine may confer analgesic benefit with a low risk of addiction but is unlikely to yield psychological or functional improvement.[68] Therefore, the long-term prescription of opioids is likely to be most beneficial to patients with a predominantly nociceptive element to their pain, although patients with neuropathic pain or a combination of both types also benefit.[60] These latter patients should not be excluded from a trial of opioid therapy provided that the general conditions (see below) are met.

A major problem concerns the poor knowledge

base relating to the neurochemical basis of drug dependence and addiction. Drug addiction is a chronic disorder characterized by the compulsive use of a substance resulting in physical, psychological or social harm to the user and continued use despite that harm. Psychological dependence is the emotional state of craving of a drug either for its positive effects or to avoid the negative effects associated with abstinence. Physical dependence is a physiological state of adaption to a drug, usually characterized by the development of tolerance to drug effects and the emergence of a withdrawal syndrome during prolonged abstinence or the administration of an antagonist. Cancer patients can exhibit physical but not psychological opioid dependence.[16] However, in chronic pain patients, it is conceded that a greater proportion of patients will display addiction in addition to physical dependence.[16] Therefore, the use of opioids to treat severe pain associated with non-terminal disease should not be considered as a first-line treatment.[60] These patients should undergo a full assessment of the physical, psychological and socioeconomic components of the pain complaint in a multidisciplinary pain relief unit and all non-invasive treatments should be given a reasonable trial.[33] The pain must be opioid sensitive; it must have a major effect on the quality of life of the patient; medical confirmation of the diagnosis must have been obtained; a full explanation to and agreement from the patient must be obtained; and the patient's general practitioner must be agreeable. The lowest clinically effective opioid dose should be used.[69] The concurrent use of non-opioid analgesics may allow lower opioid usage.[69] Patients with predominantly nociceptive pain can be considered for long-term opioid therapy if the psychological assessment reveals no drug-seeking behaviour in an otherwise psychologically stable patient.[60] The drug, dose route of administration and possible drug delivery devices can then be considered. Guidelines covering the conditions under which opioids will be prescribed, ongoing assessments, goals of therapy and frequency of therapeutic drug monitoring will require detailed attention. Some physicians consider that patients with neuropathic pain should not be considered for long-term opioid administration.[60] If agreed goals are not being met, physicians must be prepared to terminate the agreement. In this case, the opioid dose should be tapered to reduce the possibility of an abstinence syndrome.

The treatment goals are a reduction in the severity of symptoms, suffering and environmental reinforcers of pain behaviour, as well as functional improvement, a decreased dependency on the health care system and a return to work.[67] Analgesics are only part of this treatment, which includes graduated exercise programmes, the encouragement of activity and cognitive, behavioural and/or supportive measures to provide functional restoration despite continuing pain.[67]

The diagnosis of patients usually maintained on long-term opioids is most frequently back and neck pain, but chronic pancreatitis, renal colic and haematuria loin pain syndrome are not infrequently represented.[60] The preferred route of administration is orally. Mu receptor agonists (morphine, methadone, hydromorphone and fentanyl and its derivatives for spinal administration) should be selected in preference to weak opioids that are only effective against pain of low severity and have no advantages in terms of their side-effect profile.[60] Morphine is probably considered to be the opioid drug of choice. Oral methadone is a viable alternative because of its long terminal half-life, providing prolonged analgesia.[60] Neuropathic pain and severe pain on movement and weight-bearing can be effectively treated by the neuraxial administration of local anaesthetic (lignocaine or bupivacaine) and opioid (morphine or fentanyl).[60] With morphine, the position of the catheter tip is relatively unimportant, assuming greater importance if fentanyl is used and being critical to the success of the procedure if local anaesthetics are used in the combination. The nature of the drug delivery system (repeated bolus doses versus infusion) will be dictated by the type of opioid used. Transdermal therapeutic systems (e.g. TTS-fentanyl) are presently undergoing evaluation in the chronic non-cancer pain group (Pain Relief and Research Unit, Hillbrow Hospital, University of the Witwatersrand, South Africa). A legitimate cause for concern would be the possible diversion, for illicit purposes, of the remaining amount of fentanyl in used patches by some patients in the chronic pain group.[60] The American and New Zealand Pain Societies have published guidelines.[1,60] Rheumatologists and general practitioners are more likely to prescribe long-term opioids than are surgeons, neurologists or psychiatrists.[70] Until more randomized controlled studies are undertaken, the efficacy of opioids in chronic non-malignant pain will remain scientifically unproven.

Opioid poorly responsive pain

This is discussed at length in Chapter 1. It can be defined 'as pain inadequately relieved by opioids in a dose which causes intolerable side-effects (despite controlling measures)'.[24] The most common causes are neuropathic pain (pain initiated or caused by a primary lesion or dysfunction of the nervous system), usually from nerve compression or destruction.[36] Other causes in the cancer pain patient include incident bone pain, bladder and rectal tenesmus, perineal and pancreatic pain and superficial ulcer pain.[24,71] A variety of alternative strategies is required for these difficult pain problems, inflammatory pains often being accompanied by an increased sensitivity to opioids.[5]

A loss of opioid receptors (e.g. as seen after nerve section) can contribute to a reduction in opioid sensitivity.[5] The exogenous application of the non-opioid peptides FLFQPQRFamide and CCK, either spinally or supraspinally, acts as a negative influence on opioid actions.[5] Levels of CCK in the cord can determine the potency of morphine. The NMDA receptor is a strong candidate for the generation of hyperalgesic states in inflammatory, neuropathic and ischaemic pain models, with a reduction in opioid effect.[5] There are no opioid receptors on the central terminals of the A fibres. Pain transmission can, however, occur via these normally innocu-ous fibres as a result of pathological changes in the peripheral and/or central processes.[5]

The morphine metabolite morphine-3-glucuronide has no affinity for the mu receptor and, being unable to bind to the receptor, has no opioid actions.[5] In the rat, it has only a minor effect on the spinal antinociceptive actions of morphine.[72] Nevertheless, it contributes to reduced opioid sensitivity.[5] Its role in opioid poorly responsive pain remains to be determined.

Metabolism

Levorphanol and methadone have a higher bio-availability than morphine but probably few other advantages.[16] Pethidine gives rise to the toxic metabolite norpethidine. A decrease in the renal clearance and elimination rate of norpethidine results in metabolite accumulation and toxicity.[73] This argues against its chronic use, although it can be given both orally and parenterally. Diamorphine is rapidly metabolized into the active 6-monoacetyl morphine, morphine and morphine-6-glucuronide (Figure 3.4).[25]

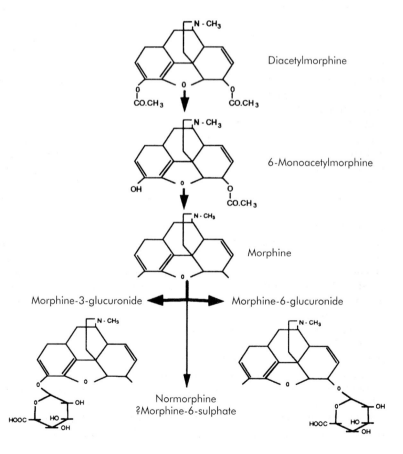

Figure 3.4 Diamorphine, morphine and metabolites.

During chronic oral morphine therapy, plasma concentrations of morphine-3-glucuronide and morphine-6-glucuronide markedly exceed those of morphine itself since hepatic metabolism converts approximately 70 per cent of the morphine into morphine-3-glucuronide (55 per cent) and morphine-6-glucuronide (15 per cent).[74] Morphine-6-glucuronide is the active metabolite of morphine that is clinically important. It has an avid affinity for the mu receptors, to which it binds stereospecifically with an affinity similar to that of morphine, exerting a potent analgesic effect.[41,73] In rats, morphine-6-glucuronide has a greater analgesic effect than morphine on both subcutaneous (3.7 times) and intracerebral (45 times) injection.[75] It also has double the duration of action of morphine and an LD_{50}/ED_{50} ratio three times that of morphine.[75] In man, intrathecal morphine-6-glucuronide has approximately double the potency of intrathecal morphine,[75] its systemic analgesic potency being 2.5–10 times that of morphine.[75] Its volume of distribution is small (less than 0.5 L/kg), and its clearance rate is low.[41] In a person with normal renal function, its elimination half-life is approximately 2 hours.[76] Morphine-6-glucuronide seems to have fewer respiratory depressant effects than morphine.[41] The morphine-6-glucuronide-to-morphine ratio is higher with oral than with parenteral administration (4–9 : 1).[73] The difference in analgesic effect between single and repeated oral doses of morphine is the result of the contribution made by morphine-6-glucuronide.[77] With severely reduced renal function, the clinical effects and duration of codeine, dihydrocodeine and morphine are increased.[25] This is thought to be caused by morphine-6-glucuronide. Its elimination half-life is prolonged in patients with impaired renal function,[41] which may produce toxicity in these patients, particularly in relation to respiratory depression.[73] The dose should thus be titrated to effect and reduced if the creatinine clearance falls below 30 mL per 24 hours.[25] However, an elevated morphine-6-glucuronide and morphine-6-glucuronide-to-morphine ratio do not independently determine morphine-related adverse effects in patients receiving repeated doses of morphine.[78] The antinociceptive effect of morphine-6-glucuronide may be antagonized by morphine-3-glucuronide.[79] After the oral administration of slow-release morphine, there is significant passage of morphine-3-glucuronide and morphine-6-glucuronide into the CSF in the concentration range at which they may have an influence on analgesia.[74]

With morphine in liver disease, glucuronidation is spared in cirrhosis.[80] However, in severe liver disease, there is a high level of oral bio-availability, lower plasma clearance and a long elimination half-life.[80]

Side-effects

The most common side-effects exhibited by opioids are nausea, vomiting, constipation and drowsiness. Others include pruritus, urinary retention, respiratory depression, tolerance and dependence.[81] If one agonist does not work for a patient, or if its side-effects are troublesome, other agonists can be tried. Often the patient does not develop the same side-effects when taking other agents, or a more favourable balance between analgesia and side-effects can be obtained.[41] Other ways of managing side-effects include dose reduction of the opioid and changing the route of administration (e.g. from oral to epidural).[81] Nausea and vomiting occur in 50–66 per cent of patients taking oral morphine.[71] They are easy to control and, in many patients, resolve with continued use. In a recent study, subcutaneous fentanyl was successfully used in cancer pain patients who were intolerant of the intractable side-effects of subcutaneous morphine.[82]

Constipation is the most common adverse effect encountered during chronic opioid therapy.[31] It is almost invariable with morphine and should be treated prophylactically using the combination of a stool softener (danthron or docusate) and a peristaltic stimulant (senna, bicosodyl or phenolphthalein). An osmotic laxative (lactulose or magnesium sulphate) can be added if necessary.[71] Rarely, oral naloxone (0.8–1.2 mg once or twice daily), acting selectively on gut opioid receptors, is used, providing there is no bowel obstruction.[31]

Opioids may produce nausea through medullary chemoreceptor trigger zone stimulation, enhanced vestibular sensitivity and increased gastric antral tone.[31] If associated with early satiety, bloating or postprandial vomiting (delayed gastric emptying), metoclopromide or cisapride is used. Patients with movement-induced nausea or vertigo are treated with scopolamine or meclizine.[31] With no signs of gastroparesis or vestibular dysfunction, treatment is started with a dopamine antagonist (prochlorperazine or metoclopromide). Other options include an alternative opioid, an antihistamine (diphenhyramine or hydroxycine), alternative neuroleptics (haloperidol, chlorpromazine and droperidol), dexamethasone or serotonin antagonists (ondansetron and tropisetron).[31]

Day-time drowsiness, dizziness or mental clouding commonly occurs at the start of treatment but usually resolves within a few days. Psychomotor skills (driving skills) are not significantly impaired in cancer patients receiving chronic morphine therapy after the initial period of drowsiness and sedation.[71] Somnolence and cognitive failure are common in far-advanced cancer and AIDS.[31] Elderly patients may develop hallucinations and confusion with morphine. Morphine is most likely to produce central adverse effects (sedation, confusion and respiratory depression) when pain is absent.[71] Respiratory depression is uncommon when the opioid dose is carefully titrated.[31] If significant, it is accompanied by other signs of CNS depression (somnolence, mental clouding and bradypnoea). Naloxone should be withheld if the patient is arousable and the T_{max} (the time taken for the drug to reach maximal concentration in the plasma) has been reached. Unarousable patients with severe respiratory depression should be given dilute naloxone (0.4 mg in 10 mL saline) titrated against the respiratory rate. Long half-life opioids (slow-release morphine, TTS-fentanyl and methadone) may require a naloxone infusion.[31] Opioids cause vasodilatation, which may result in the development of orthostatic hypotension and syncope.[69]

Myoclonus is dose related (especially with pethidine) and is treated by dose reduction, alternative opioids, clonazepam, dantrolene or valproate.[31] Opioid-induced urinary retention is infrequent but is usually observed in elderly males. Tolerance develops rapidly, and catheterization is occasionally necessary. Pruritus with epidural opioids in general, but morphine in particular, is frequently seen after the initiation of therapy but usually subsides within a short period.[60] The medullary 'scratch centre' is likely to be the medullary dorsal horn located close to the bottom of the fourth ventricle.[83] Sub-hypnotic doses of propofol (10 mg) have recently been found to relieve opioid-induced pruritus.[84] Data from the methadone maintenance programme showed a significant incidence of sexual dysfunction with long-term opioid therapy.[60] Altered prolactin secretion results in gynaecomastia in some male patients.

Direct organ toxicity is not a major problem associated with long-term opioid administration, an exception being pethidine-associated neurotoxicity (from norpethidine) with repeated doses, particularly in patients with renal insufficiency.[60] Cases of severe CNS toxicity have been reported with high-dose hydromorphone.[85] Enhanced methadone and carbamazepine clearance occurs in combination with opioids.[60]

The use of opioids in pregnancy may result in neonatal withdrawal symptoms.[69] Newborns and infants in the first 3 months of life may have increased sensitivity to opioid-induced respiratory depression and should receive opioids only in the setting of a highly monitored care area, to support respiration if necessary.[86]

The consensus is that tolerance to opioid effects other than analgesia, constipation and miosis develops rapidly.[60] The question of subtle changes in neuropsychological function remain unresolved. In the few patients who find this side-effect intolerable, another type of analgesia (e.g. nerve block) may have to be considered. In a recent study, 2 mg transnasal butorphanol impaired psychomotor performance for up to 2 hours.[87]

Opioid selection

The optimal use of opioids requires a sound understanding of opioid pharmacology and administration principles, including drug selection, routes of administration, dosing and dose titration, side-effects and their management. Patients with moderate pain have conventionally been treated with a combination product containing paracetamol or aspirin plus an opioid (codeine, dihydrocodeine, hydrocodone, oxycodone or propoxyphene).[31] These have a duration of 3–4 hours. Dose escalation is limited by the maximum dose of the non-opioid (e.g. 4000 mg paracetamol). New approaches include the use of tramadol, low-dose formulations of sustained-release morphine and new sustained-release formulations of dihydrocodeine and oxycodone.[31] Severe pain is usually treated with morphine, hydromorphone, oxycodone, oxymorphone, fentanyl, methadone or levorphanol.

Methadone and levorphanol, with their long half-lives, are not considered to be first-line therapy. They are difficult to titrate and require a longer period to approach steady state concentrations and delayed toxicity can develop as plasma concentrations gradually rise following dose increments.[31] The short half-life opioid agonists (morphine, hydromorphone, fentanyl, sufentanil, oxycodone and oxymorphone) are generally favoured as they are easier to titrate. Among these, morphine is preferred since it has a short half-life and is easy to titrate in its immediate-release form; it is also available as a controlled-release preparation that allows an 8–12 hour dosing interval.[31] Pethidine is generally not used, owing to norpethidine accumulation with repeat dosing.

A switch to an alternative opioid is considered if

there are dose-limiting toxic side-effects, if a specific formulation of another drug is needed or if sustained use is highly likely to be associated with adverse effects (as with pethidine and pentazocine).[31] Because of easier dose titration and the lesser risk of delayed toxicity from dose accumulation, the short half-life opioid agonists (morphine, hydromorphone, fentanyl, oxycodone and oxymorphone) are usually preferred. Some patients will require sequential trials of different opioids before a drug that is effective and well tolerated is identified.[31] If systemic opioids are unable to achieve adequate analgesia without excessive side-effects despite switching opioids, consideration is then given to neuraxial opioids or other regional anaesthetic or neuroablative therapies.[31]

Route selection

New routes of opioid administration have been developed. Opioids can now be given transdermally (fentanyl and buprenorphine), buccally (morphine), sublingually (buprenorphine and phenazocine), transnasally (sufentanil and butorphanol), inhalationally (morphine), epidurally, intrathecally and into the cerebral ventricles.[88] These new routes constitute an improvement only if they can achieve the required concentrations more simply, conveniently and more reliably.[89] This remains to be seen. When changing routes, the dose of the opioid must be adjusted.

Routinely, the oral route remains the most appropriate. Dextromoramide, methadone, phenazocine, levorphanol, morphine, diamorphine and papaveretum can all be given orally. Alternatives are needed for patients with impaired swallowing or gastrointestinal obstruction, and those who require a rapid onset of analgesia. Repeated parenteral bolus injections, if required, are most comfortably accomplished with an indwelling intravenous or subcutaneous infusion device.[31] To deliver repeated subcutaneous injections, a 27 gauge infusion device (a 'butterfly') can be left under the skin for up to a week.[31] Toxicity and pain breakthroughs are treated by adjusting the bolus size, the rapidity of administration and the dose interval. Continuous intravenous or subcutaneous infusions can be used. For subcutaneous infusions, opioids (morphine, hydromorphone, fentanyl and oxymorphone) must be soluble, well absorbed and non-irritant, and administered at a rate not exceeding 5 mL per hour.[31] For nausea, anxiety and agitation, opioid infusions have been combined with metoclopramide, haloperidol, scopolamine, cyclizine,

methotrimeprazine, chlorpromazine, ondansetron and midazolam.[31] Continuous intravenous infusions are appropriate with large solution volumes or when using methadone. A permanent central port is recommended for long-term continuous infusions.

For patients not requiring high doses or rapid analgesia and unable to use the oral route, the rectal and transdermal routes can be used. The opioid potency rectally approximately equals that of oral dosing.[31] Suppositories containing morphine, hydromorphone or oxymorphone are available, but controlled-release morphine tablets are often more acceptable. Transdermal opioid delivery involves a patch that adheres to the skin. The opioid diffuses through the skin and to the blood at a rate dependent on the design of the patch.[90] The aim is to provide a steady concentration without the need for venous access or syringe pumps.[90] A patch containing fentanyl (TTS-fentanyl) has been used effectively in the treatment of postoperative pain but can cause respiratory depression as it takes 18–24 hours to achieve steady state concentrations.[91] It must therefore be applied long before surgery. Since peak analgesia is not approached until 8–12 hours after the initial administration, it is essential to provide alternative analgesia during this phase.[31,91] To minimize the risk of overdose during the hours of sleep, the patch should be applied early in the morning so that the patient can be observed as blood levels rise over the ensuing 12 hours. Doses can be titrated on a daily basis. The device can produce prolonged, stable plasma levels for up to 72 hours.[91] The dosage range available is 25, 50, 75 and 100 µg per hour.[91] Plasma concentrations fall only slowly after the patch is removed and significant concentrations can remain for up to 24 hours because of delayed release from tissue and subcutaneous depots.[90] TTS-fentanyl can provide complete analgesia for a small number of patients after surgery (adults and children), but, in general, they require opioid supplementation.[91–93] TTS-fentanyl has also been used in the management of cancer pain.[94] Patients are first titrated with oral morphine (or with intravenous fentanyl using PCA) to a stable dose and then converted to TTS-fentanyl.[94] Unfortunately, proper dose finding may be difficult and episodes of breakthrough pain requiring rescue medication may occur. A recent multicentre study in cancer pain patients showed that they can be converted from oral morphine to TTS-fentanyl on a morphine-to-fentanyl ratio of 100:1 (which slightly underestimates the true ratio of 70:1).[95,96] Special indications may occur in patients with dysphagia or vomiting.

Buprenorphine has also been administered transdermally. Maximal and effective blood concentrations are observed after 9 hours.[97] It cannot, however, be reversed completely by naloxone in overdosage. Sufentanil is also readily absorbed through the skin.[80]

The more lipid-soluble drugs (buprenorphine, fentanyl, sufentanil, methadone and diamorphine) are absorbed more effectively sublingually than the less lipid-soluble drugs (morphine, oxycodone and hydromorphone).[80] The pH of the mouth is an important factor in absorption. The advantage is that the tablets may be removed from the mouth in the event of overdosage.[98] Sublingual buprenorphine has a systemic bio-availability of approximately 55 per cent.[26] For postoperative pain, $400\,\mu g$ of sublingual buprenorphine is analgesically equivalent to $300\,\mu g$ intramuscular buprenorphine.[25] In chronic nociceptive pain, sublingual buprenorphine has been found to have a similar efficacy with respect to analgesia as controlled-release morphine.[99]

The synthetic opioid fentanyl has been compounded in a hardened matrix form on a stick (oral transmucosal fentanyl), which is sucked as a lozenge (Figure 3.5).[100] The oral mucosa is moist, contains no stratum corneum (like the skin) and has a rich blood supply.[97] It has been shown to be an effective non-threatening pre-anaesthetic medication for paediatric surgical patients by inducing sedation and facilitating the inhalational induction of anaesthesia.[101,102] It may, however, reduce respiratory rate and haemoglobin oxygen saturation, as well as increasing postoperative nausea and vomiting.[102] Oral transmucosal fentanyl has been found to give effective analgesia in paediatric cancer patients undergoing bone marrow biopsy or lumbar puncture.[101] It is also a useful adjunct for the management of breakthrough pain caused by cancer.[92,100] Nasally administered sufentanil $(1.5–3\,\mu g/kg)$ has been used effectively for premedication in both children and adults.[101] The absorption of morphine via the buccal route is poor, resulting in lower plasma concentrations and inadequate preoperative sedation and postoperative pain relief.[80]

In opioid-responsive pain, if intolerable side-effects are experienced with high doses of oral or parenteral opioids, or if it is difficult to maintain effective plasma opioid concentrations, the placement of epidural or intrathecal catheters becomes a practical solution.[90] Hydrophilic drugs (morphine and hydromorphone) have a prolonged CSF half-life and significant rostral distribution. Much smaller doses (of morphine, e.g. approximately 10 per cent of the oral dose epidurally, or in the region of 1 per cent of the oral dose intrathecally) can be given, reducing the number of side-effects and improving the quality of life.[24] A Individualized Epidural Morphine Conversion Tool has recently been developed to help in the conversion of systemic to epidural morphine.[103] Lipophilic opioids (fentanyl and sufentanil) have less rostral distribution and may be preferable for segmental analgesia at the level of the spinal infusion.[31] The addition of a local anaesthetic (bupivacaine/ropivacaine 0.125–0.25 per cent) to neuraxial opioids increases analgesia without increasing toxicity.[31] The Ommaya reservoir (for intermittent injections) or an implanted pump (for continuous infusions) can be used for intraventricular opioids for the upper body and head, or for diffuse pain.[31]

Dose schedule selection and dosing

ACUTE POSTOPERATIVE PAIN

In acute postoperative pain, oral opioids may be of use when gastric function recovers and the pain is less severe.[90] Large doses may be needed because of the high first-pass metabolism. Although it is generally accepted that oral opioids are not applicable in acute postoperative pain, some physicians switch their patients to oral opioid administration on a time-contingent basis as soon as possible.[104,105] As the pain decreases, it is often appropriate to switch patients to an 'as needed' schedule.[31] Morphine, pethidine and methadone have all been used in this way. As postoperative pain becomes less severe, it is appropriate to administer less-potent opioids (codeine and dextropropoxyphene) with non-opioid analgesics (aspirin, paracetamol and NSAIDs).[105] These less potent analgesics and their combinations with opioids are discussed in Chapter 4.

CHRONIC PAIN

Patients with continuous or frequent pain are given a fixed, scheduled dose to prevent the pain from becoming recurrent and to provide continuous

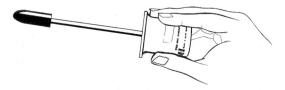

Figure 3.5   Oral transmucosal fentanyl citrate.

relief.[31] In opioid-naive patients, opioids used for severe pain are given at a dose equivalent to 5–10 mg intramuscular morphine every 3–4 hours. In opioid-naive patients and those on drugs with long half-lives, vigilance is required to detect delayed toxicity developing as the plasma concentration rises towards steady state. Controlled-release preparations lessen the inconvenience of 'around-the-clock' drug administration.[31] For maintenance, if twice daily administration is preferred to 4-hourly doses, a controlled-release tablet can be used. Maximum plasma concentrations occur 2–4 hours after administration and last about 12 hours.[26] The total daily oral dose (in mg) is divided by two to give the controlled-release dose (in mg).

All patients who receive an 'around-the-clock' opioid regimen should be offered a 'rescue dose' given on an 'as-needed' basis.[31] The size of the rescue dose should be equivalent to approximately 5–15 per cent of the 24-hour baseline dose.[31] Its frequency depends on the T_{max} for the drug and the administration route (e.g. oral rescue doses can be offered every 60 minutes and parenteral rescue doses up to every 15 minutes).[31] In the opioid-naive patient, when rapid dose escalation is needed or a long half-life drug (methadone) is given, or if there is renal impairment, an 'as needed' dosing regimen alone can be recommended.[31]

To switch to another opioid, an equi-analgesic table is required as a starting guide. When morphine is used, an intramuscular-to-oral potency ratio of 1:3 is generally recommended. The persistence of inadequate pain relief should be addressed through a step-wise dose escalation (30–50 per cent usually being safe) until analgesia is adequate or unmanageable side-effects supervene.[31] Dose-limiting side-effects require another analgesic approach or a technique to reduce opioid toxicity. Patients with very severe pain can be managed with parenteral dosing every 15–30 minutes.[31]

PATIENT-CONTROLLED ANALGESIA (PCA)

PCA is a technique of parenteral drug administration in which the patient controls a pump that delivers bolus doses of an analgesic according to parameters set by the physician. It allows patients to titrate opioids against their individual pain needs (see Chapter 7). This maintains their plasma opioid concentrations close to their minimum effective analgesic concentrations.[90] The marked peak and trough plasma levels associated with intermittent intramuscular doses are avoided. The risk of respiratory depression with peak levels and inadequate analgesia with trough levels is minimized. The more technically advanced devices have programmable variables including infusion rate, rescue dose and lock-out intervals. The involvement of patients in their pain management has substantial psychological benefits.[106] Patients are, in fact, willing to tolerate more pain when they are on PCA. The physical advantages compared with conventional intramuscular therapy include less pain in the recovery room, the ward and at home (after discharge from hospital), a more rapid recovery of normal minute ventilation, normal body temperature and the ability to walk, a reduced need for postoperative antibiotics, an earlier return to solid food, earlier discharge from hospital and a decrease in the amount of nursing time dedicated to analgesia.[90] PCA is contraindicated in patients with significant cognitive impairment.[31]

Most opioids have been used for PCA; none offers any clear-cut advantages.[90] PCA is rarely associated with a significant depression of ventilation.[90] PCA devices can infuse via various routes (e.g. intravenous, subcutaneous and epidural). The use of a constant background infusion of opioid to augment analgesia may allow the patient to sleep without being awakened by pain but has not always been shown to improve the overall quality of analgesia.[90] PCA may be used in many acute pain settings, including postoperative pain, burns and trauma cases, and for labour.[106] PCA ensures that postoperative analgesia is actively managed by the patient in cooperation with an acute pain relief service. Whether PCA improves pain relief compared with other conventional techniques is often debated, but it is generally accepted that patients treated with PCA experience less anxiety and discomfort.[104] PCA (intravenous or subcutaneous) is a major advance, providing analgesia comparable to spinal opioids with fewer major and minor side-effects.[90]

Summary

CHOICE OF OPIOID

Morphine is the standard opioid agonist, but drug availability, prescriber preference or decreased dependence liability (e.g. partial agonists or mixed agonists–antagonists) may dictate choice.[36] Unacceptable side-effects at high doses (codeine and dihydrocodeine) can also limit opioid choice. The ceiling to efficacy (found in partial agonists) is only clinically restrictive for nalbuphine.[36] Using equi-analgesic doses, there is little difference in efficacy between morphine and other strong opioids.[25]

To choose another opioid (one other than morphine), the side-effects should be considerably less at equi-analgesic doses,[25] but comparative evidence suggests that this does not occur. A high incidence of dysphoria occurs with mixed agonist–antagonists (pentazocine, nalbuphine and butorphanol).[34] The toxic metabolite norpethidine causes CNS stimulation, especially with multiple dosing and impaired renal function.[73]

The speed of onset of intramuscular opioids depends on their inherent lipophilicity.[36] Intravenously, there is little difference in speed of onset for different opioids.[36] Disparity can exist between the effect half-life and the pharmacokinetic half-life (e.g. for methadone).[25] Patient self-titration provides the safety factor in such discrepancies. Oral sustained-release preparations (morphine) lead to a slow onset of effect and time to peak effect.[24]

CHOICE OF ROUTE

If opioids are given in the appropriate dosage, efficacy seems not to be dependent on route.[24] The route may, however, be chosen out of clinical necessity. This includes cancer patients unable to swallow and the avoidance of injections in children or in patients with bleeding tendencies.[36] Sublingual (or buccal) opioid administration provides pharmacokinetic logic to the choice of route by increasing systemic bio-availability (avoiding the variable first-pass metabolism) (e.g. buprenorphine).[25] There is little pharmacokinetic logic to this choice of route with low-clearance drugs (methadone).

Patients with absorption problems may benefit from continuous subcutaneous infusions with soluble opioids (e.g. diamorphine) via portable syringe drivers. This is preferable to continuous intravenous infusions in the home-care setting, unless a permanent vascular access device is in place.[107] The spinal route is been dealt with in Chapter 9. It seems that epidural administration of the short-acting lipophilic opioids (fentanyl, sufentanil, butorphanol and nalbuphine) does not result in substantially superior analgesia or fewer side-effects than are seen with simple parenteral use.[37] New routes being explored include the transdermal, intranasal and inhalational routes.

REFERENCES

1. **Puig, M.M.** 1995: Update on opiates and their receptors. *European Society of Anaesthesiologists Refresher Course Lectures*, vol. 17, 87–92.

2. **Pleuvry, B.J.** 1991: Opioid receptors and their ligands: natural and unnatural. *British Journal of Anaesthesia* 66, 370–80.

3. **Dickenson, A.H.** 1991: Mechanisms of the analgesic actions of opiates and opioids. *British Medical Bulletin* 47(3), 690–702.

4. **Fukuda, K.** 1996: Molecular biology of the opioid receptor. *International Symposium of Regional Anaesthesia*, Auckland, New Zealand, 9–11 April, 58–61.

5. **Dickenson, A.H.** 1994: Where and how do opioids act? In Gebhart, G.E., Hammond, D.L. and Jensen, T.S. (eds) *Proceedings of the 7th World Congress on Pain – progress in pain research and management.* Seattle: IASP Press, 525–52.

6. **Sullivan, A.F. and Dickenson, A.H.** 1988: Electrophysiological studies on the spinal effects of dermorphin, an endogenous mu opioid agonist. *Brain Research* 461, 182–5.

7. **Dickenson, A.H., Sullivan, A.F., Knox, R.J., Zajac, Z. and Rogues, B.P.** 1987: Opioid receptor types in the rat spinal cord: electrophysiological studies with mu and delta receptor agonists in the control of nociception. *Brain Research* 413, 649–52.

8. **Shipton, E.A.** 1992: The spinal route – quo vadis? *South African Medical Journal* 81,1–3.

9. **Stevens, C.W. and Yaksh, T.L.** 1990: Studies of morphine and D-ala^2-D-leu^5-enkephalin (DADLE) cross-tolerance after continuous intrathecal infusion in the rat. *Anesthesiology* 76, 596–603.

10. **Dickenson, A.H.** 1992: Opioid receptors. In Kaufman, L. (ed.) *Anaesthesia Review 9.* Edinburgh: Churchill Livingstone, 65–79.

11. **Tejwani, G.A., Rattan, A.K. and McDonald, J.S.** 1992: Role of spinal opioid receptors in the antinociceptive interactions between intrathecal morphine and bupivacaine. *Anesthesia and Analgesia* 74, 726–34.

12. **Miaskowski, C., Sutters, K.A, Taiwo, Y.O. and Levine, J.D.** 1992: Antinociceptive and motor effects of delta/mu and kappa/mu combinations of intrathecal opioids. *Pain* 49, 137–44.

13. **Shipton, E.A.** 1997: Peripheral action of the opioids and the central action of the non-steroidal anti-inflammatory drugs (NSAIDs). *South African Journal of Anaesthesiology and Analgesia* 3(3), 1–2.

14. **Brooks, J.H.J., Rattan, A.K., Gupta, B. and Tejwani, G.** 1991: Opioid peptides in human peripheral nerves. *Anesthesiology* 75(3A), A591.

15. **Stein, C. and Yassouridis, A.** 1997: Peripheral morphine analgesia. *Pain* 71, 119–21.

16. **Hill, R.G.** 1994: Pharmacological considerations in the use of opioids in the management of pain associated with nonterminal disease states. *Pain Reviews* 1, 47–61.

17. **Kayser, V., Gobeaux, D., Lombard, M.C., Guilbaud, G. and Besson, J.M.** 1990: Potent and longlasting antinociceptive effects after injection of low doses of a mu-opioid agonist, fentanyl, into the brachial plexus sheath of the rat. *Pain* 42, 215–225.

18. **Dickenson, A.H.** 1995: Spinal cord pharmacology of pain. *British Journal of Anaesthesia* 75, 193–200.

19. **Wildsmith, J.A.W.** 1989: Developments in local anaesthetic drugs and techniques for pain relief. *British Journal of Anaesthesia* **63**, 159–64.

20. **Kalso, E., Tramer, M.R., Carroll, D., McQuay, H.J. and Moore, A.** 1997: Pain relief from intra-articular morphine after knee surgery: a qualitative systematic review. *Pain* **71**, 127–34.

21. **Stein, C.** 1995: Morphine – a local analgesic. *IASP Clinical Updates* **3**(1), 1–4.

22. **Shipton, E.A.** 1994: Pain care – new developments. *South African Medical Journal* **84**, 188–9.

23. **Berde, C.B.** 1996: Peripheral, spinal and supraspinal targets of opioids and NSAIDs. *IASP Newsletter*, (May/June), 3–4.

24. **Hanks, G.W.** 1991: Opioid-responsive and opioid-non-responsive pain in cancer. *British Medical Bulletin* **47**(3), 718–31.

25. **McQuay, H.J.** 1991: Opioid clinical pharmacology and routes of administration. *British Medical Bulletin* **47**(3), 703–17.

26. **McQuay, H.J.** 1989: Opioids in chronic pain. *British Journal of Anaesthesia* **63**, 213–26.

27. **Hug, C.C.** 1991: Opioids, pharmacokinetics and anesthetic effects. *American Society of Anesthesiologists Annual Refresher Course Lectures* **134**, 1–7.

28. **Galer, B.S., Coyle, N., Pasternak, G.W. and Portenoy, R.K.** 1992: Individual variability in the response to different opioids, report of five cases. *Pain* **49**, 87–91.

29. **Mather, L.E.** 1990: Pharmacokinetic and pharmacodynamic profiles of opioid analgesics, a sameness amongst equals? *Pain* **43**, 3–6.

30. **Schafer, S.L.** 1991: Pharmacokinetics, pharmacodynamics, and rational opioid selection. *Anesthesiology* **74**, 53–63.

31. **Cherny, N.I.** 1996: The medical treatment of pain in the terminal stages of cancer and other illnesses. In Campbell, J.N. (ed.) *Pain 1996 – an updated review*. Seattle: IASP Press, 469–84.

32. **Atcheson, R. and Rowbotham, D.J.** 1998: Pharmacology of acute and chronic pain. In, Rawal, N. (ed.) *Management of acute and chronic pain*. London: BMJ Books, 23–50.

33. **Shipton, E.A.** 1990: The management of intractable pain. *Hospital Medicine* (Aug), 30–4.

34. **Rosow, C.** 1989: Agonist–antagonist opioids theory and clinical practice. *Canadian Journal of Anaesthesia* **36**(3), S5-S8.

35. **Ding, Y. and White, P.F.** 1992: Comparative effects of ketorolac, dezocine and fentanyl as adjuvants during outpatient anesthesia. *Anesthesia and Analgesia* **75**, 566–71.

36. **McQuay, H.J.** 1992: Opioid clinical pharmacology. *SA Society of Anaesthetists' Annual Refresher Course Lectures* (Mar), 1–10.

37. **Camann, W.R., Loferski, B.L., Fanciullo, G.J., Stone, M.L. and Datta, S.** 1992: Does epidural administration of butorphanol offer any clinical advantage over the intravenous route? *Anesthesiology* **76**, 216–20.

38. **Aldermann, E.L., Barry, W.H., Graham, A.F. and**

Harrison, D.C. 1972: Hemodynamic effects of morphine and pentazocine differ in cardiac patients. *New England Journal of Medicine* **27**, 623–7.

39. **Popio, K.A., Jackson, D.H., Ross, A.M., Schreiner, B.F. and Yu, P.N.** 1978: Hemodynamic and respiratory effects of morphine and butorphanol. *Clinical Pharmacology and Therapeutics* **23**, 281–7.

40. **McQuay, H.J. and Moore, R.A.** 1998: *An evidence-based resource for pain relief*. Oxford: Oxford University Press, 22, 187–92.

41. **Hanna, M.H., Peat, S.J., Knibb, A.A. and Fung, C.** 1991: Disposition of morphine-6-glucuronide and morphine in healthy volunteers. *British Journal of Anaesthesia* **66**, 103–7.

42. **Grace, D. and Fee, J.P.H.** 1996: A comparison of intrathecal morphine-6-glucuronide and intrathecal morphine sulphate as analgesics for total hip replacement. *Anesthesia and Analgesia* **83**, 1055–9.

43. **Arkinstall, W., Sandler, A., Goughnour, B., Babul, N., Harsanyi, Z. and Darke, A.** 1995: Efficacy of controlled-release codeine in chronic non-malignant pain, a randomised, placebo-controlled clinical trial. *Pain* **62**, 169–78.

44. **McQuay, H.J. and Moore, R.A.** 1998: *An evidence-based resource for pain relief*. Oxford: Oxford University Press, 132–7.

45. **Hays, H., Hagen, N., Thirlwell, M.** *et al.* 1994: Comparative clinical efficacy and safety of immediate release and controlled release hydromorphone in chronic severe cancer pain. *Cancer* **74**, 1808–16.

46. **Katz, J.A.** 1996: Opioids and nonsteroidal antiinflammatory analgesics. In Raj, P.P. (ed.) *Pain medicine – a comprehensive review*. St Louis, C.V. Mosby, 126–40.

47. **Raffa, R.B., Friderichs, E., Reiman, W., Shank, R.P., Codd, E.E. and Vaught, J.L.** 1992: Opioid and non-opioid components independently contribute to the mechanism of action of tramadol, an 'atypical' opioid analgesic. *Journal of Pharmacology and Experimental Therapeutics* **260**(1), 275–85.

48. **Vickers, M.D., O'Flaherty, D., Szekely, S.M., Read, M. and Yoshizumi, J.** 1992: Tramadol pain relief by an opioid without depression of respiration. *Anaesthesia* **47**, 291–6.

49. **Houmes, R.J.M., Voets, M.A., Verkaaik, A., Erdmann, W. and Lachmann, B.** 1992: Efficacy and safety of tramadol versus morphine for moderate and severe post-operative pain with special regard to respiratory depression. *Anesthesia and Analgesia* **74**, 510–14.

50. **Grond, S., Meuser, T., Zech, D., Hennig, U. and Lehmann, K.A.** 1995: Analgesic efficacy and safety of tramadol enantiomers in comparison with the racemate, a randomised, double-blind study with gynaecological patients using intravenous patient-controlled analgesia. *Pain* **62**, 313–20.

51. **Budd, K.** 1994: Tramadol, a step towards the ideal analgesic. In *South African lecture tour*. Johannesburg: Boerhinger Mannheim, 1–4.

52. **Lehmann, K.A.** 1994: Tramadol in the management of acute pain. *Drugs* **47**(supplement 1), 19–32.

53. **James, M.F.M., Heijke, S.A.M. and Gordon, P.C.** 1996: Intravenous tramadol versus epidural morphine for postthoracotomy pain relief, a placebo-controlled double-blind trial. *Anesthesia and Analgesia* **83**, 87–91.

54. **McQuay, H.J. and Moore, R.A.** 1988: *An evidence-based resource for pain relief.* Oxford, Oxford University Press, 138–46.

55. **Gourlay, G.K., Plummer, J.L., Cherry, D.A. and Onley, M.M.** 1994: A comparison of Kapanol (a new sustained-release morphine formulation), MST Continus and morphine solution in cancer patients: pharmacokinetic aspects of morphine and morphine metabolites. In Gebhart, G.E., Hammond, D.L. and Jensen, T.S. (eds) *Proceedings of the 7th World Congress on Pain – progress in pain research and management.* Seattle: IASP Press, 631–43.

56. **Gourlay, G.K., Plummer, J.L. and Cherry, D.A.** 1995: Chronopharmacokinetic variability in plasma morphine concentrations following oral doses of morphine solution. *Pain* **61**(3), 375–81.

57. **Bruera, E.B., Fainsinger, R., Spachynski, K., Babul, N., Harsanyi, Z. and Darke, A.C.** 1995: Clinical efficacy and safety of a novel controlled release morphine suppository and subcutaneous morphine in cancer pain: a randomised evaluation. *Journal of Clinical Oncology* **13**(6), 1520–7.

58. **Kim, L., Murdande, S., Gruber, A. and Kim, S.** 1996: Sustained-release morphine for epidural analgesia. *Anesthesiology* **85**(2), 331–8.

59. **Elliot, K., Hynansky, A. and Inturrisi, C.E.** 1994: Dextromethorphan attenuates and reverses analgesic tolerance to morphine. *Pain* **59**, 361–8.

60. **Gourlay, G.K.** 1994: Long-term use of opioids in chronic pain patients with nonterminal disease states. *Pain Reviews* **1**, 62–76.

61. **Mayer, D.J., Mao, J. and Price, D.D.** 1995: The development of morphine tolerance and dependence is associated with translocation of protein kinase C. *Pain* **61**, 365–74.

62. **Basbaum, A.I.** 1995: Insights into the development of opioid tolerance. *Pain* **61**, 349–52.

63. **Portenoy, R.K.** 1994: Opioid tolerance and responsiveness: research findings and clinical observations. In Gebhart, G.E., Hammond, D.L. and Jensen, T.S. (eds) *Proceedings of the 7th World Congress on Pain – progress in pain research and management.* Seattle: IASP Press, 595–619.

64. **Mao, J., Price, D.D., Mayer, D.J.** 1995: Mechanisms of hyperalgesia and morphine tolerance: a current view of their possible interactions. *Pain* **62**, 259–74.

65. **Smith, G.D.** 1995: Morphine-3-glucuronide: evidence to support its putative role in the development of tolerance to the antinociceptive effects of morphine in the rat. *Pain* **62**, 51–60.

66. **Joranson, D.E.** 1994: Global opioid consumption, trends, barriers and diversion. *IASP Newsletter* (Sep/Oct), 4–5.

67. **Stein, C.** 1997: Opioid treatment of chronic non-malignant pain. *Anesthesia and Analgesia* **84**, 912–14.

68. **Moulin, D.E., Iezzi, A., Amireh, R., et al.** 1996: Randomised trial of oral morphine for chronic non-cancer pain. *Lancet* **347**, 143–7.

69. **Aronoff, G.M., Evans, W.O.** 1992: Pharmacological management of chronic pain: a review. In Aronoff, G.M. (ed.) *Evaluation and treatment of chronic pain*, 2nd edn. Baltimore, Williams & Wilkins, 358–68.

70. **Turk, D.C., Brody, M.C. and Okifuji, E.A.** 1994: Physicians' attitudes and practices regarding the long-term prescribing of opioids for non-cancer pain. *Pain* **59**, 201–8.

71. **Hanks, G.W.** 1996: Principles of systemic opioid pharmacotherapy. In Campbell, J.N. (ed.) *Pain 1996 – an updated review.* Seattle: IASP Press, 239–45.

72. **Hewett, K., Dickenson, A.H. and McQuay, H.J.** 1993: Lack of effect of morphine-3-glucuronide on the spinal antinociceptive actions of morphine in the rat: an electrophysiological study. *Pain* **53**, 59–63.

73. **Portenoy, R.K., Foley, K.M., Stulman, J. et al.** 1991: Plasma morphine and morphine-6-glucuronide during chronic morphine therapy for cancer pain: plasma profiles, steady-state concentrations and the consequences of renal failure. *Pain* **47**, 13–19.

74. **Wolff, T., Samuelsson, H. and Hedner, T.** 1995: Morphine and morphine metabolite concentrations in cerebrospinal fluid and plasma in cancer pain patients after slow-release oral morphine administration. *Pain* **62**, 147–54.

75. **Peat, S.J., Hanna, M.H., Woodham, M., Knibb, A.A. and Ponte, J.** 1991: Morphine-6-glucuronide: effects on ventilation in normal volunteers. *Pain* **45**, 101–4.

76. **Bigler, D., Broen Christenson, C., Eriksen, J. and Jensen, N.H.** 1990: Morphine, morphine-6-glucuronide and morphine-3-glucuronide concentrations in plasma and cerebrospinal fluid during long-term high-dose intrathecal morphine administration. *Pain* **41**, 15–18.

77. **Poulain, P., Moran Ribon, A., Hanks, G.W., Hoskin, P.J., Aherne, G.W. and Chapman, D.J.** 1990: CSF concentrations of morphine-6-glucuronide after oral administration of morphine. *Pain* **41**, 115–16.

78. **Tiseo, P.J., Thaler, H.T., Lapin, J., Inturrisi, C.E., Portenoy, R.K. and Foley, K.** 1995: Morphine-6-glucuronide concentrations and opioid-related side effects: a survey in cancer patients. *Pain* **61**, 47–54.

79. **Faura, C.C., Olaso, M.J., Garcia Cabanes, C. and Horga, J.F.** 1996: Lack of morphine-6-glucuronide antinociception after morphine treatment: is morphine-3-glucuronide involved? *Pain* **65**, 25–30.

80. **Kaufman, L.** 1991: Pain. In Kaufman, L. (ed.) *Anaesthesia Review 8.* Edinburgh: Churchill Livingstone, 231–53.

81. **Budd, K.** 1989: The pain clinic – chronic pain. In Nunn, J.F., Utting, J.E. and Brown, B.R. (eds.) *General anaesthesia*, 5th edn. London, Butterworth, 1349–69.

82. **Paix, A., Coleman, A., Lees, J. et al.** 1995: Subcutaneous fentanyl and sufentanil infusion substitution for morphine intolerance in cancer pain management. *Pain* **63**, 263–9.

83. **Magerl W.** 1996: Neural mechanisms of itch sensation. *IASP Newsletter* (Sep/Oct) 4–7.

84. **Borgeat, A., Wilder-Smith, H.G., Salah, M. and Rifat, K.** 1992: Subhypnotic doses of propofol relieve pruritus induced by epidural and intrathecal morphine. *Anesthesiology* **76**, 510–12.

85. **Macdonald, N., Der, L., Allan, S. and Champion, P.** 1993: Opioid hyperexcitability, the application of alternate opioid therapy. *Pain* **53**, 353–5.

86. **Berde, C.** 1992: Chronic pain in pediatrics. In Aronoff, G.M. (ed.) *Evaluation and treatment of chronic pain*, 2nd edn. Baltimore: Williams & Wilkins, 349–57.

87. **Zacny, J.P., Lichtor, J.I., Klafta, J.M., Alessi, R. and Apfelbaum, J.L.** 1996: The effects of transnasal butorphanol on mood and psychomotor functioning in healthy volunteers. *Anesthesia and Analgesia* **82**, 931–5.

88. **Shipton, E.A.** 1991: Recent advances in intractable pain control. *South African Medical Journal* **79**, 119–20.

89. **Black, A.M.S. and Alexander, J.I.** 1992: Analgesia for postoperative pain. In, Atkinson R.S. and Adams A.P. (eds.) *Recent advances in anaesthesia and analgesia 17.* Edinburgh: Churchill Livingstone, 119–35.

90. **Shipton, E.A.** 1992: Postoperative pain – an update. *South African Journal of Surgery* **30**(1), 2–5.

91. **Sandler, A.N.** 1992: Update on postoperative pain management. *Canadian Journal of Anaesthesia* **39**(5), R53-R56.

92. **Gourlay, G.K., Kowalski, S.R., Plummer, J.L.** *et al.* The efficacy of transdermal fentanyl in the treatment of postoperative pain, a double-blind comparison of fentanyl and placebo systems. *Pain* **40**, 21–8.

93. **Paut, O., Camboulives, J., Tillant, D., Levron, J.C. and Viard, L.** 1992: Pharmacokinetics and tolerance of transdermal fentanyl in young children. *Anesthesiology* **77**(3A), A1203.

94. **Zech, D.F.J., Grond, S.U.A., Lynch, J., Dauer, H.G., Stollenwerk, B. and Lehmann, K.A.** 1992: Transdermal fentanyl and initial dose-finding with patient-controlled analgesia in cancer pain, a pilot study with 20 terminally ill cancer patients. *Pain* **50**, 293–301.

95. **Donner, B., Zenz, M., Tryba, M. and Strumpf, M.** 1996: Direct conversion from oral morphine to transdermal fentanyl, a multicentre study in patients with cancer pain. *Pain* **64**, 527–34.

96. **Ahmedzai, S., Allen, E., Fallon, M.** *et al.* 1994: Transdermal fentanyl in cancer pain. *Journal of Drug Development* **6**(3), 93–7.

97. **Zech, D., Lehmann, K.A. and Rupreht, J.** 1991: Current developments in pain treatment 1. *Pain Clinic* **4**(3), 177–81.

98. **Smith, G.** 1989: Management of postoperative pain. *Canadian Journal of Anaesthesia* **36**(3), S1-S4.

99. **Bach, V., Kamp-Jensen, M., Jensen, N.H. and Eriksen, J.** 1991: Buprenorphine and sustained release morphine – effect and side-effects in chronic use. *Pain Clinic* **4**(2), 87–93.

100. **Fine, P.G., Marcus, M., De Boer, A.J. and Van Der Oord, B.** 1991: An open label study of transmucosal fentanyl citrate (OTFC) for the treatment of breakthrough cancer pain. *Pain* **45**, 149–53.

101. **Davis, P.J.** 1992: Opioid use in pediatric anesthesia. In Barash, P.G. (ed.) *American Society of Anesthesiologists.* Philadelphia: J.B. Lippincott **20**, 69–75.

102. **Friessen, R.H. and Lockhart, C.H.** 1992: Oral transmucosal fentanyl citrate for preanesthetic medication of pediatric day surgery patients with and without droperidol as a prophylactic anti-emetic. *Anesthesiology* **76**, 46–51.

103. **Du Pen, S.L. and Williams, A.R.** 1994: The dilemma of conversion from systemic to epidural morphine: a proposed conversion tool for the treatment of cancer pain. *Pain* **56**, 113–8.

104. **Commission on the Provision of Surgical Services.** 1990: *Report of the working party on pain after surgery.* London: Royal College of Surgeons of England/College of Anaesthetists, 1–36.

105. **Barash, P.G., Bruce, F.C. and Stoelting, R.K.** 1991: Pain – acute and chronic. In Barash, P.G. (ed.) *Handbook of clinical anesthesia.* Philadelphia: J.B. Lippincott, 410–19.

106. **Upton, P.M., Beeton, A.G. and Shipton, E.A.** 1992: Patient-controlled analgesia. *South African Medical Journal* **81**, 58.

107. **Patt, R.B.** 1992: Control of pain associated with advanced malignancy. In Aronoff, G.M. (ed.) *Evaluation and treatment of chronic pain*, 2nd edn. Baltimore: Williams & Wilkins, 313–39.

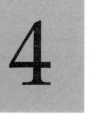

4 PRIMARY ANALGESICS:
Non-steroidal anti-inflammatory drugs (NSAIDs) and others

Primary analgesics are defined as those drugs which have a pain-relieving property as the primary nature of their clinical activity. They include aspirin and the NSAIDs, paracetamol and the opioids. The opioids are discussed in Chapter 3.

NSAIDs

Cyclic prostanoids play important physiological roles in inflammation and maintaining the normal function of several organ systems.[1] Two enzymes, cyclo-oxygenase (COX) and 5-lipoxygenase, act upon arachidonic acids to produce prostaglandins and leukotrienes.[2] Prostaglandin production requires the conversion of arachidonate to the intermediate prostaglandin H_2, by the two-step cyclo-oxygenation and peroxidation catalysed by the enzyme COX (or prostaglandin H synthetase).[1] Aspirin and the NSAIDs block the production of cyclic prostanoids by binding in different ways to this enzyme and blocking the active site.[1] This results in decreased inflammation, but it can also produce side-effects in the gastrointestinal tract, kidney and platelet system. Recent data demonstrate that there are two isoforms of the COX enzyme (the constitutive isoform, COX-1, and the inducible isoform, COX-2).[1,3] These isoforms of COX have been identified, sequenced and cloned.[4] They are similar in size, substrate specificity and kinetics but vary in their expression and distribution.[1] COX-1 is produced under normal conditions and is present in normal cells.[5] It is important in the regulation of prostaglandin synthesis in the gastric mucosa and the renal vascular bed.[5] Normal physiological functions appear to be maintained by COX-1.[1] COX-1 activation leads to the production of prostacycline, which when released by the endothelium is antithrombogenic, and when released by the gastric mucosa is cytoprotective.[3] COX-1 is thus involved in regulating normal cellular processes, such as gastrointestinal tract cytoprotection, vascular homeostasis and renal function.[4] The inducible form, COX-2, discovered 7 years ago, is undetectable in most tissues.[3] It is induced by hypoxia, epidermal growth factor, benzopyrene, transforming growth factor beta-1, inflammatory stimuli and cytokines (interleukin-1) in migratory and other cells.[2,3] Therefore, during inflammation, endothelial cells, fibroblasts and macrophages produce COX-2.[4,5] It is probable that the relative inhibition of these two isoenzymes will be related to the likelihood of side-effects.[5] Differences in efficacy and side-effects between drugs may thus reflect variability against COX.[5] It is attractive to suggest that the anti-inflammatory actions of the NSAIDs are due to the inhibition of COX-2, whereas the unwanted side-effects, such as irritation of the stomach lining, are the result of inhibition of COX-1.[3] A drug that specifically inhibits COX-2 without affecting COX-1 would, theoretically, reduce inflammation without leading to side-effects (e.g. on the gastrointestinal tract).[4] Pharmacokinetic differences contribute to significant interpatient variability in response.[5] X-ray crystal structures of COX-1 and COX-2 have provided valuable information regarding the structural basis for the COX-2 selectivity of NSAIDs.[6]

Classification and pharmacokinetics

The chemical families of the NSAIDs are a heterogeneous group of compounds containing an aromatic ring and, in all but the phenol derivatives, an acidic functional group.[7] NSAIDs are divided into the carboxylic acids, the pyrazones (e.g. phenylbutazone) and the oxicams (e.g. tenoxicam and piroxicam).[8,9] The carboxylic acid group is divided into the salicylates (e.g. aspirin, diflunisal and sodium salicylate), the acetic acids (e.g. indomethacin, tolmetin and sulindac, which may be safer in renal impairment, diclofenac and tiaprofenic acid), the propionic acids (e.g. ibuprofen, flurbiprofen, fenbufen, naproxen, ketoprofen, fenoprofen and pirprofen) and the fenamates (e.g. mefenamic acid and flufenamic acid).[5]

With the exception of the phenol derivatives (paracetamol), all the clinically useful NSAIDs are weak organic acids (pK_a 3.0–3.5), which bind extensively to plasma albumin (95–99 per cent) and may displace other highly bound drugs (oral hypoglycaemics, anticonvulsants, warfarin and sulphonamides).[5,7] Total body clearance is similar for all NSAIDs (typically 0.01–0.05 L/kg per minute), and the volumes of distribution range from 10 to 15 L in normal adults.[7] Most NSAIDs are extensively metabolized in the liver and have a low renal clearance (under 10 per cent).[7] The pharmacokinetic properties of each agent have an important bearing on its activity. Pharmacokinetic properties are reflected by differences in their half-lives and influence dosing regimens and drug accumulation. Some NSAIDs (e.g. indomethacin and diclofenac) will be effective longer than their half-lives suggest because they tend to remain within inflamed tissue.

NSAIDs are rapidly and almost completely absorbed from the upper gastrointestinal tract and, to a lesser degree, from the stomach, peak plasma concentrations mostly being reached within 2 hours.[5] The absorption of oral NSAIDs is reduced when they are taken with food but is faster when a salt rather than a poorly soluble acid is administered.[5,7] Many oral NSAIDs are prepared as the sodium salt, or as tablets containing weak bases plus acidic NSAIDs, which together produce salts on the addition of water. Most NSAIDs cannot be easily formulated as solutions for parenteral use because they have bulky hydrophobic structures. Solubilization with hydrophilic bases allows the preparation of solutions; for example ketorolac is prepared as the trometamol salt dissolved in aqueous alcohol.[7]

Some NSAIDs (e.g. many of the 2-propionic acid derivatives, known as profens) contain a chiral centre and are used as a racemate.[7] Metabolic processes alter racemic drugs (e.g. R-profen to S-profen, which is a more potent inhibitor of prostaglandin synthesis).[7] Recently, pure enantiomers of 2-propionic acid derivatives have been isolated. It is already clear that the R and S enantiomers act differently peripherally and centrally.[7] It may be possible to develop clinically useful analgesics that are free from significant peripheral prostaglandin inhibition and thus free from gastrointestinal and renal toxicity.

A ceiling on their analgesic effects exists for NSAIDs,[5] further dose escalation increasing only the adverse effects.[5] For some NSAIDs, this ceiling is much higher than for aspirin or paracetamol.[10] Some NSAIDs have time–effect curves comparable to those of aspirin and paracetamol;[10] others have a longer duration of action. The optimal dose regimen of NSAIDs for analgesia is not necessarily appropriate for their antirheumatic effects,[10] and some antirheumatic NSAIDs are not appropriate for use as analgesics. The plasma half-lives of NSAIDs vary, as illustrated by a few examples. Oral naproxen sodium is rapidly absorbed, peak plasma concentrations being obtained in 20–40 minutes.[11] Its plasma half-life is about 14 hours, with a duration of clinical action of about 8 hours.[11] Diflunisal is a fluorinated salicylic acid derivative with a plasma half-life of 10–11 hours,[10] and piroxicam is an oxicam derivative with a plasma half-life of about 50 hours.[10] However, the relative duration of effective analgesia produced by NSAIDs is not necessarily predictable on the basis of differences in their half-lives.[10] NSAIDs with long half-lives may produce toxicity in elderly patients with renal and hepatic dysfunction.[10] Most NSAIDs have inactive metabolites, but some (fenbufen, meclofenamic acid, nabumetone, sulindac and phenylbutazone) produce active metabolites.[5]

Mode of action of NSAIDs

PERIPHERAL ACTIONS, PERIPHERAL AFFERENTS AND CHEMICAL SIGNALLING

Following trauma, nociceptive stimulation occurs from damage (both mechanical and thermal) to nerve endings.[12] The substance P released causes localized oedema (from vasodilatation and increased vascular permeability).[12] This, together with the release of algogenic substances (prostaglandins, leukotrienes, bradykinin, serotonin and histamine),

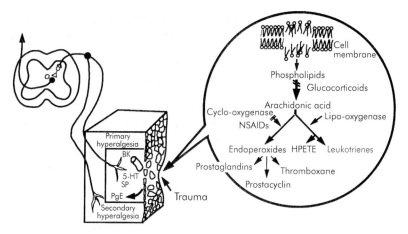

Figure 4.1 Trauma leads to the release of substance P (SP), bradykinin (BK), serotonin (5-HT), histamine and arachidonic cascade metabolites, giving rise to vasodilatation, an increase in vascular permeability and sensitization of the nociceptors (primary hyperalgesia). Secondary hyperalgesia occurs from functional changes in the peripheral and central nervous systems. Arachidonic acid can be metabolized to the prostaglandin endoperoxides (PgE) by the enzyme cyclo-oxygenase, or to hydroperoxy derivatives (HPETE) and leukotrienes by the lipo-oxygenase pathway. NSAIDs, non-steroidal anti-inflammatory drugs.

leads to nociceptor sensitization and hyperalgesia (Figure 4.1).[12] Sympathetic efferent activity may increase the inflammation by increasing the vascular permeability and indirectly increasing the release of prostanoids and leukotrienes.[12] All cells (except for non-nucleated erythrocytes) can synthesize prostaglandins in response to trauma.[12] Bradykinin and the products of arachidonic acid metabolism enhance the pain and hyperalgesia of the inflammatory response.[12] COX metabolizes arachidonic acid to the prostaglandin endoperoxides (prostaglandins, prostacyclins and thromboxanes), and lipo-oxygenase metabolizes arachidonic acid to the hydroperoxy derivatives[12] (Figure 4.1).

The NSAIDs comprise a very important analgesic

group. The inhibition of COX is generally felt to be the major mechanism of action of these drugs. The NSAID drugs inhibit the biosynthesis of prostaglandins by the reversible acetylation and inactivation of COX.[13] By blocking the formation of prostaglandins, the NSAIDs obtund the sensitization of tissues to the algesic action of kinins, resulting in depression of the inflammatory response, and analgesia.[13] Dampening of the inflammatory response is related to the degree of COX inhibition (Figure 4.2). Other mechanisms add to the production of analgesia. Some NSAIDs (e.g. indomethacin) increase intracellular cyclic AMP by inhibiting phosphodiesterase.[12] This stabilizes polymorphonuclear leucocyte membranes and decreases the generation of phagocyte superoxide.[12] Arachidonic acid (plus metabolites) may regulate neurotransmitter release.[13] This release may thus be influenced by NSAIDs, resulting in analgesia (similar to that of the tricyclic antidepressants).[13] NSAID drugs disrupt interactions within biological membranes and have recently been found to have effects that have nothing to do with prostaglandin synthesis. NSAIDs interfere with stimulus–response coupling in human neutrophils by inhibiting the cell–cell adhesion of neutrophils.[9] Neutrophils are the most abundant cells of acute inflammation. NSAIDs have also been found to interfere in particular with signals that depend on G proteins for transduction through cell membranes.[9] NSAIDs have also been found to inhibit the aggregation of marine sponge cells (which cannot make prostaglandins), just as they do to neutrophils.[9]

NSAID	Analgesic efficacy	Cyclo-oxygenase inhibition (µmol/l)
Diclofenac		1.6
Piroxicam		2.3
Indomethacin		5.6
Naproxen		5.7
Ibuprofen		39.0
Phenylbutazone		490.0
Acetyl salicylic acid		3300.0

Figure 4.2 Cyclo-oxygenase inhibition and the analgesic efficacy of various non-steroidal anti-inflammatory drugs (NSAIDs). The depression of the inflammatory response is directly related to the degree of cyclo-oxygenase inhibition, while analgesia appears to be mediated via a number of pathways.

Besides the stimulation of peripheral nerve fibres to induce pain, several other important features are associated with inflammation. There are changes in local blood flow and vascular permeability, the activation and migration of immune cells and the release of growth and trophic factors from surrounding tissues.[14] Manifold and complex changes in afferent fibres can be produced, ranging from overt activation, or sensitization to other stimuli, to alterations in the phenotype and structure of sensory nerves.[14] Mediators are released during inflammation. These are chemicals released either directly from the tissues or as a result of antidromic neuronal activity.[15] Although some mediators [e.g. protons and 5-hydroxy tryptamine (5-HT)] can act directly on membrane ion channel proteins to change permeability and cell excitability, most activate membrane receptors via G proteins and second messengers. Directly acting mediators that bind to receptors associated with ion channels to alter the polarization state of the membrane are protons, capsaicin, 5-HT and adenosine triphosphate (ATP).[14] Molecules that activate nociceptors include protons (causing membrane depolarization because of inward cation movement), 5-HT (released from platelets and mast cells during inflammation) and ATP (released in large quantities during tissue damage), which allows the entry of a wide range of cations that depolarize the cell.[14] Indirectly acting mediators (via second messengers) include 5-HT, ATP, bradykinin, eicosanoids, histamine, neutrotrophins and cytokines.[14] Molecules that activate receptors include 5-HT and bradykinin.[15] 5-HT binds to $5\text{-}HT_{1C}$ or $5\text{-}HT_2$ receptors and activates phospholipase C to produce the second messengers diacylglyceride and inositol triphosphate. Depolarization then results from activation of protein kinase C. Bradykinin (BK), a potent algogenic substance, produced on tissue damage by the cleavage of high-molecular weight kininogens by kallikrein (itself activated by inflammation), exerts its effects via actions on the BK_1 and BK_2 receptors. The binding of bradykinin to the BK_2 receptors evokes the activation of phospholipase C. BK_2 receptors are particularly located on sensory nerve terminals and dorsal root ganglia. Molecules capable of sensitizing nociceptors include 5-HT, bradykinin, ATP, eicosanoids, histamine, cytokines, neural growth factor, adrenergic agents and opioid receptors.[15] 5-HT binds to $5\text{-}HT_{1C}$ or $5\text{-}HT_2$ receptors and brings about peptide release as a result of the increase in intracellular calcium ions caused by phospholipase C activation. In addition, binding to the $5\text{-}HT_1$ or $5\text{-}HT_4$ receptors activates adenylate cyclase to increase cyclic adeno-

sine monophosphate (cAMP) and to activate protein kinase A. The metabolite des-arg-BK, the ligand of choice at BK_1 receptors, stimulates the release of tumour necrosis factor-alpha, interleukin-1 and various prostanoids in inflammation.[15] The BK_1 receptor is involved in chronic inflammatory pains and in hyperalgesia. The binding of bradykinin to the BK_2 receptors stimulates phospholipase C, with depolarization and peptide release. Phospholipase A_2 is activated to increase the production of arachidonic acid and its derivatives. ATP binds to macrophage receptors, causing the release of prostanoids and cytokines.

The most important pain eicosanoids (substances derived from arachidonic acid) are the prostaglandins and leukotrienes. These are products of the COX and lipo-oxygenase enzymes.[15] Both are produced at the site of tissue injury, although they do not themselves invoke pain when administered to man. As previously stated, prostaglandins are made by at least two isoenzymes of COX, COX-1 (the constituted form) and COX-2 (the inducible form seen in inflamed tissue). The leukotrienes LT_{D4} and LT_{B4} are implicated in nociception. In addition, LT_{D4} is thought to stimulate basophils to increase their production and the release of prostanoids. LT_{B4} seems to act by increasing the release of the hydroxy-acid (8R, 15S)-di HETE from polymorphonuclear leucocytes.[15] This may then act via the activation of protein kinase C.

The inflammatory release of histamine provokes vasodilatation, hyperaemia and plasma extravasation. Cytokines (interleukins tumour necrosis factors and interferons) are released by cells of the immune system at the site of inflammation. Interleukin-1β has been shown to produce delayed hyperalgesia *in vivo*.[15] Cytokines probably act by their ability to increase prostaglandin release and inhibit potassium ion channels.

An upregulation in the neurotrophin, neural growth factor (NGF), provoked by the increase in cytokines, occurs.[16] NGF might be an important factor in sensitizing nociceptors to the effects of algogenic substances (bradykinin) when mast cell degranulation takes place. The stimulation of alpha receptors on sympathetic neurones causes the release of prostanoids that sensitize the nociceptors.[15] In inflammatory conditions, opioid receptors found on sympathetic terminals, immune cells and primary afferents are stimulated by endogenous opioids to produce analgesia and modulate chemotaxis and degranulation.[15] Recent data suggest that the cumulative effect of mechanically removing inflammatory mediators during coronary surgical bypass by ultrafiltration may be clinically beneficial in paediatric cardiac surgical patients.[17]

CENTRAL ACTIONS OF THE NSAIDs[18]

Current evidence suggests that some, if not all, NSAIDs, in addition to their peripheral actions, may exert an important central action, especially in hyperalgesic states.[19,20] The inhibition of central prostaglandins may be important in certain pain models,[7] as prostaglandins facilitate nociceptive signal transmission in the CNS.[21] NSAIDs may also inhibit neuronal excitability, thus affecting neuronal transmission.[13] In the rat, NSAIDs produce a dose-dependent depression of C fibre evoked activity in single neurones of the thalamus.[21] Intracerebroventricular microinjections of NSAIDs abolish reperfusion hyperalgesia in the rat's tail and inhibit nociceptive responses in arthritic rats.[21,22] Sodium salicylate increases the nociceptive threshold in rats to stimulation of the lateral hypothalamus, while, in the monkey, microinjections of aspirin into the preoptic hypothalamus depress nociceptive responses.[21] This depends on an intact catecholaminergic function.

Recent clinical surveys and new *in vivo* evidence strongly suggest that, for some of these agents, centrally mediated analgesia may be achieved by additional mechanisms, which are independent of prostaglandin synthesis inhibition.[7,23,24] There are several other possible targets. This is clearly an area requiring further investigation.

A greater understanding of enantiomer pharmacology may lead to the development of safer drugs.[25] The discovery of an inducible COX offers additional insight into NSAID activity.[7] NSAIDs may vary quantitatively in terms of which prostaglandins they may inhibit, their physicochemical differences, their potency of COX inhibition and their relative affinity for COX-1 or COX-2.[26] Great interest is currently being placed on the potential for COX-2 inhibitors, which might avoid the adverse effects of damage to the gastric mucosa and kidney, while retaining their analgesic properties.[15] NSAIDs with selective inhibitory activity on the COX-2 isoform should, theoretically, decrease inflammation while maintaining normal physiological prostaglandin levels (e.g. reducing gastrointestinal toxicity).[1] *In vitro* testing has shown that individual NSAIDs possess different relative inhibitory effects in various tissues.[4] A number of compounds showing selectivity towards COX-2 relative to COX-1 have been described. The clinical relevance of the differential inhibition of COX isoenzymes may soon be known. Compounds that may be 100–300 times more effective inhibitors of COX-2, and therefore may have lower risks of toxicity as well as more potent anti-inflammatory effects, have been developed.[4] These NSAIDs are currently undergoing clinical trials in the hope of demonstrating good analgesia with few side-effects.[5] These drugs include meloxicam, flosulide, DuP-697, NS-398, SC-58125 and L-745,337.[27] DuP-697, NS-398, L-745,337 and SC-58125 are all potent anti-inflammatory agents, which have few effects on physiological prostaglandin production in the gastrointestinal tract or kidney and produce little gastrointestinal toxicity.[27] All are highly selective COX-2 inhibitors, with a COX-2:COX-1 ratio of less than 0.005 found for L-745,337 (a sulphonamide) and SC-58125 (a tricyclic methyl sulphone derivative) in a whole human blood assay and with human recombinant enzymes, respectively.[6] These compounds show fewer gastrointestinal complications in animal experiments.[6] Celecoxib inhibits COX-2 with a 375-fold selectivity over COX-1 (Schwartz, 1997, unpublished data). Both nabumetone (a prodrug whose active metabolite has a long elimination half-life) and etodolac more selectively lock COX-2 prostaglandins.[5,28] R-ketoprofen reduces gastrointestinal side-effects when compared with racemic ketoprofen. These findings need to be thoroughly investigated, particularly in relation to some intriguing new findings in 'knockout' mice with non-functioning genes for COX-1 and COX-2.[27]

Side-effects

The most common side-effects of NSAIDs are gastritis, peptic ulceration and the reduction of renal function. These drugs can cause problems in any part of the gastrointestinal tract, from the oesophagus to the rectum.[29] Owing to the relatively few doses needed in the perioperative period, the most frequent problems will relate to idiosyncratic 'allergic reactions'.[13] Skin rashes and anaphylactoid reactions (resembling hereditary angioneurotic oedema) predominate.[12,13] Rare reactions include blood dyscrasias, pulmonary and hepatic reactions and anaphylaxis.[12]

HAEMATOLOGICAL EFFECTS

Platelet aggregation, and hence haemostatic plug formation, is modulated by the balance between two substances synthesized from the unstable prostaglandin endoperoxides PGG_2 and PGH_2.

Thromboxane-A$_2$, synthesized from platelet phospholipid (also in neutrophils, macrophages and lung fibroblasts) by thromboxane synthase stimulates platelet aggregation and constricts large blood vessels.[26] Prostacyclin (PGI$_2$) synthesized from endothelial cell phospholipid by prostacyclin synthase, is a vasodilator and the most powerful inhibitor of platelet aggregation. These effects are mediated through opposing actions on cAMP.[26] The selective inhibition of thromboxane synthase should result in vasodilatation and protection against thrombosis. Aspirin inactivates COX irreversibly and completely with a dose as low as 160 mg per day.[26] Low-dose aspirin (30–75 mg per day) may partially spare endothelium-synthesized prostacyclin. Nevertheless, as doses of aspirin that suppress vascular prostacyclin do exert an antithrombotic effect, the emphasis on the balance between the two enzymes would seem to be relative rather than absolute.[26] Other NSAIDs inhibit the COX enzyme competitively. Their effect on platelet function is less profound and is related to the plasma half-life of the drug, but it takes five times the half-life of the agent to get rid of the COX inhibitory effect.[26,30] Thus, long-acting drugs such as the oxicams carry a more significant risk of haemostasis than do shorter-acting drugs such as diclofenac or ketorolac.[30] Some protection against thrombosis is anticipated, depending on the dosage and the degree of COX suppression. Agents developed to inhibit COX-2 selectively might well produce profound antinociception without affecting clotting mechanisms, as COX-1 mediates the synthesis of thromboxane by platelets.[26] Novel NSAIDs that release nitric oxide (NO) appear to have an enhanced antiplatelet activity.[26]

NSAIDs generally alter *in vitro* tests of platelet function, and, as such, there seems to be merit in checking bleeding times, with an upper limit of 10 minutes. Links between coagulation tests and clinical outcomes (e.g. increased blood loss or epidural haematoma) are not clear cut.[26] Bleeding time is typically increased in patients taking aspirin or NSAIDs but not usually beyond normal limits.[26] NSAIDs do not affect prothrombin times or partial thromboplastin times. Long-term dosing adverse effect data where gastrointestinal bleeding is the main concern rate ibuprofen as the safest.[31] In acute pain, NSAIDs can cause a significant lengthening (up to 30 per cent) of bleeding time, but it still usually remains within the normal range.[31] This can last for days with aspirin and for hours with non-aspirin NSAIDs.[31] Significantly increased blood loss has been reported in patients taking NSAIDs in some studies but not on others.[26] Problems are more likely in conjunction with other orders of haemostasis (e.g. von Willebrand's disease, pre-eclampsia if the patient is taking aspirin, haemophilia and thrombocytopaenia), and the risk-to-benefit ratio needs to be individualized.

NSAID-INDUCED GASTROINTESTINAL TRACT DAMAGE

NSAIDs can induce damage throughout the entire gastrointestinal tract.[32] Nausea, vomiting and epigastric pain are common, but dyspepsia predicts neither severe gastric mucosal damage nor intestinal blood loss.[5] In a clinical economics review, misoprostol prophylaxis was shown to result in a small but significant reduction in major gastrointestinal side-effects at the expense of an increase in minor but unpleasant ones.[28,33] Proton pump inhibitors also appeared to offer the same degree of gastroprotection as misoprostol, with the additional benefit of symptom relief.[33] Patients taking diclofenac/misoprostol combinations showed significantly less of a decline in haemoglobin and up to 50 per cent fewer clinically significant gastrointestinal side-effects than patients receiving diclofenac alone.[34] However, the Arthritis, Rheumatism and Aging Medical Information System Prospective Post Marketing Surveillance Programme of over 11 000 arthritis patients has shown that:[35]

- rheumatoid and osteoarthritis patients are 2.5–5.5 times more likely to be hospitalized for NSAID-related gastrointestinal events;
- the absolute risk for serious NSAID gastrointestinal toxicity remains constant and that cumulative risk increases over time;
- there are no reliable warning signs (80 per cent of patients with serious gastrointestinal complications having no prior gastrointestinal symptoms);
- independent factors for serious gastrointestinal events were age, prednisone use, NSAID dose, disability level and previous NSAID-induced gastrointestinal symptoms;
- antacids and histamine$_2$ (H$_2$) antagonists [as shown by several randomized controlled trials (RCTs)] do not prevent NSAID-induced gastric ulcers;[28]
- high-risk NSAID users who take gastroprotective drugs are more likely to have serious gastrointestinal complications than patients not taking such medications.

Limiting NSAID use is the only way to decrease the risk of NSAID-related gastrointestinal events, both by rational prescribing and by using non-pharmacological methods of controlling symptoms.[33,35] Most patients who have peptic ulcers without *Helicobacter pylori* infection are taking NSAIDs.[36] If Helicobacter infection is present in a patient who develops an ulcer while taking NSAIDs, it seems advisable to eradicate the infection in case the ulcer has been caused by the infection in that particular patient.[36] The proton pump inhibitor, omeprazole may be the treatment of choice for healing NSAID-associated ulcers on the basis of its efficacy and tolerability, and the optimal dose appears to be 20 mg once daily.[37]

NSAIDs affect the gastric mucosa by direct toxicity and indirectly by central prostaglandin inhibition.[26,30] NSAIDs chelate divalent and/or multivalent metallic cations in the gastrointestinal mucus and mucosa.[38] All NSAIDs are weak acids and tend to accumulate within cells of the gastric mucosa (ion trapping), destroying the barrier to acid back-diffusion and causing further mucosal damage. Given parenterally, their effect on the mucosa is more indirect.[30] The inhibition of endogenous prostaglandin suppresses their mucosal protective properties. PGI_2 and PGE_2 modulate mucosal blood flow, inhibit gastric secretion and increase bicarbonate and mucous production.[30] Thus, conventional NSAIDs inhibit the synthesis of cytoprotective prostaglandins by COX-1 in the gastrointestinal tract.[2] Surplus arachidonic acids accumulate and enhance the generation of leukotrienes by the lipoxygenase pathway, inducing neutrophil adhesion to endothelium and vasoconstriction.[2] The NSAIDs harbouring a carboxyl group also inhibit oxidative phosphorylation, lowering ATP generation and leading to loss of mucosal tight junctions and increased mucosal permeability.[2]

The administration of site-specific probes is a non-invasive technique for assessing the functional integrity of the gastrointestinal mucosa.[32] Non-invasive tests of gastric, intestinal and colonic permeability have shown promise in identifying patients who would benefit from endoscopy.[32]

Old age, female gender, dyspepsia, prior peptic ulcer disease or gastrointestinal tract haemorrhage, concomitant corticosteroid usage, smoking and excessive alcohol intake, anticoagulants (warfarin and heparin) and/or previous NSAID intolerance increase the risk of gastrointestinal complications.[5,30,39] The gastrointestinal toxicity of NSAIDs carries high morbidity and mortality rates and is the most worrying adverse effect associated with their long-term use in rheumatology.[26] Using data from four randomized trials, taking NSAIDs for more than 2 months carries a risk of gastrointestinal

bleeding or perforation of 1 in 228, a relative risk of 2.8 and an absolute risk of 0.69 per cent.[40] COX-1 may be more important than COX-2 in the maintenance of cytoprotective prostaglandins. In animal studies, relatively selective COX-2 inhibitors appear to cause less damage to the gastric mucosa.[26] Highly buffered, enteric-coated and non-acidic NSAIDs may be less harmful to the gastric mucosa. About one third of patients will have some gastrointestinal symptoms during a 3 month course of therapy,[26] but fewer than 1 per cent of users (although especially the elderly) will suffer serious gastrointestinal bleeding or perforation.[26] It has been estimated that there is a 1 in 8.3 (12 per cent) risk that patients with bleeding or perforation will die.[40]

Pharmaco-epidemiological studies suggest that the risk of upper gastrointestinal bleeding is dose-related.[30] Aspirin and naproxen are more prone to induce gastric bleeding, while the risk is less for ibuprofen, indomethacin and diclofenac.[26] Gastropathy is not prominent in the literature describing the perioperative use of NSAIDs beause of their short-term use and the paucity of large-scale studies.[26] For perioperative use, should the use of protective co-therapy be considered, prostaglandin analogues (misoprostol), non-prostaglandin protective agents (colloidal bismuth subcitrate), proton pump inhibitors (omeprazole) and H_2-receptor antagonists (in the perioperative setting to add protection against aspiration pneumonitis) may be used.

EFFECTS ON RENAL FUNCTION

Data from rheumatological patients suggest that a relatively low proportion of all adverse events associated with NSAIDs involve the kidney.[26] In the kidney, prostaglandins act as local tissue hormones – PGI_2 in the cortex and PGE_2 in the medulla – maintaining blood flow, regulating tubular processes involving electrolytes and modulating the effects of other renal hormones.[30] Vasoconstrictor hormones (renin, angiotensin, noradrenaline and vasopressin) produce a compensatory increase in the renal synthesis of vasodilatory prostaglandins by inducing phospholipase. With surgery and activation of the sympathetic nervous system, renal blood flow can become prostaglandin-dependent and NSAIDs may elicit acute adverse effects.[30] In normal conditions, renal blood flow and glomerular filtration are not prostaglandin dependent, but prostaglandins play a significant role if volume depletion, reduced renal function or congestive heart failure are present. In these situations, NSAIDs should not be used. NSAIDs may cause sodium, water and potassium to be retained to varying degrees, with the possible development of oedema, oliguria, hyperkalaemia and hyponatraemia. Fluid and electrolyte status should be monitored during NSAID therapy after all major surgery. NSAIDs should be prescribed with care perioperatively, especially in conjunction with nephrotoxic medications (e.g. aminoglycosides) or in the presence of any pre-existing renal impairment (in diabetes, hypertension, atherosclerosis and old age).[30] This is a time of haemodynamic instability and increased renin, angiotensin, adrenaline and renal prostaglandin activity.[30] The four main forms of renal insufficiency occurring in association with NSAIDs are acute tubular necrosis, papillary necrosis and chronic interstitial nephritis (aspirin, and NSAIDs alone or combined with paracetamol), idiosyncratic acute interstitial nephritis (with proteinuria) and generalized vasculitis (with glomerulonephritis).[26] The mechanism of renal papillary necrosis with NSAIDs is still controversial.[41] Some NSAIDs selectively target the medullary interstitial cells.[41] Many papillotoxins have the potential to undergo prostaglandin hydroperoxidase-mediated metabolic activation, specifically in the renal medullary interstitial cells.[41] These reactive metabolites, in the presence of large quantities of polyunsaturated lipid droplets, result in localized and selective injury of the medullary interstitial cells.[41] Prostaglandin analogue protection (misoprostol) has been limited by its side-effects, but when used in conjunction with NSAIDs has been found to reduce renal adverse effects.[26,28] In acute pain, acute renal failure can be precipitated in patients with pre-existing heart or kidney disease, those on loop diuretics and those who have lost more than 10 per cent of their blood volume.[31]

The clearance of most NSAIDs is reduced by decreased renal function in the elderly. Patients with chronic renal failure are dependent on vasodilatory prostaglandins to maintain renal function.[42] The use of NSAIDs in these patients may be particularly hazardous.[42] The clearance of texoxicam is relatively unaffected by age or mild changes in renal function.[26] NSAIDs should, however, be used in appropriate doses, for appropriate indications and with the appropriate management of fluids and electrolytes, which includes suitable screening and monitoring of renal biochemistry.

OTHER SIDE-EFFECTS AND DRUG INTERACTIONS

The pharmacokinetic or pharmacodynamic effects of NSAIDs may produce significant drug interactions.[5]

NSAIDs are strongly albumin bound and compete with other acidic drugs for albumin binding sites.[5] NSAIDs can reduce lithium clearance and reduce the effectiveness of any class of cardiac failure therapy as a result of sodium and water retention.[5]

Aspirin and the NSAIDs can precipitate acute bronchospasm in between 8 and 20 per cent of adult asthmatics.[26,30] The 'aspirin triad' comprises asthma, aspirin intolerance and nasal polyps. Existing asthma may become more severe with NSAIDs. An allergic mechanism appears unlikely. The mechanism may involve shunting the arachidonic acid metabolism away from the (bronchodilator) prostaglandins to the (bronchoconstrictor) leukotrienes.[26] Adult asthma is a relative contraindication for the use of NSAIDs.

With NSAIDs, there are many differences in the incidence, histological pattern and mechanisms of toxicity between, as well as within, chemical classes.[43] NSAIDs (including aspirin) have been associated with asymptomatic and transient increases in liver enzyme activity (the most common effect) to mild reversible hepatitis or fatal acute hepatic necrosis.[26] NSAIDs should be avoided in patients with known altered hepatic functions. Most hepatocellular reactions occur because of individual patient susceptibility (idiosyncrasy).[43] Aspirin, however, is a dose-related intrinsic hepatotoxin.[43]

Neurological and psychiatric reactions of NSAIDs include, dizziness, headache, tremor, somnolence, confusion, depression, hallucinations, anxiety and delirium.[26] NSAIDs should be stopped in elderly patients if they become confused. Ocular adverse effects include conjunctivitis, blurred vision and allergic reactions.

NSAIDs impair various leucocyte functions *in vitro*.[26] When reduced immune competence arising from their use is associated with alcoholism, malnutrition, diabetes, severe systemic illness or long-term steroid treatment, patients may possibly be at risk of developing acute necrotizing fasciitis.[26] The use of NSAIDs is relatively contraindicated in these patients.

Diclofenac can produce thrombosis on intravenous administration and local tissue damage on intramuscular administration.[26] Parenteral formulations of other NSAIDs (ketorolac and tenoxicam) appear to be free from this local tissue toxicity.

NSAIDs are not generally associated with teratogenesis and have been given to many breast-feeding mothers with no apparent harm to either mother or fetus.[26] Although NSAIDs (indomethacin) are used to treat premature labour and encourage closure of a patent ductus arteriosus in premature infants, renal failure has been reported in the newborns of mothers treated with NSAIDs.[26] In infants and young children, an acute viral illness followed by mitochondrial damage can give rise to an acute metabolic encephalopathy (Reye's syndrome) with acute microvascular hepatic stenosis and hyperammonaemia.[26] The role of aspirin in this aetiology remains controversial.

In the presence of inflammation, NSAIDs may be protective to cartilage.[26] Loosening of cement hip prostheses does not appear to be increased by NSAID therapy.

Drug interactions with NSAIDs include those with (especially potassium-sparing) diuretics, causing circulatory volume depletion and hyperkalaemia. Antihypertensive therapy (specifically with beta-blockers) may become less effective. Glomerular filtration is reduced with the combination of angiotensin-1 converting enzyme inhibitors and NSAIDs.[26] Angiotensin is involved in efferent vasoconstriction, and prostaglandins in afferent arteriolar dilatation. If given with angiotensin-converting enzyme inhibitors, hyperkalaemia may result.[5] The risk of bleeding is increased with the combination of NSAIDs and warfarin. NSAIDs may increase the unbound concentration of many protein-bound drugs (antidepressants, methotrexate and barbiturates).[30] Cimetidine reduces the clearance of many NSAIDs. NSAIDs do not significantly alter the protein binding of other NSAIDs (such as salicylates, naproxen and piroxicam).[30]

In summary, restrictions to NSAID use include:[30]

- a history of renal disease;
- hypovolaemia;
- a history of haematological or coagulation diseases;
- a history of gastroduodenal ulcer disease;
- a history of 'allergic' reactions to other NSAIDs;
- asthma;
- nasal polyposis;
- pulmonary hypertension.

NSAIDs may cross the placenta and should be avoided in pregnancy and lactation.[5] Side-effects can be reduced by careful attention to the dose and the duration of therapy, concomitant risk factors and the combined use of more specific drugs to reduce disease activity.[44]

Routes of administration

NSAIDs can be given orally, as transdermal gels (ketoprofen, diclofenac and indomethacin), intra-muscularly, intravenously, rectally, intra-articularly and as a topical ophthalmic solution.[10,45] In renal colic, there is evidence that NSAIDs act most quickly when given intravenously, which may have clinical relevance.[46] In all other pain conditions, there is no evidence of any difference in analgesic efficacy between routes.[46] In pain conditions other than renal colic, there is a strong argument to give NSAIDs orally rather than by injection.[47] Randomized controlled trials have shown that the topical application of NSAIDs is effective in relieving pain in acute (musculoskeletal) and chronic conditions.[48] Most NSAIDs have poor aqueous solubility with substantial tissue irritation, giving pain and inflammation at the injection site and limiting repeat dosage.[10] Ketorolac, diclofenac and tenoxicam can be given by injection. With diclofenac, thrombophlebitis can occur around the injection site.[49] Ketorolac has good aqueous solubility and is relatively non-irritating to the tissues. The intravenous regional administration of ketorolac has been reported, in a few recent studies, to benefit patients with postoperative pain or complex regional pain syndromes, although further studies are needed before this route of administration can be widely recommended.[50] Ketorolac given at induction provides significant analgesia evident in the later recovery period following minor laparoscopic surgery.[51] Sustained-release preparations of NSAIDs (ibuprofen, indomethacin and diclofenac) are available. For lower abdominal gynaecological surgical procedures, sustained-release ibuprofen has recently been successfully used as an adjunct to morphine PCA.[52]

The intrathecal route is being researched in animal models.[53] PGE_2 is released spinally with injury, and the spinal administration of PGE_2 is algesic.[50] The spinally administered NSAIDs exert impressive analgesic/antihyperalgesic effects.[50] It is not clear whether intrathecal or epidural NSAID administration will be safe and clinically useful. It is also unknown whether intrathecal or epidural NSAIDs have a ceiling effect and whether their maximum efficacy differs from that of systemic NSAIDs.[50] A theoretical advantage of neuraxial NSAIDs, particularly in postoperative use, would be to diminish the gastric, antiplatelet, renal and hepatic problems commonly associated with systemic NSAID use. Concerns have been raised regarding the effects of high local concentrations of NSAIDs on bleeding in the neuraxial spaces. Synergism has been demonstrated among the other classes of analgesic administered neuraxially.[50] It may be that neuraxial NSAIDs will be most useful in small doses as part of a multimodal analgesic regimen with other recognized neuraxial drugs, including opioids, adrenergics and local anaesthetics.

Advantages of NSAIDs

NSAIDs do not produce the CNS side-effects characteristic of opioids. The lack of opioid side-effects (especially sedation, cardiovascular and respiratory depression, urinary retention and dependence) is a distinct advantage.[54–56] There is also no evidence that tolerance develops to their analgesic effects.[10] Unlike opioids, NSAIDs have little effect on biliary tract pressure.[57] Other advantages include the variety of formulations (and pharmacokinetic profiles) available, allowing a rapid onset of action, good oral bio-availability and a long duration of action.[10]

Uses of NSAIDs

NSAIDs are used in rheumatic diseases, where they form the basis for treatment of inflammation in and around the joint.[44] Furthermore, NSAIDs are being increasingly used for non-rheumatic conditions, including acute and chronic pain, biliary and ureteric colic, and dysmenorrhoea.[44]

EFFICACY OF NSAIDs IN THE PERIOPERATIVE SETTING

Prostaglandins and other eicosanoids are implicated in the development of primary and secondary hyperalgesia and central sensitization. NSAIDs attenuate the febrile response to surgery and postoperative nitrogen excretion.[26] NSAIDs may vary quantitatively in terms of which prostaglandins they inhibit, their physicochemical differences, the potency of COX inhibition, their relative affinity for COX-1 and COX-2, and their dosage.[26] In major surgery, most studies using NSAIDs have shown a reduction in opioid requirements, better analgesia, reduced nursing difficulty, less pain on ambulation, earlier recovery of gastrointestinal function and better preservation of respiratory function and aspects of respiratory mechanics.[20] NSAIDs have proved particularly effective in dental pain, postoperative pain, dysmenorrhoea and pain associated with acute musculoskeletal trauma.[8,10] Large-scale surveillance studies of the side-effects of NSAIDs, when used specifically in the preoperative setting, are lacking. Studies have supported the use of NSAIDs in ambulatory surgery (orthopaedic, oral, minor gynaecological and breast surgery), showing that adequate analgesia can be achieved without the use of opioids or regional blockade.[26] In laparoscopic surgery, NSAIDs given after deflation of a pneumoperitoneum are probably safe.[26] The addition of NSAIDs in PCA can provide better analgesia than seen with opioids alone, demonstrating opioid-sparing, typically of about 30 per cent.[26] In postoperative pain, when diclofenac 50 mg (NNT = 2.3) was compared directly with ibuprofen 400 mg (NNT = 2.7), there was no significant difference between the two treatments.[58] Ibuprofen showed a clear dose response with a relative efficacy similar to that of diclofenac.[58] Both drugs work well.[58] Choosing between them is an issue of dose, safety and cost.[58]

There is no doubt that NSAIDs have considerable analgesic efficacy. The timing of administration is important, especially before major surgery, in which the risks of COX inhibition may be increased if an unexpected volume loss occurs intraoperatively. Details of dosage, trial design and patient models confound attempts to generalize from the studies done thus far. No NSAID can yet truly rival opioids for efficacy in severe pain (except for colic). However, NSAIDs exert no significant cardiorespiratory depression, do not suppress bowel motility, have no effect on biliary pressure and induce less sedation compared with morphine.[30] The improvement of psychomotor function benefits patients, especially in day surgery. In acute pain, the main concerns are renal and coagulation problems. The most important consideration is to establish how NSAIDs should be used: alone or in combination (e.g. with paracetamol), in which patients, and for which indications. What regimen will optimize analgesia (in a given group of patients)? Additional questions will involve the dosage and timing of administration. Appropriate patient selection, dosage and monitoring are essential if these drugs are to used safely and effectively. Short half-life drugs are not free from the problem of renal failure.[26] No NSAID is free from adverse effects (e.g. gastritis). It is not so much the drug, but how it is used that is important. Research into the clinical benefit and cost–benefit of preoperative treatment with NSAIDs is needed.[7]

At present, it is probably better to offer preoperative oral NSAIDs only to patients undergoing minor surgery and to reserve the injectable NSAIDs for postoperative use, when NSAIDs cannot be given orally.[7] Because of their relatively low analgesic efficacy, NSAIDs are not suitable as the sole analgesic immediately after major surgery, when the pain is severe.[34] They may be of considerable value 24–48 hours later, especially after orthopaedic and thoracic surgery.[59] NSAIDs have, however, been used as the sole agent for lesser degrees of postoperative pain.[60,61] NSAIDs should be given orally whenever possible.[31] Paracetamol in combination is also effective.[31] As the pain wanes, the prescription should be paracetamol based, supplemented if necessary by NSAIDs.[31] Preoperatively, NSAIDs with high anti-COX activity (naproxen, diflunisal and azapropazone) may be given 12–24 hours prior to the procedure to utilize their antiprostaglandin properties.[13] Postoperatively, NSAIDs with low COX inhibitory activity but high analgesic efficacy (ketorolac, tenoxicam, piroxicam and diclofenac) should be given.[13]

NSAIDs FOR CANCER PAIN

The WHO method for cancer pain relief recommends the following: 'NSAIDs (or other non-opioid analgesics) as the sole treatment for mild to moderate pain, combined with weak opioids for moderate to severe pain, and in conjunction with strong opioids for more severe pain'.[62] The non-opioid analgesics include acetylsalicylic acid, other NSAIDs and paracetamol.[63] Acetylsalicylic acid, paracetamol, ibuprofen, and indomethacin are all included in the 'Model list of essential drugs'. NSAIDs (including acetylsalicylic acid) are used to treat pain from bone metastases, where there is a high concentration of prostaglandins in the affected bone produced by the tumour cells. They are also helpful for pain caused by soft tissue and muscle infiltration.[63] Drugs in this group display a 'ceiling effect'. If pain is not adequately relieved, an opioid should be added'.[63]

In a recent meta-analysis, the existing clinical data from 25 randomized controlled trials in 1545 patients using NSAIDs for cancer pain have been examined.[64] Single doses of NSAIDs were found to produce a peak pain relief of 60 per cent even though pain intensity was moderate to severe (stage 2) in the majority of patients.[64] On the basis of these findings, it has been asked whether the WHO second analgesic step is an optimal treatment protocol or whether it should be modified so that treatment would proceed directly from NSAIDs to strong opioids in the face of unrelieved pain.[62] To date, however, there is no convincing evidence suggesting that NSAIDs have specific efficacy in malignant bone pain; neither do they have specificity in relieving visceral or somatic pain.[64] If inflammation

is involved in the pathogenesis of malignant nerve pain, NSAIDs may play a role in relieving this type of pain, even if it is opioid resistant.[64] NSAIDs induce dose-dependent analgesia up to a ceiling.[64] It might be good practice to increase the dose of an NSAID gradually, but in the case of persistent pain to switch to a more potent analgesic drug rather than to exceed the recommended dose of that particular drug. As the incidence of adverse effects tends to increase in a dose-dependent fashion without a ceiling effect, especially with multiple dosing, cautious dose titration and ongoing evaluation of each patient are required.[64] The use of long-term continuous NSAID infusions has been suggested but needs further investigation.

There is a wealth of information that NSAIDs can prevent colorectal cancer.[65] COX is constitutively expressed in normal colonic epithelium and the surrounding stroma, and could catalyse the generation of malondialdehyde, which is a known mutagen and could initiate colorectal carcinogenesis.[65] Other proneoplastic effects of COX include changing the action of transforming growth factor-beta from antiproliferative to pro-proliferative, reducing adherence to extracellular matrix and promoting metastasis and angiogenesis.[65] These properties of COX suggest that the inhibition of both isoforms may have important protective effects against colorectal cancer.[65] NSAIDs may have a role in reducing the incidence of Alzheimer's disease.[66]

USE OF NSAIDs IN CHRONIC PAIN

Few trials on the use of NSAIDs in chronic pain meet the minimum criteria for well-controlled clinical trials of analgesic efficacy.[10] Most are single-dose studies in cancer or arthritic pain.[10] There is great need for repeat-dose trials of NSAIDs in chronic pain in order to establish efficacy, to compare one against another and to compare them to the weak opioids. NSAIDs have been used in the treatment of osteo- and rheumatoid arthritis, ankylosing spondylitis and chronic back pain.[8,10,67] Their contribution in chronic pain is probably underrated as they are probably as effective as both weak opioids and small oral doses of strong opioids.[10] However, taking NSAIDs for more than 2 months carries a risk of a gastrointestinal bleeding or perforation, and in turn a risk of death.[40] Thus, if paracetamol is sufficient to control the pain, it should be chosen above NSAIDs because of its long-term safety at recommended doses.[40]

Newer NSAIDs

KETOROLAC TROMETAMOL

Ketorolac is an NSAID with strong analgesic activity. After major abdominal, orthopaedic or gynaecological surgery, or ambulatory laparoscopic or gynaecological procedures, ketorolac provides relief from mild to severe pain in the majority of patients and has an analgesic efficacy similar to that of the standard dosages of morphine and pethidine (meperidine) as well as the less frequently used opioids and other NSAIDs.[68] The analgesic effect of ketorolac may be slightly delayed but often persists for longer than that of opioids.[68] It is used in combination with opioids for more severe pain, leading to a marked reduction in their consumption.[55,69] Combined therapy with ketorolac and an opioid results in a 25–50 per cent reduction in opioid requirement, this in some patients being accompanied by a concomitant decrease in the number of opioid-induced adverse events, a more rapid return to normal gastrointestinal function and a shorter hospital stay. It has been used to treat breakthrough pain in perioperative patients receiving transdermal fentanyl.[67] In children undergoing myringotomy, hernia repair, tonsillectomy or other surgery associated with mild to moderate pain, ketorolac provides analgesia comparable to that of paracetamol (acetaminophen) and to morphine and pethidine.[68] In the emergency department, ketorolac attenuates moderate to severe pain in patients with renal colic, migraines, musculoskeletal pain or sickle cell crisis, and is usually as effective as the frequently used opioids such as morphine and pethidine.[68] Subcutaneous ketorolac reduces cancer pain and seems particularly beneficial in pain resulting from bone metastases. The acquisition cost (compared to morphine, pethidine) is offset in reduced hospital stay.[68]

The tolerability profile of ketorolac parallels that of other NSAIDs; most clinically important adverse events affect the gastrointestinal tract and/or renal or haematological functions. The reported incidence of serious or fatal adverse events has decreased with revision of the dosage guidelines. Results from a large retrospective post-marketing surveillance study in more than 20 000 patients demonstrated that the overall risk of gastrointestinal or operative site bleeding related to parenteral ketorolac therapy was only slightly higher than that seen with opioids. However, the risk increased markedly when high dosages were used for more than 5 days, especially in the elderly.[68] Acute renal failure may occur after treatment with ketorolac, but it is usually reversible on drug discontinuation. In common with other NSAIDs, ketorolac has also been implicated in 'allergic' or hypersensitivity reactions. It can be used as a sole agent for pain of moderate intensity.[56] In a retrospective review of 167 patients receiving ketorolac after spinal instrumentation surgery, 29 non-unions occurred, leading the authors to recommend its avoidance in the early postoperative period after spinal fusion.[70] It can be given orally, intramuscularly, intravenously or topically (e.g. ophthalmic solution).[10]

Ketorolac is a strong analgesic with a tolerabiliy profile resembling that of other NSAIDs. When used in accordance with current dosage guidelines, this drug provides a useful alternative, or adjuvant, to opioids in patients with moderate to severe pain.[68]

MELOXICAM

Meloxicam is an NSAID that is 98 per cent absorbed following oral administration.[71] It is extensively metabolized, and less than 5 per cent is excreted unchanged in the faeces. Meloxicam is eliminated from the body with a mean elimination half-life of 20 hours, ideal for once-daily dosing.[71] Neither hepatic nor mild or moderate renal insufficiency substantially affects its pharmacokinetics. It is indicated for both the short- and long-term treatment of rheumatoid and osteoarthritis. Cross-sensitivity to aspirin and other NSAIDs can occur. Its relative contraindications, side-effects and special precautions are similar to those of other NSAIDs.[71] Elderly, frail or debilitated patients may tolerate side-effects less well. The concomitant use of other NSAIDs may increase the adverse effects. It has not yet been indicated for children and adolescents aged less than 15 years. The use of meloxicam during pregnancy and lactation has not been established.[71]

A COX-2:COX-1 ratio of 0.33 was obtained with meloxicam (compared with 2.2, 15, 33 and 20 obtained for diclofenac, tenoxicam, piroxicam and indomethacin, respectively), indicating that meloxicam is a more potent inhibitor of COX-2 than COX-1.[71] In doses equipotent to standard doses of NSAIDs such as piroxicam, diclofenac and naproxen, meloxicam would appear to have a better gastrointestinal safety profile, showing on average a 6–9-fold and a 2–3-fold risk reduction compared with diclofenac 100 mg slow release and piroxicam 20 mg, respectively.[71] Non-serious gastrointestinal adverse events (dyspepsia, abdominal pain, nausea and diarrhoea) occurred in 18.2 per cent of the 5500 patients treated with meloxicam.[71] Clinical studies have shown that, in doses of 7.5 mg and 15 mg daily, meloxicam is comparable in efficacy to standard NSAIDs such as piroxicam, diclofenac and naproxen in both rheumatoid and osteoarthritis.[71]

TENOXICAM

This is a new thienothiazine derivative of the oxicam class of NSAIDs. For postoperative analgesia, it has the advantage of an intravenous formulation and a long plasma half-life (60–75 hours).[72] Its analgesic and anti-inflammatory efficacy, and the frequency of side-effects, compares favourably with other NSAIDs when used orally in the treatment of arthritic conditions.[72,73] Like ketorolac, it appears to have little potential for renal damage in healthy, well-hydrated patients.[72]

Combinations

Aspirin and the other NSAIDs are subject to pharmacokinetic interactions that may produce an increase in the number of adverse effects without providing superior analgesia.[10] Because of its different mechanism of action and adverse effect profile, paracetamol is sometimes found in combination preparations with NSAIDs and a weak opioid.[10] However, the risk of hepatotoxicity from paracetamol overdosage must always be guarded against. The rationale of combining an NSAID with an opioid is that each drug exerts its analgesic effect via a different mechanism, resulting in additive or synergistic analgesia.[12] The dose of each constituent can then be reduced, with a concomitant lessening of adverse effects (see Chapter 16). With chronic administration, the development of tolerance and dependence should also be reduced.[10] The combination of an optimal dose of NSAID with an opioid produces an additive analgesic effect greater than that obtained by doubling the dose of each constituent administered alone.[12]

The combination of an NSAID (e.g. ibuprofen) with a weak opioid is part of the WHO's 'analgesic ladder' for cancer pain relief. Weak opioids added include propoxyphene (about two thirds as potent as codeine), codeine, hydrocodone (6–8 times more potent than codeine) and oxycodone (9–10 times more potent than codeine).[10] Codeine, hydrocodone and oxycodone have good oral efficacy.[10] Oral opioids are most effective when given in combination with a full regimen of an NSAID.[10] A recent study has shown that, in cancer patients, diclofenac does not modify morphine bio-availability.[74] In a recent repeat dose model of arthritic pain,

the analgesic efficacy of ibuprofen and codeine was significantly superior to that of ibuprofen alone.[75] NSAIDs have recently been successfully used in combination with oral tricyclic antidepressants in the treatment of the pain of sickle cell disease vaso-occlusive crises.[76] A strategy now used (in cancer and arthritic pain) is to add an oral opioid to one of the newer NSAIDs if a full daily dose of an NSAID alone cannot provide adequate analgesia.[10] The dose is titrated to the individual's needs.

The future

Selective inhibitors of COX-2 are newer, promising drugs.[2] The intrathecal administration of NSAIDs causes inhibition of the late-phase behavioural and electrophysiological responses to formalin.[7] Low intrathecal doses of NSAIDs also reverse the thermal hyperalgesia elicited by intrathecal NMDA or substance P administration.[7] The neuraxial effects of selective COX-2 inhibitors have not yet been reported.[7] The discovery of a second form of COX offers potential for the development of a novel, safe and effective antihyperalgesic agent, even though a COX-2 inhibitor will produce only the same analgesic relief as the current NSAIDs, which clearly show a ceiling effect in their analgesic action in humans.[77] There is still a major requirement for the development of more efficacious analgesics to treat arthritic pain. The successful management of cancer-related pain often requires the use of NSAIDs, either alone or in combination with other analgesic drugs.[64] NSAIDs do have some efficacy in malignant neuropathic pain. Inhibitors of the lipooxygenase pathway products (leukotrienes), such as CP-105,696, have been lacking in analgesic activity (although they do reduce the symptoms and signs of inflammation).[15] CP-105,696 (the novel leukotriene B_4 antagonist) attenuates the progression of collagen-induced arthritis. Unanswered questions include those of the use of neuraxial NSAIDs, and the development of NSAIDs with a better profile than that of existing agents.

NSAIDs also work by inhibiting nuclear transcription factor kB, which is critical for cytokine gene expression, for example, for interleukin-1 and interleukin-6, during inflammation.[78] The development of inhibitors to this and related transcription factors could provide the anti-inflammatory and analgesic benefits of NSAIDs without their common side-effects. Cytokine-suppressive anti-inflammatory drugs such as SKF-86002 inhibit the production of interleukin-1 and tumour necrosis factor-alpha, and show analgesic activity in acute and chronic pain models.[79] SKF-86002 blocks the activity of serine/threonine protein kinases.[79] Cytokine-suppressive anti-inflammatory drugs, by blocking the activity of these kinases, may provide new analgesic/anti-inflammatory drugs for clinical use.

ASPIRIN

Aspirin (or acetylsalicylic acid) has been found to be an effective analgesic in headaches, dysmenorrhoea, dental pain, acute musculoskeletal pain, cancer pain and rheumatoid and osteoarthritis.[10] It is hydrolysed to salicylic acid, with a plasma half-life of 2–3 hours.[5] At low doses of 300–600 mg, it is well tolerated.[5] In the treatment of chronic arthritis, the dose of aspirin must exceed 3.6 g per day to achieve a satisfactory effect, with an increased incidence of, mainly, gastrointestinal side-effects.[5,8] Lesser doses of 600 mg 4–6 times daily are required for pain alone. The principal therapeutic disadvantage of aspirin is its short duration of action,[8] effective analgesia requiring dosing at 3–4 hour intervals. Its dose–response curve has a shallow slope with a ceiling of analgesic effect in the 650–1300 mg dose range.[10] The plasma half-life of salicylic acid is dose dependent (3–30 hours) because of rate-limiting hepatic conjugation.[5]

Mechanisms of action as well as the adverse effects of aspirin are discussed above under NSAIDs. Recent studies indicate that salicylate suppresses the expression of the genes involved in inflammation.[6] Aspirin is not recommended other than in single doses for children under 1 year of age because of the danger of metabolic acidosis and fatal poisoning, which may follow repeated doses.[8] Significant drug interactions, particularly the potentiation of warfarin anticoagulants and oral antidiabetic agents, can occur with aspirin.[8]

Lysine acetylsalicylic acid is an injectable preparation of aspirin but is not consistently effective in relieving postoperative pain.[8] Aspirin is often formulated in combination with other analgesics, such as codeine, paracetamol and dextropropoxyphene. Diflunisal, the difluorophenyl derivative of salicylic acid, is more potent, lasts longer and gives rise to no tinnitus and fewer platelet and gastrointestinal side-effects.[5] The non-acetylated salicylate sodium salicylate shares many of the analgesic properties of aspirin but fails to inhibit prostaglandin synthesis in disrupted cell preparations at concentrations that can be achieved in the body.[9] It neither inhibits platelet function nor causes bleeding.[9] The development of choline magnesium trisalicylate has been shown to cause much less gastrointestinal tract irritation and is being evaluated for use in chronic pain.[10]

PARACETAMOL (OR ACETAMINOPHEN)

Paracetamol has an analgesic potency equal to that of aspirin in single-dose studies.[8] The dose–response and time–effect curves are almost superimposable.[10] It is widely prescribed as an analgesic for mild to moderate pain, including headache, toothache, dysmenorrhoea and rheumatic and cancer pain, as well as an antipyretic for colds and influenza.[8] While paracetamol is a peripherally acting analgesic, it does not inhibit peripheral COX.[8] It has, however, been found to decrease swelling after acute tissue trauma.[9] Paracetamol inhibits COX activity directly in the CNS (which perhaps explains its antipyretic effect).[8,9] Compared with aspirin and the other NSAIDs, paracetamol has fewer adverse effects when given over a long time. It does not produce gastrointestinal tract irritation and ulceration,[9] nor does it inhibit platelet function or cause bleeding.[9] In addition, it does not cause salicylism. If repeat-dose studies in chronic pain show an analgesic potency equal to that of aspirin, it will provide a good alternative.[10]

Paracetamol is rapidly and almost completely absorbed in the small bowel, has a plasma binding of 20–50 per cent, reaches a peak plasma concentration within an hour and has a plasma half-life of 2–3 hours.[5] It mainly undergoes hepatic conjugation with glucuronic and sulphuric acids, and the products are excreted in the urine.[5] A daily dosage of 4–6 g paracetamol is well tolerated.[10] However, caution must be exercised in prescribing paracetamol on a long-term basis, especially in combination with other analgesics.[80] Paracetamol is frequently offered as a component of proprietary analgesic preparations (e.g. with dextropropoxyphene and caffeine). It should not be prescribed for patients with liver or renal damage, as doses in excess of 10 g per day may cause potentially fatal liver necrosis.[8] In paracetamol overdose, the depletion of glutathione is responsible for the accumulation of the toxic metabolite N-acteyl-bezoquinoneimine and hepatic necrosis.[5] This necessitates treatment with sulphydryl donors, such as oral carboxycysteine or intravenous N-acetylcysteine.[8] Although the majority of paracetamol metabolism occurs in the liver, renal metabolism is essential in the development of nephrotoxicity and is also related to the generation of toxic paracetamol metabolites.[80] When the cellular protective mechanisms (e.g. glutathiones) cannot detoxify the reactive paracetamol metabolites, tissue damage and subsequent acute tubular necrosis occur.[80] An occasional skin rash and hypersensitivity reaction may occur, but cross-hypersensitivity with aspirin is rare.[5] In randomized controlled studies of acute pain, it has been found that paracetamol is an effective analgesic, and that codeine 60 mg added to the paracetamol produces worthwhile additional pain relief even after single doses.[81]

OTHER ANALGESICS

Nefopam

Nefopam is a non-opioid analgesic that does not inhibit prostaglandin synthesis. Its mechanism of action is unclear.[8] It has anticholinergic activity and can prevent the neuronal reuptake of serotonin, dopamine and, to a lesser extent, noradrenaline.[82] It is not sedative and has little depressant effect on the cardiovascular or respiratory systems in normal doses. Reports on its potency vary considerably.[8] Perioperative pain relief for moderate pain is feasible by the oral route.[8] Nefopam is available in tablet and injection form. The most frequently reported side-effects are nausea, nervousness, dry mouth and light-headedness.[82]

REFERENCES

1. **Bjorkman, D.J.** 1998: The effect of aspirin and non-steroidal anti-inflammatory drugs on prostaglandins. *American Journal of Medicine* **105**(1B), 8S-12S.
2. **Fossalien, E.** 1998: Adverse effects of nonsteroidal anti-inflammatory drugs on the gastrointestinal system. *Annals of Clinical and Laboratory Science* **28**(2), 67–81.
3. **Vane, J.R. and Botting, R.M.** 1998: Mechanism of action of nonsteroidal anti-inflammatory drugs. *American Journal of Medicine* **104**(3A), 2S-8S.
4. **Bolten, W.W.** 1998: Scientific rationale for specific inhibition of COX-2. *Journal of Rheumatology* **51**(supplement) 2–7.
5. **Atcheson, R. and Rowbotham, D.J.** 1998: Pharmacology of acute and chronic pain. In Rawal, N. (ed.) *Management of acute and chronic pain.* London: BMJ Books, 23–50.
6. **Wu, K.K.** 1998: Biochemical pharmacology for non-steroidal anti-inflammatory drugs. *Biochemical Pharmacology* **55**(5), 543–7.
7. **Ballantyne, J.C. and Dershwitz, M.** 1995: The pharmacology of non-steroidal anti-inflammatory drugs for acute pain. *Current Opinion in Anaesthesiology* **8**: 461–8.
8. **Shipton, E.A.** 1987: Non-opiate analgesics in pain. *South African Journal of Continuing Medical Education* **5**, 69–75.
9. **Weissmann, G.** 1991: Aspirin. *Scientific American* **264**(1), 58–64.
10. **Beaver, W.T.** 1992; Non-steroidal anti-inflammatory analgesics and their combinations with opioids. In Aronoff, G.M. (ed.) *Evaluation and treatment of chronic pain.* Baltimore: Williams & Wilkins, 369–83.
11. **Comfort, V.K., Code, W.E., Rooney, M.E. and Yip, R.W.** 1992: Naproxen premedication reduces postoperative tubal ligation pain. *Canadian Journal of Anaesthesia* **39**(4), 349–52.
12. **Dahl, J.B. and Kehlet, H.** 1991: Non-steroidal anti-inflammatory drugs: rationale for use in severe postoperative pain. *British Journal of Anaesthesia* **66**, 703–12.
13. **Budd, K.** 1992: Non-steroidal anti-inflammatory drugs in the treatment of acute pain. *South African Society of Anaesthetists' Refresher Course Lectures*, Johannesburg: South African Society of Anaesthetists, 1–12.
14. **Dray, A.** 1995: Inflammatory mediators of pain. *British Journal of Anaesthesia* **75**, 125–31.
15. **Jagger, S.I. and Rice, A.S.C.** 1996: Novel vistas in analgesic pharmacology for the treatment of chronic pain. *Anaesthetic Pharmacology and Physiology Review* **4**, 66–73.
16. **Rueff, A. and Mendell, L.M.** 1996: Nerve growth factor and inflammatory pain. *IASP Newsletter*, (Jan/Feb), 3–4.
17. **Herskowitz, A. and Mangano, D.T.** 1997: Inflammatory cascade: a final common pathway for perioperative injury? *Anesthesiology* **86**, 957–60.
18. **Shipton, E.A.** 1997: Peripheral action of the opioids and the central action of the non-steroidal anti-inflammatory drugs (NSAIDs). *South African Journal of Anaesthesiology and Analgesia* **3**(3), 1–2.
19. **Code W.** 1996: Non-opiate centrally acting analgesics. In Keneally, J.P. and Jones, M.J. (eds) *150 Years on – a selection of papers presented at the 11th World Congress of Anaesthesiologists.* Rosebery, NSW: Bridge Printery, 89–95.
20. **Fleetwood-Walker, S.M.** 1995: Nonopioid mediators and modulators of nociceptive processing in the spinal horn as targets for novel analgesics. *Pain Reviews* **2**, 153–73.
21. **Jurna, I. and Brune, K.** 1990: Central effect of the

non-steroid anti-inflammatory agents, indometh-acin, ibuprofen and diclofenac, determined in C-fibre-evoked activity in single neurones of the rat thalamus. *Pain* **41**, 71–80.

22. **Gelgor, L., Cartmell, S. and Mitchell, D.** 1992: Intra-cerebroventricular micro-injections of non-steroidal anti-inflammatory drugs abolish reperfusion hyper-algesia in the rat's tail. *Pain* **50**, 323–9.

23. **McCormack, K.** 1994: Non-steroidal anti-inflammatory drugs and spinal nociceptive processing. *Pain* **59**, 9–43.

24. **Wall, P.D.** 1995: Inflammatory and neurogenic pain: new molecules, new mechanisms. *British Journal of Anaesthesia* **75**(2), 123–14.

25. **Barrett, D.H.** 1998: Stereoisomers and anaesthetics. *South African Journal of Anaesthesiology and Analgesia* **4**(3), 24–30.

26. **Merry, A. and Power, I.** 1995: Perioperative NSAIDs: towards greater safety. *Pain Reviews* **2**, 268–91.

27. **Pairet, M.** 1996: Selective COX-2 inhibitors: a phar-macological profile. *Eighth APLAR Congress of Rheumatology Abstract Book*, 13–17.

28. **Bensen, W. and Zizzo, A.** 1998; Newer, safer non-steroidal anti-inflammatory drugs: rational NSAID selection for arthritis. *Canadian Family Physician* **44**, 101–2.

29. **Cryer, B. and Kimmey, M.B.** 1998: Gastrointestinal side effects of nonsteroidal anti-inflammatory drugs. *American Journal of Medicine* **105**(1B), 20S-30S.

30. **Camu, F.** Peripherally acting analgesics. In Keneally, J.P. and Jones, M.J. (eds) *150 Years on – a selection of papers presented at the 11th World Congress of Anaesthe-siologists*. Rosebery, NSW: Bridge Printery, 83–8.

31. **McQuay, H.J. and Moore, R.A.** 1998: An evidence-based resource for pain relief. Oxford: Oxford Uni-versity Press, 22, 187–92.

32. **Davies, N.M.** 1998: Review article: Non-steroidal anti-inflammatory drug-induced gastrointestinal permeability. *Alimentary Pharmacology Therapeutics* **12**(4), 303–20.

33. **Haslock, I.** 1998: Clinical economics review: Gas-trointestinal complications of non-steroidal anti-inflammatory drugs. *Alimentary Pharmacology and Therapeutics* **12**(2), 127–33.

34. **Shield, M.J.** 1998: Diclofenac/misoprostol: novel findings and their clinical potential. *Journal of Rheumatology* **51**(supplement), 31–41.

35. **Singh, G.** 1998: Recent considerations in non-steroidal anti-inflammatory gastropathy. *American Journal of Medicine* **105**(1B), 31S-38S.

36. **Calam, J.** 1998: Clinical science of *Helicobacter pylori* infection: ulcers and NSAIDs. *British Medical Bulletin* **54**(1), 55–62.

37. **Yeomans, N.D.** 1998: New data on healing of non-steroidal anti-inflammatory drug-associated ulcers and erosions. Omeprazole NSAID Steering Commit-tee. *American Journal of Medicine* **104**(3A), 56S-61S.

38. **Wang, X.** 1998: Aspirin-like drugs cause gastrointesti-nal injuries by metallic cation chelation. *Medical Hypotheses* **50**(3), 227–38.

39. **Griffin, M.R.** 1998: Epidemiology of nonsteroidal anti-inflammatory drug-associated gastrointestinal injury. *American Journal of Medicine* **104**(3A), 23S-29S.

40. **McQuay, H.J. and Moore, R.A.** 1998: *An evidence-based resource for pain relief.* Oxford: Oxford University Press, 251–7.

41. **Bach, P.H. and Nguyen, T.K.** 1998: Renal papillary necrosis – 40 years on. *Toxicology and Pathology* **26**(1), 73–91.

42. **Harris, K.** 1992: The role of prostaglandins in the control of renal function. *British Journal of Anaesthesia* **69**(3), 233–5.

43. **Tolman, K.G.** 1998: Hepatotoxicity of non-narcotic analgesics. *American Journal of Medicine* **105**(1B), 13S-19S.

44. **Brooks, P.** 1998: Use and benefits of nonsteroidal anti-inflammatory drugs. *American Journal of Medicine* **104**(3A), 9S-13S.

45. **Monahan, S.J., Johnson, C.J., Downing, J.E., Fontenot, K.J. and Buhrman, W.C.** 1992: Post arthroscopy analgesia with intra-articular ketorolac. *Anesthesiology* **77**(3A), A854.

46. **Tramer, M.R., Williams, J.E., Carroll, D., Wiffen, P.J., Moore, R.A. and McQuay, H.J.** 1998: Comparing analgesic efficacy of non-steroidal anti-inflammatory drugs given by different routes in acute and chronic pain: a qualitative systematic review. *Acta Anaesthesi-ologica Scandinavica* **42**(1), 71–9.

47. **McQuay, H.J. and Moore, R.A.** 1998: *An evidence-based resource for pain relief.* Oxford: Oxford University Press, 11, 94–101.

48. **Moore, R.A., Tramer, M.R., Carroll, D., Wiffen, P.J. and McQuay, H.J.** 1998: Quantitative systematic review of topically applied non-steroidal anti-inflam-matory drugs. *British Medical Journal* **316**(7128), 333–8.

49. **Gopinath, R.** 1991: Venous sequelae after IV diclofenac. *British Journal of Anaesthesia* **67**, 803.

50. **Berde, C.B.** 1996: Peripheral, spinal, and supraspinal targets of opioids and NSAIDs. *IASP Newsletter*, (May/Jun), 3–4.

51. **Murrell, G.C., Leake, T. and Hughes, P.J.** 1996: A comparison of the efficacy of ketorolac and indomethacin for postoperative analgesia following laparoscopic surgery in day patients. *Anaesthesia and Intensive Care* **24**, 237–40.

52. **Plummer, J.L., Owen, H., Ilsley, A.H. and Tordoff, K.** 1996: Sustained-release ibuprofen as an adjunct to morphine patient-controlled analgesia. *Anesthesia and Analgesia* **83**, 92–6.

53. **Wang, B.C., Hiller, J.M., Simon E.J., Li, D., Rosen-berg, C. and Turndorf, H.** 1992: Analgesia following subarachnoid sodium ibuprofen in rats. *Anesthesiol-ogy* **77**(3A), A862.

54. **Perttunen, K., Kalso, E., Heinonen, J. and Salo, J.** 1992: IV diclofenac in post-thoracotomy pain. *British Journal of Anaesthesia* **68**, 474–80.

55. **Hommeril, J.L., Bernard, J.M., Gouin, F. and Pinaud, M.** 1992: IV ketoprofen versus epidural morphine for postoperative analgesia. *Anesthesiology* **77**(3A), A848.

56. **Kenny, G.N.C.** 1990: Ketorolac trometamol – a new non-opioid analgesic. *British Journal of Anaesthesia* **65**(4), 445–7.

57. **Krimmer, H., Bullingham, R.E.S. and Lloyd, J.** 1992: Effects on biliary tract pressure in humans of intravenous ketorolac tromethamine compared with morphine and placebo. *Anesthesia and Analgesia* **75**, 204–7.

58. **McQuay, H.J. and Moore, R.A.** 1998: *An evidence-based resource for pain relief.* Oxford: Oxford University Press, 10, 78–83.

59. **Shipton, E.A. and Van Der Merwe, C.** 1993: The perioperative pain care of patients – an update. *South African Journal of Continuing Medical Education* **11**(3), 459–66.

60. **Wong, H., Carpenter, R., Fragen, R., Kopacz, D. and Thompson, G.** 1992: An evaluation of ketorolac as sole analgesic after outpatient surgery. *Anesthesiology* **77**(3A), A6.

61. **Newton, P.T., Morley-Forster, P.K. and Cook, M.J.** 1992: Intramuscular ketorolac and rectal indomethacin are equally efficacious for the relief of minor postoperative pain. *Anesthesiology* **77**(3A), A14.

62. **Eisenberg, E., Berkey, C., Carr, D.B., Chalmers, T.C. and Mosteller, F.** 1994: NSAIDs for cancer pain: meta-analysis of efficacy. In Gebhart, G.E., Hammond, D.L. and Jensen, T.S. (eds) *Proceedings of the 7th World Congress on Pain – progress in pain research and management.* Seattle: IASP Press, 697–707.

63. **WHO Expert Committee on Cancer Pain Relief and Active Supportive Care** 1996: Choice of analgesic. In *Cancer pain relief,* 2nd edn. Singapore: Publications Office, World Health Organisation, 17–37.

64. **Eisenberg, E. and Birkhan, J.** 1995: Non-steroidal anti-inflammatory drugs for cancer-related pain. *Current Opinion in Anaesthesiology* **8**(5), 469–72.

65. **Watson, A.J.** 1998: Chemopreventive effects of NSAIDs against colorectal cancer: regulation of apoptosis and mitosis by COX-1 and COX-2. *Histology and Histopathology* **13**(2), 591–7.

66. **Silverstein, F.E.** 1998: Improving the gastrointestinal safety of NSAIDs: the development of misoprostol – from hypothesis to clinical practice. *Digestive Diseases and Sciences* **43**(3), 447–58.

67. **Ventafridda, V., De Conno, F., Panerai, A.E., Maresca, V. and Monza, G.C.** 1990: Non-steroidal anti-inflammatory drugs as the first step in cancer pain therapy: a double-blind within patient study comparing nine drugs. *Journal of International Medical Research* **18**(1), 21–9.

68. **Gillis, J.C. and Brogden, R.N.** 1997: Ketorolac: a reappraisal of its pharmacodynamic and pharmacokinetic properties and therapeutic use in pain management. *Drugs* **53**(1), 139–88.

69. **Kenny, G.N.C., McArdle, C.S. and Aitken, H.H.** 1990: Parenteral ketorolac: opiate-sparing effect and lack of cardiorespiratory depression in the perioperative patient. *Pharmacotherapy* **10**(6), 127S–131S.

70. **Glassman, S.D., Rose, S.M., Dimar, J.R., Puno, R.M., Campbell, M.J. and Johnson, J.R.** 1998: The effect of postoperative nonsteroidal anti-inflammatory drug administration on spinal fusion. *Spine* **23**(7), 834–8.

71. **Snyman, J.R. and Pope, A.I.** 1996: Meloxicam: a new non-steroidal anti-inflammatory (NSAID). In *MIMS product focus* (May), 1–14.

72. **Merry, A.F., Wardall, G.J., Cameron, R.J., Peskett, M.J. and Wild, C.J.** 1992: Perspective, controlled, double-blind study of IV tenoxicam for analgesia after thoracotomy. *British Journal of Anaesthesia* **69**, 92–4.

73. **Jeunet, F., Enz, W. and Guentert, T.** 1989: Tenoxicam used as a parenteral formulation for acute pain in rheumatic conditions. *Scandinavian Journal of Rheumatology* **80**, 59–61.

74. **De Conno, F., Ripamonti, C., Bianchi, M., Ventafridda, V. and Panerai, A.E.** 1992: Diclofenac does not modify morphine bioavailability in cancer patients. *Pain* **48**, 401–2.

75. **Quiding, H., Grimstad, J., Rusten, K., Stubhaug, A., Bremnes, J. and Breivik, H.** 1992: Ibuprofen plus codeine, ibuprofen, and placebo in a single- and multidose cross-over comparison for co-arthrosis pain. *Pain* **50**, 303–7.

76. **Pollack, C.V., Sanders, D.Y. and Severance, H.W.** 1991: Emergency department analgesia without narcotics for adults with acute sickle cell pain crisis: case reports and review of crisis management. *Journal of Emergency Medicine* **9**(6), 445–52.

77. **Birch, P.J.** 1995: Clinical relevance of receptor pharmacology in the nociceptive pathway. *Pain Reviews* **2**, 13–27.

78. **Goudas, L.C. and Carr, D.B.** 1996: Postoperative pain control: a survey of promising drugs and pharmacoeconomic criteria for purchasing them. In Campbell, J.N. (ed.) *Pain 1996 – an updated review.* Seattle: IASP Press, 189–94.

79. **Rang, H.P. and Urban, L.** 1995: New molecules in analgesia. *British Journal of Anaesthesia* **75**, 145–56.

80. **Walker, R.J.** 1991: Paracetamol, non-steroidal anti-inflammatory drugs and nephrotoxicity. *New Zealand Medical Journal* **104**(911), 182–3.

81. **McQuay, H.J. and Moore, R.A.** 1998: *An evidence-based resource for pain relief.* Oxford: Oxford University Press, 9, 58–77.

82. **Du Plooy, N.** 1993: *Drugs in anaesthesia.* Pretoria: Specialist Publications, 45–6.

5 SECONDARY ANALGESICS (PART I)

Secondary analgesics are defined as those agents having a pain-relieving property as a secondary aspect of their clinical activity. They can, however, be used as sole analgesic agents to treat various types of pain states. For example, in the management of cancer pain, they are used:[1]

■ to treat specific types of pain that do not respond to opioids;
■ to ameliorate other symptoms that commonly occur in cancer pain.

They are usually classified according to their mode of action.

CLASSIFICATION OF SECONDARY ANALGESICS

Secondary analgesics can be classified into (see also Chapter 6):

■ psychoactive agents
■ muscle relaxants
■ cardiovascular drugs
■ ketamine and other NMDA antagonists
■ enzyme inhibitors
■ cytotoxic agents
■ miscellaneous

PSYCHOACTIVE AGENTS

These are divided into three groups:

1. antidepressants
2. anticonvulsants
3. anxiolytics.

Antidepressants

MECHANISM OF ANTIDEPRESSIVE ACTION OF TRICYCLIC AND TETRACYCLIC ANTIDEPRESSANTS

These block α_1-adrenergic, H_1-histaminergic and muscarinic receptors and inhibit uptake-1 to presynaptic stores of the neurotransmitter catecholamines (serotonin, dopamine and noradrenaline) in the central nervous system (CNS).

Theories for their modes of action in pain are as follows:

■ *Masked depression hypothesis.* Antidepressants decrease pain through an alleviation of a masked depression.
■ *Manifest depression hypothesis.* The alleviation of depression induces an increase in the tolerance of pain, and this brings about analgesia.
■ *Sedation hypothesis.* Pain reduction is an epiphenomenon of a more general sedating effect accompanying the antidepressant effect.
■ *Placebo hypothesis.* The analgesic effects of antidepressants are considered to be a placebo artefact.
■ *Biochemical hypothesis.*

The evidence for their mechanism of action is as follows:

- Analgesic properties are already manifest in doses smaller than those usually effective in depression. The effective plasma levels are lower than those required for an antidepressant effect.[2]
- The analgesic response seems to come into action earlier (within the first week) than the antidepressant response (usually after 2 weeks).[2]
- Analgesic effects are observed in animals and humans in acute pain.[2] Tricyclics induce antinociceptive effects in rats rendered neuropathic by ligatures on the sciatic nerve.[3]
- Drugs inhibiting monamines less selectively do better as analgesics than do more selective drugs. This points to both serotonin and noradrenaline being involved in the analgesic effects of the antidepressants.[2]

There is a balance between the functions of serotonin and noradrenaline in the periventricular areas of the brain.[4] Activity in the encephalinergic cells of the peri-aqueductal grey area excites serotonergic cells in the dorsal raphe nucleus.[5] These activate a series of cells in the midline structure of the lower brain stem and medulla. The axons of the serotonergic cells travel in the dorsal lateral columns of the spinal cord and terminate in the dorsal horns, where they, in turn, excite encephalinergic interneurones.[5] These inhibit other cells that form part of the afferent pain neuronal train. The finding that drugs inhibiting monoamines less selectively do better than selective drugs is in line with pharmacological evidence that both serotonin and noradrenaline may be involved in the analgesic effects of the antidepressants.[2] Effective antidepressants ultimately increase CNS serotonergic function. The analgesic properties of the tricyclic agents depends on interrelated central serotonergic and opioid mechanisms. Tricyclic antidepressants appear to produce analgesia by potentially decreasing the serotonergic link in the endogenous opioid-mediated antinociception system, the site of which is likely to be at the level of the spinal cord.[6] Descending inhibitory serotonin and noradrenaline are entirely separate, opioid linkage only occurring in the former.[6]

Antidepressants have been reported to relieve pain in a number of different pain syndromes (e.g. myofascial pain), but only in diabetic neuropathy pain and in post-herpetic neuralgia has there been enough work to outline the principles of their analgesic pharmacology[1,7–9]. Pain relief is usually partial and accompanied by side-effects. All tricyclics that relieve neuropathic pain block noradrenaline (e.g. amitriptyline, nortriptyline, imipramine, clomipramine and desipramine).[8] In neuropathic pain, selective noradrenaline reuptake blockers are effective and may be used as alternatives to amitriptyline or imipramine.[9]

A *peripheral* action of the antidepressants via the inhibition of prostaglandin synthetase has been suggested because of their efficacy in arthritis.[10]

The analgesic effects of antidepressants have recently been investigated using four antidepressants (imipramine, citalopram, amitriptyline and maprotiline) after single-dose, 21-day long administration in rats.[11] The results obtained indicated:[11]

- a disparate sensitivity to antidepressant treatment of differently evoked behavioural reactions to the nociceptive stimuli;
- that the most potent effects of the administered antidepressants occurred in the model of visceral pain;
- that there was no relationship between the analgesic and antidepressant-like effects.

It has also been suggested that alterations in serum levels of aspartate, asparagine, serine, threonine and taurine might predict the subsequent response to treatment with antidepressants, and that the latter might modify the serum levels of excitatory amino acids and taurine.[12]

GUIDELINES FOR THE USE OF TRICYCLIC AND TETRACYCLIC ANTIDEPRESSANTS[1,4]

- Use tricyclics with serotonergic and noradrenergic effects (amitriptyline or doxepin).
- Use these in depressive patients with pain complaints.
- Use antidepressants in patients with pain on an organic basis when all other treatments have failed.
- Use these drugs in patients with pain in the head region.

Treatment should start with lower doses in non-depressive patients (because tricyclics might cause distressing anticholinergic side-effects in higher doses).[2] With sleeping problems (frequently related to chronic pain), a sedative antidepressant (amitriptyline or doxepin) should be used. This improves the patient's sleeping pattern and enables hypnotics to be discontinued.[2]

ANTIDEPRESSANT DRUGS

Tricyclic antidepressants

The most often reported tricyclic agents for pain care are the tertiary end-chain tricyclics. Amitriptyline is the tricyclic most commonly used.[1] Dothiepin is often more suited to the elderly and more debilitated patient. Other tricyclics used include imipramine, clomipramine, butriptyline, trimipramine and amoxapine,[1] which are more lipophilic than the secondary tricyclics (nortriptyline, desipramine and protriptyline). The greater intrinsic analgesic activity of tertiary amine tricyclics has been attributed to their increased lipophilicity.[13] A modified tricyclic, maprotiline, can also be used. Desipramine, with its selective noradrenergic action, can relieve neuropathic pain (e.g. painful diabetic neuropathy and post-herpetic neuralgia).[13] It has a better side-effect profile than amitriptyline with the fewest anticholinergic and sedative effects of the first-generation tricyclics.[7] Doxepin, trimepramine and amoxapine can give rise to tardive dyskinesia.

Selective serotonin reuptake inhibitors

In recent years, more specific serotonin reuptake inhibitors (SSRIs) – zimelidine, fluvoxamine, fluoxetine, paroxetine and trazodone – have been introduced. The role of SSRIs as analgesics is controversial. Fluoxetine was ineffective in the management of diabetic neuropathic pain, but paroxetine did have an effect.[8] This suggests that serotonin uptake blockade alone is insufficient to relieve pain. Further work is needed to see whether SSRIs are effective at all.[9] Prospective concentration–response studies are almost lacking. Such studies are needed in at least one other chronic pain condition besides neuropathic pain to determine whether the results can be generalized to other chronic pain syndromes. A recent randomized controlled trial (RCT) showed no difference with sertraline in pain or functional disability in women with chronic pelvic pain.[14]

Amitriptyline, fluvoxamine and paroxetine have their effects mainly on serotonin, while desipramine is biased towards noradrenaline.[6] Their acute potentiation of morphine analgesia will later be reduced as a result of the downregulation of opioid and serotonin receptors. Venlafaxine and nefazodone are novel antidepressants inhibiting the uptake of both serotonin and noradrenaline, with minimal anticholinergic activity and a adrenergic blocking activity.[8] Efficacy has not been established in randomized controlled trials, but two reports have shown SSRIs to be less effective analgesics than the tricyclics.[15] In fact, acutely administered SSRIs (fluoxetine and fluvoxamine) may exacerbate an acute type of pain.[16] With SSRIs, the rate of major side-effects is half that seen with tricyclic antidepressants.[15] Combinations of SSRIs/bupropion and noradrenergic tricyclics are especially effective in treating refractory depression.[17] Could the same be true of pain? Sustained-release bupropion, with a better side-effect profile, is now available.[18]

Tetracyclic antidepressants

Tetracyclic antidepressants have reduced cardiotoxicity compared with the tricyclic agents.[19]

Mianserin is an example of a tetracyclic antidepressant used clinically. Its tetracyclic structure ensures fewer anticholinergic side-effects, but it is sedative. Because of this, it is given an hour before bedtime, starting with 10–30 mg nightly and increasing step by step to 60–120 mg.[1] Mianserin occasionally gives rise to paradoxical aggression and agranulocytosis.

Monoamine oxidase inhibitors

These agents benefit some patients whose depression and pain do not respond to tricyclic antidepressants. A previous drug history needs to be carefully evaluated, and a tyramine-free diet needs to be followed. There are two types of monoamine oxidase inhibitor (MAOI):

- the hydrazines, for example phenelzine;
- the non-hydrazines, for example tranylcrypromine.

Monoamine oxidase is an enzyme present in the CNS, adrenergic nerve endings, liver and gastrointestinal tract. It degrades noradrenaline, adrenaline, dopamine and serotonin. The inhibition of monoamine oxidase increases the vesicular stores of noradrenaline, serotonin and dopamine within the neurones in the brain.

MAOI interactions with opioids take two forms:[20]

1. Type I (excitatory) interactions from central serotonergic overactivity, leading to agitation, hypertension, hypotension, rigidity, hyperpyrexia, convulsions and coma. Pethidine is the only commonly used opioid to have elicited the excitatory response.
2. Type II (depressive) effects from the inhibition of hepatic microsomal enzymes, which in turn increases the free opioid concentration. This leads to respiratory depression, hypotension and coma. Morphine is the opioid of choice to be used with MAOIs.

It is believed that an MAOI specific for monoamine

oxidase A, which is irreversibly bound to this enzyme and displaceable by tyramine, will be an antidepressant that will not cause a rise in blood pressure when tyramine-containing foods are ingested.[21] Many different reversible inhibitors of monoamine oxidase A (e.g. moclobemide) have recently become available, and many different candidate antidepressants with site-specific actions are being developed.[19] Their analgesic role needs testing.

Others

Viloxazine and lithium are used in patients with gross behavioural changes.

Results

Tricyclic antidepressants are effective in relieving neuropathic pain, yet a significant difference between them has not yet been shown, making a first choice still unclear.[15] Of a 100 patients prescribed antidepressants for neuropathic pain, 30 will obtain more than 50 per cent pain relief, 30 will have minor adverse reactions, and 4 will stop treatment because of major adverse effects.[15] Paroxetine and mianserin are less effective than imipramine.[15] Low-dose amitriptyline is effective in ankylosing spondylitis.[22]

Compared with placebo, in 6 out of 13 diabetic neuropathy studies, the combined relative benefit of using antidepressants was shown to be 1.9, with a numbers-needed-to-treat (NNT) for benefit of 3.[15] In three post-herpetic neuralgia studies, the combined relative benefit was 4.8, with an NNT of 2.3.[15] In two atypical facial pain studies, the combined relative benefit was 2, the NNT being 2.8.[15] In a central pain study, the NNT was 1.7.[15]

Anticonvulsants

MECHANISM OF ACTION AND USE

Anticonvulsants have membrane-stabilizing properties and act by the suppression of spontaneous neuronal firing.[1] They are used to stabilize the abnormal conduction of pain tracts, the lowest blood concentration necessary to control epilepsy usually being that needed for the control of pain. Anticonvulsants are used in lancinating neuropathic pain as a result of nerve damage, entrapment or changed function resulting from endocrine disorders.[8,23,24] These conditions include trigeminal neuralgia, post-herpetic neuralgia, phantom limb pain, causalgia, malignant infiltration of nerves and the denervation dysaesthesias in general.

GABAnergic mechanisms appear to be involved in the antinociceptive process. GABA-A agonists

(valproic acid and 3-benzyl-3-ethyl-2-piperidinone) enhance GABA-A synthesis and block its degradation to modulate nociceptive neurones.[25,26] In the spinal cord, there are at least three different GABA-A receptors responsible for spinally mediated antinociception caused by intrathecal midazolam, muscinol and 5-hydroxy-tryptamine.[27] (Baclofen, a GABA-B agonist, acts at both supraspinal and spinal sites.[28]

DRUGS USED

Carbamazepine is probably regarded as the drug of first choice. It is a potent drug with unpleasant side-effects (unsteadiness of gait, disorientation, nausea and vomiting). When carbamazepine is used, the starting dose is 100 mg a day for an adult, increasing by 100 mg every 4 days to a maximum of 400 mg a day. The target therapeutic blood level is at least $4\,\mu g/mL$. The drug can depress haematopoiesis.

Clonazepam is a benzodiazepine with a wide therapeutic index, and monitoring of drug levels in the blood is not necessary for therapeutic control. A side-effect is sedation, and treatment should begin with a small dose of 0.5 mg twice a day, working up to 1 mg three times a day over 4 weeks. Another benzodiazepine, clobazam, can also be used.[4]

Sodium valproate, if employed, is given in a dose of 200 mg 2–4 times a day in adult patients, aiming for a therapeutic blood level of $60\,\mu g/mL$. With phenytoin sodium, the initial dose is 100 mg per day in adults, increasing in 25 mg increments to a maximum of 300 mg per day. The therapeutic blood level aimed for is at least $10\,\mu g/mL$.

Low initial doses are appropriate for carbamazepine, oxycarbazepine, phenytoin, valproate, clobazam and clonazepam. Dose escalation should ensue until a favourable effect occurs, intolerable side-effects supervene or the plasma drug concentration has reached a predetermined level, which is customary at the upper end of the therapeutic range for seizure management.[29] Clinical experience is greatest with carbamazepine, but its use is limited in the cancer population by its potential to produce bone marrow suppression, particularly leukopaenia.[30] When any of these drugs are used, blood counts and liver function tests should be obtained before treatment and at regular intervals thereafter.

COMBINATIONS

A low-dose combination of anticonvulsants augments the efficacy of low-dose antidepressants.[31,32]

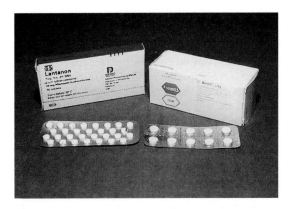

Figure 5.1 Antidepressant–anticonvulsant combinations: a combination of antidepressant mianserin (Lantanon®) and the anticonvulsant clonazepam (Rivotril®) to treat patients with combinations of burning and stabbing pains.

For better effect, tricyclics are often combined with phenothiazines (e.g. as amitriptyline and per-phenazine, amitriptyline and fluphenazine). An antidepressant-anticonvulsant combination (e.g. mianserin and clonazepam, nortriptyline and sodium valproate, or amitriptyline and oxycarb-azepine) can also be used (Figure 5.1).[1] An anti-depressant (e.g. a tricyclic agent) is useful for continuous dysaesthesia, and/or an anticonvulsant if the pain is lancinating or paroxysmal.[33] It is still necessary to determine the relative risk and benefit of the best and most appropriate anticonvulsant/antidepressant combination and compare them directly in neuropathic pain before a definite decision can be made regarding combination aug-mentation.[15]

NEWER ANTICONVULSANTS

New anticonvulsants exhibit limited drug interac-tions with fewer adverse effects, although there are few data in women of child-bearing age taking oral contraceptives.[34,35] These newer drugs include val-proyl glycinamide, fosphenytoin (a parenteral pro-drug of phenytoin that is more tolerable than parenteral phenytoin) and zonisamide.[34–36] For pain control, two major groups of drug have emerged, of which felbamate, gabapentin, lamotrigine, oxycarb-azepine, topiramate and vigabatrin are the most promising.[34,36] Vigabactrin (and tiagabine) act by enhancing brain GABA activity through the inhibi-tion of reuptake and catabolism, respectively.[34,35] The second group (e.g. lamotrigine, felbamate and topiramate) may have multiple mechanisms yet probably inhibit excitatory amino acids.[34,35] Lamot-rigine and its analogues can block sodium channels in a use-dependent manner, and can inhibit gluta-mate release in the rat striatum and cortex.[37] Oxcar-bazepine acts with similar efficacy to carbamazepine, with fewer side-effects and drug interactions.[38,39] These agents may represent a new class of analgesics in chronic pain conditions, where hypersensitivity exists and where conventional analgesics are ineffective.

Gabapentin and vigabatrin exhibit relatively ideal pharmacokinetic properties as they are not bound to proteins, are excreted mainly unchanged in the urine and show linear pharmacokinetics.[35] Lamotrigine has a variable elimination half-life depending on any co-medication.[35] Tiagabine is highly protein bound, and zonisamide shows non-linear pharmacokinetics; both are extensively metabolized.[35] Tiagabine is a mild drug with a favourable side-effect profile.[39] Fel-bamate may cause aplastic anaemia and fulminant hepatic failure, yet it remains useful because of its lack of sedative effects and high efficacy.[35,39] How-ever, in cases of pain, a trial of felbamate should only be considered in extreme cases because of its poten-tial for causing aplastic anaemia and for increasing seizure frequency on withdrawal.[40] Lamotrigine is non-sedating but prone to cause skin rash, headaches, drowsiness, nausea, vomiting, malaise and lassitude, and oxcarbazepine may cause symp-tomatic hyponatraemia.[35,39,41] Topiramate and vigaba-trin are highly effective in epilepsy, although each is associated with a variety of cognitive or psychiatric side-effects that may limit its utility.[39] Topiramate and zonisamide cause renal stones.[35]

Gabapentin is remarkable for its favourable side-effect profile, lack of interactions and straightfor-ward pharmacokinetics.[39] Although the cellular mechanisms of its pharmacological actions remain incompletely described, several hypotheses have been proposed:[42,43]

- Gabapentin crosses several membrane barriers in the body via a specific amino acid transporter (system L) and competes with leucine, isole-ucine, valine and phenylalanine for transport.
- Gabapentin increases the concentration and probably the rate of synthesis of GABA in the brain, which may enhance non-vesicular GABA release during seizures.
- Gabapentin binds with a high affinity to a novel binding site in brain tissues that is associated with an auxiliary subunit of the voltage-sensitive calcium ion current.
- Gabapentin reduces the release of several mon-amine neurotransmitters.

- Gabapentin increases the level of serotonin in human whole blood, which may be relevant to its neurobehavioural actions.
- Gabapentin prevents neuronal death by the inhibition of glutamate synthesis by branched-chain amino acid aminotransferase.
- Gabapentin and S (+)-3-isobutyl-gamma amino-butyric acid act at a common spinal locus to modulate selectively a facilitated state of nociceptive processing.

In the animal model, felbamate, gabapentin and lamotrigine appear to have the potential to be effective analgesics in neuropathic pain.[5,44] In humans, gabapentin is a useful adjunct for treating neuropathic pain, with a minimum of side-effects.[45] Examples include post-herpetic and trigeminal neuralgia, direct peripheral nerve injuries with lancinating neuropathic pain, immunotherapeutically induced (anti-GD ganglioside) allodynia, neuropathic pain of the head and neck, and HIV neuropathy.[8,30,43,45–50] Rarely, it may induce a polyneuropathy.[51]

Lamotrigine reduces post-operative analgesic requirements.[52] It is also effective in trigeminal neuralgia, migraine prophylaxis, pain with hyperalgesia, and central pain.[41,53–55]

RESULTS

Three placebo-controlled studies of carbamazepine found that in:[56,57]

- trigeminal neuralgia there was a combined NNT for effectiveness of 2.6 and for adverse effects of 2.5;
- diabetic neuropathy, the combined NNT for effectiveness was 3 and that for adverse effects 2.5;
- migraine, a combined NNT for effectiveness of 2.4 and for adverse effects of 2.4 was seen.

Carbamazepine had little effect on post-stroke pain.[56] Clonazepam was effective in one study of temporomandibular dysfunction,[56] whereas phenytoin has no effect in irritable bowel syndrome.[56] Few randomized controlled trials have shown analgesic effectiveness, and none has compared different anticonvulsants.[56]

Anxiolytics

PHENOTHIAZINE DERIVATIVES

Phenothiazine derivatives exert their effects by central dopaminergic blockade,[4] part of the molecule of clinically effective agents resembling that of dopamine. These agents are used for their analgesic and anxiolytic properties; they act as antiemetics and hypnotics and potentiate opioid analgesia.[4] Such drugs include chlorpromazine, perphenazine, fluphenazine, flupenthixol, pericyazine, prochlorperazine and methotrimeprazine. Methotrimeprazine has significant analgesic activity.[58] It allows for a decrease in tolerance to opioids by permitting a reduction of the opioid dose while still providing adequate analgesia. It is used in acute abdominal obstruction so that the opioid dosage can be reduced, thus not adding to the problem of obstruction.[1]

Controlled studies are few in number, although fluphenazine has been found to be effective chronic tension headache, cancer pain and in chronic osteoarthritis.[20] Orthostatic hypotension, sedation, parkinsonism and eprapyramidal side-effects can occur with these medications.[59]

BUTYROPHENONES

Haloperidol and droperidol also produce their effects by central dopaminergic blockade.[1] They are particularly used for their hypnotic, antiemetic and analgesic effects. They are useful agents to combine with opioids for long-term use but can, however, give marked postural hypotension and hallucinations. Haloperidol is used for patients in an agitated confusional state. Droperidol is used for its antiemetic and hypnotic effects with the administration of chemotherapy.

BENZODIAZEPINES

Benzodiazepines are useful in ameliorating the affective component of acute pain, possibly as a result of their anxiolytic action,[60] as anxiety presenting in patients with pain often diminishes once the pain is controlled.[1] Diazepam and midazolam are used to manage acute anxiety and panic states.

The use of benzodiazepines as hypnotics and anxiolytics in pain is becoming less and less. There is some evidence that benzodiazepines are beneficial for chronic tension headache, temporomandibular joint disorders and tic douloureux, but there is also evidence that diazepam may be antanalgesic (K. Budd, personal communication, 1998).[60]

Midazolam has been found to have analgesic effects when given intrathecally.[61,62] Intrathecal midazolam (2 mg) has been found to be as efficacious as epidural methyl prednisolone (80 mg) in the treatment of chronic mechanical low back pain, giving improvement in pain and activity for up to 2 months.[63] Intrathecal midazolam has also been found to be effective in the treatment of acute post-operative somatic pain, but its benefit is short-lived.[63,64] In rats, this effect has been demonstrated to be caused by an interaction of the drug with the GABA-A complex in the spinal cord, which causes activation of a spinal cord non-mu opioid pathway, possibly involving delta opioid receptor activation.[65] In the rat, intrathecal midazolam produces reversible, segmental, spinally mediated antinociception sufficient to provide balanced anaesthesia for abdominal surgery.[61] In the rabbit, intrathecal midazolam attenuates renal sympathetic activity,[66] but is intrathecal midazolam safe?[62] Neurotoxic effects have generally not been found in animals.[63] Histological spinal cord changes do occur following the epidural injection of acidic midazolam in neonatal rabbits.[67] Adding midazolam and bupivacaine to human CSF in glass test tubes neither decreased the pH below 7.0 nor reduced transparency.[68] The subject remains controversial, and the future of the neuraxial use of the benzodiazepines is uncertain at this stage.[59]

ANTIHISTAMINES

These include drugs such as diphenhydramine and hydroxyzine. These may be more effective as sedative medications than are the benzodiazepines or barbiturates. They do not lead to addiction or withdrawal crises on discontinuation of the drug. Hydroxyzine has anxiolytic, antihistaminic, antispasmodic and antiemetic properties. Additive analgesic effects occur when they are combined with opioids.[69] There is, however, limited evidence supporting the analgesic effects of the antihistamines, for example cluster headaches where clinical evidence suggests histamine involvement.[70]

Guidelines for the general use of psychoactive agents[1,4]

1. Use them to treat specific pain syndromes. Roles in malignant disease include the following:
   - for nerve destruction or neuropathic pain – an antidepressant/anticonvulsant combination (valuable, for example, for brachial, lumbar or sacral plexus infiltration, or for postsurgery neuropathic pain);
   - for superficial dysaesthetic pain – antidepressants;
   - for intermittent stabbing pain – anticonvulsants;
   - for nerve pressure pain – anticonvulsants and corticosteroids;
   - for muscle spasm pain – diazepam;
   - for pain and depression – antidepressants;
   - for pain and anxiety – benzodiazepines and phenothiazines;
   - for rectal and bladder tenesmus pain – chlorpromazine.
2. Use psychoactive agents to treat patients with a psychological component to their illness.
3. Use them when there is a lack of patient response to primary analgesics.
4. Use these drugs to treat specific responsive pathology (e.g. trigeminal neuralgia).
5. Use them to treat possible responsive pathology (e.g. atypical facial pain and postherpetic neuralgia).
6. Use them after a bizarre or paradoxical patient response to analgesic therapy.
7. Use psychoactive agents on the presentation of patients with bizarre symptomatology.

MUSCLE RELAXANTS

Conditions in which a painful lesion produces an associated muscular spasm (e.g. low back pain or

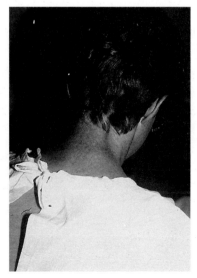

Figure 5.2 Patient with muscle spasm of her trapezius muscle needing relaxant agents.

chronic muscle tear) may be treated by the use of relaxant agents.[71] The relief of spasm will allow a more normal posture and gait, thereby reducing pain (Figure 5.2).

Diazepam

This benzodiazepine increases the efficiency of GABAnergic synapses by acting on specific benzodiazepine receptors in the CNS. In addition, it causes muscle relaxation by the inhibition of polysynaptic reflexes in the spinal cord.[1] The dosage is 2–5 mg three times a day. It should be used only for a short period of time. Other benzodiazepines that are occasionally used are nitrazapam and ketazolam.

Baclofen

Baclofen, a GABA-B agonist, has been used to treat spinal spasticity resulting from multiple sclerosis or spinal cord injury (Figure 5.3).[72] It acts presynaptically by preventing the influx of calcium ions and inhibiting transmitter release. It has efficacy in trigeminal neuralgia and is sometimes useful for other neuropathic pain syndromes.[8,29] The principal adverse side-effects are sedation and confusion. The potential for withdrawal syndromes necessitates tapering upon discontinuation.[23] It has been found to enhance the efficacy of management of postoperative dental pain. If there is no response to oral baclofen, intrathecal baclofen can be used by continuous infusion (50–800 μg per day).[72] The dose

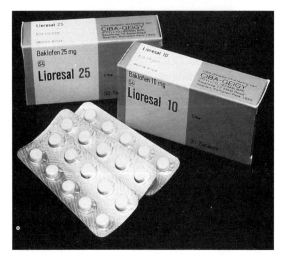

Figure 5.3 Baclofen (Lioresal®) a GABA$_B$ agonist used to treat spinal spasticity.

of oral baclofen is between 30 and 75 mg daily, starting with 5 mg three times daily and slowly working upwards. Analgesia caused by baclofen is increased by tolazoline, propranolol and nadolol.[72]

Dantrolene

This decreases the release or increases the sequestration of calcium ions from the lateral sacs of the sarcoplasmic reticulum.[1] It is contraindicated in acute hepatic disease. The dose is between 25 and 50 mg daily.

Orphenadrine

Orphenadrine blocks muscarinic cholinergic receptors and is given in a dosage of 100 mg twice daily. It has anticholinergic side-effects.

CARDIOVASCULAR DRUGS

Certain primary cardiovascular drugs are used in treating chronic pain.

Calcium channel blockers

Numerous experiments have shown that the neural processing of a painful stimulus is dependent on the movement of calcium.[73] Recent evidence suggests that N-type calcium channels located in the dorsal horn are involved in the processing of nociceptive stimuli. The intrathecal administration of SNX-III (a calcium channel blocker) produces antinociceptive effects in the rat.[73] These agents have the potential to reduce the amount of opioid required to produce an optimal analgesic effect. It has been found that some of the mechanisms involved in tolerance to morphine can be disrupted by sustained calcium channel blockade.[74]

Both nifedipine and diltiazem are used to control the pain of peripheral vascular disease. They have also been found to be of use in some of the more obscure peripheral neuralgic conditions.[75] Although diltiazem (60–120 mg three times daily) is less potent than nifedipine (10–20 mg three times daily), it shows fewer side-effects than nifedipine and is preferred.[75] Extensive clinical trials are needed to determine the analgesic efficacy and side-effect profile of these agents.

β-Adrenergic blockers

Certain β-adrenergic blocking agents (propranolol and metoprolol) are used in the prophylactic treatment of migraine.[75]

Local anaesthetics

Lignocaine and mexelitine, by blocking sodium channels, appear to suppress spontaneous injury and neuroma discharge in A delta and C fibres.[76] Systemic and oral local anaesthetics suppress ectopic neural pacemaker sites at lower concentrations than are required for conduction block along the nerve and may therefore have a prolonged duration of action.[8] An intravenous infusion of lignocaine of 5 mg/kg over 30–60 minutes may produce analgesia lasting several hours. This response has been the basis for starting an oral sodium channel blocker such as mexilitine although there are no randomized controlled trials to support the contention that intravenous lignocaine predicts the analgesic response to oral agents.[8] Two derivatives of lignocaine – tocainide and flecainide – are also used in neuropathic pain. Mexilitine is the safest of the local anaesthetics, and is preferred over flecainide and tocainide, although serious side-effects, including cardiac arrhythmias, liver damage and blood dyscrasias, are rare. All these drugs should be avoided in patients with cardiac rhythm disturbances and those on antiarrhythmic drugs.[29] The subcutaneous administration of lignocaine using an ambulatory infusion pump has been successfully used for the treatment of neuropathic cancer pain.[77]

Clonidine

The α_2-adrenergic agonists, such as clonidine, will be discussed in Chapter 6.

Adenosine

Adenosine receptors of the A_1 subtype are associated with a modulatory effect on pain transmission at the spinal cord level.[78] Animal studies have repeatedly demonstrated adenosine- and adenosine analogue-mediated inhibitory influences on nociceptive reflex responses in acute and inflammatory, as well as neuropathic, pain on both systemic and intrathecal administration.[78,79] Antinociception results from the inhibition of intrinsic neurones by an increase in potassium ion conductance and the presynaptic inhibition of sensory nerve terminals to inhibit the release of substance P and perhaps glutamate.[79]

There are observations suggesting some involvement of the spinal adenosine A_2 receptors in pain processing, but no data on any adenosine A_3 receptor involvement.[79] Endogenous adenosine systems contribute to antinociceptive properties of caffeine, opioids, noradrenaline 5-HT, tricyclic antidepressants and transcutaneous electrical nerve stimulation (TENS).[79] Purinergic systems exhibit the potential for development as therapeutic agents.

Other agents

Guanethidine and bretylium are used in the isolated limb for sympathetic dystrophy (see Chapter 10).[80]

Ketanserin (a 5-HT$_2$ antagonist) has been of some value in the treatment of algodystrophy and certain collagen diseases (e.g. Raynaud's disease).[80]

KETAMINE AND OTHER NMDA ANTAGONISTS

There is considerable evidence that NMDA receptor antagonists can abolish nociceptor hypersensitivity in animals.[81] Among the different sites of action, NMDA receptor antagonism is considered to be a most important central mechanism contributing to analgesic, amnesic, anaesthetic, psychomimetic and neuroprotective effects.[82–84] Ketamine has effects on ligand-operated and voltage-operated transmembrane ion channels, G protein-coupled receptors, transmitter uptake and the NO-cGMP system in neurones.[83] Moreover, the involvement of non-NMDA glutamate receptors, muscarinic and nicotinic cholinergic transmission, interactions with 5-HT receptors and L-type calcium channels accounts for some of its anaesthetic and neuroprotective properties.[83]

Until recently, ketamine was a racemic mixture containing equal amounts of two enantiomers, S(+) and R(−) ketamine, the main problems being psychological dysfunction and a prolonged period of arousal.[82,85] With the availability of S(+) ketamine, the analgesic and anaesthetic potency is 2–3 times higher, allowing up to a 50 per cent dose reduction to achieve comparable clinical results.[82] A faster elimination means a reduced drug load along with a more rapid recovery.[86] On a neuropharmacological basis, the clinical superiority of S(+) ketamine results from its effects on the NMDA receptors in the CNS, on opioid receptors at both central and peripheral levels, and on noradrenergic, dopaminergic and serotoninergic mechanisms.[85]

In rats, intrathecal preservative-free S(+) ketamine is effective for treating both inflammatory and neuropathic pain, offering future neuraxial administration in different pain states.[87,88] In abdominal surgery, pre-emptive ketamine decreases postoperative opioid requirements long after the normal expected duration of ketamine.[89] Oral ketamine is used as an analgesic and sedative for wound care procedures in the paediatric patient with burns.[90] Ketamine is effective in acute orofacial pain, adding to the evidence that the NMDA receptors are important for the perception of acute nociceptive pain in humans.[91] Long-term epidural ketamine, morphine and bupivacaine provide effective pain relief in chronic regional pain syndrome type 1.[81] Ketamine and gabapentin (an inhibitor of the neuronal synthesis of L-glutamate) can cure chronic migraine.[92] It has also been suggested that NMDA antagonists may play a role in treating very severe non-opioid analgesic drug dependence.[93] Dextropropoxyphene acts as a non-competitive NMDA antagonist.[94] Although consistently effective drug therapy for all neuropathic and sympathetically maintained pain is not yet available, the probability of the new NMDA antagonists being introduced offers promise.[95]

NMDA receptor activation is considered to be one of the mechanisms involved in postoperative pain and hypersensitivity.[96] The NMDA antagonist magnesium is the physiological blocker of the NMDA receptor complex-associated calcium ionophore, yet a perioperative magnesium infusion may or may not improve postoperative analgesia.[96,97] However, in chronic pain, NMDA antagonists such as MK801 delay the development of morphine tolerance.[97] In rats, the intrathecal coinfusion of magnesium with morphine over 7 days provided better analgesia than morphine alone.[97]

ENZYME INHIBITORS

ENKEPHALINASE INHIBITORS

A series of (4S)-4-[(2S)-benzyl-3-mercaptopropionylamino]-4-(N-phenylcarbamoyl)-butyric acids have been identified as potent systemically active enkephalinase inhibitors.[98] Prodrug analogues include 5b (ONO-9902).[98]

ANTICHOLINESTERASES

These agents, including pyridostigmine and physostigmine, reduce the dose of opioid needed to produce analgesia as well as somnolence.[4] Intrathecal neostigmine (100 μg) was recently found to be unsuitable for postoperative analgesia because of its side-effects of nausea and vomiting.[99]

ALDOSE REDUCTASE INHIBITORS

These agents include sorbinil and alrestatin. In the polyol pathway, glucose is converted to sorbitol under the enzymatic influence of aldose reductase. In uncontrolled diabetes, an excess of sorbitol accumulates in the nervous tissue and produces neuropathic changes.[4] The inhibition of aldose reductase by agents such as sorbinil and alrestatin will limit sorbitol formation, hence reducing pain and improving neurological function.[4] These drugs are, however, not yet commercially available.

NITRIC OXIDE (NO) SYNTHETASE INHIBITORS

Recent studies have suggested that the L-arginine/NO/cyclic GMP pathway is involved in the modulation of pain perception. The agents involved include NG-nitro-L-arginine methyl ester (L-NAME), NG-nitro-L-arginine (N-ARG) and 2-amino-4-methylpyridine.[100,101]

CYTOTOXIC AGENTS

Malignant conditions

Chemotherapy has an important role in palliating pain in different tumour types.[12] In germ cell tumours and non-Hodgkin's lymphoma, chemotherapy can be curative. In advanced breast cancer, chemotherapy is generally reserved for endocrine-resistant or rapidly progressing, life-threatening visceral disease.[102] Chemotherapy in prostate cancer is controversial. Mithramycin has been shown to have analgesic activity in pain from disseminated bone metastases.[75]

Endocrine therapy is often effective in relieving the bone pain of breast and prostate cancer.[102] In breast cancer, tamoxifen has become the treatment of choice in postmenopausal women with advanced breast cancer. Aromatase inhibitors (aminoglutethidione) are often used as second-line treatments. Premenopausal women can be treated using luteinizing hormone releasing agonists, which are also used in prostatic cancer. Other effective agents in prostatic cancer include cyproterone acetate, flutamide and ketoconazole.[102] More recently, the concept of total androgen blockade has been advocated. These agents may obviously decrease pain from the effects of malignant tissue.

Non-malignant conditions

Methotrexate is used for treating rheumatoid arthritis (both systemically and intra-articularly).

Mithramycin (50 μg/kg intravenously daily for 5 days) is used in Paget's disease to reduce pain.[23] Any relapse is treated with a single intravenous bolus dose as and when required.

MISCELLANEOUS DRUGS

Psychostimulants

Caffeine appears to have a direct analgesic effect in patients with headaches.[103] Its mechanism of action is unknown. In addition to CNS effects, it has anti-inflammatory, antipyretic and vasoconstrictive effects. Its use in postdural puncture headache may be a consequence of vasoconstriction.[103] High caffeine use may be embedded in the context of other unhealthy lifestyle behaviours.[104]

Dextroamphetamine, methylphenidate and cocaine have potent euphoric and antidepressant properties, and can produce spectacular short-term benefits in problem pain. Their use should be short term in terminal cancer patients where opioids result in excessive sedation.[59]

The potent analgesic effects of cannabis-like drugs and the presence of CB1-type cannaboid receptors in the pain-processing areas of the brain indicate that endogenous cannaboids (such as anandamide) attenuate pain behaviour by interacting with CB1-like cannaboid receptors located outside the CNS.[105]

Bromocriptine

Bromocriptine and danazol, evening primrose oil and tamoxifen have all been used successfully in the treatment of cyclical and non-cyclical mastalgia.[106]

Pyridoxine

Pyridoxine (vitamin B_6) is used in some pain clinics. Although not proven, it is thought to increase enkephalin release and dampen pain. It is given in a dose of 25 mg twice a day.

TRIPTANS (sumatriptan, zolmitriptan, naratriptan), Fenfluramine and Buspirone

It has been known for some time that intravenous serotonin will bring an abrupt end to a migraine, but its use as a practical therapy has been precluded by its other wide-ranging unwanted effects.[107] When investigators found that the blood vessels in the head contained almost exclusively one type of receptor (5-HT$_1$), agents were developed to bind to this receptor and no other, thereby mitigating serotonin's unwanted side-effects.[107] Sumatriptan is one such agent that selectively binds to 5-HT$_1$ receptors and increases serotonin's effects by constricting the meningeal vessels and reducing carotid blood flow.[107] Analgesia is induced by increasing cholinergic neurotransmission through the stimulation of 5-HT$_{1A}$ receptors.[108] Because it is selective, it has few side-effects. It can be administered orally in a 50 mg or 100 mg tablet form, intranasally in a 20 mg dose form or via the patient's own subcutaneous injection in a 6 mg dose.[59] Intravenous sumatriptan has been found to relieve the symptoms of severe migraine without affecting heart rate or blood pressure.[107] The autoradiographic distribution of [3H] sumatriptan binding sites in the human brain shows remarkable binding levels in the nucleus tractus solitarius and the nucleus trigeminalis caudalis, suggesting that, in migraine, sumatriptan could exert its specific antiemetic effects and, partly at least, induce analgesia by directly acting over these brain nuclei.[109]

Fenfluramine, a selective serotonin releaser, has been found to increase the analgesic potency of morphine but does not alter the intensity of typical opioid side-effects.[110]

Buspirone, a nonbenzodiazepine anxiolytic, is claimed to have antinociceptive properties, and, its analgesic efficacy has been demonstrated in experimental animal studies.[59] It acts as a serotonin agonist and may therefore possess antinociceptive properties.

Aminoglycosides

Streptomycin injected locally has recently been successfully used to treat intercostal neuralgia and scar pain,[111] and streptomycin has been used in dentistry for the treatment of facial pain.[112] Streptomycin–lignocaine injections have been found to be initially effective in the treatment of trigeminal neuralgia.[112]

The mode and site of action of streptomycin is unknown. It does, however, cause axonal swelling and disintegration of the myelin of large and small fibres respectively.[112] It stabilizes the nerve cell membrane and inhibits acetyl choline release at nerve endings.[112] The duration of contact with the nerve may contribute to pain relief.

Capsaicin

Topical capsaicin (8-methyl-N-vanillyl-noneamide) is known to be a safe and effective pain management adjunct for rheumatoid arthritis, osteoarthritis and post-herpetic and diabetic neuropathy.[113,114] It is also helpful for the itching and pain of the postmastectomy pain syndrome, oral mucositis, cutaneous allergy, loin pain/haematuria syndrome, neck pain, post-surgical neuropathic pain, stump pain and skin tumours, and may be beneficial for neural dysfunction [detrusor hyperreflexia, complex regional pain syndrome (CRPS) type 1 and rhinopathy].[113] High-dose capsaicin (5–10 per cent) administered with regional anaesthesia may effectively minimize CRPS and neuropathic pain.[115]

REFERENCES

1. **Shipton E.A.** 1991: Secondary analgesics in the treatment of pain from malignant disease. *Continuing Medical Education* **9**(6), 723–8.
2. **Onghena, P. and Van Houdenhove, B.** 1992: Antidepressant-induced analgesia in chronic non-malignant pain: a meta-analysis of 39 placebo-controlled studies. *Pain* **49**, 205–19.
3. **Archid, D. and Guilbaud G.** 1992: Antinociceptive effects of acute and chronic injections of tricyclic antidepressant drugs in a new model of mononeuropathy in rats. *Pain* **49**, 279–87.
4. **Budd, K.** 1989: The pain clinic – chronic pain. In Nunn, J.F., Utting, J.E. and Brown, B.R. (eds) *General Anaesthesia*, 5th edn. London: Butterworths, 1349–69.
5. **Bond, M.** 1984: *Pain – Its nature, analysis and treatment*, 2nd edn. Edinburgh: Churchill Livingstone, 3–20.
6. **Budd, K.** 1994: Monoamine function and analgesia. *Pain Reviews* **1**, 3–8.
7. **Kerrick, J.M., Fine, P.G., Lipman, A.G. and Love, G.** 1993: Low-dose amitriptyline as an adjunct to opioids for postoperative orthopaedic pain: a placebo-controlled trial. *Pain* **52**, 325–30.
8. **Moulin, D.E.** 1996: Medical management of chronic nonmalignant pain. In Campbell, J.N. (ed.) *Review Papers at 8th World Pain Congress*. Seattle: IASP Press, 485–92.
9. **Max, M.B.** 1994: Antidepressants as analgesics. In Fields, H.L. and Liebeskind, J.C. (eds) *Progress in pain research and management*. Seattle: IASP Press, 229–46.
10. **Archid, D., Eschalier, A. and Lavarenne, J.** 1991: Evidence for a central but not peripheral analgesic effect of clomipramine in rats. *Pain* **45**, 95–100.
11. **Korzeniewska-Rybicka, I. and Plaznik, A.** 1998: Analgesic effect of antidepressant drugs. *Pharmacological Biochemical Behaviour* **59**(2), 331–8.
12. **Maes, M., Verkerk, R., Vandoolaeghe, E., Lin, A. and Scharpe, S.** 1998: Serum levels of excitatory amino acids, serine, glycine, histidine, threonine, taurine, alanine and arginine in treatment-resistant depression: modulation by treatment with antidepressants and prediction of clinical responsivity. *Acta Psychiatrica Scandinavica* **97**(4), 302–8.
13. **Max, M.B, Kishore-Kumar, R., Schafer, S.C.** *et al.* 1991: Efficiency of desipramine in painful diabetic neuropathy: a placebo-controlled trial. *Pain* **45**, 3–9.
14. **Engel, C.C., Walker, E.A., Engel, A.L., Bullis, J. and Armstrong, A.** 1998: A randomised, double-blind crossover trial of sertraline in women with chronic pelvic pain. *Journal of Psychosomatic Research* **44**(2), 203–7.
15. **McQuay, H.J. and Moore, R.A.** 1998: *An evidence-based resource for pain relief*. Oxford: Oxford University Press, 31, 231–41.
16. **Dirksen, R., Van Luijtelaar, E.L. and Van Rijn, C.M.** 1998: Selective serotonin reuptake inhibitors may enhance responses to noxious stimulation. *Pharmacological Biochemical Behaviour* **60**(3), 719–25.
17. **Nelson, J.C.** 1998: Augmentation strategies with serotonergic-noradrenergic combinations. *Journal of Clinical Psychiatry* **59** (suppl. 5), 65–8.
18. **Settle, E.C.** 1998: Bupropion sustained release: side effect profile. *Journal of Clinical Psychiatry* **59** (suppl. 4), 32–6.
19. **Lynch, S. and Curran, S.** 1996: Antidepressants. *Psychiatry* **1**(2), 5–8.
20. **Stack, C.G., Rogers, P. and Linter, S.P.K.** 1988: Monamine oxidase inhibitors. *British Journal of Anaesthesia* **60**, 222–7.
21. **Harfenist, M., McGee, D.P.C., Reeves, M.D. and White, H.L.** 1998: Selective inhibitors of monoamine (MAO).5. 1-Substituted phenoxathiin inhibitors containing no nitrogen that inhibit MAO A by binding it to a hydrophobic site. *Journal of Medical Chemistry* **41**, (12), 2118–25.
22. **Koh, W.H., Pande, I., Samuels, A., Jones, S.D. and Calin, A.** 1997: Low dose amitriptyline in ankylosing spondylitis: a short term, double blind, placebo controlled study. *Journal of Rheumatology* **24**(11), 2158–61.

23. **Budd, K.** 1989: The pain clinic – chronic pain. In Nunn, J.F., Utting, J.E. and Brown, B.R. (eds) *General anaesthesia,* 5th edn. London: Butterworths, 1349–69.

24. **Agular, J.L., Montes, A. and Vidal, F.** 1992: Combined neurogenic and visceral pain in metastatic rectal cancer. *Pain Clinic* **5**(2), 81–4.

25. **Cutrer, F.M. and Moskowitz, M.A.** 1996: The actions of valproate and neurosteroids in a model of trigeminal pain. *Headache* **36**(10), 579–85.

26. **Hill, M.W., Reddy, P.A., Covey, D.F. and Rotham, S.M.** 1998: Inhibition of voltage-dependent sodium channels by the anticonvulsant gamma-aminobutyric acid type A receptor modulator, 3-benzyl-3-ethyl-2-piperidinone. *Journal of Pharmacology and Experimental Therapeutics* **285**(3), 1303–9.

27. **Nadeson, R., Guo, Z., Porter, V., Gent, J.P. and Goodchild, C.S.** 1996: Gamma-aminobutyric acid A receptors and spinally mediated nociception in rats. *Journal of Pharmacology and Experimental Therapeutics* **27**(2), 620–6.

28. **Sawynok, J.** 1984: GABAergic mechanisms in antinociception. *Progress in Neuropsychopharmacology Biology and Psychiatry* **8**(4–6), 581–6.

29. **Cherny, N.I. and Portenoy, R.K.** 1995: Systemic drugs for cancer pain. *Pain Digest* **5**, 245–63.

30. **Portenoy, R.K.** 1996: Nontraditional analgesics in the management of cancer pain. In Campbell, J.N. (ed.) *Review Papers at 8th World Pain Congress.* Seattle: IASP Press, 559–66.

31. **Dietrich, D.E. and Emrich, H.M.** 1998: The use of anticonvulsants to augment antidepressant medication. *Journal of Clinical Psychiatry* **59**(suppl. 5), 51–8.

32. **Sussman, N. and Joffe, R.T.** 1998: Antidepressant augmentation: conclusion and recommendations. *Journal of Clinical Psychiatry* **59**(suppl. 5), 70–3.

33. **Martin, L.A. and Hagen, N.A.** 1997: Neuropathic pain in cancer patients: mechanisms, syndromes, and clinical controversies. *Journal of Pain Symptom Management* **14**(2), 99–117.

34. **Emillien, G. and Maloteaux, J.M.** 1998: Pharmacological management of epilepsy: mechanism of action, pharmacokinetic drug interactions, and new drug discovery possibilities. *International Journal of Clinical Pharmacology and Therapeutics* **36**(4), 181–94.

35. **Natsch, S., Hekster, Y.A., Keyser, A., Deckers, C.L., Meinardi, H. and Renier, W.O.** 1997: Newer anticonvulsant drugs: role of pharmacology, drug interactions and adverse reactions in drug choice. *Drug Safety* **17**(4), 228–40.

36. **Curry, W.J. and Kulling, D.L.** 1998: Newer antiepileptic drugs: gabapentin, lamotrigine, felbamate, topiramate and fosphenytoin. *American Family Physician* **57**(3), 513–20.

37. **Nakamura-Craig, M. and Follenfant, R.L.** 1994: Lamotrigine and analogs: a new treatment for chronic pain. In Gebhart, G.F., Hammond, D.L. and Jensen, T.S. (eds) *Progress in pain research and management.* Seattle: IASP Press, 726–30.

38. **Beydoun, A.** 1997; Monotherapy trials of new antiepileptic drugs. *Epilepsia* **38**(suppl. 9), S21-S31.

39. **Blum, D.E.** 1998: New drugs for persons with epilepsy. *Advances in Neurology* **76**, 57–87.

40. **Welty, T.E., Privitera, M. and Shukla, R.** 1998: Increased seizure frequency associated with felbamate withdrawal in adults. *Archives of Neurology* **55**(5), 641–5.

41. **Steiner, T.J., Findley, L.J. and Yuen, A.W.** 1997; Lamotrigine versus placebo in the prophylaxis of migraine with and without aura. *Cephalalgia* **17**(2), 109–12.

42. **Taylor, C.P., Gee, NS., Su, T.Z. et al.** 1988: A summary of mechanistic hypotheses of gabapentin pharmacology. *Epilepsy Research* **29**(3), 233–49.

43. **Partridge, B.J., Chaplan, S.R., Sakamoto, E. and Yaksh, T.L.** 1998: Characterization of the effects of gabapentin and 3-isobutyl-gamma-aminobutyric acid on substance P-induced thermal hyperalgesia. *Anesthesiology* **88**(1), 196–205.

44. **Hunter, J.C., Gogas, K.R., Hedley, L.R. et al.** 1997: The effect of novel anti-epileptic drugs in rat experimental models of acute and chronic pain. *European Journal of Pharmacology* **324**(2–3), 153–60.

45. **Rosenberg, J.M., Harrell, C., Ristic, H., Werner, R.A. and de Rosayro, A.M.** 1997: The effect of gabapentin on neuropathic pain. *Clinical Journal of Pain* **13**(3), 251–5.

46. **McCaffery M.** 1998: Gabapentin for lancinating neuropathic pain. *American Journal of Nursing* **98**(4), 12.

47. **Gillin, S. and Sorkin, L.S.** 1998:Gabapentin reverses the allodynia produced by the administration of anti-GD2 ganglioside, an immunotherapeutic drug. *Anesthesia and Analgesia* **86**(1), 111–16.

48. **Newshan, G.** 1998: HIV neuropathy treated with gabapentin. *AIDS* **12**(2), 219–21.

49. **Carrazana, E.J. and Schachter, S.C.** 1998: Alternative uses of lamotrigine and gabapentin in the treatment of trigeminal neuralgia. *Neurology* **50**(4), 1192.

50. **Sist, T.C., Filadora, V.A., Miner, M. and Lema, M.** 1997: Experience with gabapentin for neuropathic pain in the head and the neck: report of ten cases. *Regional Anesthesia* **22**(5), 473–8.

51. **Gould, H.J.** 1998: Gabapentin induced polyneuropathy. *Pain* **74**(2–3), 341–3.

52. **Bonicalzi, V., Canavero, S., Cerutti, F., Piazza, M., Clemente, M. and Chio, A.** 1997: Lamotrigine reduces total postoperative analgesic requirement: a randomised double-blind, placebo-controlled study. *Surgery* **122**(3), 567–70.

53. **Zakrzewska, J.M., Chaudhry, Z., Nurmikko, T.J., Patton, D.W. and Mullens, E.L.** 1997: Lamotrigine (lamictal) in refractory trigeminal neuralgia: results from a double-blind placebo controlled crossover trial. *Pain* **73**(2), 223–30.

54. **Harbinson, J., Dennehy, F. and Keating, D.** 1997: Lamotrigine for pain with hyperalgesia. *Irish Medical Journal* **90**(2), 56.

55. **Canavero, S. and Bonicalzi, V.** 1996:. Lamotrigine control of central pain. *Pain* **68**(1), 179–81.

56. **McQuay, H.J. and Moore, R.A.** 1998: *An evidence-*

based resource for pain relief. Oxford: Oxford University Press 30, 221–30.

57. **McQuay, H., Carroll, D., Jadad, A.R., Wiffen, P. and Moore, A.** 1995: Anticonvulsant drugs for management of pain: a systematic review. *British Medical Journal* 311(7012), 1047–52.

58. **Foley, K.M. and Inturrisi, C.E.** 1987: Analgesic drug therapy in cancer pain: principles and practice. *Medical Clinics of North America* 71, 207–32.

59. **Murphy, T.M.** 1994: Psychoactive drugs for pain control. *Pain Reviews* 1, 9–14.

60. **Dellemijn, P.L.I. and Fields, H.L.** 1994: Do benzodiazepines have a role in chronic pain management? *Pain* 57, 137–52.

61. **Bahar, M., Cohen, M.L., Grinshpon, Y. and Chanimov, M.** 1997: Spinal anaesthesia with midazolam in the rat. *Canadian Journal of Anaesthesia* 44(2), 208–15.

62. **Malinovsky, J.M.** 1997: Is intrathecal midazolam safe? *Canadian Journal of Anaesthesia* 44(2), 1321–2.

63. **Serrao, J.M., Marks, R.L., Morley, S.J. and Goodchild, C.S.** 1992: Intrathecal midazolam for treatment of chronic mechanical low back pain: a controlled comparison with epidural steroid in a pilot study. *Pain* 48, 5–12.

64. **Valentine, J.M., Lyons, G. and Bellamy, M.C.** 1996: The effect of intrathecal midazolam on post-operative pain. *European Journal of Anaesthesiology* 13(6), 589–93.

65. **Goodchild, C.S., Guo, Z., Musgreave, A. and Gent, J.P.** 1996: Antinociception by intrathecal midazolam involves endogenous neurotransmitters acting at spinal cord delta opioid receptors. *Britsh Journal of Anaesthesia* 77(6), 758–63.

66. **Hashimoto, K., Karasawa, F. and Satoh, T.** 1997: Intrathecal midazolam attenuates renal sympathetic nerve activity in rabbits. *Masui* 46(8), 1059–65.

67. **Bozkurt, P., Tunali, Y., Kaya, G. and Okar, I.** 1997: Histological changes following epidural injection of midazolam in the neonatal rabbit. *Paediatric Anaesthetics* 7(5), 385–9.

68. **Nishiyama, T., Sugai, N. and Hanaoka, K.** 1998: In vitro changes in the transparency and pH of cerebrospinal fluid caused by adding midazolam. *European Journal of Anaesthesiology* 15(1), 27–31.

69. **Swerdlow, M. and Ventafridda, V.** 1987: *Cancer pain.* Lancaster: MTP Press, 83–8.

70. **Neubauer, D., Kuhar, M. and Ravnik, I.M.** 1997: Antihistamine responsive cluster headache in a teenaged girl. *Headache* 37(5), 296–8.

71. **Shipton, E.A.** 1989: Low back pain and the postlaminectomy pain syndrome. *South African Medical Journal* 76, 20–3.

72. **Kaufman, L.** 1991: Pain: In Kaufman, L. (ed.) *Anaesthesia review 8.* Edinburgh: Churchill Livingstone, 231–53.

73. **Miaskowski, C.** 1996: Pain assessment and management in nursing. In Campbell, J.N. (ed.) *Review Papers at 8th World Pain Congress.* Seattle: IASP Press, 9–12.

74. **Santillan, R., Maestre, J.M., Hurle, M.A. and Florez, J.** 1994: Enhancement of opiate analgesia by

nimodipine in cancer patients treated with morphine: a preliminary report. *Pain* 58, 129–32.

75. **Budd, K.** 1989: Recent advances in the treatment of chronic pain. *British Journal of Anaesthesia* 63, 207–212.

76. **Chabal, C., Russel, L.C. and Burchiel, K.J.** 1989: The effect of intravenous lidocaine, tocaimide, and mexilitine on spontaneously active fibres originating in rat sciatic neurones. *Pain* 38, 333.

77. **Brose, W.G. and Cousins, M.J.** 1991: Subcutaneous lidocaine for treatment of neuropathic cancer pain. *Pain* 45, 145–8.

78. **Sollevi, A.** 1997: Adenosine for pain control. *Acta Anaesthesiologica Scandinavica Supplement* 110, 135–6.

79. **Sawynok, J.** 1998: Adenosine receptor activation and nociception. *European Journal of Pharmacology* 347(1), 1–11.

80. **Shipton, E.A.** 1991: Recent advances in intractable pain control. *South African Medical Journal* 79, 119–20.

81. **Lin, T.C., Wong, C.S., Chen, F.C., Lin, S.Y. and Ho, S.T.** 1998: Long-term epidural ketamine, morphine and bupivacaine attenuate reflex sympathetic dystrophy neuralgia. *Canadian Journal of Anaesthesia* 45(2), 175–7.

82. **Adams, H.A. and Werner, C.** 1997: From the racemate to the eutomer: (S)-ketamine. Renaissance of a substance? *Anaesthetist* 46(12), 1026–42.

83. **Kress, H.G.** 1997: Mechanisms of action of ketamine. *Anaesthetist* 46 (suppl. 1), S8-S9.

84. **Wenk, G.L., Baker, L.M., Stoehr, J.D., Hauss-Wegrzyniak, B. and Danysz, W.** 1998: Neuroprotection by novel antagonists at the NMDA receptor channel and glycine B sites. *European Journal of Pharmacology* 347(2–3), 183–7.

85. **Hempelmann, G. and Kuhn, D.F.** 1997: Clinical significance of S(+) ketamine. *Anaesthetist* 46 (suppl. 1), S3-S7.

86. **Adams, H.A.** 1997: S(+) ketamine. Circulatory interactions during total intravenous anaesthesia and analgesia-sedation. *Anaesthetist* 46(12), 1081–7.

87. **Klimscha, W., Horvath, G., Szikszay, M., Dobos, I. and Benedek, G.** 1998: Antinociceptive effect of the S(+) enantiomer of ketamine on carrageenan hyperalgesia after intrathecal administration in rats. *Anesthesia and Analgesia* 86(3), 561–5.

88. **Sonoda, H. and Omote, K.** 1998: Suppressive effects of ketamine on neuropathic pain. *Masui* 47(2), 136–44.

89. **Fu, E.S., Miguel, R. and Scharf, J.E.** 1997: Preemptive ketamine decreases postoperative narcotic requirements in patients undergoing abdominal surgery. *Anesthesia and Analgesia* 84(5), 1086–90.

90. **Humphries, Y., Melson, M. and Gore, D.** 1997: Superiority of oral ketamine as an analgesic and sedative for wound care procedures in the pediatric patient with burns. *Journal of Burn Care and Rehabilitation* 18, 34–36.

91. **Mathisen, L.C., Skjebred, P., Skoglund, L.A. and Oye, I.** 1995: Effect of ketamine, an NMDA receptor

inhibitor, in acute and chronic orofacial pain. *Pain* **61**(2), 215–20.

92. **Nicolodi, M. and Sicuteri, F.** 1998: Negative modulators of excitatory amino acids in episodic and chronic migraine: preventing and reverting chronic migraine. *International Journal of Clinical Pharmacology* **18**(2), 93–100.

93. **Nicolodi, M., Del Bianco, P.L. and Sicuteri, F.** 1997: Modulation of excitatory amino acids pathway: a possible therapeutic approach to chronic daily headache associated with analgesic drugs abuse. *International Journal of Pharmacology Research* **17**(2–3), 97–100.

94. **Ebert, B., Andersen, S., Hjeds, H. and Dickenson, A.H.** 1998: Dextropropoxyphene acts as a noncompetitive N-methyl-D-aspartate antagonist. *Journal of Pain and Symptom Management* **15**(5), 269–74.

95. **Lipman, A.G.** 1996: Analgesic drugs for neuropathic and sympathetically maintained pain. *Clinial Geriatric Medicne* **12**(3), 501–15.

96. **Wilder-Smith, C.H., Knopfli, R. and Wilder-Smith, O.H.** 1997: Perioperative magnesium infusion and postoperative pain. *Acta Anaesthesiologica Scandinavica* **41**(8), 1023–7.

97. **McCarthy, R.J., Kroin, J.S., Tuman, K.J., Penn, R.D. and Ivankovitch, A.D.** 1998: Antinociceptive potentiation and attenuation of tolerance by intrathecal co-infusion of magnesium sulfate and morphine in rats. *Anesthesia and Analgesia* **86**(4), 830–6.

98. **Senokuchi, K., Nakai, H., Nagao, Y., Sakai, Y., Katsube, N. and Kawamura, M.** 1998: New orally active enkephalinase inhibitors: their synthesis, biological activity, and analgesic properties. *Bioorganic Medical Chemistry* **6**(4), 441–63.

99. **Lauretti, G.R., Mattos, A.L., Gomes, J.M. and Pereira, N.L.** 1997: Postoperative analgesia and antiemetic efficacy after intrathecal neostigmine in patients undergoing abdominal hysterectomy during spinal anaesthesia. *Regional Anesthesia* **22**(6), 527–33.

100. **Pavone, F., Capone, F., Populin, R. and Przewlocka, B.** 1997: Nitric oxide synthetase inhibitors enhance the antinociceptor effects of oxotremorine in mice. *Polish Journal of Pharmacology* **49**(1), 31–6.

101. **Pettipher, E.R., Hibbs, T.A., Smith, M.A. and Griffiths, R.J.** 1997: Analgesic activity of 2-amino-4-methylpyridine, a novel NO synthase inhibitor. *Inflammation Research* **46**(suppl. 2), S135-S136.

102. **Houston, S.J. and Rubens, R.D.** 1994: Metastatic bone pain. *Pain Reviews* **1**, 138–52.

103. Ward, N., Whitney, C., Avery, D. and Dunner, D. 1991: The analgesic effects of caffeine in headache. *Pain* **44**, 151–2.

104. **Currie, S.R., Wilson, K.G. and Gauthier, S.T.** 1995: Caffeine and low back pain. *Clinical Journal of Pain* **11**(3), 214–19.

105. **Calignano, A., La Rana, G., Guiffrida, A. and Piomelli, D.** 1998: Control of pain initiation by endogenous cannabinoids. *Nature* **394**(6690), 277–81.

106. **Gateby, C.A. and Mansel, R.E.** 1990: Breast pain. *Pain Clinic* **3**(4), 207–12.

107. **Overmyer, R.H.** 1990: The clinical use of serotonin receptors in migraine, emesis, and other presentations. *Modern Medicine of South Africa* (Sep), 33–9.

108. **Ghelardini, C., Galeotti, N., Nicolodi, M., Donaldson S., Sicuteri, F. and Bartolini, A.** 1997: Involvement of central cholinergic system in antinociception induced by sumatriptan in mouse. *International Journal of Pharmacological Research* **17**(2–3), 105–9.

109. **Pascual, J., Arco, C., Romon, T., del Olmo, E., Castro, E. and Pazos, A.** 1996: Autoradiographic distribution of [3H] sumatriptan-binding sites in post-mortem human brain. *Cephalalgia* **16**(5), 317–22.

110. **Coda, B.A., Hill, H.F., Schaffer, R.L., Luger, T.J., Jacobson, R.C. and Chapman, C.R.** 1993: Enhancement of morphine analgesia by fenfluramine in subjects receiving tailored opioid infusions. *Pain* **52**, 85–91.

111. **Gallagher, J. and Hammann, W.** 1989: Chronic neuropathic pain: aminoglycosides, peripheral somatosensory mechanisms and painful disorders. In Atkinson, R.S. and Adams, A.P. (eds) *Recent Advances in Anaesthesia and Analgesia* **126**, 191–205.

112. **Stajcic, Z.** 1992; The effects of streptomycin on autotomy. *Pain* **48**, 257–9.

113. **Hautkappe, M., Roizen, M.F., Toledano, A., Roth, S., Jeffries, J.A. and Ostermeier, A.M.** 1998: Review of the effectiveness of capsaicin for painful cutaneous disorders and neural dysfunction. *Clinical Journal of Pain* **14**(2), 97–106.

114. **Ellison, N., Loprinzi, C.L., Kugler, J.** *et al.* Phase III placebo-controlled trial of capsaicin cream in the management of surgical neuropathic pain in cancer patients. *Journal of Clinical Oncology* **15**(8), 2974–80.

115. **Robbins, W.R., Staats, P.S., Levine, J.** *et al.* Treatment of intractable pain with topical large-dose capsaicin: preliminary report. *Anesthesia and Analgesia* **86**(3), 579–83.

6 SECONDARY ANALGESICS (PART II)

CLASSIFICATION OF SECONDARY ANALGESICS[1]

The remaining classes secondary analgesics are:

- hormones
- catecholamine precursors
- catecholamine antagonists
- opioid antagonists.

HORMONES

Corticosteroids

Corticosteroids (Figure 6.1) are of greatest value in

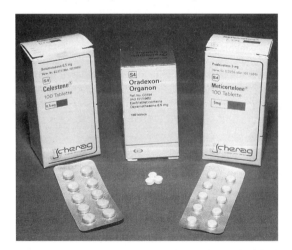

Figure 6.1 Corticosteroids used as secondary analgesics.

peripheral nerve trauma, malignant disease and rheumatoid and degenerative arthritis.

PERIPHERAL NERVE TRAUMA

Peripheral nerve trauma is caused by entrapment or direct nerve damage. The traumatized area is treated with a mixture of a local anaesthetic (lignocaine, bupivacaine or ropivacaine) and a corticosteroid (hydrocortisone, methylprednisolone or triamcinolone).[2] The efficacy of epidural corticosteroid injections for low back pain and sciatica has not yet been established in the long term,[3] the best studies having shown only inconsistent results.[3] The benefits of epidural corticosteroids, if any, seem to be of short duration only.[3] Future research efforts concentrating on trial methodology are warranted. Cervical epidural corticosteroid injections have produced excellent and complete long-term results in 70.8 per cent of patients suffering from chronic radicular pain unrelated to a compressive or malignant origin.[4] However, using epidural corticosteroids for sciatica, the short-term numbers-needed-to-treat (NNT) (of 50 per cent pain relief) is just under 3, the long-term NNT being 13.[5] For patients with chronic painful disease, interventions may be attractive even if their success rate is far lower than would be acceptable in postoperative pain.[5]

MALIGNANT DISEASE

Corticosteroids have a membrane stabilizing effect and block C and A delta fibre transmission.[6] Corticosteroids have anti-inflammatory properties and relieve pain associated with nerve and spinal cord compression.[7] They lessen headache from raised intracranial pressure and reduce pain produced by tumour pressure as they reduce tumour size and surrounding tissue oedema.[8] Prednisolone, betamethasone and dexamethasone are all effective. Corticosteroids also enhance the mood and improve the appetite. They prevent the release of prostaglandins by their stabilizing effect on cell membranes, making them useful for bone pain.[7] They are of use in both nociceptive and neuropathic pain.

High doses are often required initially, for example prednisolone 60 mg daily or dexamethasone 4 mg 6-hourly, which can be maintained for a week.[8] If the corticosteroid does not help, it should be discontinued. If there is a response, the dose should be reduced to the lowest possible maintenance dose.[8] Misoprostol prophylaxis seems protective for patients receiving high doses of corticosteroids and for those with a previous history of peptic ulceration.[9] One large survey of acceptably low-dose corticosteroid therapy in patients with advanced cancer suggests that the actual risk of serious side-effects is acceptably low.[10]

There have been no systemic studies to evaluate the possibility of drug-selective differences, the dose–response relationships for the various effects, the predictors of efficacy or the durability of favourable effects.[10]

The painful conditions that usually respond to corticosteroids include raised intracranial pressure, acute spinal cord compression, superior vena cava syndrome, metastatic bone pain, neuropathic pain resulting from infiltration or compression by tumour, symptomatic lymphoedema and hepatic capsular distension.[11, 12]

RHEUMATOID AND DEGENERATIVE ARTHRITIS

Corticosteroids are either given orally (pulse dosing, where possible, being increasingly preferred to chronic daily dosing; P. Dessein, E.A. Shipton, personal research data, 1999), intravenously or intramuscularly, or are injected into trigger points, joints or the epidural space.

Calcitonin

Calcitonin is secreted by the parafollicular cells of the thyroid gland. Calcitonin has been shown to have analgesic effects in Paget's disease, in patients with osteoclastic metastases, in phantom limb pain and in complex regional pain syndrome (type 1).[10,13,14] Although it is known to be an osteoclast

inhibitor,[10] the exact mechanism by which it inhibits or modulates pain perception is unknown.[15] Its analgesic actions can be reversed by serotonin-blocking agents (methysergide) so it probably produces its effects via a serotonergic mechanism.[13]

Three forms of calcitonin – porcine, salmon and human – are available. The optimal dose, route of administration and dosing frequency of calcitonin are unknown, and the durability of favourable effects has not been evaluated systematically.[10] To date, therapy has involved daily or twice daily subcutaneous administration. Following skin testing with 1 i.u., a low starting dose such as 25 i.u. daily is gradually increased to 100–200 i.u. per day.[10] When used to treat the pain of Paget's disease, 50–100 i.u. daily for 3–6 months is recommended.[9] It can be used combined with disodium etidromate. For the acute treatment of pain from bone metastases, 200–400 i.u. 6–12 hourly for 48 hours is advised.[15] Intranasal salmon calcitonin (1000 i.u. given three times daily) has been found to decrease pain (at rest and on movement) when added to physical therapy in patients with complex regional pain syndromes (type 1).[10] An infusion of calcitonin can be used.[13] Salmon calcitonin appears to be more potent than betablockers, antidepressants, neuroleptics and transcutaneous electrical nerve stimulation (TENS) in alleviating phantom limb pain.[13]

Randomized controlled trials have found that calcitonin reduces the acute pain associated with osteoporotic fractures and is useful in treating chronic back pain following vertebral fractures in spinal osteoporosis.[16] It can prevent bone loss and may be effective in preventing fractures.[16] Side-effects are dose related and are usually mild; they include gastrointestinal, vascular and dermatological conditions that can be treated symptomatically or by varying the dosage.[16] Most side-effects can be avoided with nasal administration.[16]

Biphosphonates

The biphosphonates are enzyme-resistant analogues of pyrophosphate, the naturally occurring inhibitor of bone mineralization.[17] Etidronate, clodronate and pamidronate are among those that have been synthesized.[18] Oral biphosphonates have a low bio-availability and produce gastrointestinal side-effects.[8] The intravenous route gives the best analgesia. Biphosphonates exert their effect by inhibiting osteoclast-mediated bone resorption. The exact mechanism of inhibition of bone resorption is unclear, but direct biochemical effects on the osteoclast, the prevention of osteoclast attachment to the bone matrix and the inhibition of osteoclast differentiation and recruitment have all been implicated.[8] It is clear that biphosphonates have analgesic properties when used alone.

Bone metastases in patients with cancer cause extensive morbidity, much of it attributable to hypercalcaemia. The growing recognition of hypercalcaemia has particularly focused attention on the crucial importance of the osteoclast as a mediator of neoplastic damage in bone.[18] The interruption of osteoclastic absorption is rapidly followed by a reduction of local hyperaemia, pain and even sclerosis of lytic bone lesions.[19] Biphosphonates thus reduce the pain in patients with hypercalcaemia of malignancy or with bone metastases. With breast and prostate osteolytic bone metastases, 50 per cent of patients show pain relief, and 25 per cent show radiological evidence of bone healing.[8] A reduction in pain and hypercalcaemia occurs in multiple myeloma patients.[8] Biphosphonates are used to treat Paget's disease.[8, 19] They can also be used in the long-term modulation of bone remodelling in osteoporosis, osteogenesis imperfecta and steroid-induced osteoporosis.[19] In future, biphosphonates will routinely be prescribed because of their ability to reduce considerably the morbidity associated with bone metastases. Their use in delaying the development of bone metastases is currently being evaluated.[8]

Gallium nitrate is another osteoclast inhibitor that may be analgesic for multifocal malignant bone pain.[10]

Radiopharmaceuticals

Site-directed radiotherapy using radionucleotides with differing properties is currently under investigation.[8,9,10,20] The agents concerned are all beta emitters (with or without also being gamma emitters for post-therapy imaging) and deposit their ionizing radiation within a short range, thereby avoiding damage to healthy tissue. Most work has been undertaken in prostate and breast bone metastases using strontium-89 (with a half-life of 50.5 days), samarium-153 (with a half-life of 46.8 hours) and rhenium-186.[8] In 10–15 per cent of patients, a 'flare' response in pain may occur in the first week. All radiopharmaceuticals can cause myelosuppression, and regular haematological monitoring is essential.

Somatostatin and octreotide

SOMATOSTATIN

Small peptides are thought to be involved in nociception.[21] Substance P, vasoactive intestinal peptide,

CCK and neuropeptide Y have all been implicated in the perpetuation of chronic pain states.

Somatostatin 1–14 is a naturally occurring neuropeptide. Somatostatinergic neurones exist in central and peripheral pathways related to the transmission of nociceptive information.[22] A high concentration is present in the substantia gelatinosa.[22] It may also be released in bulbospinal neurones, which descend through the spinal cord white matter mediating the descending inhibition of nociceptive neurones.[22] Somatostatin exerts modulatory effects (usually inhibitory) on peptides and cyclic AMP-mediated transmission.[21] However, its role in the transmission of nociceptor information is still under discussion.

Intrathecal somatostatin is a potent analgesic.[23] It may have neurotoxic effects when given in the rat or cat, but this is a species-dependent effect.[23,24] Intrathecal or epidural somatostatin administration in man is associated with potent analgesia without adverse effects.[23] The major drawback in the clinical use of somatostatin has been its very short half-life. It needs to be given by continuous infusion. Intrathecally, it decreases plasma levels of growth hormone and insulin.[24] Epidurally, somatostatin has been found to be effective in controlling intractable cancer pain. Epidural somatostatin (125 μg per hour) also provides sustained perioperative pain relief in patients undergoing upper abdominal surgery.[22] Respiratory depression is not evident.[24,25]

OCTREOTIDE

Octreotide is a long-acting analogue of somatostatin to which 14 amino acids are attached. This prolongs its analgesic effects. Octreotide may inhibit and/or modulate the actions of peripheral neuromodulators, possibly by desensitizing C receptors.[21]

In cancer patients with pain unrelieved by opioids, intrathecal octreotide (5–20 μg) administered for 13–91 days decreases pain scores and the dose of oral opioids used.[26] In patients with burning pain and hyperaesthesia from degenerative disease of the spine or post-herpetic neuralgia, the topical application (150–500 ng) of octreotide to a skin surface of 100–500 cm^2 results in the specific disappearance of the burning pain and hyperaesthesia.[21]

A novel method of administering octreotide has been used.[27] More research needs to be undertaken to validate this approach. In patients with various types of pain, octreotide has been applied to both eyeballs or both sphenopalatine ganglia, or given as an aerosol to the nose. Slight vertigo may occur, but no changes were observed in blood pressure and heart rhythm. The analgesic effects are said to last between 12 and 18 hours.[27]

Octreotide is known to have a powerful inhibitory effect on gastrointestinal secretion and motility.[28] Patients with refractory pain from bowel obstruction or with diarrhoea from an autonomic neuropathy following coeliac plexus blockade can be controlled with octreotide.[10,28]

5-Hydroxy tryptamine (5-HT) antagonists (also see below)

Given intrathecally, 5-HT3 and the 5-HT3 receptor agonist 1-(m-chlorophenyl) biguanide (mCPBG) have antinociceptive effects.[29] This spinal serotonin-induced analgesia is differentially reversed by 5-HT3 receptor antagonists (granisetron and tropisetron).[29]

CATECHOLAMINE PRECURSORS

L-TRYPTOPHAN

This is a serotonin precursor that has some analgesic benefit in chronic facial pain and in migraine but not in postoperative pain.[30] It has recently been banned in several countries because of suspected toxic side-effects.[30] It is given in a dose of 500–1000 mg four times a day.

L-DOPA

L-Dopa is a precursor of dopamine. It is a powerful analgesic in the treatment of bone metastases of cancer of the breast and prostate.[31]

CATECHOLAMINE ANTAGONISTS

Beta-adrenergic blocking agents

Propranolol, metoprolol and labetalol have been used in resistant migraine, atypical facial pain and pain following spinal cord transection.[32]

Serotonin (5-HT) antagonists

Cyproheptadine and pizotifen have proved to be of value in the prophylaxis and treatment of migraine.[32]

Noradrenaline antagonists

Guanethidine and bretylium deplete noradrenaline from nerve endings. Relief from sympathetically maintained pain can be obtained with a chemical sympathectomy using intravenous guanethidine and bretylium in the isolated limb.[15,31]

α_1-Adrenergic agonists

α_1-Agonists (phenylephrine and methoxamine), when given as systemic injections, produce analgesia in the animal formalin test model.[33] Alpha$_1$ receptors contribute to adrenergic analgesia by an undefined action on sensory processing mechanisms.

α_2-Adrenergic agonists in analgesia

α_2-Adrenergic agonists have recently been introduced into the clinical practice of anaesthesia for their analgesic, sedative, anxiolytic, anaesthetic-sparing and haemodynamic stabilizing properties.[34] Initially, their modest anaesthetic-sparing actions dominated the clinical area, but now their efficacy in pain management, regional anaesthesia and organ protection is coming to the fore.[35]

RECEPTOR LOCATION

Human molecular genetic cloning studies have shown that three genes encode distinct α_2-adrenergic receptor subtypes.[36] Pharmacological studies have defined four subtypes – α_{2A}, α_{2B}, α_{2C} and α_{2D}, the latter representing a homologue of α_{2A}.[36] Localization of the subtypes within the nervous system has been assessed by:[36]

- competitive binding of semiselective α_2 ligands;
- immunochemistry with a polyclonal antibody for the α_2 subtype;
- reverse transcriptase polymerase chain reaction for mRNA encoding α_2-adrenoceptor subtypes;
- *in situ* hybridization with oligonucleotide probes for mRNA of the α_2 subtypes.[36]

α_{2A} is the most prevalent and ubiquitous of the three, while α_{2B} is only present at a few discrete sites.[36] The α_{2A} subtype mediates the nociceptive action of systemic α_2 agonists and accounts for 80–90 per cent of the α_2-adrenoceptors in the spinal cord.[36]

α_2-Adrenergic receptors are present in the CNS and may be found in both presynaptic and postsynaptic locations.[37] Prejunctional receptors are not restricted to the adrenergic system but occur on nerve terminals that release other transmitters, such as acetylcholine and 5-HT.[38] Postsynaptic sites are mostly found on the autonomic ganglia and central neurones. α_2-adrenergic binding sites are densely distributed in the dorsal horn, particularly in the substantia gelatinosa and lamina X. The CNS anatomical target sites at which α_2-adrenergic ligands may influence pain processing and perception include the dorsal horn and the brain stem nuclei (the locus coeruleus and the A5 and A7 noradrenergic nuclei, all expressing only the α_{2A} subtype, the A7 nuclei being an important relay site for noradrenergic input into nociceptive processing at the spinal cord level).[36]

MECHANISMS OF ACTION

The α_2-adrenergic receptor is a glycoprotein with a single polypeptide chain that weaves back and forth through the cell membrane (Figure 6.2). The ability of α_2-adrenergic receptors rapidly to stimulate an effector system is transduced by a pertussis toxin-sensitive G protein.[39] However, more than one mechanism is involved in the analgesic effects of the α_2-agonists. Peripherally administered, they cause behavioural analgesia in animal models, partly because of their action in inhibiting cyclic AMP generation.[40] In sympathetically maintained pain, topical clonidine provides analgesia by the presynaptic inhibition of noradrenaline release from α_2-adrenergic autoreceptors.[40] There may also be a minor A delta and C fibre-selective degree of axonal blockade at the periphery.[40] The central actions of the α_2-adrenergic agonists produce primary neural blockade and may provide analgesia by supraspinal mechanisms, yet the spinal cord is their main site of action via activation of cholinergic neurones. Neuraxial clonidine selectively increases acetylcholine in the dorsal horn, a response that is enhanced in humans by neostigmine.[41] This interaction is not fully understood and is likely to be mediated by activation of the spinal muscarinic (M_2) receptors.[42] It is further dependent on the local synthesis of NO since it has been shown to be antagonized by the neuraxial administration of N-methyl-L-arginine, an NO synthetase inhibitor.[40,42]

The presynaptic mechanism of the α_2-adrenergic agonists inhibits the N-type calcium channel and reduces substance P and excitatory amino acids release (glutamate) following noxious peripheral nerve stimulation.[36] The α_2-agonists effectively suppress convergent dorsal horn neuronal

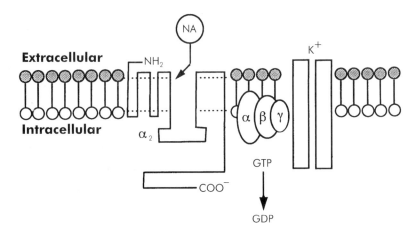

Figure 6.2 Structure of the α_2-adrenergic receptor. The α_2-agonist (e.g. noradrenaline [NA]) binds to the receptor protein, instituting a conformational change that facilitates contact with the pertussis toxin-sensitive G protein (its three subunits being α, β and γ). Transmembrane signalling is mediated by a decreased affinity of guanine diphosphate (GDP) for the α subunit and its replacement with guanine triphosphate (GTP). One of several effector mechanisms activated by the G protein is hyperpolarization and outward opening of the 4-aminopyridine-sensitive potassium (K^+) channel.

responses to noxious stimuli, with the selective presynaptic inhibition of smaller-diameter primary afferents.[36] The α_{2C} and α_{2D} subtypes mediate the α_2 presynaptic inhibition of neurotransmitter release.[36] The spinal antinociceptive effect is primarily caused by postsynaptic inhibition.[36] Postsynaptic α_2-adrenergic agonists hyperpolarize dorsal horn neurones. This is via the efflux of potassium ions through an activated channel, which can hyperpolarize the excitable membrane and provide an effective means of suppressing neuronal firing,[43] rendering the neurones less responsive to afferent input.[40] These agents also mimic the release of noradrenaline from neurones extrinsic to the spinal cord and with cell bodies in the pons and medulla.[40] The α_{2A} subtype is responsible for about 80 per cent of the autoinhibition of noradrenaline from sympathetic postganglionic neurones.[36]

The α_2-adrenergic agonists are also able to combine in the CNS with non-adrenergic 'imadazolin-preferring' receptors, whose stimulation determines a central hypotensive and antiarrhythmogenic action.[44] Their analgesic, sympathoinhibitive and anaesthetic-sparing effects are exclusively determined by their α_2-adrenergic properties.[44]

PHYSIOLOGICAL EFFECTS

Activation of the α_2-adrenergic receptors produces many physiological effects, including analgesia, anxiolysis, sedation, decreased salivary secretion, bradycardia, lowered blood pressure (reduced sympathetic flow), hypothermia and mydriasis.[45] Given their desirable physiological profile, α_2-adrenergic agonists are useful analgesic adjuvants.

AGONISTS

α_2-Adrenergic agonists include drugs such as clonidine, medetomidine, azepexole, mivazerol, tizanidine and oxymetazoline.[46]

Clonidine

Clonidine has an α_2:α_1 selectivity ratio of approximately 200:1.[47] It is highly lipid soluble. Orally, the T_{max} occurs after 1.5 hours. Oral and injectable forms are available. Clonidine has a relatively long elimination half-life (between 9 and 12 hours),[44] and the major fraction is excreted unchanged in the urine.[48] It is 10–100 times less selective for the α_2-adrenergic receptor than is dexmedetomidine and is known to have a ceiling effect that limits its anaesthetic actions.[49] This may be because of its α_1-agonist properties, which manifest themselves at higher doses.

Medetomidine

Medetomidine is a 1:1 racemic mixture of optical isomers of which the *d*-isomer, dexmedetomidine, is pharmacologically active.[50] Dexmedetomidine is a more specific α_2-adrenergic agonist (α_2:α_1 of 1620:1),[44] with a shorter duration than clonidine. It is more potent than clonidine, but no specific clinical data exist to show the superiority of the one agent over the other.[44] When given orally, it has a shorter elimination half-life, of 1.0–2.3 hours (compared with clonidine), a more rapid onset of action (less than 5 minutes) and a T_{max} of 15 minutes. Another selective α_2 agonist, azepexole, has anaesthetic properties similar to those of dexmedetomidine.[51] Mivazerol is another new α_2-adrenergic agonist under development for perioperative use.[44]

ANTAGONISTS

The effects of α_2-agonists can be reversed by α_2-antagonists such as idazoxan, atipamezole and yohimbine.[48] Yohimbine is not very selective, idazoxan being more so. But the most selective is atipamezole.[48]

DYNAMICS AND SIDE-EFFECTS

α_2-Agonists have two main biphasic effects on the cardiovascular system.[38] First is a transient, hypertensive or pressor effect from vascular smooth muscle constriction (especially if the drug has been given in high doses intravenously) because of a peripheral α_2- or α_1-adrenergic vasoconstriction.[44] This is followed by a central hypotensive or depressor and bradycardic effect associated with a decrease in sympathetic nerve outflow in the CNS. This decreased sympathetic outflow is manifested via a profound decrease in plasma catecholamines. There is a reflex, baroreceptor-mediated bradycardia in the pressor phase, and a falling heart rate with the fall of sympathetic outflow in the second phase. Thus cardiac output decreases during both phases.[38] Clonidine (unlike β-adrenergic blockers) reduces but does not totally suppress the sympathetic responses of baroreceptor activation.[44]

Hypotension can occur. The dose of α_2-agonist must be carefully titrated. α_2-Agonists may decrease cardiac conduction velocity.[52] Caution is needed in patients with pre-existing conduction system disturbances. Patients receiving drugs that cause bradycardia (beta-blockers and digoxin) or patients suffering from sick sinus syndrome are at risk of bradycardia from α_2-agonists. Patients dependent upon sympathetic tone to maintain circulatory integrity (with hypovolaemia, poor left ventricular function and congestive heart failure) should be given α_2-agonists with great caution.[49] Thus, α_2-agonists diminish sympathetic outflow and decrease heart rate, systemic arterial pressure and also plasma catecholamine levels.

The sympatholysis induced by the α_2-adrenergic agonists may result in potentially adverse clinical effects such as a fall in blood pressure and hypotension.[44] However, the haemodynamic effects elicited by the α_2-adrenergic agonists in the perioperative period appear to be more useful than deleterious.[44] There is a low incidence of major side-effects with clonidine, and it is apparent that α_2-adrenergic agonists are being used for more specific indications and via a variety of routes for their sympatholytic effect.[44] They counteract the sympathetic stimulation (tachycardia and hypertension) seen with the initial titration of desflurane. A clonidine premedication of 300 μg orally significantly attenuates these undesirable haemodynamic effects of desflurane, and because desflurane has a rapid wash-out, the post-anaesthetic sedation caused by clonidine is avoided.[35] Clonidine has been found to be as effective as esmolol or fentanyl at attenuating the sympathoexcitatory response to desflurane.[35] The need to pre-empt sympathoexcitatory responses in high-risk patients undergoing general anaesthesia is likely to become an important future clinical indication for these drugs.[35]

The discrepancy between the effective α_2-agonist analgesia seen in animal studies and the inability of low-dose clinical trials to demonstrate analgesia probably reflects the inadequate systemic doses used in the clinical trials.[36] α_2-Subtype specific agonists are unlikely to provide effective systemic clinical analgesia for acute nociceptive pain without side-effects.[36] Unless new strategies are developed to overcome the dosage ceiling imposed by the adverse side-effects, the use of systemic α_2-agonists for chronic pain may be limited.[36] The development of subtype-selective agonists, peripherally acting hydrophilic agonists and combinations of α_2-agonists with other analgesics may be a way of overcoming this problem.[36]

ADVANTAGES AND DISADVANTAGES

Studies confirm the minor respiratory effects of clonidine compared with those of opioids.[48,53] Additionally, there is no synergism between the respiratory depressant effects of opioids and α_2-agonists.[54] The advantages of α_2-agonists include a lack of respiratory depression and addiction, and a lack of other opioid side-effects such as nausea, vomiting and pruritus.[34] Disadvantages include hypotension, bradycardia and a drop in cardiac output.[34]

PREMEDICATION

Given as premedicants, α_2-agonists have been found to reduce the sleep dose of induction agents (thiopentone and methohexitone) needed, as well as that of the volatile inhalational agents.[50,53] A combination of oral clonidine (3.0–4.5 μg/kg) and a clonidine transdermal patch (7.0–10.5 cm^2) results in less volatile anaesthetic being required to maintain haemodynamic stability and less morphine being needed for postoperative analgesia.[47]

A single dose of clonidine (300 μg) has the same pharmacokinetic and pharmacodynamic profile whether administered orally or sublingually.[55] The rectal administration of 2.5 μg/kg clonidine in children approximately 20 minutes before the induction of anaesthesia achieves plasma concentrations within the range known to be clinically effective in adults.[56] Atropine was able to increase the heart rate in each case of children pretreated with clonidine 2 or 4 μg/kg orally.[57] In clonidine-premedicated hypotensive patients, the restoration of blood pressure can be achieved with relatively small doses of ephedrine or phenylephrine.[35]

α_2-AGONISTS AND OPIOIDS

Animal and clinical data indicate a synergistic or additive analgesic effect between α_2-agonists and opioids with systemic administration.[36] This may allow the use of very low systemic doses without sedation or cardiovascular complications.[36] α_2-Agonists augment the perioperative analgesia/anaesthesia produced by opioids.[54] Opioid doses can thus be reduced. Both agents also cause a marked decrease of central sympathetic outflow.[48] Opioids modulate responses to nociceptive stimuli partly by activating descending serotonergic and noradrenergic inhibitory pathways. Opioid-produced antinociception results in part from the activation by descending noradrenergic neurones of spinal α_2-adrenergic receptors regulating the responses of primary afferent neurones to nociceptive stimuli. Systemically, there is an additive reaction between medetomidine and opioids;[58] spinally, there is a synergistic reaction.[58] The therapeutic advantage of combinations of opioids and α_2-agonists is the increased analgesia with reduced respiratory depression and haemodynamic effects. In the rat, yohimbine attenuates the antinociceptive effect of both clonidine and morphine, furthering the evidence for interactions between the two systems.[59]

Dexmedetomidine can induce skeletal muscle relaxation and may be clinically effective in preventing the muscle rigidity produced by moderate to high doses of opioids.[45] This effect is mediated in the brain stem.[35] Intrathecal clonidine has been used to treat patients who have become tolerant after receiving continuous intrathecal morphine.[43]

TOXICOLOGY

Of the α_2-agonists, only clonidine has been examined rigorously for toxicity following intraspinal use. Intraspinally administered clonidine does not alter spinal cord blood flow or produce evidence of local neurotoxicity (in sheep), but it does substantially decrease spinal cord blood flow (in conscious rats).[60] It does not, however, produce a flow-metabolism imbalance that leads to ischaemia.[60] It also does not produce signs of sensory or motor blockade.[38] Twenty-eight days of epidural clonidine administration in dogs induced no change in CSF composition, the spinal cord or other organs, illustrating the safety of long-term administration of α_2-adrenergic agonists.[61] Phase III clinical trials with clonidine are currently being undertaken. Clonidine is preservative-free and isotonic, making it suitable for epidural administration. The combination of morphine, bupivacaine and clonidine retains its physical and chemical stability when the components are stored together.[62]

EPIDURAL/INTRATHECAL ADMINISTRATION

Pharmacokinetics

The lipid solubility and rapid absorption and elimination in the CSF of the α_2-agonists limit their rostral spread. Clonidine has an octanol-to-water partition coefficient 10 times greater than that of morphine and comparable to that of pethidine.[49] Rapid dural transfer (10 per cent of the dose) of clonidine following epidural administration occurs, giving a rapid onset of effective analgesia within 15–20 minutes.[49,50] Clonidine's short elimination half-life in CSF (43 minutes) suggests a brief duration of analgesia and that CSF accumulation is unlikely.[63] Epidural clonidine has an onset and duration of analgesia similar to that of epidural fentanyl.[52] The duration of analgesia may be prolonged by injecting large doses.[52] It is slowly absorbed into the systemic circulation (perhaps because of its slow release from the epidural fat). Peak plasma concentrations may not occur until more than 1 hour following injection.[64] The pharmacokinetics of clonidine in the CSF were studied after a controlled epidural clonidine infusion in volunteers.[64] The data showed the maintenance of a steady concentration of clonidine over a prolonged period.[64] After chronic α_2-adrenergic agonist administration, the analgesic properties persist after the hypnotic response has been attenuated.[44]

Dosage

Epidural clonidine (600 μg or more) is effective for acute postoperative pain,[52] analgesia lasting 4–6 hours. A continuous epidural infusion of clonidine (20 μg per hour) produces analgesia, although supplemental opioids are still required.[65] CSF clonidine concentrations of 100–150 ng/ml are needed for maximal analgesia.[65] Epidural clonidine (800 μg bolus, then 20 μg per hour) after caesarean section decreases the need for supplemental morphine.[66]

Side-effects

Dose-dependent sedation (from α_2-receptor stimulation in the brain stem) follows doses of over 300 μg. It lasts 2–4 hours. Clonidine decreases the heart rate, but its most common side-effect is hypotension. This occurs from the inhibition of neuronal firing in the locus coeruleus and direct spinal inhibition of preganglionic sympathetic outflow.[49] It is more likely to occur following intrathecal administration in patients with pre-existing hypertension (e.g. the elderly) or with hypovolaemia.[52] Because clonidine may increase blood pressure by a peripheral (α_1) action, hypotension is again lessened by increasing plasma concentrations (e.g. following bolus doses of over 500 μg).[63] Hypotension will occur within 30 minutes and responds to intravenous fluid administration or, if necessary, to ephedrine.[65] Epidural clonidine in pregnant ewes does not adversely affect the fetuses, nor does it alter uterine blood flow.[65] The successful relief of pain with epidural clonidine has thus been widely reported.[38]

Prolongation of spinal local anaesthesia

It is now possible both qualitatively and quantitatively to enhance conduction blockade by α_2-adrenergic agonists by various routes of administration. Unfortunately, the mechanism for understanding these local anaesthetic-enhancing qualities is not completely understood.[35] Oral clonidine effectively prolongs sensory and motor blockade from lignocaine neuraxial anaesthesia. Intrathecal clonidine seems to be more effective than adrenaline at prolonging the duration of intrathecal or epidural anaesthesia.[60] The addition of clonidine (1:100 000 to 1:200 000) to lignocaine (2 per cent) for epidural anaesthesia provides a sedative effect and relatively stable haemodynamics but tends to increase the plasma lignocaine concentration. This may be related to an altered metabolism of lignocaine caused by clonidine.[67] It has been suggested that spinal vasoconstriction may contribute to clonidine's ability to prolong spinal anaesthesia.[60] Oral clonidine (75–300 μg) as premedication has been found to prolong tetracaine spinal anaesthesia.[68] When intrathecal clonidine was used to supplement bupivacaine, the mean time for two-segment regression was considerably longer than that with either saline or adrenaline-supplemented bupivacaine.[38] Clonidine 5 μg/mL is a useful additive to lignocaine 1.5 per cent for cervical plexus block to reduce the incidence of tachycardia.[69]

MISCELLANEOUS ASPECTS

Tourniquet pain

Spinal clonidine has been used with bupivacaine to prevent tourniquet pain.[70] Tourniquet pain persisting after spinal anaesthesia with bupivacaine may be successfully decreased by the additional administration of intrathecal clonidine. Intravenous medetomidine (25 μg doses) in healthy subjects attenuated the unpleasantness of tourniquet-induced ischaemic pain without changing the estimate of pain magnitude.[71] In animal models of visceral pain, the antinociceptive action of clonidine has been demonstrated.[35]

Nitrogen Balance

Perioperative infusions of clonidine have been found to increase growth hormone levels.[72] Such a positive effect on nitrogen balance may be of future use in the severely ill patients in intensive care units.[35]

DRUG COMBINATIONS

Spinal α_2-agonists and opioids

The close complementarity between α_2-adrenergic agonists and opioids in anaesthesia and pain relief has been confirmed by many studies.[44] When combined with opioids (clonidine, morphine or fentanyl), either epidurally or intrathecally, there is a shift of the opioid dose–response curve to the left (Figure 6.3).[58,73] The combination produces greater analgesia than either drug alone, thereby reducing

dose requirements and delaying the onset of tolerance. It has been found that low doses of both clonidine and morphine do not reduce wide dynamic range (WDR) neuronal activity (in cats), whereas the combination of the two produces a significant reduction. This is borne out clinically as subanalgesic concentrations of clonidine and morphine will potentiate one another. A continuous epidural infusion of clonidine (450 μg per 24 hours) and epidural morphine (6 -mg per 24 hours) has been found to provide more effective pain relief than epidural bolus injections after major abdominal surgery.[75] A combination of epidural sufentanil (25 μg) with clonidine (1 μg/kg) was found to produce a longer-lasting and better quality of pain

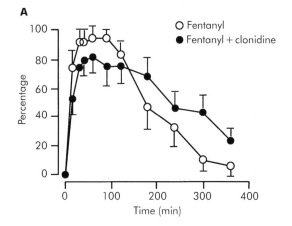

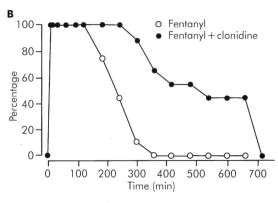

Figure 6.3　Effect on postoperative analgesia of the combination of epidural fentanyl and clonidine. Following abdominal surgery, 20 patients were randomly allocated to receive either epidural fentanyl 100 μg or epidural fentanyl 100 μg plus epidural clonidine 150 μg. (A) Percentage reduction in visual analogue pain scale rating in the two groups. (B) Percentage of patients not requesting analgesia after epidural fentanyl, or fentanyl plus clonidine. A log-rank test indicated that the two curves are significantly different.

relief with less arterial desaturation than sufentanil alone.[75] Patients who received epidural clonidine and morphine had an earlier onset and a longer duration of analgesia than when morphine alone was used.[76] However, the addition of clonidine to epidural butorphanol for postoperative pain did not enhance its analgesic effect.[77]

Reports on the intrathecal route of administration are somewhat less enthusiastic. The intrathecal route increases the reduction in mean blood pressure afforded by bupivacaine without additional analgesic benefit.[35] In parturients, the use of α_2-adrenergic agonists alone for postsurgical analgesia does not seem to be useful, except in extremely high doses.[35] A cat model has shown the complex modification of the somatoadrenal reflex that is differentially inhibited by spinal opioids (morphine), benzodiazepines (midazolam) and α-adrenergic receptor systems (clonidine).[78] It does, however, appear that intrathecal clonidine has an important role in the treatment of spasticity (as a single agent or adjuvant) when intrathecal baclofen alone is ineffective or when there is increasing tolerance to baclofen.[79]

Spinal α_2-agonists, opioids and local anaesthetics

Combinations of α_2-agonists, opioids and local anaesthetic agents (e.g. clonidine, fentanyl/sufentanil, and bupivacaine/ropivacaine) are now used for perioperative anaesthesia and analgesia.[73,80] Pain is then inhibited by three different mechanisms, resulting in a decrease in the dose of α_2-agonist, opioid and local anaesthetic agent needed.[81] With the manufacture of microcatheters (28–32 gauge), the intermittent or continuous intrathecal delivery of these combinations is now a reality.[82]

SHIVERING

α_2-Agonists diminish shivering in postoperative patients.[38,47] They have also been found to suppress shivering after epidurals with local anaesthetic agents.[65,83] In addition, clonidine 150 μg intravenously suppresses shivering during labour.[35]

CLINICAL USES

Acute pain

Clonidine enhances epidural opioid and local anaesthetic analgesia and anaesthesia, and is frequently combined with these agents for obstetric and paediatric, as well as intraoperative and postoperative uses.[35,40] In acute perioperative pain, epidural clonidine improves analgesia and decreases opioid requirements and side-effects.[44] Neuraxially, the effective analgesic dose of clonidine is lower after intrathecal (100–300 μg) than epidural (700–900 μg) administration.[40] The duration of pain relief is longer after intrathecal (12–18 hours) than epidural (4–6 hours) administration. Continuous epidural infusion (10–40 μg per hour) is required for sustained analgesia. Epidural clonidine is an adequate alternative to opioids in prolonging analgesia from local anaesthetics in children and in pregnancy.[44] Epidural clonidine (75 μg) improves labour analgesia when combined with bupivacaine and has no adverse effects on mothers or neonates.[44]

When patients (having undergone major orthopaedic surgery) are additionally allowed to self-administer epidural or intravenous clonidine as the sole neuraxial analgesic agent, the epidural route is associated with a significant reduction in the amount of self-administered clonidine.[44] In post-caesarean section patients, the addition of clonidine to epidural sufentanil decreased the number of PCA sufentanil administrations.[84] Following a combined epidural morphine and clonidine technique for post-gastrectomy patients, patients required less systemic PCA morphine when clonidine was added.[85]

Both clonidine and mivazerol alleviate angina pectoris and reduce myocardial ischaemia in patients undergoing cardiac revascularization surgery.[44]

Intractable pain

Neuraxial administration may not predict analgesic responses to systemic α_2-agonists in chronic pain states, as α_2-agonists may simultaneously induce both spinally mediated analgesia and peripherally mediated hyperalgesia.[36] Controlled clinical trials with α_2-adrenergic agonists in neuropathic pain patients have used topical, epidural and oral clonidine.[36]

Epidural clonidine (100–900 μg bolus or 30 μg per hour) has been found to be effective in treating neuropathic pain in up to 55 per cent of cancer patients with it, but chronic systemic administration (with daily doses of 3–5 μg/kg) has been ineffective in most neuropathic pain patients.[36,40,64,86] Effective analgesia can also be produced in the cancer patient tolerant to opioids or resistant to intrathecal morphine.[74] Epidural clonidine/morphine infusions (or epidural PCA) have been successfully administered to cancer patients at home for up to 5 months.[58] Epidural clonidine has been successfully used in treating the pain of arachnoiditis and proctalgia fugax, as well as in treating neuropathic pain following spinal cord injuries or peripheral nerve injuries.[87,88] Oral clonidine doses have proven effective in post-therpetic neuralgia.[89] Transdermal clonidine has value in treating the pain of diabetic neuropathy.[90] Oral clonidine has long been used in the treatment of migraine, where it may have an effect on 5-HT. Sustained analgesia has been obtained in patients with complex regional pain syndromes (type 1) from a continuous epidural clonidine infusion (10–50 μg per hour) for weeks.[40] Clonidine attenuates the hypertensive response to ketamine, which is useful in the analgesic use of this NMDA antagonist.[44] Controlled clinical trial data with systemic α_2-agonists in chronic soft tissue pain states are not available.[36] Future studies need to show that the analgesic effects of α_2-adrenergic agonists in chronic pain are durable and without long-term complications.

SUMMARY

The prior limited clinical success with α_2-agonist analgesia for the treatment of chronic pain indicates a need for new approaches to harness the powerful noradrenergic system.[36] One such approach would be to identify a sensitive chronic pain state to effectively use systemic doses too low to trigger significant side-effects.[36] Another is to develop and use α_{2B} and α_{2C} subtypes for responsive neuropathic pain or soft tissue injury pain states.[36] This allows for the use of high systemic doses for analgesia without the problems associated with α_{2A}-adrenoceptor-mediated side-effects.[36] Also, a peripheral analgesic site would allow the use of high doses of less lipophilic α_2-agonists (ST-91 and 4-hydroxyclonidine), which could not cross the blood–brain barrier and cause the supraspinally and spinally mediated sedation, hypotension and bradycardia.[36] The systemic use of a peripherally acting α_2-antagonist (L659.066) combined with a systemic α_2-agonist can be used to identify a peripheral site of α_2-adrenoceptor-mediated analgesia in various pain states.[36] The role of intradermal α_2-adrenoreceptor-mediated hyperalgesia should be considered in some pain states.[36] Systemic α_2-agonists may have a simultaneous central analgesic effect and a peripheral hyperalgesic effect in some pain states.[36] The combination neuraxial administration of opioids, neostigmine and serotonin enhances α_2-analgesia with large reductions in the doses of each.[36] The α_2-

agonists have properties of great potential benefit to pain control. The clinical introduction of the second generation of α_2-adrenergic agonists and formulations allowing different routes of administration (e.g. transdermal and neuraxial) will further extend their clinical use.[35] However, their advantages and limitations require further definition. The present confusion regarding the sensitivity, site of action, receptor subtypes and analgesic versus hyperalgesic effects of α_2-agonists in different chronic pain states remains a challenge to unravel.[36]

OPIOID ANTAGONISTS

General use

Opioid antagonists have traditionally been used to reverse not only the CNS depressant effects of opioids, but also the peripheral side-effects (e.g. itching and urinary retention). Certain opioids (e.g. dextropropoxyphene and buprenorphine) may require larger than normal doses of antagonist to reverse their effects fully.[91] Large doses of antagonist may be necessary to reverse the side-effects of opioids generated by activity at a receptor other than the mu receptor (e.g. to reverse the dysphoria engendered by sigma or kappa receptor stimulation).[91]

Naloxone has a short half-life (of about 20 minutes) and can only be given intravenously or intramuscularly (Figure 6.4). Should the opioid being antagonized have a half-life significantly longer than that of naloxone, naloxone should be given in repeated doses or by infusion.[91] If the patient is able to tolerate orally administered drugs, one of the longer-acting antagonists should be given by mouth.

Opioid antagonists have side-effects. Because of a massive release of catecholamines from the adrenal medulla in response to the pain resulting from acute opioid reversal, naloxone may generate hypertensive crises, cardiac arrhythmias and arrest.[92] Facilities for resuscitation should be available when opioid antagonists are given.

Opioid antagonists have also been used for non-opioid reversal (benzodiazepines, alcohol and nitrous oxide) and in spinal injury and spinal shock.[93–96]

Types of opioid antagonists

Other than naloxone, opioid antagonists include naltrexone, nalmephene and the new family of naltrexone-derived antagonists.

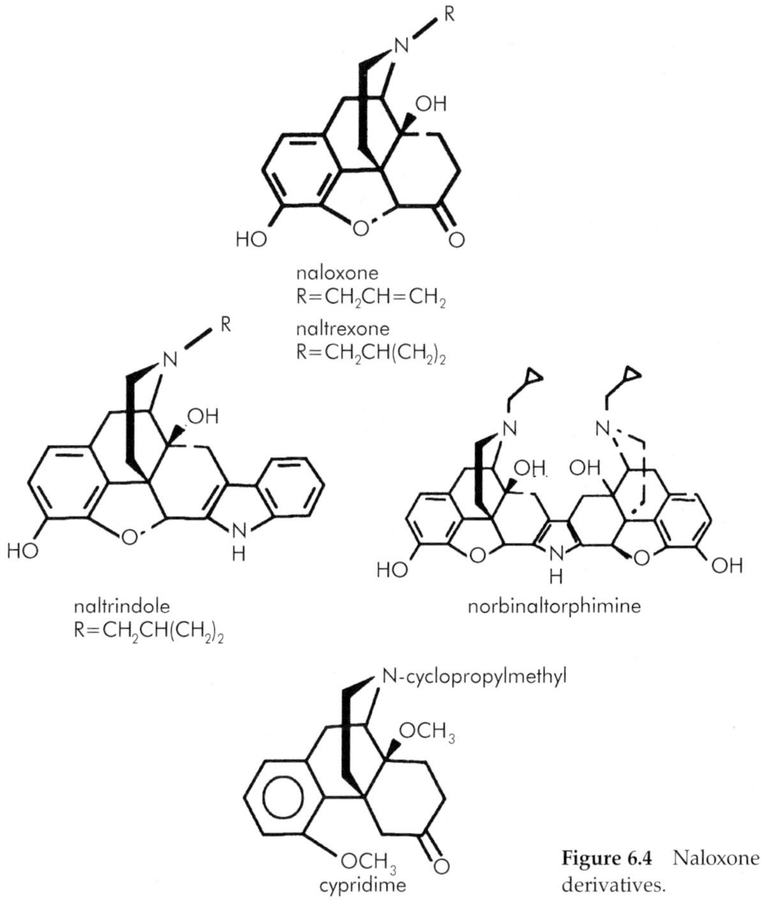

Figure 6.4   Naloxone and the newer opioid antagonist derivatives.

Naltrexone is rapidly and almost completely absorbed from the gastrointestinal tract, peak plasma concentrations being reached in 1 hour. The plasma concentration declines in a biexponential manner up to 24 hours, corresponding to an elimination half-life of 7 hours. There then follows a third phase of slow decline with an estimated half-life of 96 hours, indicating a high degree of tissue absorption from which the drug is slowly released into the systemic circulation.[92] Beta-naltrexol is the major metabolite of naltrexone, which also has opioid antagonist activity and persists in large amounts in the plasma, with a half-life of some 13 hours.[97]

Nalmephene in a single oral dose will produce opioid receptor blockade for up to 72 hours.[91] Other workers specifically studying the reversal of respiratory depression give its duration of effect as 4–6 hours.[98,99]

A new family of naltrexone-derived opioid antagonists has been synthesized. Of these, naltrindole shows the best combination of potency and selectivity. It shows 152- and 256-fold higher affinity for delta than for mu and kappa receptor subtypes, respectively.[100]

The bimorphinan compound nor-binaltorphimine has recently been found to have a high affinity as well as selectivity for the kappa receptor subtype. It should possess good central activity when given peripherally and is a pure antagonist with a kappa preference of 300- and 380-fold over mu and delta sites, respectively.[101]

Cypridime is one of a series of 14-hydroxy-codeine derivatives showing less potency but a greater selectivity for mu receptors than naloxone.[101]

Use as secondary analgesics

Patients who suffer a cerebrovascular accident might develop post-stroke pain. The usual components of this syndrome are transient flaccid hemiparesis or hemiplegia followed by permanent impairment of superficial and deep sensation, severe pain, usually dysaesthetic or shocking in nature, choreoathetotic movements, ataxia and tremor.[102] It has been observed that a symptom common to all post-stroke pain patients is a disturbance of temperature sensibility. A particular problem is the spontaneous pain occurring in paroxysms of often excruciating intensity. It is now clear that all such pain is not always of thalamic origin.[102] It is associated with sensory abnormalities in the painful body part.[103] Hyperalgesia or allodynia is an essential part of this syndrome. Consequently, the syndrome is termed 'central post-stroke pain'. Central post-stroke pain is thus a neuropathic pain syndrome characterized by constant or intermittent pain in a body part occurring after a stroke. Eight per cent of stroke patients suffer from central post-stroke pain, and the pain is severe in 5 per cent.[104] After a stroke, 63 per cent of patients develop pain within a month, 19 per cent within 6 months and 19 per cent after 6 months.[103]

It is very difficult to determine the exact anatomical lesion present. A vascular lesion is assumed to be responsible for the pain.[103,105] The pain is usually caused by ischaemic or haemorrhagic lesions, but less commonly it is due to tumours, trauma, arteriovenous malformations and surgical intervention.[102]

Concentrations of endogenous opioids in the CSF are raised in these patients, and it is believed that these opioids are released as a result of cerebral ischaemia. They are thought to inhibit the activity of the locus coeruleus, which is located in the forward end of the sulcus limitans on the floor of the fourth ventricle, and whose cells synthesize catecholamines. It is involved in maintaining cerebrovascular tone, a function mediated by the release of noradrenaline, with a consequent drop in cerebral blood flow. This intensifies the neurological injury and symptoms.[106] The most likely mechanism, however, is a central sensitization of third (or higher)-order CNS neurones that have lost part of their afferent input.[104]

Opioid antagonists also have a role as secondary analgesics in the treatment of central pain, particularly in central post-stroke pain. The final common pathway by which opioid antagonists act is most likely to be an effect on the vascular system of the CNS via β-endorphinergic receptors, neuropeptide Y and delta opioid receptors, either singly or in combination.[91]

Naloxone (in relatively large doses), naltrexone and nalmephene have all been shown to be of value,[91,102] although naloxone has occasionally been found to be ineffective.[107] Clinically, the doses of naloxone given frequently exceed the standard dose used in order to produce a lasting analgesic effect.[92] This may well be because of the need for mu receptor saturation before the clinical effect is exerted on a delta receptor. The maintenance of therapy has been made much easier with the introduction of the oral formulations naltrexone and nalmephene. Naltrexone can cause loss of appetite, and the risk of liver damage makes routine liver function tests mandatory.[102] Cross-reactivity is not always seen, and patients who respond to naloxone may not necessarily continue to obtain analgesia with naltrexone or nalmephene.[91]

CONCLUSION

The use of secondary analgesics has revolutionized the way in which various pain conditions, especially neuropathic pain, are now treated.

REFERENCES

1. **Shipton, E.A.** 1997: Secondary analgesics. *Current Anaesthesia and Critical Care* **8**, 68–76.
2. **Perry, H. and Nash, T.P.** 1992: Scar neuromata. *The Pain Clinic* **5**(1), 3–7.
3. **Koes, B.W. Scholten, R.J.P.M., Mens, J.M.A. and Bouter, L.M.** 1995: Efficacy of epidural steroid injections for low-back pain and sciatica: a systematic review of randomised clinical trials. *Pain* **63**, 279–88.
4. **Castagnera, L., Maurette, P., Pointillart, V., Vital, J.M., Erny, P. and Senegas, J.** 1994: Long-term results of cervical epidural steroid injection with and without morphine in chronic cervical radicular pain. *Pain* **58**, 239–43.
5. **McQuay, H.J. and Moore, R.A.** 1998: *An evidence-based resource for pain relief.* Oxford: Oxford University Press 27, 216–18.
6. **Johannson, A., Hao, J. and Sjolund, B.** 1990: Local corticosteroid application blocks transmission in nociceptive C-fibres. *Acta Anaesthesiologica Scandinavica* **34**, 335–8.
7. **Twycross, R.G.** 1989: The management of pain in cancer: In Nimmo, W.S. and Smith, G. (eds) *Anaesthesia.* Oxford: Blackwell Scientific, 1216–29.
8. **Houston, S.J. and Rubens, R.D.** 1994: Metastatic bone pain. *Pain Reviews* **1**, 138–52.
9. **Cherny, N.I. and Portenoy, R.K.** 1995: Systemic drugs for cancer pain. *Pain Digest* **5**, 245–63.
10. **Portenoy, R.K.** 1996: Nontraditional analgesics in the management of cancer pain. In Campbell, J.N. (ed.) *Pain 1996 – an updated review.* Seattle: IASP Press, 559–66.

11. **Shipton, E.A.** 1991: Secondary analgesics in the treatment of pain from malignant disease. *South African Journal of Continuing Medical Education* **9**(6), 723–8.

12. **Hanks, G.W., Trueman, T. and Twycross, R.G.** 1983: Corticosteroids in terminal cancer. *Postgraduate Medical Journal* **59**, 702.

13. **Jaeger, J. and Maier, C.** 1992: Calcitonin in phantom limb pain: a double blind study. *Pain* **48**, 21–7.

14. **Chiang, M.F., Weigel, K., Mutze, M. and Brock, M.** 1990: Long-term follow-up of three patients with chronic non-malignant pain treated with a continuous infusion of salmon calcitonin. *Pain* (suppl. 5), 5240.

15. **Budd, K.** 1989: The pain clinic – chronic pain. In Nunn, J.F., Utting, J.E. and Brown, B.R. (eds) *General anaesthesia*, 5th edn. London: Butterworths, 1349–69.

16. **Siminoski, K. and Josse, R.G.** 1996: Prevention and management of osteoporosis: concensus statements from the Scientific Advisory Board of the Osteoporosis Society of Canada. *Canadian Medical Association Journal* **155**(7), 962–5.

17. **Dodwell, D.J., Howell, A., Morton, A., Daley-Yates, P.T. and Hoggarth, C.R.** 1990: Pamidronate (APD) treatment of skeletal metastases from breast cancer. In Rubens, R.D. (ed.) *The management of bone metastases and hypercalcaemia by osteoclast inhibition.* Toronto: Hogrefe & Huber, 62–75.

18. **Coleman, R.E. and Rubens, P.D.** 1987: 3 (amino-1, 1-hydroxypropylidene) biphosphonate (APD) for hypercalcaemia of breast cancer. *British Journal of Cancer* **56**, 465–9.

19. **Bijvoet, O.L.M.** 1990: Pamidronate (APD) in cancer therapy – the pharmacological background. In Rubens, R.D. (ed.) *The management of bone metastases and hypercalcaemia by osteoclast inhibition.* Toronto: Hogrefe & Huber, 13–27.

20. **Hoskin, P.J.** 1995: Radiotherapy for bone pain. *Pain* **63**, 137–9.

21. **Ellis, W.V.** 1990: Octreotide, a small peptide alleviates burning pain and hyperaesthesia: a preliminary study. *The Pain Clinic* **3**, 239–42.

22. **Taura, P., Planella, V., Balust, J.** *et al*. 1994: Epidural somatostatin as an analgesic in upper abdominal surgery: a double-blind study. *Pain* **59**, 135–40.

23. **Mollenholt, P., Post, C., Paulsson, I. and Rawal, N.** 1990: Intrathecal and epidural somatostatin in rats – can antinociception, motor effect, and neurotoxicity be separated? *Pain* **43**, 363–70.

24. **Desborough, J.P., Edlin, S.A., Burrin, J.M., Bloom, S.R., Morgan, M. and Hall, G.M.** 1989: Hormonal and metabolic responses to cholecystectomy: comparison of extradural somatostatin and diamorphine. *British Journal of Anaesthesia* **63**, 508–15.

25. **Carli, P., Eaffey, C., Chrubasik, J., Benlabed, M., Cross, J.B. and Samii, K.** 1989: Spread of analgesia and ventilatory response to carbon dioxide following epidural somatostatin. *European Journal of Anaesthesiology* **6**, 257–63.

26. **Penn, R.D., Paice, J.A. and Kroin, J.S.** 1992: Octreotide: a potent new non-opiate analgesic for intrathecal infusion. *Pain* **49**, 13–19.

27. **Mocavero, G.** 1991: Novel method of analgesia either by nasal aerosol of somatostatin, morphine, and lidocaine or by installation on conjunctiva and sphenopalatine ganglion: a preliminary report. *The Pain Clinic* **4**, 239–42.

28. **Mercadante, S.** 1995: Octreotide in the treatment of diarrhoea induced by coeliac plexus block. *Pain* **61**, 345–6.

29. **Bardin, L., Jourdan, D., Alloui, A., Lavarenne, J. and Eschalier, A.** 1997: Differential influence of two serotonin 5-HT receptor antagonists on spinal serotonin-induced analgesia in rats. *Brain Research* **765**(2), 267–72.

30. **Ekblom, A., Hansson, P. and Thomsson, M.** 1991: L-tryptophan supplementation does not affect postoperative pain intensity or consumption of analgesics. *Pain* **44**, 249–54.

31. **Shipton, E.A.** 1991: Recent advances in intractable pain control. *South African Medical Journal* **79**, 119–20.

32. **Bond M.** 1989: *Pain – its nature, analysis and treatment*, 2nd edn. Edinburgh: Churchill Livingstone, 3–20.

33. **Tasker, R.A.R., Connell, B.J. and Yole, M.J.** 1992: Systemic injections of alpha$_1$ adrenergic agonists produce antinociception in the formalin test. *Pain* **49**, 383–91.

34. **Shipton, E.A.** 1991: Alpha adrenergic agonists in anaesthesia and analgesia. *South African Medical Journal* **79**, 578–80.

35. **Kamibayashi, T. and Maze, M.** 1996: Perioperative use of alpha-2 adrenergic agonists. *Current Opinion in Anaesthesiology* **9**, 323–7.

36. **Kingery, W.S., Davies, M.F. and Maze, M.** 1997: Molecular mechanisms for the analgesic properties of alpha-2 adrenergic agonists. In Borsook, D. (ed.) *Molecular neurobiology of pain.* Seattle: IASP Press, vol. 9, 275–304.

37. **Zornow, M.H., Fleischer, J.E., Schneller, M.S. Nakakimura, K. and Drummond, J.C.** 1990: Dexmedetomidine, an alpha$_2$-adrenergic agonist decreases cerebral blood flow in the isoflurane-anesthetised dog. *Anesthesia and Analgesia* **70**, 624–30.

38. **Flacke, J.** 1990: Opioid anaesthesia and the alpha$_2$-agonists. *American Society of Anesthesiologists Annual Refresher Course Lectures* **235**, 1–7.

39. **Maze, M.** 1991: Clinical uses of alpha$_2$ agonists. *American Society of Anesthesiologists Annual Refresher Course Lectures* **245**, 1–7.

40. **Eisenach, J.C.** 1996: Physiology and pharmacology of blockade: alpha$_2$ and other agonists. In *Congress Manual of International Society of Regional Anaesthesia*, Auckland, 30–4.

41. **Hood, D.D., Mallak, K.A., Eisenach, J.C. and Tong, C.** 1996: Interaction between intrathecal neostigmine and epidural clonidine in human volunteers. *Anesthesiology* **85**(2), 315–25.

42. **Goudas, L.C.** 1995: Clonidine. *Current Opinion in Anaesthesiology* **8**, 455–60.

43. **Maze, M.** 1991: Cardiovascular pharmacology in the 1990's: the role of alpha₂ adrenergic agonists in anaesthesia. *International Anaesthesia Research Society Review Course Lectures* 1991, 68–76.

44. **De Kock, M.** 1996: Alpha₂ adrenoceptor agonists: clonidine, dexmedetomidine, mivazerol. *Current Opinion in Anaesthesiology* **9**, 295–9.

45. **Weinger, M.B., Segal, I.S. and Maze, M.** 1989: Dexmedetomidine acting through central alpha₂ adrenoceptors prevents opiate-induced muscle rigidity in the rat. *Anesthesiology* **71**, 242–9.

46. **Kauppila, T., Kemppainen, P., Tanila, H. and Petovarra, A.** 1991: Effect of systemic medetomidine, an alpha₂ adrenoceptor agonist on experimental pain in humans. *Anesthesiology* **74**, 3–8.

47. **Segal, I.S., Jarvis, D.J., Duncan, S.R., White, P.F. and Maze, M.** 1991: Clinical efficacy of oral–transdermal clonidine combinations during the perioperative period. *Anesthesiology* **74**, 220–5.

48. **Flacke, J.** 1990: Opioid anaesthesia and the alpha₂-agonists. *American Society of Anesthesiologists Annual Refresher Course Lectures* 1990, **235**, 1–7.

49. **Shipton, E.A.** 1991: Alpha₂ adrenergic agonists in anaesthesia and analgesia. Hospital Medicine (Jul), 7–13.

50. **Aantaa, R.E., Kanto, J.H., Scheinin, M., Kallio, A.M.I. and Scheinin, H.** 1990: Dexmedetomidine premedication in minor gynaecologic surgery. *Anesthesia and Analgesia* **70**, 407–13.

51. **Nagasaka, H. and Yaksch, T.L.** 1990: Pharmacology of intrathecal adrenergic agonists: cardiovascular and nociceptive reflexes in halothane-anesthetised rats. *Anesthesiology* **73**, 1198–207.

52. **Eisenach, J.C., Lysak, S.Z. and Viscomi, C.M.** 1989: Epidural clonidine analgesia following surgery: phase I. *Anesthesiology* **71**, 640–6.

53. **Kallio, A., Salonen, M., Forssell, H., Scheinin, H., Scheinin, M. and Touminen, J.** 1990: Medetomidine premedication in dental surgery – a double blind cross-over study with a new alpha₂ adrenoceptor agonist. *Acta Anaesthesiologica Scandinavica* **34**(3), 171–5.

54. **Bailey, P.L., Perry, R.J., Johnson, G.K.** *et al.* 1991: Respiratory effects of clonidine alone and combined with morphine in humans. *Anesthesiology* **74**, 43–8.

55. **Cunningham, F.E., Baughman, V.L., Peters, J. and Laurito, C.E.** 1994: Comparative pharmacokinetics of oral versus sublingual clonidine. *Journal of Clinical Anesthetics* **6**, 430–3.

56. **Lonnqvist, P.A., Bergendahl, H.T. and Eksborg, S.** 1994: Pharmacokinetics of clonidine after rectal administration in children. *Anesthesiology* **81**, 1097–101.

57. **Nishina, K., Mikawa, K., Maekawa, N. and Obara, H.** 1995: Oral clonidine premedication blunts the heart rate response to intravenous atropine in awake children. *Anesthesiology* **825**, 1126–30.

58. **Ossipov, M.H., Harris, S., Lloyd, P. Messineo, E., Lin, B.S. and Bagley, J.** 1990: Antinociceptive interaction between opioids and medetomidine: systemic additivity and spinal surgery. *Anesthesiology* **73**, 1227–35.

59. **Van Essen, D.J., Boville, J.G. and Ploeger, E.J.** 1991: Extradural clonidine does not potentiate analgesia produced by extradural morphine after menisectomy. *British Journal of Anaesthesia* **66**, 237–41.

60. **Crosby, G., Russo, M.A., Szabo, M.D. and Davies, K.R.** 1990: Subarachnoid clonidine reduces spinal cord blood flow and glucose utilisation in conscious rats. *Anesthesiology* **73**, 1179–85.

61. **Yaksh, T.L., Rathbun, M., Jage, J., Mirzai, T., Grafe, M. and Hiles, R.A.** 1994: Pharmacology and toxicology of chronically infused epidural clonidine HCL in dogs. *Fundamentals of Applied Toxicology* **23**, 319–35.

62. **Wulf, H., Gleim, M. and Mignat, C.** 1994: The stability of mixtures of morphine hydrochloride, bupivacaine hydrochloride, and clonidine hydrochloride in portable pump reservoirs for the management of chronic pain syndromes. *Journal of Pain and Symptom Management* **9**, 308–11.

63. **Eisenach, J.C., Rauck, R.L., Buzzanell, C. and Lysak, S.Z.** 1989: Epidural clonidine analgesia for intractable cancer pain: phase I. *Anesthesiology* **71**, 647–52.

64. **Eisenach, J.C., Hood, D.D., Tuttle, R., Shafer S., Smith, T.** 1995: Computer-controlled epidural infusion to targeted cerebrospinal fluid concentrations in humans: clonidine. *Anesthesiology* **83**, 33–47.

65. **Eisenach, J.** 1990: Alpha₂ adrenergic agonists. *American Society of Anesthesiologists Annual Refresher Course Lectures* **126**, 1–4.

66. **Mendez, R., Eisenach, J.G. and Kashtan, K.** 1990: Epidural clonidine analgesia after cesarean section. *Anesthesiology* **73**, 848–52.

67. **Nishikawa, T. and Dohi, S.** 1990: Clinical evaluation of clonidine added to lidocaine solution for epidural anesthesia. *Anesthesiology* **73**, 853–9.

68. **Ohta, K., Takahashi, I., Iwasaki, H., Matsumoto, M. and Namiki, A.** 1991: Dose–response relationship of oral clonidine in tetracaine spinal anaesthesia. *Anesthesia and Analgesia* **72**, S204.

69. **Molnar, R.R., Davies, M.J., Scott, D.A., Silbert, B.S. and Mooney, P.H.** 1997: Comparison of clonidine and epinephrine in lidocaine for cervical plexus block. *Regional Anesthesia* **22**(2), 137–42.

70. **Bonnet, F., Diallo, A., Saada, M., Belon, M., Guilbaud, M. and Boico, O.** 1989: Prevention of tourniquet pain by spinal isobaric bupivacaine with clonidine. *British Journal of Anaesthesia* **63**, 93–6.

71. **Kauppila, T., Kemppainen, P., Tanila, H. and Petovarra, A.** 1991: Effect of systemic medetomidine, an alpha₂ adrenoceptor agonist on experimental pain in humans. *Anesthesiology* **74**, 3–8.

72. **De Kock, M., Merello, L., Pendeville, P., Maiter, D. and Scholtes, J.L.** 1994: Effects of intravenous clonidine on the secretion of growth hormone in the peri-

operative period. *Acta Anaesthesiologica Belgica* **45**, 167–74.

73. **Kitahata, L.** 1989: Spinal analgesia with morphine and clonidine. *Anesthesia and Analgesia* **68**, 191–3.

74. **Motsch, J., Graber, E. and Ludwig, K.** 1990: Addition of clonidine enhances postoperative analgesia from epidural morphine – double blind study. *Anesthesiology* **73**, 1067–73.

75. **Vercauteren, M., Lauwers, E., Meert, T., De Hert, S. and Adriaensen, H.** 1990: Comparison of epidural sufentanil plus clonidine with sufentanil alone for postoperative pain relief. *Anaesthesia* **45**, 531–4.

76. **Rockemann, M.G., Seeling, W., Brinkmann, A.** *et al.* 1995: Analgesic and hemodynamic effects of epidural clonidine, clonidine/morphine, and morphine after pancreatic surgery – a double-blind study. *Anesthesia and Analgesia* **80**, 869–74.

77. **Tan, P.H., Chou, A.K., Perng, J.S., Chung, H.C., Lee, C.C. and Mok, M.S.** 1997: Comparison of epidural butorphanol plus clonidine with butorphanol alone for postoperative pain relief. *Acta Anaesthesiologica Singapore* **35**(2), 91–6.

78. **Gaumann, D.M., Yaksh, T.L. and Tyce, G.M.** 1990: Effects of intrathecal morphine, clonidine, and midazolam on the somato-sympathadrenal reflex response in halothane-anesthetised cats. *Anesthesiology* **73**, 425–32.

79. **Middleton, J.W., Siddall, P.J., Walker, S., Molloy, A.R. and Rutkowski, S.B.** 1996: Intrathecal clonidine and baclofen in the management of spasticity and neuropathic pain following spinal cord injury. *Archives of Physical Medicine and Rehabilitation* **77**(6), 824–6.

80. **Bonnet, F., Brun-Buisson, V., Saada, M., Boico, O., Rostaing, S. and Touboul, C.** 1989: Dose-related prolongation of hyperbaric tetracaine spinal anesthesia by clonidine in humans. *Anesthesia and Analgesia* **68**, 619–22.

81. **Eliasen, K., Ejlersen, E. and Mogensen, T.** 1990: Epidural clonidine enhances postoperative analgesia of a combined low-dose epidural bupivacaine and morphine regimen. *Proceedings of European Society of Regional Anaesthesia (IX Annual Congress)*, 5–8 September, Berne, 1990.

82. **Hurley, R.J. and Lambert, D.H.** 1990: Continuous spinal anaesthesia with a microcatheter technique: preliminary experience. *Anesthesia and Analgesia* **70**, 97–102.

83. **Tryba, M., Zenz, M. and Pern, U.** 1990: Clonidine suppresses postepidural shivering – a double blind study. *Anesthesiology* **73**(3A), A788.

84. **Vercauteren, M.P., Vandeput, D.M., Meert, T.F. and Adriaensen, H.A.** 1994: Patient-controlled epidural analgesia with sufentinil following caesarean section: the effect of adrenaline and clonidine admixture. *Anaesthesia* **49**, 767–71.

85. **Anzai, Y. and Nishikawa, T.** 1995: Thoracic epidural clonidine and morphine for postoperative pain relief. *Canadian Journal of Anaesthesia* **42**, 292–7.

86. **Eisenach, J.C., DuPen, S., Dubois, M., Migue, I.R. and Allin, D.** 1995: Epidural clonidine analgesia for intractable cancer pain. *Pain* **61**, 391–9.

87. **Coventry, D.M. and Todd, D.M.** 1989: Epidural clonidine in lower limb deafferentation pain. *Anesthesia and Analgesia* **69**, 424–5.

88. **Glynn, C.J., Jamous, M.A. and Teddy, P.J.** 1992: Cerebrospinal fluid kinetics of epidural clonidine in man. *Pain* **49**, 361–7.

89. **Gordon, N.C., Heller, P.H. and Levine, J.D.** 1992: Enhancement of pentazocine analgesia by clonidine. *Pain* **42**, 167–9.

90. **Zeigler, D., Lynch, S., Muir, J., Benjamin, J. and Max, M.B.** 1992: Transdermal clonidine versus placebo in painful diabetic neuropathy. *Pain* **48**, 403–8.

91. **Budd, K.** 1991: Antagonists in anaesthetic practice. In Atkinson, R.S. and Adams, A.P. (eds) *Recent advances in anaesthesia and analgesia*. London: Churchill Livingstone, vol. 17, 161–71.

92. **Budd, K.** 1987: Clinical use of opioid antagonists. In Budd, K. (ed.) *Clinical anaesthesiology*, vol. **1**. London: Baillière Tindall, 993–1011.

93. **Bell, E.F.** 1975: The use of naloxone in the treatment of diazepam poisoning. *Journal of Pediatrics* **87**, 803–4.

94. **Moss, L.M.** 1973: Naloxone reversal of non-narcotic induced apnea. *Journal of the American College of Emergency Physicians* **1**, 46.

95. **Jefferys, D.B., Flanagan, R.J. and Volans, G.N.** 1980: Reversal of ethanol induced coma with naloxone. *Lancet* **1**, 308–9.

96. **Berkonitz, B.A., Finck, A.D. and Ngai, S.H.** 1977: Nitrous oxide analgesia: reversal by naloxone and development of tolerance. *Journal of Pharmacology and Experimental Therapeutics* **203**, 539–47.

97. **Crabtree, B.L.** 1984: Review of naltrexone, a long acting opiate antagonist. *Clinical Pharmacology* **3**, 273–80.

98. **Konieczko, K.N., Jones, J.G., Barrowcliffe, M.P.** *et al*. 1988: Antagonism of morphine induced respiratory depression with nalmefene. *British Journal of Anaesthesia* **61**, 318–23.

99. **Barsan, W.G., Seger, D., Danzl, D.F.** *et al*. 1989: Duration of antagonistic effects of nalmefene and naloxone in opiate induced sedation for emergency department procedures. *American Journal of Emergency Medicine* **2**, 155–61.

100. **Portoghese, P.S., Sultana, M. and Takemori, A.E.** 1988: Naltrindole – a highly selective and potent non-peptide delta opioid receptor antagonist. *European Journal of Pharmacology* **146**, 185–6.

101. **Haynes, L.** 1990: Opioid receptors and signal transduction. *Trends in Pharmacological Science* **9**, 309–11.

102. **Gauci, C.A. and Thorp, T.A.S.** 1991: The long-term management of central post-stroke pain with the orally administered opiate antagonist naltrexone. *The Pain Clinic* **4**, 47–51.

103. **Andersen, G., Vestergaard, K., Ingeman-Nielsen, M. and Jensen, T.S.** 1995: Incidence of central post-stroke pain. *Pain* **61**, 187–93.

104 **Jensen, T.S. and Lenz, F.A.** 1995: Central post-stroke pain: a challenge for the scientist and the clinician. *Pain* **61**, 161–4.

105 **Vestergaard, K., Nielsen, J., Anderson, G., Ingeman-Nielsen, M., Arendt-Nielsen, L. and Jensen, T.S.** 1995: Sensory abnormalities in consecutive, unselected patients with central post-stroke pain. *Pain* **61**, 177–86.

106. **Strahlendor, F.** 1980: Endorphin mediated intubation of locus coeruleus. *Brain Research* **191**, 284–86.

107. **Bainton, T., Fox, M., Bowsher, D., and Wells, C.** 1992: A double-blind trial of naloxone in central post-stroke pain. *Pain* **48**, 159–62.

7 DRUG DELIVERY

New drug delivery systems have emerged. Determining the drug delivery system most suitable for a particular drug may improve its therapeutic ratio.[1] Most drugs act by a concentration-dependent, reversible interaction at specific receptor sites.[2] To maximize the desired response, an appropriate amount of the drug must be transported to the receptor and the required concentrations maintained for as long as the effect is desired.[2] Drugs for the relief of pain may be given by routes providing direct access to receptors by diffusion and/or bulk flow (e.g. epidural, intrathecal and intracerebroventricular) and by those requiring blood carriage (e.g. intravenous, intramuscular, subcutaneous and oral), thereby having indirect access.[3] Optimum delivery is thus dependent on the amount, rate, route, site of absorption and selectivity of distribution.[4] In addition, the concentration–response relationship should be known.

BLOOD–BRAIN BARRIER

An increased understanding of the pharmacology of the brain and its blood supply, and methods for rational drug design, are leading to potential new drug therapies based on highly specific actions on particular target sites, such as neurotransmitter receptors and uptake systems.[5,6] The major obstacle to targeting the brain with therapies is the presence of the blood–brain barrier, which controls the concentration and entry of solutes into the central nervous system (CNS).[7] The binding to albumin in plasma reduces the amount of compound free to diffuse across the blood–brain barrier.[8] This amount may be determined directly or indirectly by the following methods:[8–11]

- direct measurements of blood–brain ratios;
- direct measurements of brain penetration using an *in situ* brain perfusion model (in the rat) to measure the amount of drug crossing the blood–brain barrier;
- indirectly using warfarin, which dose-dependently competes for the albumin binding sites;
- non-empirical parameters for estimating the cerebrovascular penetration of drugs;
- magnetic resonance imaging (MRI) to track the transport of paramagnetic contrast markers in the brain, employing a mathematical model;
- a tridimensional blood–brain barrier cell culture model in which human endothelial cells exposed to intraluminal flow form a barrier to ions and proteins following prolonged co-culturing with glia.

Pharmacokinetic considerations for drug equilibration based on the microdialysis method with special emphasis on hydrophilic drugs have demonstrated the following:[12]

1. Equilibration across the blood–brain barrier is rapid.
2. The half-life is similar in brain and blood for most drugs.
3. Unbound brain concentrations seldom reach the level of unbound blood concentrations.

These results are more in line with recent findings on the presence of P glycoprotein and other transport mechanisms at the site of the blood–brain barrier.[12] Non-passive transport across the blood–brain barrier is the case for almost all drugs studies with microdialysis thus far.[12] Ageing alters the blood–brain barrier in terms of select carrier-mediated transport systems, including those for choline, glucose, butyrate and tri-iodothyronine.[13] These age-related changes are the result of an alteration in either the carrier molecules or the physicochemical properties of the cerebral microvessels.[13]

Peptides are generally polar in nature, do not easily cross the blood–brain barrier by diffusion and, except for a small number, do not have specific transport systems.[7] Peptides can also undergo metabolic deactivation by peptidases of the blood, the brain and the endothelial cells that comprise the blood–brain barrier.[7] Recent strategies have been used to promote peptide stability and entry into the brain.[7] Specific transport systems found on the brain endothelial cells can be targeted.[7] The microencapsulation of neuroactive compounds and living cells producing such substances may also overcome the blood–brain barrier.[14] Hyperosmolar blood–brain barrier disruption (with mannitol) transiently increases the delivery of water-soluble compounds by trapping the drug within the blood–brain barrier.[15]

ORAL ROUTE

The bio-availability of opioids is low and often unpredictable when they are given orally.[4] The oral route cannot be used in patients who are unable to swallow, are unconscious, have a bowel obstruction or are suffering from persistent nausea and vomiting. It also depends on patient compliance.

Controlled-release oral formulations (e.g. of morphine) extend drug action and smooth the fluctuations in plasma concentrations (see Chapter 3).[2] A recently available morphine sulphate sustained-release preparation (20 mg, 50 mg and 100 mg capsules) gives sustained levels for a full 24 hours with a single dose. Modern formulations have release properties independent of food, pH and gastric emptying.[2] This method is potentially useful to sustain the plasma concentrations and duration of all analgesics with shorter half-lives, including the NSAIDs (e.g. ketoprofen).[3]

INTRAMUSCULAR ROUTE

Problems with this route include pain on injection, accidental intravenous injection, local tissue irritation, infection and absorption (which is highly dependent on perfusion factors).[4] Contraindications include anticoagulation and severe thrombocytopaenia. Intramuscular opioids are often administered in inadequate doses because of the variability in their kinetic and dynamic properties. Convenience and time factors, as well as fear of respiratory depression and addiction, often result in suboptimal administration, resulting in peaks and troughs of opioid concentration.[4]

INTRAVENOUS ROUTE

The intravenous route offers rapid and dependable drug action, and doses can be titrated to effect. Constant-rate or programmable infusion devices are available, powered by a variety of different energy sources. For chronic states, they may be implantable. Route limitations include venous access and the inability to retrieve what has been given. The wide peak and trough concentrations obtained with opioids with periodic intravenous dosing can result in toxic concentrations followed shortly by ineffective levels.[1] This can be effectively overcome with intravenous PCA, but this requires special equipment and monitoring. A target-controlled infusion (using computer-assisted infusion technology) can be designed to achieve a predicted target concentration based on population kinetics. Although the actual concentration may be greater or less than the target selected, it provides the closest approximation for any individual patient.[4,16]

RECTAL ROUTE

With the rectal route, systemic absorption is often slow, irregular and incomplete.[1] Faecal blockage and hepatic metabolism of that portion of the drug entering the portal system contribute to the poor systemic absorption. Other limitations include a lack of patient compliance and mucosal irritation. Rate-controlled rectal drug delivery can be achieved by using hydrogel formulations and osmotic pumps.[2] The Osmet osmotic pump is designed to be filled by the prescriber and will deliver 2 mL in 24–40 hours.[2] It has potential in analgesic drug delivery. Morphine can be incorporated into a hydrophilic hydrogel polymer.

INHALATIONAL ROUTE

The administration of morphine through the pulmonary system is short lived.[17] Inhalational morphine has a low bio-availability because of its relatively low lipid solubility. Opioids with a higher lipid solubility (fentanyl and methadone) are absorbed to a much greater extent by this route, although only about 10 per cent of the inhaled drug will reach the lungs.[4,17] Ten per cent is deposited in the oropharynx, and 50 per cent is lost on exhalation, some of the dose remaining adherent to the tubing.[17] The pharmacokinetics of fentanyl are affected by absorption, local metabolism and mucociliary transport. Fentanyl (100–300 μg) can provide postoperative analgesia when administered as a nebulized aerosol via an oxygen-driven nebulizer.[17] However, the serum concentration remains low (T_{max} = 2–3 minutes), and the duration of the mild analgesic effect is about 2 hours.[17]

A liposomal-encapsulated formulation of fentanyl in a nebulized aerosol delivery system providing a controlled, sustained release has been used to increase its absorption and prolong its duration of action.[17] The administration in volunteers of a single dose of 2000 μg (of a nebulized mixture of 50 per cent free and 50 per cent liposomal-encapsulated) fentanyl gave a C_{max} of 1.15 ± 0.36 ng/mL, a T_{max} of 16 ±8 minutes, and a bio-availability of 12 ±11 per cent.[17] Plasma concentrations at 8 and 24 hours post-inhalation were 0.25 ± 0.14 and 0.12 ±0.16 ng/mL respectively, indicating the potential of providing prolonged plasma fentanyl concentrations in the analgesic range following the inhalation of liposomal-encapsulated fentanyl.[17]

SUBCUTANEOUS ROUTE

This route is often used for long-term opioid administration. Absorption can, however, be quite variable, and only small volumes of non-irritant drugs can be injected (see the section on PCA below).[1]

TRANSMUCOSAL ROUTE

Three potential areas for transmucosal delivery exist in the mouth: sublingually, buccally (between the gum of the upper molars and the cheek) and gingivally (between the gum of the incisors and the upper lip).[1] The mouth is covered largely by stratified squamous epithelium. Optimal parameters for penetration include a small molecular weight, a greater concentration of ionized drug, and biphasic solubility (with lipid preference).[1] The potential advantages of transmucosal opioid delivery include fast absorption, less presystemic elimination, a rapid onset of action and patient comfort and convenience.[1]

The wide variability in morphine absorption by the buccal route (because at its low lipid solubility and the poor adherence to and dissolution on the buccal mucosa) makes it a poor candidate for this type of drug delivery.[1,2]

With the sublingual route, opioids with a high lipid solubility (buprenorphine, fentanyl and methadone) have better bio-availability than those with low lipid solubility (morphine).[1] Sublingual buprenorphine has been successfully used for premedication and for the management of postoperative and cancer pain.[1]

Oral transmucosal fentanyl incorporates fentanyl into a sucrose-based lozenge on a stick (see Chapter 3). The citrate salt of fentanyl is soluble on both water and a number of candy matrices and is resistant to heat (having a melting point of 152°C), which allows it to be incorporated into a buccal lozenge system.[17] Oral transmucosal fentanyl can produce dose-dependent increases in sedation in adult volunteers and has been successfully used for premedication in children.[17] It has also been used for postoperative analgesia in adults undergoing hip or knee arthroplasty:[17] Patients have achieved VAS scores similar to those of patients using PCA morphine alone, with a reduction of about half the dose in morphine supplementation.

The nasal mucosa is lined with pseudostratified columnar epithelium and has a large blood supply for easy access to the systemic circulation. A variety of drugs (sufentanil, butorphanol, ketamine, calcitonin and midazolam) have been administered via this route.[4,18] Drugs can be instilled in droplet form or in a prepacked, dose-specific swab.[4] The difficulty is in retaining a delivery system for rate-controlled delivery.[2] To enhance intranasal drug absorption, formulations using different surfactant agents (mechanism unknown), bioadhesive agents (to increase mucosal contact) and agents with vasoactive properties (to increase nasal mucosal blood flow) can be used.[1]

In one study, six spray doses (27 μg) of intranasal fentanyl (4.5 μg in 0.9 mL saline) were administered in the early postoperative period after a variety of procedures and repeated every 5 minutes until the patients were pain-free.[17] A mean of 3.7 doses (of 27 μg) achieved excellent pain scores at rest within 15–20 minutes. There were minimal respiratory effects and a less than 1 per cent incidence of nausea, vomiting and euphoria. Intranasal fentanyl (non-irritant to the nasal mucosa) performed virtually identically to intravenous fentanyl of an equal dose in terms of analgesia and side-effects.[17]

TRANSDERMAL ROUTE

Principles, apparatus and drugs used

Transdermal drug systems deliver a drug to the skin surface at a rate less than the maximum rate of transport through the skin.[2] This enables the control of drug administration to remain with the delivery system rather than the skin, and the drug is driven down a concentration gradient towards the patient. Transdermal drug absorption involves passive diffusion. The main factor modulating the speed of absorption is the penetration of the stratum corneum,[19] but the stratum corneum (15–20 cells thick) has, however, proved difficult to penetrate. In addition, a drug depot may form in the stratum corneum and prolong drug action after removal of the system.[2] Potential advantages include the elimination of peak and trough concentrations, a reduction in the variability of plasma drug concentration profiles, the avoidance of first-pass metabolism, a prolonged duration, improved compliance and a concentration-dependent selectivity of drug action.[1,2]

A simplified transdermal system consists of several strategically arranged layers (Figure 7.1).[4] The layer furthest from the patient is a non-permeable, protective cover. Under this is a highly concentrated reservoir of the drug in a gel matrix. This is followed by a rate-controlling membrane (specifically tailored to the drug), which provides for a sustained and programmed release. Closest to the patient, an adhesive allows for secure attachment.

Transdermal local anaesthesia may ultimately permit painless intravenous or intramuscular needle insertion, or superficially confined surgical procedures in both adults and children.[4] EMLA cream (lignocaine and prilocaine) provides local anaesthesia for venepuncture.[19] A transdermally applicable 10 per cent lignocaine gel mixture with 3 per cent glycyrrhetinic acid monohemiphthlate disodium as an absorption promoter is undergoing testing.[19] Skin pretreatments, such as stripping and cleaning, are useful for shortening the onset of dermal patch anaesthesia.[19]

Fentanyl is the prototypical opioid for transdermal application; its use is discussed in Chapter 3. The TTS-fentanyl patch consists of a drug reservoir formed from a shallow compartment moulded from a drug-impermeable laminate, the compartment's open surface being covered by a microporous rate-controlling membrane.[17] The outer membrane surface is coated with an adhesive polymer that is in contact with the skin. Large amounts of fentanyl (up to 10 mg) are present in a gel matrix to provide a driving force for diffusion. Different size patches (25, 50, 75 and 100 cm²) provide sustained infusion rates of about 25, 50, 75 and 100 μg per hour for 48–72 hours. The skin layers act as a secondary reservoir that must be filled before sustained systemic absorption occurs, and continued absorption takes place after the patch is removed. This has proved reasonably effective for chronic pain of neoplastic origin.[17] It has also been used successfully in treating chronic non-malignant pain of the failed back syndrome (L. Zuccherelli, D.

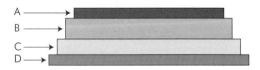

Figure 7.1 A simplified transdermal system consisting of several strategically arranged layers. A = protective, impermeable cover; B = concentrated drug in gel matrix; C = rate-controlling membrane; D = adhesive surface to patient.

Lines and E.A. Shipton, 1996, unpublished data). TTS-fentanyl should not replace intravenous PCA for postoperative pain management because of its delayed onset and prolonged residual effects.[20] It may, however, prove a useful adjunct to non-opioid analgesia in chronic pain management.[20] Transdermal nitroglycerine systems have an antianginal effect for 8–12 hours, but tolerance occurs with sustained treatment.[2]

A transdermal preparation of the α_2-adrenergic agonist clonidine has been developed for the treatment of hypertension. Three systems are available, delivering 100, 200 or 300 μg clonidine in 24 hours.[2] Steady-state concentrations are reached on the third day.[2] After patch removal, plasma concentrations remain constant for 8 hours before declining over 3 days. Transdermal clonidine successfully reduces hyperalgesia in patients with sympathetically maintained pain.[21]

Iontophoresis

The transdermal drug delivery of ionized drugs can be enhanced by iontophoresis: the active transport of ionized molecules into tissues by the application of electric current through solutions containing the ions to be delivered.[17] Thus, transfer can be facilitated by a small current across two electrodes (one above the drug reservoir and one at a distal skin site).[2] Positive ions can be introduced from the positive pole, and negative ions from the negative pole.[2] The electrically charged components are forced through the skin by the external electrical field, the rate of drug delivery being proportional to the current applied. Drugs can be delivered for 3 hours or more by using silver electrodes and chloride ion solutions of the different positively charged drugs.[1]

Electropolation describes the increased permeability of biological membranes when an electrical field is applied to them, thus increasing the diffusion coefficient across the membrane.[17] The most dominant of these processes in active transdermal drug transfer is iontophoresis, in which pure solutions are used, but as several processes are involved, the term 'electromotive drug administration' (EMDA) is used for this novel mode of administration.[17]

The electromotive administration of morphine hydrochloride has been used to reduce postoperative intravenous opioid requirement,[1] plasma morphine levels being related to the iontophoresis current. Morphine hydrochloride applied by this method postoperatively after orthopaedic procedures significantly attains serum concentrations of 20–50 ng/mL and decreases the use of PCA pethidine.[17] Larger (less mobile) electrochemically suitable counter-ions improve the efficiency of transdermal morphine transfer. Morphine sodium citrate, with the same counter-ion as fentanyl, increases the efficiency of transdermal transfer and increases serum morphine concentrations using less direct current.[17] Trials with electromotively administered morphine tricitrate are currently in progress.[17] With the electromotive administration of fentanyl, analgesic concentrations are rapidly reached (like morphine, within 15–30 minutes).[17] A PCA delivery system for the EMDA of fentanyl is currently being investigated.[17] With opioids, EMDA has the potential advantage of delivering systemic doses in which the dose delivered is dependent on the delivery current.[1] Switching off the current stops drug delivery and avoids a depot effect.

The electromotive administration of lignocaine has been used for superficial surgical procedures.[22] EMDA has also been used to deliver corticosteroids for the treatment of painful joints.[23]

Topical NSAIDs

Topical NSAIDs are effective and safe.[24,25] In acute painful conditions (soft tissue trauma, strains and sprains), placebo-controlled trials have been shown to have a relative benefit of 1.7 and an NNT of 3.9.[24,25] With analysis by drug, ketoprofen (NNT = 2.6), felbinac (NNT = 3.0), ibuprofen (NNT = 3.5) and piroxicam (NNT = 4.2) had significant efficacy.[24,25] Benzydamine and indomethacin were no differently from placebo.[24,25] In chronic pain conditions (osteoarthritis and tendinitis), placebo-controlled trials had a relative benefit of 2.0 and an NNT of 3.1.[24,25] There is no clear message on which NSAID (ketoprofen, ibuprofen or piroxicam) was best.[24]

Topical NSAIDs are not associated with the gastrointestinal side-effects seen with the same drugs taken orally.[24] Local skin reactions were rare (3.6 per cent), and systemic effects were rarer (less than 0.5 per cent), probably because of the much lower plasma concentrations obtained from similar doses applied topically as administered orally.[24] In future, it will be important to identify those patients (especially the elderly) with chronic disease who may benefit from topical rather than oral NSAIDs.[24]

INTRA-ARTICULAR ROUTE

Intra-articular corticosteroids and other rheumatological agents

Locally injected intrasynovial corticosteroids work rapidly, effectively and safely in juvenile chronic arthritis (JCA).[26] They are most useful for limited joint, tendon sheath or bursal involvement in pauciarticular JCA, or for the few most active joints in polyarticular or systemic juvenile chronic arthritis, while awaiting the onset of action of the disease-modifying antirheumatic drugs.[26] In medial epicondylitis, the local injection of corticosteroids provides only short-term benefits.[27] Important contraindications to using intra-articular corticosteroids include infection, prostheses, arthroscopy, surgical procedures, damaged joints and hypersensitivity.[26] The most common complication is subcutaneous atrophy, while serious complications include infection and damage to the joint and its surrounding structures.[26] Proper technique, the use of magnetic resonance imaging (MRI) and adequate analgesia, post-injection rest and subsequent mobilization are important.[26] Gadolinium-enhanced MRI has been used to assess the efficacy and effects on cartilage and statural growth of intra-articular corticosteroid therapy (with triamcinolone hexacetonide) for chronic arthritis in children and adolescents 13 months after the steroid therapy.[28] MRI showed a long-lasting suppression of inflammation and pannus without evidence of toxic effects on cartilage.[28] Statural growth was not affected.[28] Long-acting microcrystalline corticosteroids such as triamcinolone hexacetonide are useful for prolonged remission.[26] Repeated injections can be safe and effective.[26] Failure may be a result of incorrect technique, insufficient (e.g. less than 160 mg of methyl prednisolone) or a short-acting corticosteroid, poor general disease control or intrasynovial septa.[26] Also, the evidence that intra-articular steroid therapy for shoulder problems is worthwhile is scarce and less than compelling.[29,30]

In generalized and local osteoarthritis, intra-articular galactosaminoglucuronoglycan sulphate (GGGS) revealed a significant improvement of the articular data, with a decrease in anti-inflammatory consumption.[31] In the cat model, intra-articular sodium hyaluronate (a glycoaminoglycan) reduced nociceptive activity in inflamed joints through an elastoviscous, rheological effect on the nociceptive afferent fibres via the intercellular matrix in which these fibres were embedded.[32] In the rat model, a single intra-articular injection of liposomally conjugated methotrexate suppressed joint inflammation in antigen-induced arthritis.[33] The intra-articular injection of somatostatin has been used in the treatment of osteoarthritis and in rheumatoid arthritis, with encouraging results.[34] Its good tolerability and the absence of unwanted side-effects may lead to its use in those patients in whom other drugs are inappropriate.[34] The intra-articular injection of rifampicin in rheumatoid arthritis is effective against active synovitis, with evidence that the development of new erosions can be prevented or delayed by this treatment.[35] In acute arthritis, the intra-articular injection of a non-specific NO synthase inhibitor, NG-nitro-L-arginine methyl ester hydrochloride (L-NAME), results in a complete reversal of heat hyperalgesia and prevents any further increase in joint swelling and temperature, suggesting an important role for NO in mediating peripheral nociceptive transmission and inflammation.[36] Novel biological (e.g. intra-articular interleukin-1 receptor antagonists) show considerable promise as antirheumatic agents.[37] Also, considerable progress has been made in gene therapy to treat animal models of rheumatoid arthritis.[37]

Intra-articular morphine

Opioids may also diminish post-traumatic inflammation through acting on leucocytes, the inhibition of bradykinin formation or plasma extravasation.[38] Peripheral opioid binding sites have been shown on primary afferent neurones. The intra-articular injection of morphine in patients undergoing arthroscopic surgical procedures is thought to produce an analgesic effect of delayed onset approximately 2 hours post-injection) but of long duration (up to 2 days postoperatively).[38] However, in a systematic review of the relevant published literature on the analgesic efficacy of intra-articular morphine, only a minority of the analysed data could be regarded as valid.[39] Nevertheless, this limited amount of data has provided some evidence for the analgesic efficacy of intra-articular morphine.[39] In the confined space of the knee joint, doses of morphine (0.5–50 mg) produce very high local concentrations.[39] Following knee arthroscopy, intra-articular morphine (2 mg) and clonidine (150 μg) produce comparable analgesia, but the combination is not more effective than morphine alone.[40] In anterior cruciate ligament repairs, patients receiving a multimodal analgesic regimen of perioperative NSAIDs, intra-articular bupivacaine and external cooling did not receive any additional benefit from intra-articular morphine (5 mg).[41]

Intra-articular NSAIDs

Following arthroscopy, intra-articular tenoxicam 20 mg provides better analgesia and decreases the requirements for postoperative analgesics when compared with 20 mg intravenous tenoxicam.[42] In a recent study of day case knee arthroscopy, intra-articular tenoxicam 20 mg at the end of arthroscopy reduced oral analgesia requirements during the first day post-surgery, but it did not alter patients' perception of their pain.[43]

Intra-articular liposomal lignocaine

Both aqueous lignocaine and liposomal lignocaine have been injected into rabbit knee joints and the pharmacokinetic changes studied.[44] The peak serum concentration and the amount absorbed in 4 hours of liposomal lignocaine was significantly lower than that absorbed from the aqueous preparation.[44] This was probably because of the local accumulation of liposomal lignocaine and the slow release of lignocaine from the liposomes, giving lower systemic serum concentrations.[44] Intra-articular lignocaine is used in outpatient knee arthroscopy.[45] Although there have been several encouraging reports in animals that have shown local anaesthetic effects in general lasting up to several days, there are currently no agents (polymers or liposomes) that have given reliable and practically ultra-long-acting local anaesthesia in humans.[46]

INTERPLEURAL ROUTE

Interpleural analgesia with local anaesthetics (bupivacaine) has been used for postoperative analgesia as well as for the treatment of malignant and post-traumatic pain.[47] Subcutaneous implantable infusion systems can be used if long-term analgesia is required (Figure 7.2).[47]

ENCAPSULATION MATRICES

The action of rapidly cleared drugs (e.g. some of the local anaesthetics, and opioids) can be prolonged by incorporating them in a variety of encapsulation

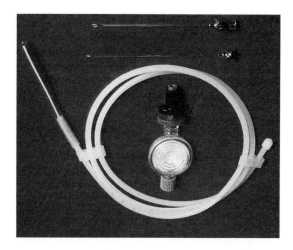

Figure 7.2 19 gauge interpleural catheter (Arrow®) for interpleural analgesia with local anaesthetics through a 17 gauge interpleural needle for acute and chronic pain.

matrices (see Chapter 16) including liposomes, iophendylate and polyanhydride polymers.[48] The duration of epidural analgesia can also be extended by using a poorly soluble fentanyl salt (fentanyl citrate), which creates a depot in the epidural space.[49]

LIPOSOMES

Liposomes are reservoirs containing an aqueous phase surrounded by phospholipid bilayers.[50] Liposome encapsulation permits the delivery of relatively large concentrations of a drug in a form that is sequestered and slowly released into the local biophase.[48] This exposes the local tissue (skin or spinal cord) to relatively steady-state concentrations of the drug over an extended period by reducing bio-availability, so high-dose effects (e.g. respiratory depression) or high-dose tissue toxicity may be reduced. Local anaesthetics have been encapsulated into liposomes for topical application around nerve structures (peripheral nerves and spinal cord) or intra-articularly to prolong their analgesic effects.[50,51] The epidural and brachial plexus administration of liposomal-encapsulated bupivacaine leads to a prolongation of human post-surgical and chronic pain relief with minimal or absent motor blockade.[50]

Liposomes made of egg yolk phosphatidyl-cholines do not produce histological lesions of the nervous system.[50] However, hydrolysis and the oxidation products of lecithin (e.g. lysophosphatidyl-choline and fatty acid free radical scavengers) have been shown to be neurotoxic and cytotoxic.[50] Liposomal formulations thus need chemical analysis before safe in vivo administration. Multilamellar bupivacaine liposomes injected intracisternally in rabbits produce spinal cord histopathological changes not significantly different from those observed with plain bupivacaine.[50]

IOPHENDYLATE

In rabbits, placing local anaesthetics in iophendylate prolongs their spinal action.[52]

TRANSFERSOMES

A new type of analgesic drug carrier, the transfersome, can penetrate rapidly down hydration gradients through the intact dermis and can reach the cutis and subcutis, thus affecting the nociceptors and other nerve endings.[53] Transfersomes are mainly vesicular particles. Each transfersome consists of at least one inner aqueous compartment. This is surrounded by a lipid bilayer.[53] In the morphological but not the functional sense, they resemble the liposomes. Transfersomal drug carriers can accommodate hydrophilic drugs (in the aqueous interior of a carrier) or lipophilic drugs (in the enveloping lipid bilayer).

In humans, complete local anaesthesia can be obtained within 30 minutes with tetracaine, or after 90 minutes with lignocaine.[53] In both cases, the local anaesthesia lasts for over 4 hours. The use of transfersomes will have far-reaching consequences for local pain therapy. The choice of agent and concentration, the transfersome composition and the best application mode still need to be optimized.

MICROSPHERES

Encapsulating bupivacaine in poly(D,L)-lactidecoglycolide microspheres prolongs analgesia and diminishes systemic toxicity.[54] In the acute inflammatory pain model in rats, bupivacaine microspheres induced a dose-dependent increase in the duration of antinociception compared with plain bupivacaine.[54] Glucocorticoids prolong neural blockade from bupivacaine microspheres in rat sciatic nerves.[55]

SPINAL IMPLANTS

The treating physician who chooses to use implantable technologies for pain control should know the appropriate and accepted use of all the 'tools of the trade' and position these tools appropriately.[56] Drug delivery systems may be categorized as follows:[57]

- percutaneously inserted epidural catheters;
- subcutaneously tunnelled epidural or intrathecal catheters;
- implanted epidural or intrathecal catheters connected to access ports;
- implanted intrathecal manual pumps;
- implanted intrathecal or epidural infusion pumps;
- external pumps.

Indications

The selection criteria in cancer- or AIDS-related pain patients with proven opioid-responsive pain who develop intolerable and intractable side-effects after sequential drug trials of strong, long-acting, orally administered opioids are candidates for a trial of an infusion of spinally administered opioids.[56] Life expectancy should be greater than 3 months to justify expensive implantable infusion systems, and there should be no tumour encroachment into the thecal sac.[56] They should be the last resort before neuroablative and destructive procedures.

The experience of giving opioids to patients with chronic non-malignant pain suggests a low incidence of tolerance, few pharmacological consequences and a low incidence of iatrogenic addiction.[56] Implantable therapies for non-malignant pain should only be used when more conservative, non-invasive methods fail to provide analgesia.[56,58]

During patient selection, the general and mental status, life expectancy, nature and the origin of the pain, skin over the implantation area, patient's environment and support systems should be considered.[57] A percutaneous catheter or a subcutaneously inserted catheter may be preferred if the patient has a life expectancy of days to weeks, while ports or pumps are considered for a life expectancy of months or years.[57] Neurogenic, neuropathic or deafferentation pain, incident pain as observed on weight-bearing, or bone pain and other pain syndromes, such as pancreatic pain, rectal tenesmus or pressure sore pain, are all types of pain less likely to respond to opioids.[57]

The area of implantation should be far from any dermatitis, infection, inflammation, skin or subcutaneous tissue metastases.[57] In patients with colostomies, the opposite side should be chosen. The implantation of a pump system on or close to a rib may cause irritation when manipulating the buttons on certain devices.[52] In obese patients and patients with subcutaneous oedema, sites with thinner subcutaneous tissue are preferred.

Contraindications

Contraindications include patient refusal, cachexia, sepsis (localized or generalized) and concomitant anticoagulant therapy.[58]

Trial of spinally administered opioids

Before implanting a drug delivery system, a preimplantation trial is essential, and a decision to implant should be made only after a positive trial response. Thus, before implantation of a device for spinal opioid treatment, the following should be undertaken. Spinal opioid sensitivity should be tested to define the patient's probable acute response to spinal infusions and to suggest the outcome likely to be anticipated from long-term administration.[59,60] The patient's response to the opioid given through a temporary catheter inserted percutaneously is observed.[61] The percutaneous catheter is usually placed intrathecally through a Tuohy needle at the L1–4 levels and advanced cephalad under fluoroscopic control until the tip is close to the spinal cord level that is processing the patient's pain.[56] Thus, the daily epidural (or intrathecal) opioid consumption, the level of activity and sleep, subjective pain scores, the need for additional analgesics and the side-effects should be recorded. In doubtful situations, the spinal administration of a placebo, or an opioid combined with a local anaesthetic, might bring clarity.[58] The trial ensures the efficacy and tolerance of the drug being infused. The procedure and potential side-effects, and the expected goals, should be explained to the patient and family. During the trial, the timed, systemically administered opioid medications are reduced, and the patient is allowed medication as needed for breakthrough pain.[56] To prevent withdrawal symptoms, 50 per cent of the calculated 24-hour prespinal opioid dose is withdrawn at the rate of 20 per cent per day using a timed schedule.[56] The remaining 50 per cent is given as spinal equivalents, being increased by 20 per cent per day. Rescue parenteral or oral opioid medication can be requested. The patient is kept under observation for at least 3

days. During the trial, the response to the spinal opioid (the initial dose and duration of analgesia), the need for the addition of local anaesthetics or other drugs, the adminstration route (epidural or intrathecal) and the success of the method can be assessed.[57] Clonidine 100–300 μg will usually reduce the side-effects of an abstinence syndrome.[56]

Side-effects are both dose independent (urinary retention, pruritus, sweating and sedation) and dose dependent (nausea, vomiting, dysphoria and euphoria, major sedation, respiratory depression, hypotension and tachyphylaxis).[57] Other side-effects include polyarthralgia, amenorrhoea and peripheral oedema.[56] An attempt should be made to manage these symptoms pharmacologically before changing to another opioid. Taking advantage of the incomplete cross-tolerance of one opioid agonist to others, side-effects may be reduced or eliminated, or analgesia restored (after tolerance), by switching opioids.[56]

Pharmacological management

With its low lipid solubility, high receptor affinity and long duration as a spinal opioid, morphine remains the prototypical agent.[57] With morphine, the placement of a catheter for intrathecal infusion anywhere in the thecal sac ensures analgesia anywhere in the body.[56] To convert systemic morphine to spinal morphine, the following formula is used:[56] 300 mg oral morphine = 100 mg parenteral morphine = 10 mg epidural morphine = 1 mg intrathecal morphine.

To convert to hydromorphone (5–10 times more potent and 8–10 times more lipid soluble than morphine), the initial dose is about 50 per cent of the equi-analgesic dose of the new drug.[56] A starting dose of one tenth of the morphine dose should be initiated in the pump. After implantation, a 24-hour intrathecal continuous opioid infusion is given, although some patients do better with a bolus or mixed continuous and bolus dosing.[56] The intrathecal route is preferred, but if it does not relieve the pain, the epidural route should be tried.[57] Pethidine (with its local anaesthetic property) in an intrathecal dose of 0.5 mg/kg has an onset of about 10 minutes and lasts up to 6 hours or longer.[56] It may corrode the inner pump tubing, but this does not preclude its use in external pumps. To convert to sufentanil (with its 1000 times higher lipid partition coefficient than morphine, and its greater affinity for the mu opioid receptors, thus delaying the development of tolerance), a dose conversion of sufentanil 1 μg to morphine 1000 μg (1 mg) is used.[56] Whenever analgesia to an ever-increasing dose of opioid (e.g. 20 mg morphine equivalent) is no longer experienced, bupivacaine starting at 3 mg per day can be added.[56] This can be increased by 20 per cent per week until analgesia or side-effects occur. Continuous intrathecal clonidine (0.7–4.0 μg per hour) can be used via implanted devices.[56] Side-effects include hypotension, a decrease in heart rate, a dry mouth, dizziness and constipation. The opioid peptide D-ala-D-leucine enkephalin can restore analgesia in morphine-tolerant patients.[56] For non-neuropathic cancer pain, octreotide 50 μg/mL (pH adjusted) can be infused intrathecally via an implanted pump at 2.5–20.0 μg/hour.[56] In clinical practice, the use of epidural morphine as a single-drug therapy has virtually been eliminated with the broad selection of oral and transdermal opioids and/or adjuvant therapies currently available.[62]

Intraspinal baclofen can be used to treat spinal spasticity secondary to multiple sclerosis and spinal cord injury (after failed oral baclofen), leading to a marked reduction in motor tone, an improvement in bladder and sphincter function, and a reduction in spasm-related pain.[52,63] Prescreening with test injections of 50, 75 or 100 μg is first employed to obtain a two-point reduction in the Ashworth muscle rigidity/tone scale and muscle spasm scores for at least 4 hours before pump implantation for a continuous infusion of baclofen.[56] The pump is filled with baclofen (500 μg/mL or 1000 μg/mL) and programmed to deliver a total dose equal to double the effective screening dose per 24 hours.[56] Oral antispasmodic medications are gradually reduced to avoid withdrawal seizures. Baclofen and morphine are compatible and stable at 37°C for at least 30 days in the pump.[56] The treatment of CNS toxicity resulting from baclofen administration (dizziness, somnolence, rostral hypotonia, seizures, respiratory depression and coma) may include airway maintenance, ventilation and physostigmine administration.[56]

Which delivery system?

In general, the delivery system is selected according to life expectancy.[58]

TEMPORARY EPIDURAL CATHETER (see Figure 7.3)

Percutaneous or subcutaneously tunnelled epidural and intrathecal catheters are selected for patients

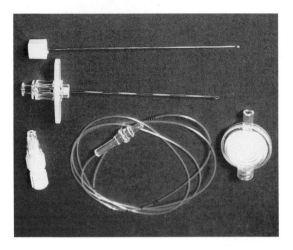

Figure 7.3　Spinal implants: an 18 gauge Tuohy epidural needle with modified Huber point for temporary catheter insertion. A 0.2 μm filter is fitted to the end of the catheter.

with a short life expectancy, inactive patients for whom occasional dislodgement and replacement are preferable to implantation, or patients with severe pain for whom the short-term catheter immediately provides quick access and rapid relief, with further device planning at a future time.[62] A lumbar epidural catheter is the most accepted means of access to the CNS because of the avoidance of dural puncture headache and the protective barrier of the dura against infection (especially with frequent injections).[64] Catheters range from polyethylene (nylon) catheters to more pliable polyurethane and Silastic catheters.[64] The more semipermanent catheters are constructed from softer materials like silicone rubber.[62] The tunnelled portion of these catheters have a dacron cuff for anchoring and an antibacterial barrier. The Du Pen catheter (Bard Access Systems) is a two-part catheter and connector system.[62] The catheter is externalized to the abdominal wall for daily to bi-weekly self-care. The catheter can be used for single bolus injections or connected to an ambulatory infusion pump.[62] Percutaneous catheters are mostly used for the preimplantation trial.

For subcutaneous tunnelling surgery, under image intensification and using a radio-opaque catheter guide, the tip of the epidural catheter can be advanced to the desired level.[63] The epidural catheter emerges from the skin over the lumbar midline. It should be tunnelled laterally for 10 cm. Drugs (opioids and local anaesthetics) can be given as intermittent boluses or via a standard portable constant infusion pump (Fresenius Injector MS26,

Travenol Infuser, Graseby Dynamics Portable Infusion Pump, or Deltec CADD-PCA).[63,64] An adhesive airtight, waterproof dressing should be placed over the catheter exit site and bacterial filters connected to the end of the catheter. These need to be changed regularly. A 'double' PALL filter technique, whereby the 'outer' filter is changed monthly and the 'inner' filter never changed is currently being studied.[62] The use of externalized intrathecal catheters for chronic drug administration has been considered to be a technique carrying too much risk of infection.[62] Disadvantages of the catheter include easy displacement, short duration, kinking or obstruction, leakage, breakage, migration, skin irritation, superficial infection and difficulty with skin cleansing.[57,58]

PERMANENTLY IMPLANTED CATHETERS

If improved pain control and decreased side-effects warrant more prolonged therapy, temporary catheters are usually replaced by permanent, implanted catheters (Figure 7.4) within days to weeks.[61] These systems have advantages in terms of sterility, comfort and freedom of movement for the patient.[64] This requires either a port (bolus injector or reservoir type) for percutaneous access, or an implanted, pump-driven, percutaneously refillable reservoir system.[64] The optimal positioning of a port is in the anterolateral chest wall on the side contralateral to the patient's dominant arm (for the insertion technique, see Figure 7.5). This allows the potential to self-inject.[63] The port should be placed against a bony landmark (e.g. a rib) and positioned so that the patient is able to lie comfortably in a

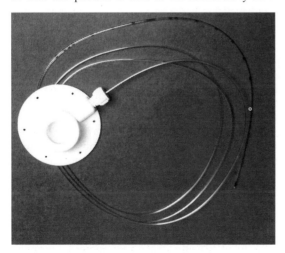

Figure 7.4 Spinal implants – permanent implanted catheters: a subcutaneous reservoir port for percutaneous access (Braun Periplant®).

supine or lateral position.[63] All this is performed under local anaesthesia. The port system has a resealable membrane capable of withstanding percutaneous injections, and a filter to prevent particulate matter being injected spinally.

There are various injection ports available (e.g. Port-a-Cath, Spinalgesic, Spinoplant, Periplant, Celsite and Pharmacia Epidural Port). These may be used for intermittent opioid administration or be connected to an external pump if the patient has a life expectancy of several months.[58] Disadvantages of such systems include numerous skin punctures, blockage of the port outlet or catheter, greater expense (than a simple catheter), the risk of infection, and surgical intervention being needed for system placement and removal.[58] Special needles are necessary for puncture of the port, and the number of injections possible through the port is limited.[57]

IMPLANTABLE INFUSION DEVICE

Implantable infusion devices are indicated in patients with a long life expectancy. They are expensive initially but have the advantage of low costs over time.[62] The device is implanted within the subcutaneous tissues of the anterior abdominal wall or subpectorally, the catheter being sited in the intrathecal (usually) or epidural space. The only significant drawback of such a system is usually the low reservoir volume.[62] Opioid requirements are much less with intrathecal (than epidural) administration because of direct access to the CNS.[61] Refilling of these devices is more difficult than with external pumps.[58]

Implanted pumps consist of a reservoir system and a pump mechanism. The pump mechanism can be driven either internally (e.g. by a lithium battery), externally (by an induction device) or mechanically (being patient operated).[64] Pumps offering continuous plus on-demand infusion rates are preferable to those with fixed infusion rates because of greater flexibility as 'tolerance' develops.[58] Tolerance seems to develop more quickly with bolus intrathecal injections than with continuous intrathecal infusions.[59]

The Infusaid is a continuous (constant-rate), freon-driven pump. A 50 mL reservoir is filled percutaneously every 14–21 days, and a constant volume of drug (2–4 mL per day) is infused continuously (Figure 7.6).[61] If necessary, bolus doses can be given via a separate port. Other pumps (e.g. the Synchromed) use microprocessor technology (Figure 7.7).[65] The hockey puck-sized, microcircuitry-controlled pump is usually implanted in the

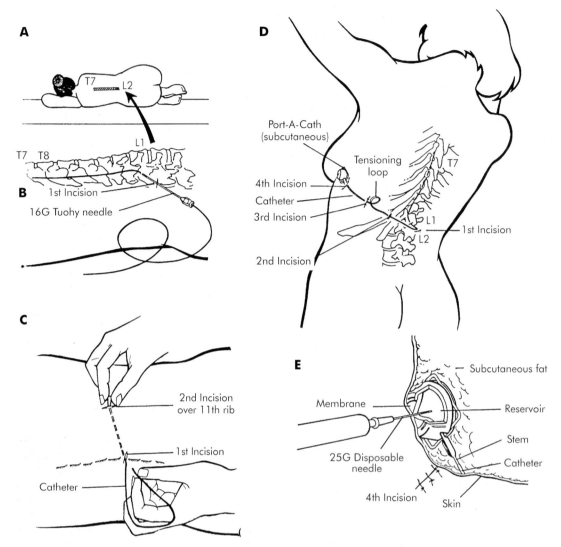

Figure 7.5   Permanent implanted catheters: insertion technique of an epidural portal system. (A) Position of patient before implantation. (B) Insertion of a 16 gauge epidural catheter through a Tuohy needle. (C) Tunnelling technique used to relocate the end of the epidural catheter to the anterior chest wall. (D) Portal attached to the inserted epidural catheter. (E) Injection technique and exposed view of the epidural portal.

subcutaneous tissue of the abdomen. The 18 mL capacity reservoir permits the drug supply to be replenished intermittently (every 1–2 months).[65] There is a port for reservoir replenishment and an accessory port for bolus injections. A portable laptop computer is used to alter infusion rates, and a programming wand transmits new information to the infusion device by telemetry.[65]

Complications

Bleeding can occur at the surgical site. Prior to implantation, a full coagulation profile should be carried out as many cancer patients may be undergoing chemotherapy (with low platelet counts) or taking NSAIDs.[57] All anticoagulant and NSAID therapy should cease 3–7 days prior to implantation. Rarely, a haematoma can develop along the course of the subcutaneous tunnelling.[57] An epidural haematoma may rarely develop as a result of coagulation disorders (e.g. leukaemias) or the use of Tuohy needles to place intrathecal catheters 'blindly' into the thecal sac.[56] Pump pocket seromas are self-limiting.

CSF leakage may occur from accidental dural rupture during the epidural approach or because of

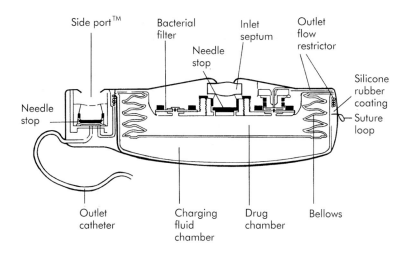

Figure 7.6 Implantable infusion devices for opioid administration. The Infusaid® continuous pump. Volatile hydrocarbon liquid (freon) in the charging fluid chamber expands and compresses the metal bellows; this discharges fluid from the drug chamber via the outlet catheter into the epidural space. Supplementary bolus doses can be given via the separate side port.

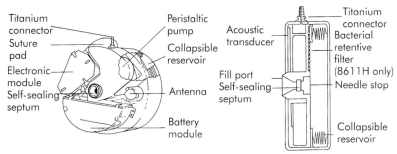

Figure 7.7 Implantable infusion devices. The Medtronic's® drug administration device with a drug reservoir, microprocessor-based circuitry, a lithium battery-driven peristaltic pump and an acoustic transducer attached to an antenna. An external programming wand transmits new information to the infusion device by telemetry.

the discrepancy between size of the intrathecal catheter and that of the needle.[57] Persistent CSF leakage can lead to a post-dural puncture headache in about 20 per cent of patients, the treatment of which is autologous epidural blood patching.[56] A subcutaneous CSF collection (a CSF hygroma) is mostly self-limiting within 1–2 weeks.

Infections can occur at the catheter exit site (in 6 per cent of patients), the pump pocket, the epidural space (abscess) or the intrathecal space (meningitis).[57] Prevention is by prescribing antibiotics during and following implantation, meticulous site care and providing aseptic conditions when changing the needle or filter and when administering the solutions.[57] If the infection involves deep subcutaneous tissues, the catheter or the implant pocket, all the foreign bodies should be removed.[56] Definitive treatment is guided by culture results. The overall incidence of epidural space infection is about 8 per cent or more.[62] It can occur without any sign of infection at the exit site, suggesting that such infections occur secondary to contamination of the infusion solution.[62] With an epidural abscess, there will be lack of analgesia despite an increased dose.[57] The patient's temperature will rise as the abscess devel-

ops. Diagnosis is by MRI with contrast. [Two cases have recently been successfully reported of sterilizing an indwelling infected (*Staphylococcal aureus*) epidural catheter with vancomycin (50 μg/mL at 3 mL per hour) over a period of 14 days.[62]] All hardware should be removed and the abscess drained. Intrathecal infections are rare.[56] The diagnosis is confirmed by CSF findings consistent with a bacterial infection. When related to catheter days, infections occurred half as frequently in the injection port group as in the group with percutaneous catheters.[57] The infection risk is higher with the epidural (about 9 per cent) than with the intrathecal route (about 4 per cent).[57]

Needle placement and intrathecal catheter advancement can damage nerve roots, the conus medullaris or the spinal cord itself, leading to radiculitis, myelitis, paralysis, paresis, loss of bowel and bladder control, and/or myelopathic pain.[56] Epidural opioid administration leads to fibrotic proliferation (in about 13 per cent of patients) within the epidural space. A resistance to flow through the epidural catheter develops initially, followed by dose escalation (pseudotolerance).[57] There is always the possibility of spinal cord damage when using high doses of potent opioids (morphine and hydromorphone) in the intrathecal space.[56] Pain on injection can occur. This is thought to be caused by pressure on the dorsal nerve roots and/or the spinal cord as the result of the formation of a fibrous sheath around the catheter tip.[66, 67]

Occlusion of the system may be caused by the catheter or the port pump. The catheter may be occluded as a result of clot formation, tip fibrosis, kinking (at the subcutaneous exit site, in the epidural space or at the access port junction) or foreign particles in the injected solution.[57] Filters should be used, and contrast dye should be diluted during injection to prevent the formation of a film layer over the filter. Pump occlusion may occur because of valve failure or pump malfunction.[57] The incidence of occlusion is higher in the epidural space than in the intrathecal space, and is less with pumps than with ports.[57] Curling up and knotting of the catheter can occur in the epidural and intrathecal spaces. Removal requires the patient's back to be flexed and steady traction applied, failing which a laminectomy may have to be performed. Catheter dislodgement is most frequently seen with a percutaneous epidural catheter but should be prevented by fastening it with a suture in the fascia at the point at which it is introduced. Catheter disconnection occurs in about 7 per cent of patients, the efficacy of the spinally administered opioid suddenly dropping.[57] Catheter misplacement can occur, the catheter entering a vein, the paravertebral space, the subdural space, on the intrathecal space when placed epidurally. Mechanical catheter problems are confirmed using imaging techniques.[56] In a pump with a side port, injecting contrast dye after aspiration of the catheter dead space, under fluoroscopy, will allow the diagnosis of minor catheter breakage, kinking, disconnections, tip obstruction and dislodgement.[56,58,60,63,68] Skin reactions may develop to percutaneous catheters. Skin necrosis at the port/pump edges may occur in the debilitated cancer patient.

Programmable pump complications include pump overfilling, battery failure (a battery may last 3–5 years), hybrid failure and torsion/flipping of a freely movable pump itself.[56] Overpressurization may damage the pump and overdose the patient. Battery or pump failure present with a loss of analgesia. Drug and pump incompatibility may lead to breakdown of the internal catheter system and workings of the pump. Hybrid failure prevents the pump receiving programmed instruction while allowing it to function as a constant rate pump.[56]

Errors of refilling, dosing and reprogramming

can lead to disaster.[23] Several pumps, including the Infusaid 400 and the Medtronic Synchromed 8165 and 8165-S, contain side ports. When accessing the reservoir port of pumps other than the Synchromed 8165-S, one must, to avoid overdosage, be certain that the needle is within the central and not the side port.[56] Incorrect drug programming can lead to under- or overdosing.

Drug delivery systems still have some disadvantages. The increasing sophistication of these systems is an attempt to decrease the incidence of complications. However, cost containment in health care will undoubtedly impact on pain interventional practice.

PATIENT-CONTROLLED ANALGESIA (PCA)

Conventional analgesic treatments do not consider either the variability of opioid dose requirements between individuals or the change in requirement for an individual over the course of his or her treatment.[69] PCA is a relatively new route of drug administration, offering great promise in both pain control and research. The PCA system was introduced in 1968[70] and is now a major component in the treatment of pain. With its proven efficacy, the range of applications for PCA has grown. It is now used in paediatric surgery, obstetrics, trauma, burns, patients receiving immunotherapy and a variety of medical conditions (acute myocardial infarction, sickle-cell crises and acute herpes zoster infection.)[71, 72] PCA has been successfully used for patient-controlled sedation in patients undergoing surgical procedures under local anaesthesia.[73] It has also been used as patient-controlled neuroleptanalgesia in patients undergoing minor surgical procedures.[74, 75] Results from the management of chronic pain show that PCA can lead to significant lifestyle improvements in ambulatory patients with cancer.[76, 77] Most patients from a wide range of ages and cultures, with varied complaints and extent of tissue damage, find PCA an appropriate method for obtaining analgesia.[78] PCA has also been used as a research tool allowing comparison between different analgesic agents and techniques.[78]

There is a wide variation in opioid requirements between similar types of patient and even within the same patient under different conditions.[78] The fundamental principle of PCA is that it allows patients to reach their own analgesic state and thereby achieve an individual balance between pain relief and the appearance of side-effects.[79]

Although most PCA is administered via the intravenous route, this has in some areas been replaced by oral, sublingual, intramuscular, subcutaneous, neuraxial and intraventricular PCA, and most recently the intranasal and pulmonary routes.[69,71,75,80–82] The use of intravenous PCA is associated with very few true failures, but there is a trend towards better efficacy with epidural PCA.[83]

Are there any predictors of efficacy? Some authors believe the size of the demand bolus to be critical.[83] During the first 24 hours after surgery, age (less being required in the elderly) has been found to be the best predictor of morphine PCA requirements.[83] In one study children aged 4–8 years had significantly higher total postoperative morphine requirements than children aged 9–15 years.[83] Subjective parameters are usually more important for efficacy than are objective criteria as most patients use PCA for comfort rather than freedom from pain.[83] Ethnicity has been found to play a major role because of the prejudice of medical staff, who have been seen to adjust PCA devices to significantly lower opioid doses for Asians and Hispanics.[83, 84]

Advantages

Prospective randomized trials have reported several advantages of PCA over conventional analgesia in the early postoperative period.[76] Although not supported by all controlled trials, the advantages include improved pain relief, less sedation, lower opioid consumption, fewer postoperative complications, greater patient satisfaction and improved pulmonary function.[76]

IMPROVED QUALITY OF ANALGESIA AND PATIENT SATISFACTION

A recent meta-analysis in postoperative patients found the use of PCA to be associated with only a small improvement in analgesia but with a large increase in patient satisfaction compared with intramuscular opioids.[79] Pain is a subjective experience, and PCA allows patients to titrate opioids against their pain, theoretically maintaining their opioid plasma concentrations close to the minimum effective analgesic concentration.[79] Opiophobia (e.g. fear of addiction) on the part of the patient and the medical and nursing staff is likely to provide fewer opioid demands.[85] However, PCA patients are almost always more satisfied with their pain control.[85]

LOWER OPIOID CONSUMPTION AND SEDATION

A general finding with PCA is that patients consume larger amounts of opioids in the early postoperative period but require fewer analgesics over time compared with patients given intramuscular opioids.[79]

FEWER POSTOPERATIVE COMPLICATIONS

The undertreatment of severe acute pain causes harmful physiological effects.[79] Several studies have shown that PCA patients, compared with those receiving intramuscular opioids, have a more rapid recovery of pulmonary function, are able to mobilize and eat solid food earlier, and have a shorter hospital stay.[79]

TIME AND COST-SAVING

Controlled studies have shown PCA to save nursing time and be more cost-effective than conventional analgesia.[79] Time spent on the administration of intramuscular injections and repeated drug register entries, and the cost incurred from disposable syringes, needles and drug wastage, is minimized with PCA.[79]

Prescribing

Informed prescribing is based on a maximum knowledge (of pharmacokinetic and pharmacodynamic factors) of the drugs involved. It seems that the success of PCA is independent of the opioid used.[85] However, the metabolites of morphine (morphine-3-glucuronide and morphine-6-glucuronide) show greater accumulation in patients with poor renal function. The chronic use of pethidine is not ideal as the propensity for norpethidine intoxication is increased after 24 hours of dosing, especially in patients with diminished renal function.[85] Fentanyl produces no known pharmacologically active metabolites and appears to be the least complex and most efficacious of the agents commonly used in the PCA setting.[85]

The point at which the patient becomes uncomfortable enough to make a demand has become known as the minimum effective (blood drug) concentration (MEC). The MEC represents that concentration which removes the distress of pain but not necessarily the sensation of pain. There are no reliable MECs for individual drugs during PCA, and intra-individual variability (of up to 30 per cent) can occur.[85] Theoretically, when using PCA, patients should load themselves to exceed their MEC and then demand to deliver the drug as needed to maintain it.[85] This demand pattern ensures that the patient maintains satisfactory pain relief without excessive sedation. If patients follow this demand pattern, the parameters of PCA (such as bolus size) should be relatively unimportant (within safe and practical limitations) as patients will demand until they exceed their MEC and then only demand if their blood drug concentration falls below the MEC.[85, 86] This is a point they will recognize as that at which they are no longer satisfied with their pain relief. While most patients seem to demand to some pattern whereby they load and then maintain at a relatively stable level, the end-point for which they are demanding is influenced by factors other than their state of pain at that time. The PCA drug demand decision is determined by the pain felt, which will in turn be dependent on any interaction of factors that influence the hierarchy of states (anatomical, physiological, biochemical, pharmacological and psychological) pertaining to the pain and its treatment.[85] The patient's fears, pain history, pain meaning, coping mechanisms and attitude to the pain determine the treatment response irrespective of the drug's pharmacokinetics. Preoperative education concerning PCA may greatly influence its postoperative use. Patients should be assured that their personal contact with the nursing or medical staff will not be reduced. The insight that pain thresholds (both subjective thresholds and objective parameters such as plasma drug concentrations) are unpredictable in individual patients is one of the greatest merits in using PCA.[83] However, not all patients want control over their analgesia, and some may not perceive that they have control.[85] This may explain why some patients do not fare well with PCA. Thus, a thorough knowledge of current advances in PCA, and clinical experience, results in safe prescribing.

Analgesic drugs

Virtually all available opioids have been tried for intravenous PCA, and no 'best' opioid has so far been defined.[83] There are no clear pharmacological reasons for selecting a particular opioid,[3] but patients do, however, seem to prefer some opioids to others.[3] Interpatient variability makes it difficult to define the maximum dose or dose rate. It is still to be determined whether there is an optimum lock-out interval for various opioids.[3] Ideally, opioids used for PCA should be potent, of rapid onset and of moderate duration, should not accumulate or give rise to tolerance and should have no ceiling effect.[79] Drugs with a very short (alfentanil) or a very long duration of action (methadone), partial agonists (buprenorphine) and agonist–antagonists (pentazocine) are not recommended.[79] Opioids used include morphine (mostly), hydromorphone, methadone, oxymorphone and fentanyl. PCA tramadol is as effective as morphine but has the same side-effects.[87] Methadone, pentazocine and pethidine have all been associated with tissue irritation and are not recommended for chronic use.[77] In addition, there is the potential of norpethidine to provoke CNS irritation. In postoperative pain relief, the comparison of morphine with fentanyl shows an improved demand-to-delivery ratio for fentanyl during the first 12 hours; afterwards the ratios become similar.[79] Morphine consumption decreases linearly over a long period of time, while that of fentanyl remains constant.[79] It might prove advantageous to start using an opioid with a rapid onset and a short T_{max} (fentanyl), and then switch to a longer-acting agent (morphine).[79] Using intravenous PCA pethidine, intrathecal morphine-6-glucuronide (100–125 μg) prolongs analgesia compared with intrathecal morphine (500 μg) after hip replacements.[83]

Multimodal analgesia (including epidural mepivacaine and morphine, systemic diclofenac, metamizol, midazolam, magnesium sulphate and clonidine) significantly reduces postoperative morphine consumption.[83] The intention is to decrease opioid requirements, improve analgesia with the combination of agents and decrease opioid side-effects. This has been demonstrated with PCA morphine and clonidine, and with PCA morphine and ketamine.[17] Alternative analgesics also have side-effects (e.g. ketorolac – platelet dysfunction and gastric irritation; clonidine – hypotension and dry mouth; and ketamine – sedation and hallucinations), but, by using small doses, the aim is to avoid these side-effects.[17] Ketamine and ketorolac tend to require opioid supplementation in patients with severe pain, whereas PCA clonidine is effective on its own but produces increased sedation.[17, 79] PCA has been used in the assessment of locoregional techniques (EMLA cream), in interpleural anaesthesia, with ropivacaine and with other NSAIDs (intravenous ketoprofen, piroxicam and sustained-release ibuprofen).[83] Perioperatively, the pre-emptive effects of PCA and PCEA may only be detectable if the prophylaxis of and protection against painful stimuli are both highly effective and extend long enough into the recovery period.[83]

PCA devices

PCA equipment ranges from simple disposable pumps (Baxter Health Care and Go-Medical) to very sophisticated microprocessor systems (the CADD-Pharmacia Deltic, the Graseby-PCA and the Abbott Pain Manager).[72, 88–90] Most consist of a microprocessor-driven syringe/reservoir that delivers a bolus of drug (usually intravenously, but the equipment can be readily adapted to the subcutaneous and the epidural routes) when a button is pressed by the patient.[78, 79] A background infusion can often be administered independently. Infusion rates and intervals are preset by the physician, but the PCA is activated by the patient by pressing the button. Programming modalities include drug concentration, bolus size, loading dose, infusion mode, lockout interval, maximum hourly dose and constant background infusion rate.[78] Other variants include an infusion demand, and a bolus demand plus variable infusion (for research purposes).[3] Options exist for the use of all or some of these modalities, and there is considerable latitude for the patient to use as much analgesic as required. Safety, however, is ensured by the use of the lock-out interval, maximum demand settings, high-pressure alarms, the detection of air in the dispensing set and antitampering devices.[78,79] A recording mode monitors the frequency and success of analgesic demands (both met and unmet attempts). A review of this information allows the physician to reprogramme the PCA device appropriately.

Patient selection

In the perioperative situation, patients undergoing major surgery are most likely to benefit from PCA. This includes those undergoing: laparotomy (for treatment of the abdominal and pelvic organs and for arterial disease); post-caesarean section; amputation; mastectomy; extensive, full-thickness burn skin grafting; thoracotomy (for conditions of the lungs, heart and oesophagus, and for arterial disease) and sternotomy; major orthopaedic surgery (open reductions, joint replacements, osteotomies, arthrodesis and bone grafts); laminectomy and discectomy; extensive free tissue flaps and tendon transfers; all microvascular surgery; and the extensive dissection of malignant tumours. Most patients, even children of 4 years or older, are suitable.[79]

Patients must, however, be able to understand the technique of PCA and be capable of being active in their own care. This will obviously exclude patients with cognitive defects (those who are confused or mentally impaired), unconscious patients, patients with organic brain syndromes and those who find the technique intimidating. Understanding and being able to push the PCA button might exclude the very young and the very old.[63] Intravenous drug abusers are excluded because of their drug-seeking behaviour and interference with PCA devices.[71] PCA should be used with care in patients with unstable cardiovascular systems (especially if they are hypovolaemic).[71] Patients physically unable to operate the pump can be considered for 'nurse-controlled PCA'. Modified apparatus with pedals or pneumatically controlled devices activated by blowing in a tube have also been described.[79] In chronic cancer pain, PCA should be considered when oral or rectal analgesics are no longer appropriate as a result of alimentary dysfunction or intractable dose-limiting side-effects, or in advanced-stage malignancies involving multiple organs or infiltrating bone or a nerve plexus.[77] Inadequate staff training will at best provide expensive poor analgesia and at worst increase the risk of complications.[79] Training programmes or the employment of a dedicated acute pain nurse are probably more effective than sophisticated technical equipment.[83]

Monitoring

Experience with PCA shows that there are few problems in clinical practice.[91] In the acute pain situation, a high dependency level of nursing care and a monitoring regimen should be used to assess efficacy and any side-effects, and avoid any complications.[92] Besides routine vital signs, the systematic recording of pain scores (visual analogue and verbal rating), sedation scores, respiratory rates and any side-effects should be undertaken at regular intervals (preferably hourly).[71,93] The use of pulse oximetry to monitor for hypoxaemia should become standard in patients with acute pain receiving PCA. The total amount of opioid delivered, the ratio of met and unmet PCA demands, and the drugs used to treat side-effects should also be recorded.[79] A clear identification of the staff responsible for pain relief must be established. The responsible physician must be available to assess and manage treatment adequacy, side-effects and indications for alterations in the treatment regimen so that the treatment is individualized and optimized.[77]

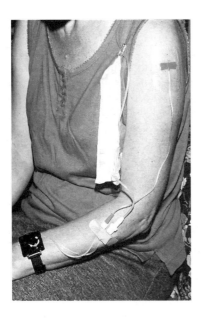
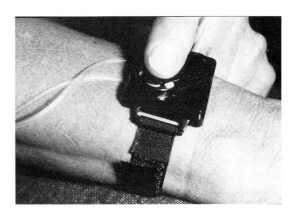

Figure 7.8 A patient using a disposable PCA infuser (Baxter Healthcare) for postoperative pain. See text for details.

Equipment

PCA equipment ranges from simple, disposable systems (to contain costs) to very sophisticated microprocessor systems. All pumps should be bench-tested and should fulfil their technical specifications.[71] A simple system for PCA made from disposable items has recently been described.[94] It uses hydrostatic pressure for its driving force. A disposable PCA infuser (Baxter Healthcare) has recently been evaluated in paediatric surgical patients (Figure 7.8).[92,95] The infuser has a (50 mL) elastometric reservoir. This empties at a constant rate into a wrist-watch-style patient-control module, which incorporates a reservoir (with a volume of 0.5 mL). There are three types of infuser, which empty at different rates (0.5, 2.0 and 5.0 mL per hour).[92] Flow occurs into the reservoir until it is full. The outlet from the reservoir is occluded by a spring-loaded push mechanism. This is released when the wristwatch button is pressed, and a bolus dose is delivered into the intravenous cannula via a one-way valve. The watch reservoir is refilled in 6 minutes (a nominal lock-out time).[92] A background infusion can be used by using two Y-pieces so that one limb bypasses the wristwatch reservoir. Care needs to be taken to fill the system with the correct drug concentration and use the correct infuser model.

The Basal-Bolus Infuser system is a non-electrical, completely disposable PCA device.[96] It has two lines

coming out of the cylinder ballooning reservoir, both with capillary resistors limiting flow. One of these goes directly to the patient-control module, and the other goes directly to the patient's intravenous line. In this way, the patient may have both PCA and a fixed rate background infusion. Another non-electrical, completely disposable PCA device is the Patient Controlled Injector (Go Medical) (Figure 7.9).[97] These disposable PCA devices are filled by injecting fluid into a large reservoir syringe. The patient line is then primed with fluid. When the patient-demand syringe is attached with the button depressed, a vacuum is created, which draws the fluid at a prescribed rate into the patient-demand syringe.[97] Safety is assured by refilling with small reservoir doses, and sudden dumping of the full reservoir dose is avoided as the only forward pumping mechanism depends on the patient pushing the button.[97] It can be used for intravenous, subcutaneous and epidural drug administration.

The Edmonton Injector has been designed for subcutaneous PCA in chronic cancer pain.[98] An opioid solution is kept in a standard 50 mL or 100 mL bag. With a simple movement, the patient fills up a specially designed 1 mL syringe, and a second movement injects the opioid subcutaneously.[98] A double-valve system prevents the solution returning to the bag when injected.[98] The whole system weighs a total of 80 g when full and is kept in a pocket pouch. A potential problem is that the

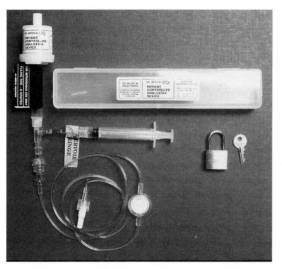

Figure 7.9 A disposable intravenous patient controlled injector (PCI) (Go-Medical Industries®). It consists of a PCI syringe, a patient demand button, a one-way valve, and a reservoir port containing a loading syringe (locked in a plastic casing). The filling time for the PCI syringe is 6 minutes.

Edmonton Injector does not have a lock-out mechanism to limit the amount of opioid that the patient can self-administer.

In recent years, commercially available, non-disposable systems have multiplied in number. Up until only a few years ago, only the Cardiff Palliator and the On-demand Analgesic Computer were available.[99] Recent advances in microprocessor control are now providing a larger choice of pumps,

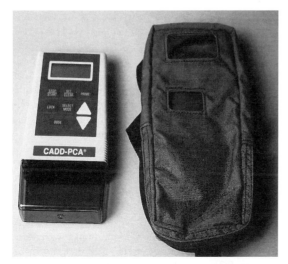

Figure 7.10 Ambulatory CADD-PCA pump with cassette attached and carrying pouch.

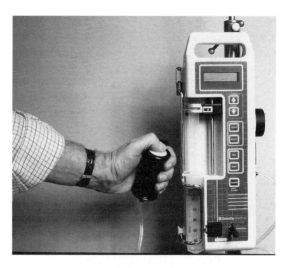

Figure 7.11 The Graseby patient controlled analgesic pump.

which are increasingly compact and user friendly, and offer more control over infusion and bolus dose variables. Some of the PCA pumps available include the CADD-PCA, the Bard Harvard PCA (PCA 1 and ambulatory), the Graseby PCA 3300, the IVAC PCA 310, the Abbott Lifecare and Provider 5500, and the Bionic MDS 110 PCA series (Figures 7.10 and 7.11).[71] Recent additions include the APM-Abbott Pain Manager PCA Infuser, and the CADD-Prizm for intravenous, subcutaneous and epidural drug delivery. The equipment for PCA comprises two components: the pump itself and the accessories (the drug reservoir, the delivery tubing and the antireflux valves).[71]

Faults and precautions

Despite the worldwide use of PCA for several years, there have been only a handful of recorded episodes of equipment malfunction leading to opioid overdose.[100] The most common problem is probably pump failure as a result of inadequate power supply (low batteries or disconnection from the main power source).[79] Occlusion of the dispensing set and of the intravenous cannula also commonly occurs.

The emptying of the PCA opioid reservoir by gravity can occur as a result of poorly seated or cracked syringes and failure to include appropriate non-return or antisyphon valves in the dispensing set.[79] In one case, a crack in a glass vial of analgesic solution allowed solution to syphon into the patient.[101] A third overdose occurred when a glass syringe from the PCA machine disengaged from the drive mechanism.[102] Probable syphoning from the syringe occurred in two patients recently reported to have received morphine overdoses from PCA pumps.[103] To prevent this, the PCA pump should be at the level of the patient, an antisyphon valve should be used, the syringe should have a big enough plunger to allow proper plunger clamping, and the plunger position should be checked to ensure its accurate placement every time the syringe is changed.[102,103] Two overdoses have occurred because of corruption of the pump's software by either mains electrical fluctuations or static electrical discharges from the patient's bed.[100,104] Errors in programming or using PCA may cause over- or underdosing.[79] Inadequate patient instruction (leading to inappropriate demands) or PCA activation by staff and friends can lead to overdosing.[79]

Some characteristics have been suggested to optimize the purchase of a PCA pump:[71,95]

- The pump should have a dual power supply (battery and mains) and be activated by a double push button.
- The pump should be specific for individual agents and the mode of delivery (e.g. by using programmed chips).
- The programme should be simple to run, with the machine scrolling the completed prescription for review before starting the infusion.
- Software protection against current surges and static interferences is essential.
- Patients should not be able to interfere with alarms, which should warn against a low battery, air in the line, line occlusion or an empty syringe.
- Pumps need to be lightweight, robust and accurate (within 10 per cent of set values).
- The use of antireflux valves (to prevent retrograde opioid flow during occlusion), and line clips when changing syringes or cassettes, is essential.
- To avoid tampering by untrained staff or patients, the analgesic reservoir should not be able to be detached from the pump during use.[105]

As the complexity of PCA pump design increases, the number of potential faults that can occur also increases. All pumps should be carefully matched to delivery systems and to drug dilutions,[71] and all pumps should be checked and maintained regularly. Electronic devices should not be operated near PCA pumps.[71] One PCA device (Infuscommand) has been developed coupled to a pulse oximeter control feedback for added safety.[106] Continuous in-service training programmes for medical and nursing staff should be undertaken.[85] A nurse educator dedicated to PCA is an advantage.

Opioid side-effects

The most frequently reported side-effects remain postoperative nausea and vomiting, having an incidence of 40–100 per cent.[79] The addition of droperidol 0.05–0.16 mg per bolus of PCA decreases postoperative nausea and vomiting but increases sedation.[79, 83] Transdermal hyoscine has proved useful in children.[79] The combination of ondansetron and droperidol is still to be tested. If nausea and vomiting are problematic, the bolus dose may need to be reduced or the patient changed to another opioid.

Pruritus occurs commonly but rarely needs to be treated with antihistamines.[79] Another side-effect is urinary retention, which may require temporary catheterization. Anticipatory treatment and patient mobilization help to alleviate constipation.

The incidence of respiratory depression varies between 0.2 and 1.2 per cent.[79] The risk of respiratory depression can be minimized if epidural morphine is injected in a small volume (1–2 mL saline), which significantly decreases the amount reaching the cerebellar medullary cistern.[69] Sedation is an early indicator of respiratory depression, as respiratory rate is not a good guide to the severity of respiratory depression.[79] A safety feature is that as the patient becomes more sedated, no further demands are made.

Use in cancer pain and home care

PCA is both practical and desirable for the care of patients with chronic pain, and its use in chronic pain is likely to increase dramatically in the future.[77] PCA is particularly successful in cancer pain, where pain is relatively constant and likely to persist. A background infusion is often given, whose rate is adjusted to provide adequate analgesia with a minimum of sedation.[77] The bolus dose provides supplemental analgesia to counteract breakthrough pain and to minimize, incident pain. Intermittent pain related to specific activity (e.g. with movement from bony metastases) can be managed with bolus doses given prior to the activity. Interestingly, intravenous PCA allows early decisions if neuropathic or chronic non-malignant pain responds to opioids.[83]

Intravenous PCA with fentanyl has been used to optimize the starting dose of transdermal fentanyl patches.[83]

Home care PCA maintains patient comfort while promoting independent functioning in familiar surroundings. Proper supervision by a family member is essential. Staff from the pain relief service must always be available for assessments and dose adjustments or for any mechanical problems.[77] With partner-controlled (or parent-assisted) analgesia, careful screening of the spouse (or parent) and frequent reassessment are necessary.[77] Only a few patients with chronic pain (usually cancer pain) require PCEA.[69]

Patient-controlled sedation

Patient-controlled sedation is another application that has attracted wide interest. Midazolam, methohexitone and propofol have been investigated in several studies of premedication – conscious sedation – during oral or cataract surgery.[83] A new disposable device (the Baxter Intermate LV250 infuser) has been developed for the more viscous fluids.[83]

Routes

SUBCUTANEOUS

Continuous subcutaneous infusions of opioids are used in patients in whom the oral route is precluded or who are poorly controlled on large doses of oral opioids (Figure 7.12). Subcutaneous morphine infusions have been shown to have great efficacy in the treatment of chronic malignant pain, with a high patient acceptability and a low side-

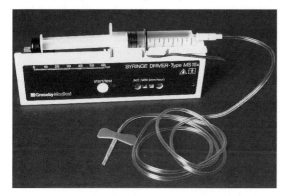

Figure 7.12 The portable battery driven Graseby Medical MS 16 syringe driver for continuous subcutaneous opioid infusion. Continuous subcutaneous infusions of opioids are used in patients where the oral route is precluded, or who are poorly controlled on large doses of oral opioids.

effect profile.[107] The treatment can be started in the hospital and then continued at home. The concentration of the opioid solution should be increased in order to deliver smaller bolus volumes and prevent swelling of the subcutaneous site. For perioperative pain relief, the subcutaneous route has been found to be as effective as the intravenous route when the same doses of morphine are used, the plasma levels reaching similar concentrations within a very short time (minutes).[79, 87] The demonstration that the subcutaneous route is safe and effective for opioid administration has made home care particularly easy.[108] A variety of infusion pumps are commercially available.[61] They are usually portable, battery driven and inexpensive, with incorporated alarm systems. Simple spring-loaded syringe drivers (the Medifuse and Springfusor Pumps) have been tested for subcutaneous infusion.[109] With subcutaneous infusions, a 27 gauge butterfly needle is inserted subcutaneously (e.g. into the chest wall) and taped flush with the patient's skin. The infusion site is checked twice daily for erythema and changed weekly or as needed.

ORAL

The use of oral bedside PCA where oral opioids are kept at the patient's bedside for swallowing when needed has been described.[110]

VENTRICULAR

A patient-controlled apparatus (the L-224) has been developed and successfully tested for the ventricular administration of opioids in patients with intractable pain.[81]

EPIDURAL

Epidural PCA (or PCEA; see Chapter 9) using fentanyl or hydromorphone has been successfully given as an alternative to intravenous PCA for post-surgical pain (e.g. caesarean section – fentanyl; post-thoracotomy – fentanyl; upper abdominal surgery – hydromorphone; vascular surgery – morphine).[111–114] Much less opioid is consumed, with similar or even improved analgesia, emphasizing the spinal action of opioids. The majority of PCEA studies have concentrated on bupivacaine/opioid (fentanyl, diamorphine or pethidine) combinations, in which the addition of the local anaesthetic has led to some improvement of efficacy and less opioid-induced pruritus, but usually also to minor cardiovascular depression.[83] If the MECs of the opioids are used, PCEA is a safe technique, incurring a low risk of dose-dependent side-effects.[69] Patients given PCEA with morphine or fentanyl seem to recover more quickly, as judged by shorter mechanical ventilatory times, higher satisfaction with analgesia and fewer postoperative complications, than patients given intravenous PCA.[69] Thus, the length of stay in hospital and intensive care units and, subsequently, hospital costs may be reduced.[69] Important considerations for opioid selection for PCEA for postoperative pain are:

- the dose requirement ratio for systemic versus epidural administration;
- the opioid concentrations achieved during the epidural dosage regimen;
- the quality of epidural versus systemic analgesia;
- the incidence of side-effects associated with the opioid.[69]

The benefit to risk ratio should be as high as possible.

Pumps for PCEA require particular infusion characteristics.[115] These include portability, the accuracy of infusion against backpressure and the ability to deliver a bolus dose without activation of the occlusion alarm, while retaining the ability to detect an occlusion. The Provider 5500 has recently been tested and found to be suitable for the safe delivery of PCEA.[115] An increase in PCEA among cancer patients is likely to be seen in the future.[76]

INTRANASAL

The use of intranasal PCA (PCINA) for perioperative pain management has recently been described[82]. The venous outflow of the nasal mucosa enters the systemic circulation, bypassing the first-pass effect. Two such devices (Go Medical® Lockout Nasal Sprays) consist of a specially designed spray bottle with a bolus spray of 0.2 mL and filling (lock-out) times of 3 and 4 minutes, respectively. The maximum volumes that can be delivered per hour are 4 and 3 mL, respectively. A study using sufentanil in these devices for perioperative paediatric pain has recently been completed (J.A. Roelofse and E.A. Shipton, 1999, unpublished data). Another such device consists of a specially designed spray bottle and includes a Baxter PCA-on-demand system consisting of a mechanically driven infuser, a flow restrictor and a patient-controlled module for bolus administration (of 0.5 mL) adapted for PCINA.[82] Using fentanyl, this device relieves postoperative pain as effectively as intravenous PCA, although the doses required are

higher and the demands more frequent.[82] Patient acceptance is high.[82] Recent studies have confirmed the rapid onset of action of intranasal fentanyl, sufentanil and butorphanol.[82] The bio-availability of intranasal fentanyl is 71 per cent, that of alfentanil 65 per cent and that of sufentanil 78 per cent.[82]

OTHER NON-INVASIVE PCA ROUTES

From the available data, which include experience with sublingual buprenorphine and submucosal (lollipops) or transdermal (iontophoretically applied) fentanyl, non-invasive PCA seems to be a valuable tool, particularly in ambulatory care (e.g. for breakthrough pain treatment in cancer patients.[83] The future development of iontophoretic delivery techniques may provide an effective and non-invasive system for PCA techniques.

LOCOREGIONAL PCA

This is a technique delivering a local anaesthetic/opioid mixture by means of a PCA device connected to a catheter and placed in a nerve trunk sheath.[79,83] This has been used successfully in interscalene PCA for shoulder surgery, and in the cervical sympathetic trunk for brachialgia.[79,83]

New research concepts on PCA technique

New approaches are aimed at improving analgesia with PCA by allowing greater flexibility and individualization of the technique. The following concepts have been tested for this purpose.[79]

CONTINUOUS BACKGROUND INFUSION

The addition of a continuous infusion to PCA increases the total dose of opioid delivered and the incidence of side-effects without improving analgesia or sleep.[46] The inherent safety of PCA is reduced as this method delivers opioid regardless of sedation levels.[46] Continuous infusions are no longer generally recommended.

CHANGING THE LOCK-OUT INTERVAL

In practice, there is no discernible difference in effect between different opioids when commonly selected lock-out intervals are used.[79] There is now the possibility of eliminating the lock-out interval and replacing it with a dose/time limit.[79] Some PCA devices offer an hourly or 4-hourly limit, which allows the patient to receive a set amount of opioid within this time. In the early postoperative period, when pain level, opioid requirement and demand-to-delivery ratio are high and changing, the patient has more flexibility to titrate pain relief with the dose/time limit, while a safety mechanism exists to prevent overdosage.[79] Large interindividual variations in opioid requirements make it difficult to predict a safe limit for all patients.

CHANGING THE OPIOID DOSE

Variable-dose PCA

The concept of variable dose PCA has emerged to improve pain relief by changing, at regular intervals, the bolus dose (e.g. 0.5, 1.0 or 1.5 mg morphine) according to patient's pain score and the occurrence of side-effects.[116] The intention is to better match supply with demand. The optimal demand dose is that which produces adequate analgesia with no undesirable side-effects.[116]

Patient-maintained, target-controlled infusion

This technique uses a target-controlled infusion under patient control.[63] A computerized device linked to an infusion pump is programmed with the patient's data (age, weight and sex) and the desired opioid concentration to be achieved according to pooled pharmacokinetic data.[79] The device calculates the bolus dose and the infusion rate (e.g. of alfentanil) required to maintain this target concentration. The target concentration may be increased by the patient pushing a button within a chosen lock-out interval.[79] If no further demands are made within a set interval, the target concentration is reset at the previous lower level until it reaches the initial baseline concentration. For chronic pain, an algorithm and computer pump system have also been developed along similar lines, allowing patients to control their own analgesic plasma concentrations.[16] This approach uses individually determined pharmacokinetic parameters to provide steady plasma opioid concentrations that can be increased or decreased by the patient in line with the need for more pain relief or fewer side-effects.[16,117]

Conclusion

Over the past decade, PCA has proved to be a safe and effective technique in the management of acute and chronic pain. PCA is still one of the best ways of achieving patient satisfaction and recuperation in the postoperative period. The challenge now is to improve the quality of pain relief further by modifying the method to suit each patient, catering for wide interindividual variations.[79] Furthermore, even if PCA devices are lacking, the PCA principle can still be applied.[83] This involves trusting the patient, providing adequate monitoring and appropriate documentation, and raising the educational level of the staff on the surgical wards.[83] PCA devices are increasingly used in ambulatory cancer care and for terminally ill patients.[83] So far, however, there is no perfect PCA analgesic agent, and our understanding of current agents remains incomplete.

DISPOSABLE INFUSION DEVICES

Several affordable, disposable infusion pumps are currently available for the intravenous and epidural infusion of analgesic medications in ambulatory outpatients experiencing chronic intractable pain.[118] Recently, three such pumps (the Baxter 2C1075, the Homepump H100020 and the Surgipeace SP500-24) were tested for their effectivity in delivering an epidural infusion of 2 mL per hour.[118] The Baxter infuser relies on a balloon reservoir to supply sustained internal pressure. The delivery tubing between the pump and the connector will not restrict flow. A Luer body houses a filter and a controlled-size orifice. The Homepump Elastomeric Infusion system is also a balloon-powered unit. The membrane consists of three layers of latex, the flow being regulated by a capillary tube orifice.[118] In addition to a micropore filter, there is a clamp present on the tubing to allow the user to stop and start the flow. The Surgipeace Pain Control System provides constant internal pressure to drive the infusion system by a metal spring, which is housed within a cylindrical, durable plastic casing.[118] A combined connector, micropore filter and flow restrictor unit is interposed within the pump tubing to the catheter. An external scale estimates the remaining volume of infusate in millilitres. All pumps initially infused at a rate above 110 per cent for the first 3–6 hours, after which a steady decline in flow rate occurred.[118]

The Drug Infusion Balloon System is composed of a silicon balloon and a ceramic microregulator. It can be used for continuous intravenous and epidural infusions.[86] The various balloon volumes range from 25 to 250 mL and the possible infusion time from 5 to 200 hours.[119] It has been used in a continuous epidural infusion method on patients undergoing open chest surgery, abdominal digestive surgery and gynaecological surgery (H. Hirota, A. Yoshioka and K. Hase, 1997, unpublished data). The primary pressure in the balloon is relatively low, the intraballoon pressure being maintained within the 70–100 mmHg range. The infusion rate is slightly lower than that reported in the manufacturer's literature. The Drug Infusion Balloon System with a three-way stopcock has been used for PCEA (by teaching patients to control the flow by means of the stopcock) in patients suffering chronic pain (musculoskeletal pain and post-herpetic neuralgia) (M. Murozono, Y. Toyohiko and H. Miyatake, 1997, unpublished data).

For a 10 mL drug infusion over 15 minutes, the Band-It Syringe Driver can be used. This simple, disposable device consists of an elastic band placed on both sides of the cylinder and plunger of a 10 mL syringe. The cost-benefits of using these pumps compared with computerized pumps warrants further improvement and development.

NON-DISPOSABLE MECHANICAL INFUSION DEVICES

The Paragon Ambulatory Pump is used for delivering constant intravenous, subcutaneous or epidural infusions.[120] It uses a mechanical spring design to drive the infusion, and the flow rate (0.5–200 mL per hour) is controlled by a precision glass orifice or microbore tubing. Its 110 mL maximum-fill volume infusion bag can deliver 100 mL over periods ranging from 0.5 hours to 8 days. It is easy to fill with a needleless syringe. The set includes a 1.2 micron air-eliminating filter. Its carrying case is designed to be worn on a belt or over the shoulder. It has recently been successfully used for continuous epidural analgesia in labour.[120]

SPINAL MICROCATHETERS

These are also discussed in Chapter 9 (see also Figure 7.13). Problems with microcatheters include

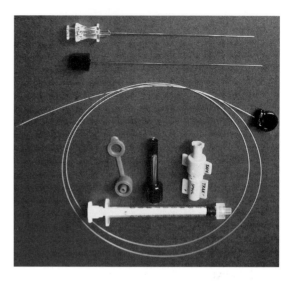

Figure 7.13 Spinal microcatheters. The Kendall Cospan® continuous spinal catheter kit.

difficulty in placement and the maldistribution of local anaesthetic.[121] A suggested cause for recently reported cases of cauda equina syndrome is the neurotoxic effect of high concentrations of local anaesthetics.[122] Straight microcatheters (TFX Med, Kendall) frequently stick to the vertebral body.[121] The placement of a pigtail catheter, however, seems quick, easy and more reliable.[121]

Catheter breakage can be problematic. Catheters should be inserted using an oblique paraspinal approach so that the catheter makes an oblique angle to the dura and does not transverse the interspinous or supraspinous ligament.[123] This enables the catheter to be carefully removed with the minimum of force. Continuous spinal anaesthesia (via a 32 gauge catheter) with incremental opioid (diamorphine) and local anaesthetic (bupivacaine) has been successfully used in labour and delivery.[124]

SPINAL NEEDLES (SEE CHAPTER 9)

Dural puncture with 29 and 30 gauge Quincke needles is associated with technical difficulties because of their small size.[125] The 27 gauge Quincke needle is easy to use through an introducer, and spinal fluid returns adequately. It is, however, associated with an incidence of post-dural puncture headache of 1.5–10.3 per cent.[126,127]

The Whitacre spinal needle is a solid-tip, pencil-point needle with a lateral eye (to spread rather than cut dural fibres).[125] A 25 gauge pencil-point Whitacre needle is also available, is technically easy to insert and is associated with an extremely low incidence of post-dural puncture headache. It is also cheaper than the 24 gauge Sprotte needle.[128] The 24 gauge Sprotte needle has a solid tip and is ogival in shape, with a lateral eye that is longer than the Whitacre needle eye. It is associated with a small incidence of post-dural puncture headache (0.02–2.0 per cent).[125] Pencil-point needles are blunter than cutting-tip needles and pierce the dura less readily.[129]

COMBINED SPINAL–EPIDURAL NEEDLES (CSEA)

There are five main varieties of CSEA: the single-needle, single-interspace method; the double-needle, double-interspace method, the double-needle, single-interspace method; the needle-beside-needle, single-interspace method; and the needle-through-needle method.[129] The single-needle, single-interspace method consists of inserting a pencil-point needle epidurally and, after injecting local anaesthetic, extending it intrathecally to administer further local anaesthetic. It is now of historical interest only. The double-needle, double-interspace method involves the insertion of an epidural catheter at one interspace followed by intrathecal injection at a separate (usually adjacent) interspace.[129] The double-needle, single-interspace method involves catheter insertion through both the intrathecal and epidural needles, producing a double-catheter, single-interspace technique.[129] The needle-beside-needle, single-interspace method involves an epidural needle with a intrathecal needle guide attached to, or built into, the wall of the epidural needle.[129,130] None of these has impacted on the international market.

Needle-through-needle technique

The needle-through-needle technique is the most popular variety of CSEA, and manufacturers have been quick to respond with a variety of customized equipment.[129] The epidural needle guides the fine intrathecal needle to the dura mater. Patients prefer

a single skin puncture. The critical measurement is the maximum protrusion of the intrathecal needle past the tip of the epidural needle where the hub abuts. Too short a protrusion can fail to penetrate the dural sac; too long a protrusion may result in the intrathecal needle passing out of the dural sac anteriorly; or if CSF is obtained while the hubs are some distance apart, it may be very difficult to stabilize the intrathecal needle within the epidural needle during the intrathecal injection.[129] Most manufacturers have settled on a maximum protrusion of about 1.2 cm. If the intrathecal needle has not pierced the dural sac after 1.2 cm, it is probably passing through the lateral part of the epidural space, and re-alignment is advisable.[129] Twenty-nine gauge intrathecal needles, guided and supported by the epidural needle, may have advantages over pencil-point needles for CSEA.[129]

ADJUSTABLE CSEA DEVICE

This device varies the length of the intrathecal needle shaft and forms part of the intrathecal needle hub.[129] It consists of two parts that slide over one another when a fine-toothed ratchet is disengaged by pressure on a plastic button. Once the epidural needle is in place, half of the device is inserted into its hub by a male Luer-slip attachment, and the intrathecal needle is inserted with the ratchet disengaged.[129] On entering the epidural space, the button is released so that the ratchet locks the intrathecal needle protrusion at that distance past the tip of the epidural needle, preventing movement during injection.

BACK-EYE EPIDURAL NEEDLES

The Tuohy needle has a hole (back-eye) punched in its curved tip for passage of the intrathecal needle, while the epidural catheter passes to the tip of the Tuohy needle and strikes the dura some distance from the hole left by the intrathecal needle.[129] A plastic sleeve can be incorporated on the intrathecal needle shaft (except near its tip) to centre the intrathecal needle in order for it to pass through the back-eye.

POTENTIAL PROBLEMS

There may be failure to obtain CSF if the epidural needle is not in the epidural space or if the intrathecal needle is occluded by nerve root or connective tissue.[129] Difficulty in introducing, or intravascular placement of, the epidural catheter may also occur.

With the patient in the lateral position with a hyperbaric solution, the delay may cause the solution to reach high levels.[129] This can be prevented by placing the patient in the usual left lateral, flexed position, with the left shoulder on an inflated 3 L bag and the head on three pillows.[129] On correctly placing the epidural catheter, the patient is turned to the identical position on the other side. When surgery is about to start, a supine position is adopted (with a lateral wedge for the obstetric patient). The best possible relief of aortocaval occlusion in the obstetric patient is provided in one or the other full lateral position. Despite epiduroscopic studies showing epidural catheters unable to pass through dural holes caused by intrathecal needles, the insertion of the epidural catheter intrathecally may still occur, emphasizing the need for a test dose in all CSEA techniques.[129] There may be difficulty in evaluating test doses in the presence of effective intrathecal analgesia.[129] Needle-tip damage and metal particulate contamination have been suggested with CSEA, but the examination of all needles under magnification show this to be unlikely.[129]

Advantages of CSEA

CSEA provides flexibility of technique and drug choice with the ability to 'kick-start' analgesia with a variety of local anaesthetics/opioids and to continue analgesia via the epidural catheter.[129]

Clinical uses of CSEA

Although the dominant use of CSEA has been in obstetrics (labour and caesarean section) and gynaecology, it is increasingly being used in orthopaedic, urological and vascular surgery.[131] For example, using CSEA techniques for walking epidurals in labour, patients may receive an intrathecal dose of bupivacaine 2.5 mg plus fentanyl 25 μg, plus epidural boluses of bupivacaine 0.1 per cent and fentanyl 2 μg/mL to maintain analgesia.[129] The ability of CSEA techniques to inject agents into the intrathecal and epidural spaces in a double-blind randomized manner has opened new avenues for research.

TRANSCRANIAL ELECTROSTIMULATION

A new transcranial electrostimulation device, the Pulsatilla, has been developed for use in acute and chronic pain.[132] Quasi-resonance produced by the pulses in the antinociceptive region of the brain induce accelerated beta-endorphin secretion (three or more times the normal level in the brain and blood). It consists of a microcontroller-based stimulus generator with resident medical software library, and a headset with electrodes. One electrode is placed on the forehead and another on the mastoid bone behind each ear. The battery-operated generator emits pulses of a fixed and controlled frequency and shape at a maximum of 4 mA strengths. Treatment sessions last up to 30 minutes. Contraindications include epilepsy, glaucoma, CNS disease, demand cardiac pacemakers and skin damage over electrode areas. A recent study in patients with chronic neck and back pain showed good pain relief in 60–80 per cent of patients for between 2 weeks and 3 months following treatment.[132]

REFERENCES

1. **Ashburn, M.A. and Stanley, T.H.** 1992: Drug delivery systems in the 1990's. *International Anesthetic Research Society Review Course Lectures*, 129–35.
2. **Nimmo, W.S.** 1991: Alternate modes of drug delivery. *International Anesthetic Research Society Review Course Lectures*, 141–5.
3. **Mather, L.E. and Cousins, M.J.** 1992: The pharmacological relief of pain – contemporary issues. *Medical Journal of Australia* **56**, 796–802.
4. **Biddle, C. and Gilliland, C.** 1992: Transdermal and transmucosal administration of pain-relieving and anxiolytic drugs: a primer for the critical care practitioner. *Heart and Lung* **21**(2), 115–24.
5. **Abbott, N.J. and Romero, I.A.** 1996: Transporting therapeutics across the blood–brain barrier. *Molecular Medicine Today* **2**(3), 106–13.
6. **Schulze, C.** 1997: Understanding the blood-brain-barrier. *Neuropathology and Applied Neurobiology* **23**(2), 150–1.
7. **Engleton, R.D. and Davis, T.P.** 1997: Bioavailability and transport of peptides and peptide drugs into the brain. *Peptides* **18**(9), 1431–9.
8. **Rowley, M., Kulagowski, J.J., Watt, A.P.** *et al.* 1997: Effect of plasma protein binding on in vivo activity and brain penetration of glycine/NMDA receptor antagonists. *Journal of Medical Chemistry* **40**(25), 4053–68.
9. **Basak, S.C., Gute, B.D. and Drewes, L.R.** 1996: Predicting blood-brain transport of drugs: a computational approach. *Pharmacological Research* **13**(5); 775–8.
10. **Kalyanasundaram, S. Calhoun, V.D. and Leong, K.W.** 1997: A finite element model for predicting the distribution of drugs delivered intracranially to the brain. *American Journal of Physiology* **273**, R1810–R1821.

11. **Stanness, K.A., Westrum, L.E., Fornaciari, E.** *et al.* Morphological and functional characterization of an in vitro blood–brain barrier model. *Brain Research* **771**(2), 329–42.

12. **Hammarlund-Udenaes, M., Paalzow, L.K. and de Lange, E.C.** 1997: Drug equilibration across the blood–brain barrier – pharmacokinetic considerations based on the microdialysis method. *Pharmacological Resaerch* **14**(2), 128–34.

13. **Shah, G.N. and Mooradian, A.D.** 1997: Age-related changes in the blood-brain barrier. *Experimental Gerontology* **32**(4–5), 501–19.

14. **Maysinger, D. and Morinville, A.** 1997. Drug delivery to the nervous system. *Trends in Biotechnology* **15**(10), 410–18.

15. **Zunkeler, B., Carson, R.E., Olson, J.** *et al.* 1996: Quantification and pharmacokinetics of blood–brain barrier disruption in humans. *Journal of Neurosurgery* **185**(6), 1056–65.

16. **Hill, H.F., Jacobson, R.C., Coda, B.A. and Mackie, A.M.** 1991: A computer-based system for controlling plasma opioid concentration according to patient need for analgesia. *Clinical Pharmacokinetics* **20**(4), 319–30.

17. **Sandler, A.N.** 1997: New drug delivery systems for acute pain management. In Jain, S., Mauskop, A. and Vietsauskop, B. (eds) *Current concepts in acute, chronic, and cancer pain management.* New York: World Foundation for Pain Relief and Research, 77–81.

18. **Theroux, M., West, D., Corddry, D., Kettrick, R. and Bachrach, S.** 1992: Efficacy of midazolam administered nasally for suturing lacerations in emergency rooms. *Anesthesiology* **77**(3A), A1172.

19. **Kano, T., Nakamura, M., Hashiguchi, A.** *et al.* 1992: Skin pretreatments for shortening onset of dermal patch anesthesia with 35 GA MHPh 2Na-10% lidocaine gel mixture. *Anesthesia and Analgesia* **75**, 555–7.

20. **Sevarino, F.B., Naulty, J.S., Sinatra, R.** *et al.* 1992: Transdermal fentanyl for postoperative pain management in patients recovering from abdominal gynecologic surgery. *Anesthesiology* **77**, 463–6.

21. **David, K.D., Treede, R.D., Raja, S.N., Meyer, R.A. and Campbell, J.N.** 1991: Topical application of clonidine relieves hyperalgesia in patients with sympathetically maintained pain. *Pain* **47**, 309–17.

22. **Petelenz, T., Petelenz, A.I., Iwinski, T.J. and Dubel, S.** 1984: Mini set for iontophoresis for topical analgesia before injection. *International Journal of Clinical Pharmacology Therapeutics and Toxicology* **22**, 152–5.

23. **Glass, J.M., Stephen, R.L. and Jacobson, S.C.** 1980: The quantity and distribution of radiolabelled dexamethasone delivered to tissue by iontophoresis. *International Journal of Dermatology* **19**, 519–25.

24. **McQuay, H.J. and Moore, R.A.** 1998: *An evidence-based resource for pain relief.* Oxford: Oxford University Press 12, 102–7.

25. **Moore, R.A., Tramer, M.R., Carroll, D., Wiffen, P.J. and McQuay, H.J.** 1998: Quantitative systemic review of topically applied non-steroidal anti-inflammatory drugs. *British Medical Journal* **316**(7128), 333–8.

26. **See, Y.** 1998: Intra-synovial corticosteroid injections in juvenile chronic arthritis – a review. *Annals of the Academy of Medicine of Singapore* **27**(1), 105–11.

27. **Stahl, S. and Kaufman, T.** 1997: The efficacy of an injection of steroids for medial epicondylitis: a prospective study of sixty elbows. *Journal of Bone and Joint Surgery* **79A** (11), 1648–52.

28. **Huppertz, H.I., Tschammler, A., Horwitz, A.E. and Schwab, K.O.** 1995: Intraarticular corticosteroids for chronic arthritis in children: efficacy and effects on cartilage and growth. *Journal of Pediatrics* **127**(2), 317–21.

29. **McQuay, H.J. and Moore, R.A.** 1998: *An evidence-based resource for pain relief.* Oxford: Oxford University Press 29, 220.

30. **Green, S., Buchbinder, R., Glazier, R. and Forbes, A.** 1998: Systematic review of randomised controlled trials of interventions for painful shoulder: selection criteria, outcome assessment, and efficacy. *British Medical Journal* **316**(7128), 354–60.

31. **Coaccioli, S., Allegra, A., Pennacchi, M.** *et al.* 1998: Galactoaminoglucuronoglycan sulphate in the treatment of osteoarthritis; clinical efficacy and tolerance of oral and intra-articular administrations. *International Journal of Clinical Pharmacology Research* **18**(1), 39–50.

32. **Pozo, M., Balazs, E.A. and Belmonte, C.** 1997: Reduction of sensory responses to passive movements of inflamed knee joints by hylan, a hyaluronan derivative. *Experimental Brain Research* **116**(1), 3–9.

33. **Williams, A.S., Camilleri, J.P., Goodfellow, R.M. and Williams, B.D.** 1996: A single intra-articular injection of liposomally conjugated methotrexate suppresses joint inflammation in rat antigen-induced arthritis. *British Journal of Rheumatology* **35**(8), 719–24.

34. **Silveri, F., Lo Barco, C. and Brecciaroli, D.** 1997: Somatostatin in peri-arthropathies of the shoulder: clinical effectiveness and tolerability after sub-acromial administration. *Clinica Terapeutica* **148**(3), 75–81.

35. **Caruso, I.** 1997: Twenty years of experience with intra-articular rifamycin for chronic arthritides. *Journal of International Medical Research* **25**(6), 307–17.

36. **Lawand, N.B., Willis, W.D. and Westlund, K.N.** 1997: Blockade of joint inflammation and secondary hyperalgesia by L-NAME, a nitric oxide synthase inhibitor. *Neuroreport* **3**(4), 895–9.

37. **Evans, C.H. and Robbins, P.D.** 1996: The promise of a new clinical trial-intra-articular IL-1 receptor antagonist. *Proceedings of the Association of American Physicians* **108**(1), 1–5.

38. **Khoury, G.F., Chen, A.C.N., Garland, D.E. and Stein, C.** 1992: Intra-articular morphine, bupivacaine, and morphine/bupivacaine for pain control after knee videoarthroscopy. *Anesthesiology* **77**, 263–6.

39. **McQuay, H.J. and Moore, R.A.** 1998: *An evidence-based resource for pain relief.* Oxford: Oxford University Press, 18, 156–63.

40. **Gentili, M., Houssel, P., Osman, M., Henel, D., Juhel, A. and Bonnet, F.** 1997: Intra-articular mor-

phine and clonidine produce comparable analgesia but the combination is not more effective. *British Journal of Anaesthesia* 79(5), 660–1.

41. **Reuben, S.S., Steinberg, R.B., Cohen, M.A., Kilaru, P.A. and Gibson, C.S.** 1998: Intraarticular morphine in the multimodal analgesic management of postoperative pain after ambulatory anterior cruciate ligament repair. *Anesthesia and Analgesia* 86(2), 374–8.

42. **Elhakim, M., Fathy, A., Elkott, M. and Said, M.M.** 1996: Intra-articular tenoxicam relieves post-arthroscopy pain. *Acta Anaesthesiologica Scandinavica* 40(10), 1223–6.

43. **Cook, T.M., Tuckey, J.P. and Nolan, J.P.** 1997: Analgesia after day-case knee arthroscopy: double-blind study of intra-articular tenoxicam, intra-articular bupivacaine and placebo. *British Journal of Anaesthesia* 78(2), 163–8.

44. **Hou, S.M. and Yu, H.Y.** 1997: Comparison of systemic absorption of aqueous and liposomal lidocaine following intra-articular injection in rabbits. *Journal of the Formosan Medical Association* 96(2), 141–3.

45. **Goranson, B.D., Lang, S., Cassidy, J.D., Dust, W.N. and McKerrel, J.** 1997: A comparison of three regional anaesthesia techniques for outpatient knee arthroscopy. *Canadian Journal of Anaesthesia* 44(4), 371–6.

46. **Kuzma, P.J., Kline, M.D., Calkins, M.D. and Staats, P.S.** 1997: Progress in the development of ultra-long-acting local anaesthetics. *Regional Anesthesia* 22(6), 543–51.

47. **Levine, C.B. and Levin, B.H.** 1992: Long-term inter-pleural analgesia using a subcutaneous implantable infusion system. *Canadian Journal of Anaesthesia* 39(4), 408.

48. **Bernards, C.M., Luger, T.J., Malmberg, A.B., Hill, H.F. and Yaksh, T.L.** 1992: Liposome encapsulation prolongs alfentanil spinal analgesia and alters systemic redistribution in the rat. *Anesthesiology* 77, 529–35.

49. **Randell, T,. Ostman, P.L., Hardy, J., Flanagan, D. and Perng, C.Y.** 1992: Prolonged analgesia after epidural injection of a poorly soluble salt of fentanyl. *Anesthesiology* 77(3A), A901.

50. **Malinovsky, J.M., Benhamou, D., Alafandy, M.** *et al.* 1997: Neurotoxicological assessment after intracisternal injection of liposomal bupivacaine in rabbits. *Anesthesia and Analgesia* 85, 1331–6.

51. **Grant, G.J.** 1997: Effect of liposomal encapsulation of bupivacaine on plasma drug levels after intraarticular administration in rabbits. *Anesthesia and Analgesia* 84, S296.

52. **Langerman, L., Grant, G.J., Zakowski, M., Ramanathan, S. and Turndorf, H.** 1992: Prolongation of spinal anesthesia: differential action of a lipid drug carrier on tetracaine, lidocaine, and procaine. *Anesthesiology* 77, 475–81.

53. **Planas, M.E., Gonzalez, P., Rodriguez, L., Sanchez, S. and Cevc, G.** 1992: Noninvasive percutaneous induction of topical analgesia by a new type of drug carrier, and prolongation of local pain insensitivity by

anesthetic liposomes. *Anesthesia and Analgesia* 75, 615–21.

54. **Fletcher, D., Le Corre, P., Guilbaud, G. and Le Verge, R.** 1997: Antinociceptive effect of bupivacaine encapsulated in poly-(D, L)-lactide-co-glycolide microspheres in the acute inflammatory pain model of carrageenin-injected rats. *Anesthesia and Analgesia* 84, 90–4.

55. **Castillo, J., Curley, J., Hotz, J.** *et al.* 1996: Glucocorticoids prolong rat sciatic nerve blockade in vivo from bupivacaine microspheres. *Anesthesiology* 85, 1157–66.

56. **Krames, E.S. and Schuchard, M.** 1995: Implantable intraspinal infusion analgesia: management guidelines. *Pain Reviews* 2, 243–67.

57. **Erdine, S. and Yucel, A.** 1995: Complications of drug delivery systems. *Pain Reviews* 2, 227–42.

58. **Chrubasik, J., Chrubasik, S., Friedrich, G. and Martin, E.** 1992: Long-term treatment of pain by spinal opiates: an update. *The Pain Clinic* 5(3), 147–56.

59. **Onofrio, B.M. and Yaksh, T.L.** 1990: Long-term pain relief produced by intrathecal morphine in 53 patients. *Journal of Neurosurgery* 72, 200–9.

60. **Hassenbusch, S.J., Pillay, P.K., Magdinec, M.** *et al.* 1990: Constant infusion of morphine for intractable cancer pain using an implanted pump. *Journal of Neurosurgery* 73, 405–9.

61. **Patt, R.B.** 1992: Control of pain associated with advanced malignancy. In Aronoff, G.M. (ed.) *Evaluation and treatment of chronic pain*, 2nd edn. Baltimore: Williams & Wilkins, 313–39.

62. **Du Pen, S.L.** 1997: Current trends in interventional drug delivery systems for cancer pain. In Jain, S., Mauskop, A. and Vietsauskop, B. (eds). *Current concepts in acute, chronic, and cancer pain management*. New York: World Foundation for Pain Relief and Research, 233–40.

63. **Cherry, D.A.** 1991: Surgical procedures for the relief of acute and chronic pain. *Medical Journal of Australia* 155, 701–4.

64. **Cousins, M.J., Cherry, D.A. and Gourlay, G.K.** 1988: Acute and chronic pain: use of spinal opioids. In Cousins, M.J and Bridenbaugh, P.O. (eds) *Neural blockade*, 2nd edn. Philadelphia: J.B. Lippincott, 955–1029.

65. **Wu, C.L. and Patt, R.B.** 1992: Accidental overdose of systemic morphine during intended refill of intrathecal infusion device. *Anesthesia and Analgesia* 75, 130–2.

66. **Cherry, D.A. and Gourlay, G.K.** 1992: CT contrast evidence of injectate encapsulation after long-term epidural administration. *Pain* 49, 369–71.

67. **North, R.B., Cutchis, P.N., Epstein, J.A., and Long, D.M.** 1991: Spinal cord compression complicating subarachnoid infusion of morphine: case report and laboratory experience. *Neurosurgery* 29(5), 778–84.

68. **Benedetti, C., McDonald, J.S, Lingham, R. and Seitz, M.** 1991: Efficacy of a Port-A-Cath epidural system for cancer pain management. *Anesthesiology* 77(3A); A841.

69. **Chrubasik, S. and Chrubasik, J.** 1995: The use of

patient-controlled epidural analgesia for acute and chronic pain. *Pain Reviews* **2**, 29–37.

70. **Welchew, E.** 1995: *Patient controlled analgesia.* In Hahn, C.E.W. and Adams, A.P. (eds) Principles and practice series. London: BMJ Publishing Group, 1–133.

71. **Kluger, M.T. and Owen, H.** 1991: Patient-controlled analgesia: can it be made safer? *Anaesthesia and Intensive Care* **19**(3), 412–20.

72. **Shipton, E.A., Minkowitz, H.S. and Becker, P.** 1993: Patient-controlled analgesia in burn injuries: the subcutaneous route. *Canadian Journal of Anaesthesia* **40**, 898.

73. **Ghouri, A.F., Terkonda, R., Taylor, E. and White, P.F.** 1992: Patient-controlled sedation: a comparison of three techniques during local anesthesia. *Anesthesia and Analgesia* **74**, S110.

74. **Hopkins, D. and Shipton, E.A.** 1992: Extending patient-controlled analgesia to patient-controlled neuroleptanalgesia. *South African Journal of Surgery* **30**(4), 168–70.

75. **Monahan, S.J., David, S.E., Finley, J.M. and Buhrman, W.C.** 1991: Patient controlled anaesthesia for prolonged conscious sedation. *Anesthesiology* **75**(3A), A32.

76. **Smythe, M.** 1992: Patient-controlled analgesia: a review. *Pharmacotherapy* **12**(2), 132–43.

77. **Patt, R.B.** 1992: PCA: prescribing analgesia for home management of severe pain. *Geriatrics* **47**(3), 69–84.

78. **Beeton, A.G., Upton, P.M. and Shipton, E.A.** 1992: Patient-controlled analgesia. *South African Medical Journal* **81**, 58.

79. **Hopkins, D.** 1998: Patient controlled analgesia: advantages, disadvantages and techniques. *Hospital Supplies* (Mar), 4–10.

80. **Shipton, E.A., Beeton, A.G. and Minkowitz, H.** 1993: An acute pain relief service – the first ten months. *South African Medical Journal* **83**, 501–5.

81. **Lu, S.L., Wang, J.L., Weng, R.Z. and Wang, Q.A.** 1991: Clinical application of a patient-controlled apparatus for ventricular administration of morphine in intractable pain: report of 28 cases. *Neurosurgery* **29**(1), 73–5.

82. **Striebel, H.W., Oelmann, T., Spies, C., Rieger, A. and Schwagmeier, R.** 1996: Patient-controlled intranasal analgesia: a method for noninvasive postoperative pain management. *Anesthesia and Analgesia* **83**, 548–51.

83. **Lehmann, K.A.** 1997: Update of patient-controlled analgesia. *Current Opinion in Anaesthesiology* **10**, 374–9.

84. **Upton, P.M., Beeton, A.G. and Shipton, E.A.** 1992: The case for patient-controlled analgesia: interpatient variation in postoperative analgesic requirements. *South African Journal of Surgery* **30**, 5–6.

85. **Mather, L.E. and Woodhouse, A.** 1997: Pharmacokinetics of opioids in the context of patient controlled analgesia. *Pain Reviews* **4**, 20–32.

86. **Shipton, E.A.** 1998: Patient controlled analgesia: quo vadis? *Hospital Supplies* (Mar), 2.

87. **Hopkins, D., Shipton, E.A., Potgieter, D.** *et al*. 1998: The comparison of tramadol and morphine by subcutaneous PCA. *Canadian Journal of Anaesthesia* **45**, 435–42.

88. **Shipton, E.A.** 1996: The relief of acute pain. *South African Journal of Surgery* **34**(1), 40–3.

89. **Shipton, E.A.** 1996: Modern use of neuraxial opioids in acute pain. *South African Journal of Surgery* **34**(4), 180–5.

90. **Irwing, G., Allwood, C.W., Levin, V. and Shipton, E.** 1996: Cancer pain: a South African perspective. In Paris, W. (ed.) *Cancer pain management: principles and practice.* Newton: Butterworth Heinemann, 561–6.

91. **MacIntyre, P., Runciman, W.B. and Webb, R.** 1990: An acute pain service in an Australian teaching hospital: the first year. *Medical Journal of Australia* **153**, 417–21.

92. **Irwin, M., Gillespie, J.A. and Morton, N.S.** 1992: Evaluation of a disposable patient-controlled analgesia device in children. *British Journal of Anaesthesia* **68**, 411–13.

93. **Shipton, E.A.** 1992: Postoperative pain – an update. *South African Journal of Surgery* **30**(1), 2–5.

94. **Martin, L.V.** 1992: A simple system for patient-controlled analgesia. *European Journal of Anaesthesiology* **9**(4), 335–9.

95. **Rowbotham, D.J.** 1992: The development and safe use of patient-controlled analgesia. *British Journal of Anaesthesia* **68**(4), 331–2.

96. **Shipton, E.A.** 1996: Patient controlled analgesia (PCA) – an update. *Hospital Supplies* (Feb), 12–16.

97. **O'Neill, G.** 1997: New patient controlled pump applications and new low cost continuous infusion pump applications. *Go Medical Industries – A description of new programmes and product catalogue.* Subiaco, Western Australia: Go Medical, 35–42.

98. **Bruera, E., MacMillan, K., Hanson, J. and MacDonald, R.N.** 1991: The Edmonton injector: a simple device for patient-controlled subcutaneous analgesia. *Pain* **44**, 167–9.

99. **Jackson, I.J.B., Semple, P. and Stevens, J.D.** 1991: Evaluation of the Graseby PCAS. *Anaesthesia* **46**, 482–5.

100. **Notcutt, W.G., Knowles, P. and Kaldas, R.** 1992: Overdose of opioid from patient-controlled analgesia pumps. *British Journal of Anaesthesia* **69**, 95–7.

101. **Thomas, D.W. and Owen, H.** 1988: Patient-controlled analgesia – the need for caution. *Anaesthesia* **43**, 770–2.

102. **Grover, E.R., and Heath, M.L.** 1992: Patient-controlled analgesia: a serious incident. *Anaesthesia* **47**, 402–4.

103. **Kwan, A.** 1996: Morphine overdose from patient-controlled analgesia pumps. *Anaesthesia and Intensive Care* **24**(2), 254–6.

104. **Notcutt, W.G.** 1992: Overdose of opioid from patient-controlled analgesia pumps. *British Journal of Anaesthesia* **68**, 450.

105. **Stevens, D.S., Cohen, R.I., Kanzaria, R.V. and Dunn, W.T.** 1991: Air in the syringe: patient-controlled analgesia machine tampering. *Anesthesiology* **75**, 697–9.

106. **Juhl, G.** 1990: A patient-controlled device using pulsoximetric bolus control. *Anaesthetist* **39**, 236–9.

107. **Cooper, I.M.** 1996: Morphine for postoperative analgesia: a comparison of intramuscular and subcutaneous routes of administration. *Anaesthesia and Intensive Care* **24**, 574–8.

108. **Bruera, E.** 1990: Ambulatory infusion devices in the continuing care of patients with advanced diseases. *Journal of Symptom Management* **5**(5), 287–96.

109. **Bruera, E., Macmillan, K., Kuehn, N., Moore, M. and Bliss, A.** 1991: Evaluation of a spring-loaded syringe driver for the subcutaneous administration of narcotics. *Journal of Pain and Symptom Management* **6**(3), 115–18.

110. **Litman, R.S. and Shapiro, B.S.** 1992: Oral patient-controlled analgesia in adolescents. *Journal of Pain and Symptom Management* **7**(2), 78–81.

111. **Parker, R.K. and White, P.F.** 1992: Epidural patient-controlled analgesia: an alternative to intravenous patient-controlled analgesia for pain relief after cesarean delivery. *Anesthesia and Analgesia* **75**, 245–51.

112. **Grant, R.P. Dolman, J.F., Harper, J.A.** *et al.* 1992: Patient-controlled lumbar epidural fentanyl compared with patient-controlled intravenous fentanyl for post-thoracotomy pain. *Canadian Journal of Anaesthesia* **39**(3), 214–19.

113. **Welchew, E.A. and Breen, D.P.** 1991: Patient-controlled on-demand epidural fentanyl: a comparison of patient-controlled on-demand fentanyl delivered epidurally or intravenously. *Anaesthesia* **46**, 438–41.

114. **Bustamante, J. Sawaki, Y. and White, P.F.** 1992: Comparison of IV-PCA vs Epidural-PCA following major vascular surgery. *Anesthesia and Analgesia* **74**, S39.

115. **Baldwin, A.M., Ilsley, A.H. Kluger, M.T. and Owen, H.** 1991: Assessment of a new infusion pump for epidural PCA. *Anaesthesia and Intensive Care* **19**(2), 246–50.

116. **Love, D.R., Owen, H., Ilsley, A.H., Plummer, J.L., Hawkins, R.M. and Morrison, A.** 1996: A comparison of variable-dose patient-controlled analgesia with fixed-dose patient-controlled analgesia. *Anesthesia and Analgesia* **83**, 1060–4.

117. **Chaudhri, S., White, M. and Kenny, G.N.C.** 1992: Induction of anaesthesia with propofol using a target-controlled infusion system. *Anaesthesia* **47**, 551–3.

118. **Valente, M. and Aldrete, J.A.** 1997: Comparison of accuracy and cost of disposable, nonmechanical pumps used for epidural infusions. *Regional Anesthesia* **22**(3), 260–6.

119. **Novacon Corporation.** 1997: *Drug Infusion Balloon System – Product Information and Clinical Evaluation.* Minnesota: Novacon Corporation, 1–12.

120. **Dotan, A., Livio, C. and Esra, S.** 1997: Continuous epidural analgesia in labour: a comparison of two techniques of administration – top-up versus continuous infusion using a new device. *South African Journal of Anaesthesiology and Analgesia* **3**(1), 14–15.

121. **Yurino, M.** 1992: Pigtail micro spinal catheter. *Anesthesiology* **77**(3), A865.

122. **Leicht, C., Vasdev, G. and Ross, B.** 1992: Microcatheter continuous spinal anesthesia: an in vitro reassessment of the potential for neurologic injury. *Anesthesiology* **77**(3A), A897.

123. **Jones, B.R. and Ley, S.J.** 1992: Strength of continuous spinal catheters. *Anesthesia and Analgesia* **74**, 778–9.

124. **Ketsin, I.G., Madden, A.P., Mulvein, J.T. and Goodman, N.W.** 1992: Analgesia for labour and delivery using incremental diamorphine and bupivacaine via a 32-gauge intrathecal catheter. *British Journal of Anaesthesia* **168**, 244–7.

125. **Mayer, D.C., Quance, D. and Weeks, S.K.** 1992: Headache after spinal anesthesia for cesarean section: a comparison of the 27-gauge Quincke and 24-gauge Sprotte needles. *Anesthesia and Analgesia* **75**, 377–80.

126. **Wiesel, S. Easdown, J. and Tessler, M.** 1992: Postdural puncture headache: 27 gauge Quincke versus 24 gauge Sprotte in young patients. *Canadian Journal of Anaesthesia* **39**(5ii), A92.

127. **Kang, S.B., Goodnough, D.E., Lee, Y.K.** *et al.* 1992: Comparison of 26- and 27-G needles for spinal anesthesia for ambulatory surgery patients. *Anesthesiology* **76**, 734–8.

128. **Campbell, D.C., Douglas, M.J., Pavy, T.J.G., Flanagan, M.L. and McMorland, G.H.** 1992: Comparison of 25G Whitacre vs 24G Sprotte needles for caesarean section. *Canadian Journal of Anaesthesia* **39**(5ii), A46.

129. **Carrie, L.E.S.** 1996: Combined spinal epidural anaesthesia (CSEA) in obstetric practice. In Carrie, L.E.S. Urmey, W.F. and Hanaoka, K. (eds) *New advances in combined spinal epidural anaesthesia – a global update.* International Symposium of Regional Anaesthesia. Auckland: Customised Medical Communications, 1996: 1–7.

130. **Eldor, J.** 1992: Combined spinal and extradural anesthesia. *Anesthesia and Analgesia* **75**, 640–1.

131. **Hanaoka, K.** 1996: Combined spinal epidural anesthesia: the Japanese experience. In Carrie, L.E.S., Urmey, W.F. and Hanaoka, K. (eds) *New advances in combined spinal epidural anaesthesia – a global update.* International Symposium of Regional Anaesthesia. Auckland: Customised Medical Communications, 13–16.

132. Vatashsky, E. 1996: Transcranial electrical stimulation in the treatment of chronic neck and low back pain. In *7th International Symposium – the Pain Clinic,* Istanbul, 289–94.

8 PERIPHERAL NEURAL BLOCKADE

Peripheral neural blockade aims to interrupt nociceptive transmission in the peripheral nervous system. Somatic and sympathetic nerve fibres can be blocked at various sites after they leave the spinal canal, from their peripheral terminals to the intervertebral foramen. Nociceptive traffic can be considered broadly as reaching the spinal cord via primary afferent receptors in somatic nerves (sensory nerve terminal, axon, plexus, dorsal root ganglion and spinal nerve root) and visceral sensory afferents in sympathetic nerves (plexuses or nerves). Such techniques can produce pain relief without any central depressant effect on consciousness or respiration. Nerve blocks with local anaesthetics are often spectacular in controlling acute perioperative pain. In some instances, they can be used to block somatomotor nerves to relieve skeletal muscle spasm.[1] They are also useful in the diagnosis and treatment of chronic pain. The relief of certain types of pain may, however, outlast the pharmacological action of the local anaesthetic by hours, days or even weeks.[1] Neural blockade may actually suppress the spinal cord changes that potentiate pain and predispose to persistent painful sequelae. Sympathetic fibres run with peripheral nerves, and intervention here may be an alternative to sympathetic blockade (especially in hard-to-block areas such as thoracic dermatomes). Corticosteroids may be added if an inflammatory component is thought to exist. They have also been shown to block C fibres directly, and reversibly in intact nerves and neuromas.[2]

Especially in day case surgery, the advantages of regional anaesthesia include the avoidance of airway instrumentation, rapid recovery, a decreased incidence of nausea and vomiting, less cardiorespiratory depression, improved perfusion via sympathetic blockade, reduced blood loss, a decreased risk of thromboembolism, and postoperative analgesia.[3] Regional techniques on their own allow intraoperative patient communication (an advantage in managing patients with brittle diabetes, unstable cardiac disease or significant cerebrovascular pathology).[3] Many patients prefer being 'awake' in order to avoid loss of autonomy. While commonly used by continuous infusion or in small boluses as required, patient-controlled sedation (with propofol) can result in high patient satisfaction. With day case surgery, routine follow-up telephone calls are necessary to detect the onset of pain or delayed neurological complications.[3]

ACTIONS OF LOCAL ANAESTHETICS

Local anaesthetics can be classified by functional group and by their physicochemical properties (e.g. relative lipophilicity and fraction ionized).[4]

Amethocaine and butamben have high lipophilicity, lignocaine has moderate lipophilicity, and bupivacaine has high lipophilicity.[4] Lipophilicity has implications for potency, onset time and duration of anaesthesia. Ionization is relevant to stability, solubility, activity and the equilibrium distribution of local anaesthetics in the various body compartments.[4] Because their ionized forms are more water soluble than their free bases, local anaesthetics are dispensed as their hydrochloride salts, the resulting solutions being acidic (pH typically 3–6). Whereas the chemical stability of the ester caines is greatest at pH 3.7, the amide caines are stable over a wide range of pH. There is no evidence of the significant enantiomeric inversion of chiral caines even at a strongly basic pH.[4] The aqueous solubility of a local anaesthetic is directly related to the extent of its ionization and inversely related to its lipid solubility. Except for benzocaine and butamben, which have no hydrophilic amino group to ionize, the ester caines are more ionized at body pH than are the amide caines.[4] Among the amide caines, bupivacaine and ropivacaine have slightly higher ionized fractions than lignocaine, prilocaine and mepivacaine, perhaps giving slightly longer onset times.[4]

Local anaesthetics disrupt the normal 'gating' behaviour of the sodium channels.[5] When a local anaesthetic binds to a channel, it perpetuates an 'inactive state' from which normal activation cannot occur. Local anaesthetics reduce the frequency rather than the duration of sodium channel opening.[6] About 80 per cent of the sodium channels must be inhibited to prevent active currents developing.[5] The length of axon exposed to the local anaesthetic is a critical factor in determining the effectiveness of blockade.[6] Other channels and receptors that are indirectly linked to channels (e.g. through G protein-mediated changes) may be involved in the therapeutic actions of intravenous local anaesthetics in relieving chronic neuropathic pain.[7] Less than 5 per cent of an injected dose of local anaesthetic reaches a blocked nerve,[6] most being absorbed by fat and muscle.[5] Adrenaline-mediated vasoconstriction slows the dispersion profile of the local anaesthetic at the nerve, thereby increasing the dose of local anaesthetic reaching the axons.[5] Small-diameter nociceptive C fibres require more local anaesthetic to achieve a block than do A beta mechano-sensitive or A delta fibres, which are larger, myelinated fibres.[6] The protein binding of local anaesthetics is a kinetic process wherein the perfused organ extracts drug molecules to a degree that is dependent on their rate of dissociation from the proteins, as well as on their free fraction.[7] The

ability of local anaesthetics to provide a differential inhibition of physiological function may reside in the different criteria for the successful transmission of 'information patterns' between the different fibre types subserving a particular functional modality rather than in any clearly differential impulse blockade.[7] There is still ignorance of the mechanisms by which very low concentrations (10^{-5} M) of intravenous lignocaine can ameliorate or abolish chronic neuropathic pain for days or weeks.[5]

Local anaesthetic activity is related to both drug distribution and intrinsic potency.[4] The non-ionized fraction is essential for drug passage through the lipoidal barriers to the site of action of the nerve membrane. In principle, decreasing ionization by alkalinization of the solution for injection will effectively raise the initial concentration gradient of diffusible drug base, thereby increasing the rate of drug transfer; once at the nerve membrane, ionization is again necessary for complete anaesthetic activity.[4] Alkalinization has not been found to be uniformly successful.[4] Sustained local anaesthetic release into the region of the nerve can be obtained by using long-acting local anaesthetics and incorporating local anaesthetics into liposomes and polymer microspheres.[4] In general, the S-enantiomers of chiral caines have greater potency in neural blockade and generally lower toxicity than the R-enantiomers.[4] S-bupivacaine (levobupivacaine) and ropivacaine promise to extend the range of regional blockade by allowing higher and more efficacious doses of local anaesthetic to be used safely.[8]

TYPES OF PERIPHERAL NEURAL BLOCKADE

There are diagnostic, prognostic, therapeutic and prophylactic indications for nerve blocks.[2]

Diagnostic neural blockade

The purposes of diagnostic blockade are as follows:

- to diagnose the site of the pain;
- to identify a contribution from the sympathetic nervous system;
- to separate somatic from visceral pain;
- to separate local disease from referred pain;
- to distinguish peripheral nerve from dermatomal input;

- to aid in the diagnosis of 'central' neuropathic pain disorders;
- to assess the prognosis of neurolytic procedures.[9]

Few blinded control studies exist that have tested the use of these alluring methods.[10] There has been no critical examination of the theoretical basis on which diagnostic blockade is founded. Diagnostic neural blockade rests on three premises. First, the pathology causing the pain is located in an exact peripheral location, and impulses from this site travel via an unique and consistent neural route.[10] Second, the injection of local anaesthetic totally abolishes the sensory function of intended nerves and does not affect other nerves. Third, pain relief after neural block is attributable solely to blockade of the target afferent pathway. The validity of these assumptions is limited by complexities of anatomy, physiology and psychology of pain perception, and the effect of local anaesthetics on impulse conduction.[10]

There is a need for precise anatomical knowledge in order to place small volumes of local anaesthetic accurately to avoid blocking neighbouring nerves.[2] The blocks must be valid and reproducible. The sensitivity and specificity of the blocks should be known by comparison against a gold standard when one exists. Patients with chronic neuropathic pain may have a placebo response up to twice that of the normal population, and controls are needed for diagnostic accuracy.[2] Diagnostic blocks may give false-positive and false-negative results. A false-positive outcome takes place if a positive result (pain relief) occurs but for a reason other than the intended interruption of transmission via particular nerves. Potential causes include the systemic absorption of local anaesthetics, the blockade of afferent pathways other than those intended, and placebo effects.[11] A diagnostic block can relieve pain when the blocked nerve is not the pain source but is distal or collateral to the nerve involved.[2] A high false-positive rate and low specificity occur in diagnostic blocks of spinal nerves in low back pain and radiculopathy.[2] A nerve block is regarded as false negative if a negative result (a lack of pain relief) is caused by an inadequate interruption of transmission via the intended nerves, usually owing to technical or anatomical factors.[11]

The improvement of techniques and instruments, and the use of nerve finders and radiological guidance, have enhanced the safety and technical feasibility of nerve block procedures. Factors used to determine proper needle positioning include:[11]

- surface or bony land marks (e.g. for intercostal nerve blocks);
- changes in tissue compliance to injection (e.g. a loss of resistance for epidurals);
- fluid identification (CSF for intrathecal injection);
- the needle position as seen by radiographic imaging (e.g. in coeliac plexus block);
- the spread pattern of the contrast agent (e.g. linear dye spread anterior to the psoas fascia for lumbar sympathetic block);
- paraesthesias (e.g. referred sensation to the hand during axillary brachial plexus block);
- the motor response to electrical nerve stimulation (e.g. twitches of the hand or forearm during brachial plexus block with a stimulator needle).

In a successful block there may be a subjective response, there may be an improvement in function of the blocked area, there should be objective evidence of the action of the block with appropriate sympathetic, sensory or motor changes, and the time course of the response should be appropriate to the agent employed.[9] Diagnostic regional blockade is usually a predictor of whether a therapeutic block may be of benefit. The diagnosis must always be based on an observed response. Because an expected response does not occur, this is insufficient for diagnostic purposes.[9] Factors associated with a significant reduction in treatment success include being out of work because of pain, being injured at work, receiving financial compensation, the involvement of legal action, previous surgery for pain, a long duration of pain, high pain severity ratings, frequent analgesic use and the use of tranquillizers.[9]

Complex physiological events may confound the simplest interpretation of diagnostic blocks. The dorsal root ganglia of injured nerves participate in abnormal impulse generation. Blockade proximal to the injured segment but distal to the dorsal root ganglion may then not relieve pain.[10] Nerve blocks distal to the primary site of nerve pathology may alter pain perception by interrupting antidromic impulses, contrary to the common assumption that axonal function must be interrupted proximal to the area of injury to provide relief.[10] Peripheral sciatic nerve blockade has been shown to provide profound pain relief in lumbosacral radiculopathies.[10] There is a sympathetic component to the inflammatory response (especially in joints).[10] Pain relief after peripheral blockade may be caused by interruption of these efferent mechanisms rather than of somatic sensory fibres. Whatever the contribution of receptor, neuropathic or sympathetic mechanisms, activity in nociceptive afferent fibres is subject to processing in the spinal cord. Single peripheral nerve injury may create allodynia in adjacent territories innervated by other nerves because of the altered central processing of afferent signals from the uninjured as well as the injured nerve.[10] Blocking the uninjured nerve relieves pain within its borders, leading to the erroneous interpretation that the blocked nerve has been injured. Denervation may produce sufficient sensitization of WDR neurones such that non-noxious stimulation, including stimuli outside the original receptive field, can produce pain.[10]

The subtle, complex and variable action of local anaesthetics should inspire caution in the interpretation of blocks. If pain continues after a diagnostic block, it cannot be certain that the injected pathway is not involved because neural blockade is often not absolute. The variable effects of local anaesthetics on fibres conveying different functions is termed 'differential block'. Problematic for the use of local anaesthetics in diagnosis is the great range of conduction speed and fibre size within a fibre type and the lack of correlation between size and anaesthetic concentration necessary for blockade within the group.[10] Anaesthetic potency and the degree of differential effects varies with the length of nerve exposed (to prevent conduction, three or more successive nodes of Ranvier must be blocked completely). The block that develops when the axon is firing at very low rates (tonic block) is less intense than the block that develops while the nerve is active (phasic block).[10] During diagnostic blockade, local anaesthetic is absorbed from the injection site, raising the question of how much systemic analgesic affects stimulated impulse generation arising from injured nerves. The principal effect of systemic local anaesthetics on neuropathic pain is peripheral.[10]

With diagnostic blocks, patients may be looking for reassurance, proof to persuade doubting family members or disability certification (for legal and financial reasons), or may wish to please the physician.[10] Patients obtain placebo relief during acute pain about a third of the time, and in chronic pain about two-thirds of the time,[10] injections and the physician's convictions being potent placebo response generators.[10] The ambiguity created by these responses is a major impediment to the valid use of diagnostic neural blockade.

Evidence indicates that anatomical uncertainties with regard to neural connections and structural variability degrades the accuracy of diagnostic information obtained by neural blockade.[10] The separation of somatic input into a discernible segmental pattern is a fundamental concept that underlies many diagnostic blocks. There is, however, variability in the formation of segmental spinal nerves and their peripheral distribution.[10] Extensive overlap between consecutive peripheral dermatomes is also evident. Because peripheral nerve trunks consist of both somatic and sympathetic fibres, the components of both types are often blocked.[2] Anatomical variability is more common in the sympathetic than in the somatic nervous system and has been implicated in cases of failure of surgical sympathectomy.[2] The extent of sympathetic blockade after regional anaesthesia is poorly understood and difficult to predict. Pain not relieved by blocks of sympathetic pathways may still be visceral in origin but may be transmitted by non-sympathetic routes.[10]

The specificity of diagnostic nerve blocks can be greatly improved if selective agents are developed that act differentially on the nerve fibres of interest (e.g. specific sodium channel blockers, N-type voltage-sensitive calcium channel blockers and more selective adrenergic agonists).[12] The challenge is to identify, using randomized controlled trials, those patients who clearly do benefit from neural blockade. The confusion and complexity that typifies diagnosis in chronic pain may justify the selective use of diagnostic blocks that make anatomical and physiological sense, even if their validity is incompletely proved.

Prognostic neural blockade

Prognostic local anaesthetic blocks purportedly determine whether the clinical results of neurolytic or neurosurgical treatment would be effective and acceptable to the patient.[2] Therapeutic blocks are generally only performed after a positive response to a prognostic block. Similar arguments apply to prognostic as to diagnostic blocks. There is no relationship between the outcome of prognostic blocks and the related therapeutic procedure.[2] Prognostic blockade frequently fails to predict the outcome of surgical procedures. The risk-to-benefit ratio of the intended procedure also requires consideration. If the therapeutic procedure has significant morbidity, reliance on a single positive prognostic block is unwarranted.[2] A negative prognostic block is likely to predict the failure of the therapeutic procedure.

Therapeutic neural blockade

Therapeutic blocks can be used directly to treat the cause of pain, as an adjunct or indirectly to provide temporary symptomatic relief in order that other treatments can be given.[2] The agents employed are either non-neurolytic (local anaesthetics, corticosteroids and opioids) or neurolytic (chemical agents, radiofrequency techniques and cryotherapy). There is little hard evidence from well-constructed trials that favours the use of therapeutic nerve blockade as a method of treatment.[9] Local anaesthetics can affect pain reduction, outlasting the conduction block by several days.[2] For sustained relief, the placement of a catheter is required. Using liposomes or 'microspheres' prolongs local anaesthetic duration and reduces systemic toxicity.[2] N-Butyl p-aminobenzoate is a long-lasting tested local anaesthetic given epidurally; when it is applied to the peripheral nerves, neurolysis may occur. Intra-articular morphine reduces postoperative knee pain, and topical morphine has been used for neuropathic eye pain.[2] Because of nerve regeneration (2–6 months later), the procedural risk-to-benefit ratio and patient selection are important prior to neurolysis. Nerves lesioned with radiofrequency techniques include the medial branches of the posterior primary rami, the spinal dorsal nerve roots and ganglia, the cranial sensory nerve roots and the gasserian ganglia. Cryolesions used to treat acute post-thoracotomy pain may be associated with a high incidence of chronic dysaesthesias.[2]

Prophylactic neural blockade

Neurobiochemical studies have shown that surgical tissue damage results in a central memory for pain via *c-fos* gene expression.[2] Much interest has been shown regarding the use of neural blockade to prevent the changes in central processing that may be initiated by acute nociception and may result in chronic pain. The efficacy of pre-emptive analgesics can be assessed as an index of *c-fos* expression.[2] Early coeliac plexus blockade for pancreatic carcinoma may improve life expectancy.[2] Early sympathetic blockade may modify the incidence of post-herpetic neuralgia and reduce the chronic phases of complex regional pain syndromes, but not conclusively so.[2]

PERIPHERAL NERVE STIMULATION AND NERVE BLOCKS

While it is not considered to be an essential item of equipment for performing peripheral nerve block-

ade, a peripheral nerve stimulator can make all the difference between success and failure because of obtaining more accurate needle placement by the objective observation of stimulated muscle contraction.[13] The peripheral nerve stimulator delivers a pulsed electric current to the tip of the exploring electrode. As the needle approaches the nerve, depolarization is produced. Efferent motor fibres (A alpha) are the most easily depolarized, giving the advantage of identifying mixed peripheral nerves by producing a muscle twitch rather than eliciting uncomfortable paraesthesias. A peripheral nerve stimulator facilitates needle placement in the following situations:

- any patient (especially in paediatrics) undergoing a nerve block during general anaesthesia (such as those who are very anxious, mentally handicapped, demented and elderly or unco-operative, and those with language problems);
- the patient sedated too heavily to respond to paraesthesia techniques;
- anyone, in whom eliciting paraesthesia is to be avoided, in order to prevent possible nerve damage.

Evidence suggests that paraesthesia can be responsible for post-block nerve lesions, as they are indicative of nerve injury by probing needles.[13] The use of peripheral nerve stimulators is contraindicated whenever a regional procedure is contraindicated. The peripheral nerve stimulator output should not come in contact with pacing catheters or lead wires, or with flammable anaesthetic gases. The technique usually requires two individuals for its safety and correct performance.

The minimum requirement of a peripheral nerve stimulator is a low-frequency, adjustable, constant current output of 0.1–10.0 mA at resistances of 500–10000 ohms (normal skin/tissue resistance). Most peripheral nerve stimulators provide an impulse lasting 0.1 milliseconds with a frequency adjusted between 1 and 2 Hz as the shorter the pulse duration, the less likelihood there is of the nerve being stimulated while the needle tip is not in proximity of the nerve.[13] Advanced peripheral nerve stimulator machines have a selectable pulse duration: 0.1 milliseconds for selective motor fibre stimulation and 1.0 millisecond for additional sensory fibre stimulation. A dual-purpose stimulator is used for performing blocks as well as for assessing neuromuscular blockade. Insulated needles allow for more precise nerve location, having a non-conductor bonding except for the last millimetre above the bevel of the needle. One peripheral nerve stimulator lead is earthed to the patient (positive, red lead) so that the current does not directly traverse a nerve path or flow through the myocardium), while the other is directly part of the needle (negative, black lead) or is applied to the needle using an alligator clip.[13] Combined with a variable voltage peripheral nerve stimulator, the precise location of motor-evoked potentials at low voltage ensures a high success rate. The new pinpoint needle electrode concentrates the entire stimulus current at the very tip. Most studies have shown less accurate needle placement using an ordinary needle, the minimum nerve stimulation current occurring when the tip is 0.1–0.8 cm past the nerve.[13]

The block needle is aimed towards the nerve or plexus in question. The peripheral nerve stimulator is turned on at an initial current of 1–10 mA (usually 3–5 mA) and a frequency of 1–2Hz (depending on nerve size), and the needle is advanced.[13] Motor-evoked contractions will increase as the nerve is approached and decrease as the needle passes beyond the nerve. A current of 2 mA produces depolarization of a motor nerve at a distance of about 1 cm. For precise localization, the current should then be decreased to a minimum that produces a muscle response.[13] This is known as the 'threshold current'. An evoked response at 1 mA is highly specific, and one at less than 0.5 mA almost 100 per cent so.[13] The local anaesthetic is a conducting hydrochloride salt, which briefly augments nerve impulses until conduction block begins before a rapid extinction occurs. If a regular needle is used, it should be inserted to the appropriate motor-evoked response, withdrawn until the response disappears, and then re-inserted until it just returns. Complications include pain (with too high a current) in an awake patient, equipment error, intraneural injection and microshock and burns in susceptible patients.[13]

INACTIVATION OF MYOFASCIAL TRIGGER POINTS

Myofascial pain syndrome is characterized by pain associated with movement of the affected muscles and the reproduction of pain on palpation of well-localized trigger points in the affected muscle.[10] Myofascial syndrome is commonly associated with other painful disorders (such as facet arthropathy and radiculopathy).

The trigger pain approach regards painful points primarily as localized phenomena – foci of hyper-irritable tissue (myofascial, cutaneous, fascial, ligamentous and periosteal), occurring as a result of compensatory overload, a shortened range or a response to activity in other trigger points.[14] They can be caused by trauma from a specific accident or chronic occupational abuse (e.g. typing and poor posture).[15] The myofascial trigger point injection of local anaesthetics is the simplest and most frequently used analgesic block in the treatment of pain. Trigger points are localized mainly by a sense of feel. They are usually located on the muscle or fascial areas of the back, neck and shoulders. By applying pressure on the point, pain is reproduced in a constant referral pattern, usually in a non-dermatomal distribution. The reproduction of pain during injection and relief afterwards for the duration of the local anaesthetic are used to indicate that myofascial pain is at least partially responsible for the pain. Weak local anaesthetic solutions (lignocaine 0.5 per cent or bupivacaine 0.25 per cent) are injected.[15] Corticosteroids are often mixed with the local anaesthetic to treat trigger points associated with neuroma formation. Saline injections may be even more effective than local anaesthetics.[2] The avoidance of frequent courses of local anaesthetic injections has been suggested because of the possibility of direct damage to muscle cells, particularly with bupivacaine,[2] yet the predictable and selective destruction of mature myocytes may be the mechanism of long-term response to trigger point injections as it encourages the growth of a new generation of myocytes.[10]

The muscle tenderness seen in fibromyalgia differs from the myofascial pain syndrome in that tender points are more diffuse, numerous and usually symmetrical. There are poor capacity for muscular exertion, sleep disturbances, brief morning stiffness and intolerance to cold, damp weather.[14] Palpation generally produces local but not referred, pain.[2] It has recently been postulated that fibromyalgia results from neuroendocrine deficiencies (decreased serotonin, growth hormone and cortisol production), which are probably genetically determined and interact with each other, thereby creating vicious circles.[16]

A crucial ingredient of myofascial pain is muscle shortening from contracture. Intramuscular stimulation by dry needling is used for the diagnosis and treatment of myofascial pain syndromes when there is no obvious injury or inflammation.[14] The needling not only produces local inflammation, which is necessary for healing, but also influences distant components of the segmental nerves by reflex stimulation.[14] This technique is safe in qualified hands and has few iatrogenic side-effects. It is effective in chronic musculoskeletal pain when muscle shortening resists conventional physical therapies, especially in those muscles normally inaccessible to the palpating finger.[14]

SUBCUTANEOUS INFILTRATION WITH LOCAL ANAESTHETIC

This technique is useful in herpes zoster, for neuroma and for other subcutaneous nodular or fibrotic pains.[17] Corticosteroids are sometimes added.

WOUND INFILTRATION WITH LOCAL ANAESTHESIA

Wound infiltration with local anaesthetics is safe and cost-effective, and may be the method of choice for surgical and postoperative analgesia, or both, for various minor to moderately sized operative procedures.[18] Local anaesthesia by field blocks or other techniques is safe, minimally invasive and cost-effective, and may be the method of choice for various surgical procedures such as inguinal herniotomy and knee arthroscopy.[18] In recent years, local anaesthetic solutions have been injected into the wound edges at the end of surgery.[19] The implantation of polyethylene catheters in the surgical wound (e.g. in the posterior rectal sheath), followed by the infusion of local anaesthetics, can also provide effective analgesia and have an opioid-sparing effect following major surgery.[20] Plain bupivacaine (0.25 per cent) is the preferred local anaesthetic.[20] The addition of adrenaline is avoided because of the theoretical risk of delayed wound healing. This is despite the fact that there is no evidence to support the fact that wound healing is delayed or infection introduced by this technique.[20]

Wound infiltration with local anaesthetics provides a clinically significant reduction in postoperative pain and analgesic requirement during the first 6–12 hours after herniotomy but contributes a minor effect on pain after more major abdominal surgery.[18] The short-lasting analgesic effect observed with intra-articular and peritonsillar local anaesthetics limits their usefulness in post-arthroscopy and post-tonsillectomy pain management.[18] More studies are needed to evaluate the optimal methods of infiltration, the efficacy of continuous wound perfusion with local anaesthetics and combinations of topical local anaesthetics with other pharmacological agents or analgesic methods. A major advantage would be the development of new local anaesthetics with an extended duration of action.

INTRAVENOUS REGIONAL ANAESTHESIA

Intravenous regional anaesthesia is an easy, reliable, safe method with few contraindications that produces anaesthesia of the distal parts of the limbs, especially for relatively short procedures of a minor nature.[21] Reported success rates have varied between 96 and 100 per cent.[21] The risk of systemic toxicity (from local anaesthetic leakage while the tourniquet is apparently inflated) is no greater than with other arm block technique.[21] Mortality with intravenous regional anaesthesia is indeed rare (all reported cases occurring with bupivacaine), and up to 45 000 treatments have been successfully performed without mortality.[21] The use of automatic gas-operated tourniquets and bupivacaine is not advised. Contraindications include disease processes in which prolonged tourniquet times can cause morbidity (e.g. sickle cell disease or trait), extensive tissue cellulitis, known sensitivity to the local anaesthetic agent and certain cardiac diseases (untreated heart block).[21]

Surgery around the elbow can be performed. A well-padded and carefully applied hand tourniquet can be used for hand surgery.[21] The ultimate is digital intravenous regional anaesthesia, in which only the finger is anaesthetized. For leg surgery, intravenous regional anaesthesia is best confined to the foot and the ankle as the knee is not easily anaesthetized, the quantity of local anaesthetic required being too great. The use of a wide cuff is desirable as narrow-cuffed double tourniquets may not occlude the artery even at pressures 100 mmHg above systolic.[21] The problem with long procedures is not diminishing block but tourniquet pain.

Over the years, all local anaesthetic agents have been tried, but by far the safest and best drug remains prilocaine 0.5 per cent, in a dose of 40–50 mL for the arm and 20–30 mL for the lower calf downwards.[21] Various additives (bicarbonate and NSAIDs) have been recommended from time to time, but their usefulness remains unproven.[21] A recent study has shown pethidine to be an effective analgesic agent for intravenous regional anaesthesia, providing sufficient anaesthesia for minor operations on the forearm and the hand.[22] However, local venous irritation and unpleasant CNS side-effects (with the danger of convulsions) may preclude the use of pethidine for intravenous regional anaesthesia in the future.[22] For the technique, non-invasive blood pressure and pulse oximetry monitoring are required, and an intravenous line should be inserted on the non-operated side.[21] Venous exsanguination should be as complete as possible. A single wide cuff should be carefully applied over adequate padding. The agent should be injected slowly. The cuff should remain inflated for a minimum of 20 minutes (this is not applicable to the forearm cuff method). The cuff's gauge should be observed throughout (and tubing not clamped). Monitoring should continue for about 10 minutes after surgery until the risk of any systemic complications has passed.

In intravenous regional sympathetic blockade, the response to intravenous guanethidine or bretyllium may help to confirm a sympathetic component to a given patient's pain, particularly if the response has been compared with an intravenous regional placebo procedure.[10]

TOPICAL LOCAL ANAESTHETIC

Lignocaine aerosol has been used to provide effective postoperative analgesia when sprayed into herniorrhaphy and tonsillectomy wounds.[20] EMLA is a mixture of lignocaine (2.5 g) and prilocaine (2.5 g) per 100 g of cream. It can be applied to the dorsum of the hand to provide local anaesthesia for venepuncture, especially in children, and for venous ulcers, where it reduces the pain during cleansing.[2,23] Lignocaine tape, a new preparation of lignocaine for cutaneous topical anaesthesia in the form of a self-adhesive tape, relieves needle insertion pain (for stellate ganglion blockade) after an application time of 7 minutes or more.[24] Topical lignocaine 5 per cent in the form of a non-woven polyethylene patch has been found to relieve post-herpetic neuralgia with minimal systemic lignocaine absorption.[25]

Topical capsaicin reversibly depletes stores of substance P and possibly other neurotransmitters from unmyelinated C fibres.[2] It is used for treating post-herpetic neuralgia, diabetic neuropathy and osteoarthritis.[2]

PERIPHERAL NERVE BLOCKS

Appropriate blocks exist for almost all areas of the body. The relief of peripheral blockade may help to predict the response to neural decompression but has unproven prognostic value in predicting the response to neuroablation. Any peripheral nerve blocks performed with long-acting local anaesthetics (e.g. bupivacaine) provide analgesia for about 12 hours.[20] Wrist, ankle and elbow blocks are easy to perform. Ilio-inguinal and ilio-hypogastric blocks can provide fairly effective analgesia after herniorrhaphy.[20] Infraorbital blocks can give effective analgesia after cleft lip repair.[26] Infrapatellar nerve blocks can be used for chronic pain following arthroscopy.[27]

Catheters can be introduced into the brachial plexus, femoral nerve lumbar plexus, and into the paravertebral and intercostal spaces.

INTRA-ARTICULAR LOCAL ANAESTHETICS

Intra-articular local anaesthetics can be used to provide postoperative analgesia. This has mostly been used after arthroscopic knee surgery with bupivacaine 0.5 per cent.[28] Intra-articular opioids such as morphine are sometimes also added.[29] In patients with rheumatoid arthritis, the intra-articular injection of local anaesthetic with a corticosteroid usually produces a temporary improvement in both the pain control and the range of motion of the involved joint.[30] It is recommended that an individual joint be injected no more than three times at intervals of 6 months or longer.[31]

Local anaesthetic injection of the sacroiliac joint is used to test whether the joint is a source of low back pain, particularly when diffuse degenerative disease involving the lumbosacral spine is present, to differentiate sacroiliac arthropathy from facet disease, myofascial pain and disc disease.[10] There are no prospective controlled evaluations of the technique. If the procedure is carried out under fluoroscopic or computed tomography (CT) control, the inferior extent of the joint can be identified and the joint space entered.

INTERCOSTAL NERVE BLOCKS

This technique can be used to provide pain relief after upper abdominal and thoracic surgery. It decreases opioid requirements and improves postoperative pulmonary function.[20,32] In chronic pain, it can provide pain relief for fractured ribs and flail chests, as well as for pleuritic pain.[33] Herpes zoster pain may also be relieved in this way. It can be used diagnostically to differentiate visceral from abdominal wall pain and to treat the entrapment of the intercostal nerves in the rectal sheath.[33] The benefits associated with repeated intercostal blocks should be weighed against the morbidity associated with repeated injections or the insertion of an intercostal catheter.[2]

At their origin, the intercostal nerves lie between the pleural and the posterior intercostal fascia,[34] and there is nothing to stop the local anaesthetic spreading extrapleurally and affecting several adjacent nerves. The upper six intercostal nerves terminate at the sternum, their branches supplying the skin of the anterior part of the thorax. The lower six intercostal nerves pass under the costal margin and supply the muscles and skin of the anterior abdominal wall.[34]

Regardless of the site of injection (mid-axillary or at the angle of the rib), the technique of needle insertion is the same. The needle point should be in close proximity to the rib if puncture of the pleura is to be avoided.[34] Intercostal block can give rise to one of the highest plasma concentrations of local anaesthetic in regional anaesthesia.[32] The dose should therefore be carefully calculated.

Continuous intercostal analgesia via an indwelling catheter has been successfully used to treat pain following upper abdominal surgery, chest trauma, sternotomy and thoracotomy.[20] This avoids multiple blocks, with their attendant risks. Its advantage over interpleural catheterization is that the local anaesthetic has direct access to the intercostal nerves. Safe, non-toxic plasma bupivacaine concentrations lasting for up to 24 hours have been attained with this method.[32] Intercostal blocks with the non-water-soluble local anaesthetic butamben appears to be a new promising method of treating post-thoracotomy pain syndrome.[35]

SUPRASCAPULAR NERVE BLOCK

The suprascapular nerve supplies 70 per cent of the sensory nerve supply to the shoulder joint.[26] A double-blind study in rheumatoid arthritics has found blocking this nerve with bupivacaine to be as effective as intra-articular injections.[2] It provides temporary analgesia in patients with persistent rotator cuff lesions who are awaiting or are not suitable for surgery.[2] A suprascapular nerve block has recently been shown to be effective for pain relief in arthroscopic shoulder surgery.[36]

FACET NERVE BLOCKS

The medial branch of the posterior primary ramus, which is the nerve supply to the facet joint, can be blocked in the groove between the pedicle and the transverse process.[37] Because each medial branch supplies part of two facets, the complete denervation of one facet requires partial blockade of the facet above and below.[10] Facet nerve blocks or intra-articular injections of local anaesthetic and corticosteroid into the facet joint have been used diagnostically, therapeutically and prognostically to assess suitability for facet denervation,[37] yet pain relief from the blocks cannot distinguish between pain originating at any of the three levels. In addition to the facet joint capsule, the medial branch of the posterior primary ramus also supplies the muscle and ligaments, and the periosteum of the neural arch.[38] Thus, pain relief after facet nerve block cannot be regarded as specific to the facet joint. The effect of intra-articular facet joint injections is dependent on adequate diffusion of the agents into the joint capsule. Any ruptures of the joint capsule will introduce infiltrate into the intervertebral foramina and may confuse the diagnosis.[38] The specificity of facet denervation thus depends on limiting local anaesthetic spread to the target site (joint space or nerves to the joint). In general, a patient's pain can be attributed to the facet if:[10]

- the pain produced by needling is similar to the usual pain;
- pain relief is noted in response to local anaesthetic injection;
- sensory examination shows no evidence of segmental spinal block.

In subjects clinically suspected of having lumbar facet pain, confirmation by injection ranges from 16 to 94 per cent.[10]

Because no standard to confirm facet pain is available for correlation with blockade findings, the ability of facet joints to validly distinguish the source of back pain has not been established. A positive bone scan may support the diagnosis of facet arthropathy.[10] Pathological facet changes are a common cause of nerve root injury and may irritate afferents on the posterolateral aspect of discs.

In the cervical region, facet nerve blocks or joint injections have been used to treat headache, neck and shoulder pain.[39] For cervicogenic headache, suggested diagnostic blocks to detect the anatomical source include a greater occipital nerve block, then a C2 block, a C2–C3 facet joint injection and finally a C3 nerve block.[2] The third occipital nerve has been found to cause chronic headaches after trauma in 53 per cent of patients.[2] The anatomy of the greater occipital nerve is well defined and the block easily confirmed, but the diagnostic meaning of a favourable response is clouded by the lack of pathophysiological understanding of cervicogenic headache.[10] Therapeutically, in chronic low back pain, neither facet joint block nor intraarticular local anaesthetic injections are superior in terms of the duration of pain relief and provide only a brief 'window' of pain relief.[37,38] Intra-articular facet joint injection with corticosteroids produces significant pain relief, outlasting the local anaesthetic in 30–54 per cent of selected patients with back pain.[10]

Facet joint treatments remain scientifically unproven, the uncertainty surrounding both their indications and the efficacy and diagnostic specificity of these techniques dictating that the findings should be interpreted cautiously.[10,38]

PARAVERTEBRAL SOMATIC SPINAL NERVE BLOCKS

Technique

The spinal nerve is blocked at its exit from the intervertebral foramen as it crosses the space between the transverse processes.[40] Various techniques of paravertebral somatic nerve block have been described. Methods for identifying the paravertebral space include positioning the needle under radiological guidance or using the loss of resistance noted on passing through the costotransverse ligament.[41] A paraesthesia may be elicited or a nerve stimulator may be used to confirm the correct needle position. After careful aspiration to exclude blood, air or CSF, a test dose of local anaesthetic (e.g. 0.5 mL bupivacaine 0.75 per cent) mixed with radiographic contrast can be given to confirm the loss of resistance and to exclude intravascular or intraneural needle placement.[41] The accuracy of spinal nerve block depends on limiting local anaesthetic spread. Only a small amount of local anaesthetic is used in order to try to limit the blockade to one or two segments.

Indications

Pain relief with blockade of a spinal nerve cannot distinguish between pathology of the proximal nerve in the intervertebral foramen and pain transmitted from distal sites by that nerve.[10] Paravertebral somatic nerve blocks can be used for the relief of perioperative thoraco-abdominal pain and for the management of painful disorders of the back of the head, neck, trunk and lower limbs (e.g. osteoporosis, metastatic fracture and lumbar spondylosis).[42] A single paravertebral injection can produce a somatosensory blockade of several nerve roots. Diagnostically, they have been used in determining the extent of spinal nerve involvement and in giving prognostic information prior to ablative procedures.[40] This technique can also be used in herpes zoster pain.

Complications

It is possible to inject into the intravascular, epidural or intrathecal space. Cervical blocks may result in vertebral artery puncture and blockade of the phrenic and vagus nerves.[33] Pneumothorax is a risk in thoracic paravertebral blocks. This can be reduced by entering the paravertebral space as medially as possible, using the loss of resistance technique.[41] Epidural or intrathecal blocks can occur at all levels if the needle is directed too far medially towards the intervertebral foramen.

The paravertebral space is not as anatomically discrete as is often described,[41] and spread of injectate to the epidural and interpleural spaces and into the psoas muscle can occur. Even the spread of a small volume of solution can be unpredictable and extensive. Accompanying sympathetic block is commonplace, especially after paravertebral block. Consequently, there is little rationale for the use of paravertebral blocks as diagnostic blocks. Spinal nerve injection is often used to plan decompressive surgery in complicated cases.[10] The accuracy of this diagnostic information has not yet been proved by controlled and blinded studies. Neuroablative procedures should not be undertaken on the basis of diagnostic paravertebral injection alone.

DORSAL ROOT GANGLION BLOCK

Segmental pain that is peripheral and circumscribed has been considered appropriate for local anaesthetic block and later for radiofrequency lesioning (in which the dorsal root is also partially lesioned).[2] The dorsal root ganglion is anatomically distinct from the motor fibres and is accessible percutaneously in the intervertebral foramen.[2]

SOMATIC PLEXUS ANAESTHESIA/ ANALGESIA FOR THE UPPER EXTREMITIES

All major plexuses (cervical, brachial, lumbar and sacral) in their formation or distribution, will pass between two muscles and be 'invested' with the fascia of these muscles. Here, the plexus can be blocked by a single injection of local anaesthetic.[42] With upper extremity blocks, patients are often ready for discharge (with their arm in a sling) while

residual sensory or motor anaesthesia is still present.[43] For prolonged local anaesthesia, catheters can be placed. In chronic pain, there is no research suggesting that somatic plexus blocks play a significant part in management other than for diagnostic and temporary therapeutic purposes in cancer pain (where catheters can be used).[2] As a diagnostic aid, brachial plexus blocks may be helpful in determining the degree of fixed shoulder deformity and also as an aid to physiotherapy, in patients with chronic shoulder pain, including 'frozen shoulder'.[2]

Upper Extremity

The brachial plexus can be blocked above and below the clavicle, and in the axilla. The perineural and perivascular space surrounding the brachial plexus from the roots to the terminal nerves may be entered at the axillary, subclavian or interscalene level.[42] The interscalene technique is appropriate for upper arm and shoulder pain or surgery. The subclavian perivascular technique can be used for pain or surgery from the shoulder distally. The axillary block is useful for pain or surgery of the hand or forearm. Retrospective reviews attest to the safety and efficacy of brachial plexus anaesthesia.[3]

Brachial plexus blocks can be used to confirm the results of cervicothoracic sympathetic blockade in patients with complex regional pain syndromes type 1 or painful peripheral vascular disorders.[17] They may even be superior to stellate ganglion blocks for the management of type 1 complex regional pain syndromes of the upper extremity.[44] They can be used to differentiate the pain of peripheral neuralgia from CNS pain (e.g. avulsion pain) and also to differentiate pain arising from reflex muscle spasm from that caused by irreversible changes in muscles and tendons.[1]

Continuous brachial plexus blockade with prolonged analgesia and sympathetic block is useful in patients who have undergone the re-attachment of a severed limb or digits and in those whose blood supply to the extremities is compromised.[17] Local anaesthetics of low toxicity (prilocaine and mepivacaine) are often used because of the large doses that may be required.[34] Ropivacaine (0.25–0.5 per cent) produces a brachial plexus block similar to that of bupivacaine in terms of onset and duration of sensory block.[45] Connective tissue septa may divide the brachial plexus into compartments but are of little clinical significance.[42]

Potentiation of the duration of lignocaine, bupivacaine, and mepivacaine in brachial plexus blockade has occurred with the local addition of the

α2-adrenergic agonist clonidine.[46] This is probably because of a direct action on neural tissue, as has been found in the animal model, which clonidine (in low doses) enhances the effects of lignocaine on C fibre action potentials.[47] Analgesia via a systemic mechanism and vasoconstriction have been suggested as other mechanisms.[46,48] The addition of α2-adrenergic agonists may be an attractive alternative to the addition of adrenaline. Also, opioids such as fentanyl, when added locally, are claimed to hasten the time of onset of the block.[49] In the animal model, fentanyl injected at very low doses into the brachial plexus sheath can induce a localized, potent and prolonged antinociceptive effect, which can be reversed by naloxone.[50] Methylprednisolone can also be added to plexus blocks with local anaesthetics in order to hasten the onset and prolong the duration of anaesthesia.[51]

AXILLARY PERIVASCULAR TECHNIQUE

Advantages of this block are its ease of performance, safety and reliability, particularly for hand and forearm surgery. A variety of approaches have been described, including the elicitation of paraesthesias, transarterial injection, sheath blocks and the use of a nerve stimulator.[3] The upper limb on the injected side should be abducted at the shoulder and flexed at right angles at the elbow so that the wrist is at the patient's head.[34] The axillary artery should be palpated and followed as high as possible into the axilla. Ultrasound will accurately identify the artery. With the index finger directly over the pulse, a 4 cm (22 gauge), short-bevelled needle (or an insulated needle with a nerve stimulator) is inserted just above the artery and directed towards the apex of the axilla. Penetration of the neurovascular sheath is usually felt as a definite 'give' or 'click', and the needle will pulsate if left untouched.[42] Paraesthesia (mechanical or cold) may be felt, confirming the correct position. The response of appropriate muscles in the hand or forearm to nerve stimulation also confirms the correct positioning. If arterial blood is seen, the needle is advanced to penetrate the posterior arterial wall. This position may provide the highest success rate.[42]

A catheter can be inserted through the needle and into the perivascular sheath. After negative aspiration, 20–50 mL (42 mL in the average adult) of local anaesthetic with adrenaline 1:200 000 is injected slowly in 4–5 mL increments, with repeated aspiration for blood between increments.[43] Little resistance should be encountered. The needle is then withdrawn to the subcutaneous tissue superfi-

cial to the pulse, and 2 mL local anaesthetic is injected to block the intercostobrachial nerve. To block the musculocutaneous nerve, the needle must be placed as high in the axilla as possible, the maximal acceptable volume used and digital pressure applied behind the needle. The nerve can, however, be blocked separately by injecting 5–8 mL local anaesthetic into the coracobrachialis muscle or as the nerve courses superficially above the interepicondylar line.[3] Complications include systemic local anaesthetic toxicity and intraneural injection. Vascular insufficiency has also been known to occur.[52] The concept of a single compartment within the neurovascular sheath has been questioned.[53] A volume of 50 mL injected with the patient's arm by his or her side lessens the risk of missing blockade of the musculocutaneous and radial nerves.[53]

INFRACLAVICULAR TECHNIQUE

This can be used when the supraclavicular and interscalene approaches are not suitable and the axillary route is inaccessible for surgery on the elbow, forearm and hand.[54] Localizing the plexus by means of a nerve stimulator is recommended. The patient lies supine with the arm at the side. The physician palpates the coracoid process with the right middle finger. When the finger is moved in a downwards direction, it falls into the groove bordered by the coracoid insertions of the pectoralis major and coracobrachialis muscles.[54] That point is marked on the skin. A 22 gauge, 50 mm insulated needle connected to a peripheral nerve stimulator (for flexion of the wrist or fingers) is inserted at an angle of about 45 degrees to the skin plane and parallel to the cutaneous depression bordered by the deltoid and pectoralis major muscles. At a depth of 25–45 mm, the tip of the needle will encounter the lateral cord of the brachial plexus, which adjoins the posterior cord.[54] Despite the medial cord being covered by the axillary artery, it can also be blocked if at least 30 ml local anaesthetic (0.5 per cent bupivacaine 1.5 mg/kg) is injected. The musculocutaneous, median, axillary and radial nerves will be involved earlier than the ulnar nerve. The injection of 20–30 mL local anaesthetic will usually result in a satisfactory block, including the axillary and musculocutaneous, and usually the intercostobrachial (T2), nerves.[53] There is no involvement of the phrenic nerve.[55]

SUBCLAVIAN PERIVASCULAR TECHNIQUE

This approach provides excellent surgical anaesthesia for the elbow, forearm and hand. To avoid the undesirable features of the classical supraclavicular approach, it is modified as follows.[42] The patient is placed supine with the head turned somewhat to the opposite side. The clavicular head of the sterno-cleidomastoid muscle is made prominent by the patient elevating his or her head. An index finger is placed posterior to the muscle on the anterior scalene muscle. The finger is rolled laterally until the interscalene groove is palpated and is then moved inferiorly down the groove as far as it can easily be palpated.

If subclavian arterial pulsations are felt, a 2.5–4.0 cm, short-bevelled needle is inserted just above this point in a directly caudad direction. It should not proceed medially, laterally or posteriorly. If no pulsations are felt, the needle should be inserted as low in the interscalene groove and as close to the middle scalene muscle as is possible, and be advanced in a directly caudad direction. It will then usually strike one of the three trunks of the brachial plexus. Any paraesthesia of the upper extremity below the shoulder, or a click as the needle perforates the enclosing fascia, indicates correct placement in the subclavian perivascular space. A similarly distributed 'pressure paraesthesia', induced by the rapid injection of 2–3 mL local anaesthetic before the main dose, will confirm an adequate needle position.[53] Otherwise, a nerve stimulator must be used. Muscular twitching in the arm or the hand to nerve stimulation also indicates correct placement. If the needle misses all three trunks, it will strike the first rib. It should then be withdrawn and the process repeated as close as possible to the artery.

With this technique, the injection is made where the perivascular space is reduced to its smallest diameter, and thus lower volumes of local anaesthetic can be used. The direction of needle insertion and the use of a short needle improve the incidence of satisfactory results and minimize the possibility of a pneumothorax.[42] After negative aspiration, the local anaesthetic is injected in increments of 4–5 mL (usually up to 30–40 mL lignocaine 1 per cent, mepivacaine 1 per cent, bupivacaine 0.5 per cent or ropivacaine 0.5 per cent). A dull aching pain often confirms the correct placement. Complications include a high incidence of transient phrenic nerve block, ipsilateral stellate ganglion block, arterial puncture, intraneural injection, pneumothorax, systemic local anaesthetic toxicity, epidural or intrathecal block and, rarely, recurrent laryngeal nerve block.[53] With supraclavicular methods, the C5–C7 segments (radial, median and musculocutaneous nerves) are usually well blocked, while the lower segments, C8–T1 (ulnar nerve), may be less reliable.[53]

INTERSCALENE TECHNIQUE

This is best suited to surgery on the shoulder, where a block of the cervical plexus is also desirable.[3] Blockade of the inferior trunk (C8–T1) is often incomplete, requiring supplementation at the ulnar nerve.[3] The use of a nerve stimulator or elicitation of paraesthesia is recommended to site the local anaesthetic accurately.[3] This block can be uncomfortable unless the patient is asleep. In shoulder surgery, it is used for immobilization following recurrent shoulder dislocation repair, for postoperative passive mobilization and for perioperative pain control.[56] The anterior scalene muscle is located at the level of C6 (cricoid cartilage) in a manner similar to that of the subclavian perivascular technique. The index and middle fingers are then rolled laterally across the muscle until the interscalene groove is located. A 3–4 cm needle is inserted between the palpating fingers into the interscalene groove. The head should be kept straight. The needle is inserted perpendicular to the skin (i.e. medially but slightly downwards and backwards) until a paraesthesia (below the shoulder) is elicited or the transverse process contacted. The needle should be walked laterally along the transverse process until paraesthesia is elicited.[34] Using a peripheral nerve stimulator, the positive (red) electrode should be placed on the deltoid muscle for shoulder surgery or over the biceps insertion for forearm surgery. With nerve stimulation, muscle twitching in the arm or hand indicates plexus proximity. If the 'stomach' starts to jump, the phrenic nerve has been stimulated. Bupivacaine 0.5 per cent 20 mL with 1:200 000 adrenaline and 10 mL plain bupivacaine 0.5 per cent are drawn up in three 10 mL syringes. After negative aspiration, an assistant injects the desired volume of local anaesthetic in 4–5 mL increments, with repeated aspirations in between. A lump felt under the skin means that the needle is superficial to the plexus sheath. A high resistance on injection may mean that the needle is not deep enough or is lying intraneurally. Complications include systemic local anaesthetic toxicity, intraneural injection (very rare), transient ipsilateral auditory dysfunction, Horner's syndrome and hoarseness, convulsions, pneumothorax, epidural or intrathecal blockade and pulmonary function changes.[56] Ipsilateral phrenic nerve block can occur in 40–100 per cent of patients.[56] This block should thus never be performed bilaterally. Raising the head end of the bed and giving oxygen by mask usually suffice in a healthy patient.

MISCELLANEOUS ASPECTS

It is recommended not to repeat an incomplete block using a needle technique as this may injure an already blocked nerve (without paraesthesia).[53] Supplementary doses can, however, be safely given via an initial, correctly inserted catheter left *in situ*. A problem with continuous blockade may be local anaesthetic leakage backwards around the catheter, or catheter dislocation. Top-up catheter doses of 4–10 mL of local anaesthetic per hour (bupivacaine 0.25 per cent), are often used. Additives include adrenaline (5 µg/mL to reduce absorption and prolong duration), and fentanyl or clonidine to modify onset and duration of the blockade.[53] The landmarks for a supraclavicular brachial plexus block are not easily determined in young children (the subclavian artery is impalpable and the scalene muscles poorly developed).[57]

NEW METHODS

A new supraclavicular approach, the intersternocleidomastoid technique, makes use of the triangle formed by the palpable sternocleidomastoid heads.[58] The catheter entry point is cephalad enough not to obscure the surgical field on the shoulder.

Another new method is to place the patient in the supine position, head slightly retroflexed, with a pillow under the shoulder.[59] The cricoid cartilage, the sternocleidomastoid muscle and the carotid artery are palpated. Two fingers are placed between the sternocleidomastoid and the trachea, and the Chassaignac tubercle on the 6th cervical transverse process is palpated. The sternocleidomastoid and the carotid artery are retracted laterally. A small area of the skin is anaesthetized at the level of the Chassaignac tubercle. A short bevelled needle with an injection tube extension leading to a nerve stimulator is used. The needle is advanced perpendicularly through the skin and fascial planes until it strikes the 6th cervical process.[59] The needle is withdrawn another 2–4 mm, angled at 60 degrees towards the trachea and advanced to the tip of the transverse process with the nerve stimulator turned on. As the needle tip passes through the origin of the scalenus anterior muscle, it will enter the brachial plexus. Stimulation of the shoulder and upper extremity muscles indicates the proper location of the needle tip in the proximity of the roots and trunks of the brachial plexus.[59] The needle is tilted 75 degrees cephalad with the bevel directed towards the mid-clavicular point and may be advanced another 1–2 mm with repeated aspiration. Radio-opaque material (0.5 mL) is injected to locate (under fluoroscopy) the position of the needle tip in the brachial plexus sheath between the two scaleni muscles. Then, 20–25 mL of local anaesthetic (bupivacaine 0.5 per cent, ropivacaine 0.5 per cent or lignocaine 2 per cent) is injected. For chronic neck pain, cervical radiculopathy, shoulder or arm pain, 5 mL bupivacaine 0.5 per cent with methyl prednisolone 40 mg are injected.

A mid-humeral approach involving the location of four nerves at the midhumeral level has recently been described.[60] In this study, a 22 gauge insulated needle connected to a nerve stimulator was used to locate the nerves as follows: musculocutaneous nerve – arm flexion; radial nerve – arm and finger extension, and supination; ulnar nerve – fourth and fifth finger flexion and thumb adduction; and median nerve – wrist, second and third finger flexion, and pronation. Lignocaine 1.5 per cent 10 mL with adrenaline 1:200 000 was used for each of the four nerves. The success rate and incidence of motor blockade were greater with the mid-humeral than the axillary approach.[60]

Lower extremity

At the level of its formation, the roots of the lumbar plexus are invested by the fascia of the quadratus lumborum and psoas major muscles.[42] The obturator nerve, lateral cutaneous nerve of the thigh and femoral nerve are derived from the lumbar plexus. In its course to the thigh and to its termination in the upper leg, the femoral nerve is enveloped by an extension of this fascia. For prolonged local anaesthesia, catheters can be placed along the femoral and sciatic nerves.[19] Peripheral neural blockade of the lower extremity is easily accomplished with the minimum of side-effects and the advantage of pain relief without urinary retention.[3] Femoral nerve blockade, as well as more peripheral blocks at the popliteal fossa and ankle, have found a place in the management of orthopaedic outpatient procedures.

The indications for lumbar sacral plexus or sciatic and femoral nerve blockade are similar to those for the brachial plexus, for example relieving acute pain, producing sympathetic blockade of the leg, or differentiating between muscle spasm pain and pain caused by irreversible changes in muscles and tendons.[17]

INGUINAL PARAVASCULAR TECHNIQUE OF LUMBAR PLEXUS THREE-IN-ONE BLOCK

A single injection into the envelope around the femoral nerve can thus provide blockade of the obturator and lateral cutaneous nerves as well.[42] When combined with the sciatic block, the entire lower limb is affected.[34] With the patient supine, the needle is inserted lateral (1.0–1.5 cm) to the femoral artery just below the inguinal ligament. It is directed cephalad at about 60 degrees from the skin until paraesthesia is elicited or nerve stimulation causes movement of the patella.[34] A click will be felt as the needle enters the femoral canal. After negative aspiration, 2 mL local anaesthetic are initially injected using a stationary needle to exclude intraneural injection.[61] The desired volume (20–30 mL) is then injected in 4–5 mL increments, with intermittent aspiration in between. A total volume of 20 mL will be required to anaesthetize the femoral and lateral cutaneous nerves, while 30 mL will be required for the obturator nerve (which provides sensation to the lower third of the medial aspect of the thigh). Firm digital pressure distal on the needle promotes cephalad spread. Complications include systemic local anaesthetic toxicity and neuropathy. By reducing the number of injections and the volume of local anaesthetic required, this technique decreases the chances of neural or systemic complications. For a femoral nerve block, an identical technique is used, but less drug (10–15 mL) is required.

SCIATIC NERVE BLOCK

There are five main approaches: one anterior, two posterior, one lateral, and one in the popliteal fossa.[34,61,62] Which is chosen will depend on the ability to turn the patient without discomfort. A nerve stimulator should be used. Complications include neuropathy and systemic local anaesthetic toxicity.

Anterior approach

The patient is placed in a supine position. One line is drawn from the anterior superior iliac spine to the public tubercle, and a parallel line is drawn from the greater trochanter across the upper thigh.[42] At the junction of the medial and middle thirds of the upper line, a line is drawn at right angles to both previous lines. Where it joins the lower line marks the position of the lesser trochanter. A long needle (12–15 cm) is inserted 1 cm medial to this point, perpendicularly downwards and slightly laterally to contact the femur.[34] The needle is then realigned

until it passes medially to the femur. The sciatic nerve is contacted about 5 cm behind the femur. With nerve stimulation, the foot will move. Local anaesthetic 15–20 mL are injected.

Posterior approach

The patient lies on his or her side in the Sim's position, the side to be injected uppermost. A line is drawn from the superior border of the greater trochanter to the posterior iliac spine.[42] A second line is drawn bisecting and perpendicular to the first line and passing inferiorly. A third line is drawn between the superior border of the greater trochanter and the sacral hiatus. Where this third line crosses the second line determines the position of the sciatic nerve. Nerve stimulation causes foot movement. Aspirating in between, 4–5 mL increments of local anaesthetic are injected, up to 20 mL. The advantage of this technique is that it locates the position of the nerve more accurately than any other technique.[42]

Posterior approach (Raj technique)

With the patient supine, the leg is raised into the lithotomy position. The sciatic nerve lies between the greater trochanter and the ischial tuberosity. An 8 cm (22 gauge) needle is inserted at right angles to the skin at the midpoint between the greater trochanter and the ischial tuberosity until paraesthesia is obtained or nerve stimulation causes foot movement.[34] Between 15 and 20 mL of local anaesthetic are injected in 4–5 mL increments, aspirating in between.

Lateral approach

Because of the discomfort, patients not asleep should be sedated and given analgesia. A 10–15 cm, 20 gauge, insulated needle connected to a peripheral nerve stimulator is inserted 3 cm distally to the greater trochanter until the lateral side of the femur is contacted. The needle is then withdrawn to the subcutaneous tissue and is directed towards the posterior side of the femur at an angle of 30 degrees to the previous plane.[61] The tip will encounter the tibial nerve (foot plantar flexion) or the common peroneal nerve (foot dorsiflexion) at a depth of 8–12 cm, and 1 mg/kg bupivacaine 0.5 per cent is given to block the sciatic nerve.[61]

Popliteal fossa (suprapopliteal block)

Blockade of the sciatic nerve in the popliteal fossa provides satisfactory analgesia for operative procedures of the foot. To locate the sciatic nerve, peripheral nerve stimulation is used. Inversion of the foot is the motor response that best predicts complete sensory blockade of the foot.[62] To assure proximity to the nerve, the local anaesthetic should only be injected if the motor response is elicited at less than 1 mA.[62] The presence of a common epineural sheath enveloping the tibial and common peroneal nerves explains why anaesthesia may be profound in both divisions, while paraesthesia or a peripheral nerve stimulator response is obtained in one division only.[63] Incomplete blockade of the sciatic nerve may be the result of its size, the separate fascial coverings of the tibial and common peroneal nerves, or the blockade of either the tibial or common peroneal nerves after branching from the sciatic nerve.[62] Continuous popliteal sciatic nerve blockade has been used to provide postoperative analgesia after foot surgery.[64] In this study, the sciatic nerve was localized with a short-bevelled needle connected to a peripheral nerve stimulator. A 20 gauge catheter was placed at the same depth as the needle with a Seldinger technique. Mepivacaine 1 per cent 30 mL with adrenaline 1:200 000 was injected, followed by a continuous infusion of bupivacaine 0.125 per cent, sufentanil 0.1 μg/mL and clonidine 1 μg/mL at 7 mL per hour for 48 hours.[64]

COMBINED LUMBOSACRAL PLEXUS BLOCK

This can be used if inguinal paravascular sciatic, epidural or intrathecal techniques are contraindicated. The patient is placed in the lateral spinal position with the side to be injected uppermost.[42] A line is drawn connecting the superior borders of both iliac crests.

A second line is drawn parallel to the spine, passing through the posterior superior iliac spine. Where the two lines cross, an 8 cm (22 gauge) needle is inserted perpendicular to the skin and advanced until paraesthesia is produced. If the transverse process (of L4) is contacted, the needle is redirected more caudally. If no paraesthesia is obtained, a nerve stimulator can be used to stimulate a response in the quadratus femoris muscle. Local anaesthetic in a dose of 40 mL is then injected.

Cervical plexus block

This block is useful for superficial surgery of the neck, thyroidectomy, carotid endarterectomy and possibly tracheostomy.[65] Bilateral deep cervical plexus blocks (for thyroidectomy and tracheostomy) should be avoided because of the risk of bilateral phrenic nerve palsies.

SUPERFICIAL CERVICAL PLEXUS BLOCK

The head is turned slightly away from the side of the block and is elevated to bring the sternocleidomastoid muscle into prominence.[65] A volume of 5 mL local anaesthetic is deposited subcutaneously at the mid-point of the posterior border of the sternocleidomastoid muscle. A further 10 mL local anaesthetic are infiltrated up and down along the posterior border of the muscle.

DEEP CERVICAL PLEXUS BLOCK

The patient is positioned as above but without head elevation.[65] A line is drawn from the tip of the mastoid process to the anterior tubercle of the transverse process of C6. A second parallel line is drawn 1 cm behind it. The C2 transverse process is the highest one palpable along this line. The C4 transverse process is palpable about 5 cm caudally. The needle is inserted at this point, perpendicular to the skin, until bony contact is made at 1.5–3.0 cm.[65] The needle is walked anteriorly or posteriorly until paraesthesia is elicited. At this point, 10 mL local anaesthetic are injected. Phrenic nerve palsy is almost inevitable but, if unilateral, is usually of no clinical significance. Cervical sympathetic blockade and laryngeal nerve block (with hoarseness) may occasionally occur. Rarely, neuraxial spread or direct vertebral arterial injection (with convulsions) occurs.[65] A mixture of lignocaine (for fast onset) and bupivacaine (for duration) is often used for carotid endarterectomy.[66] Plasma local anaesthetic concentrations can reach an early near-toxic peak.[66]

A new method to block both the superficial and deep cervical plexus has recently been described.[67] The patient is placed supine with the head in mid-extension on a fluoroscopy table. The trachea, cricoid cartilage, cricothyroid membrane, thyroid cartilages, hyoid bone and carotid artery are gently palpated. Two fingers are inserted between the sternocleidomastoid and the trachea. The Chassaignac tubercle, located at the level of the cricoid cartilage on the C6 transverse process, is palpated. The fingers are gradually slid up, and the 3rd, 4th and 5th transverse processes are felt. The 4th or 5th transverse process is placed between the two fingers. The sternocleidomastoid and carotid artery are retracted laterally from the larynx, and the overlying skin is anaesthetized. The needle is passed until it touches the transverse process of the 3rd, 4th or 5th cervical vertebrae. A short-bevelled needle with an injection set extension leading to a peripheral nerve stimulator is used. The needle is advanced perpendicular to the skin until it strikes the transverse process. It is then withdrawn 2–4 mm, and the hub is angled 60 degrees towards the trachea. As the needle is passed, an aspiration test is repeatedly performed. Using a peripheral nerve stimulator, the needle is advanced beyond the lateral edge of the transverse process until the cervical plexus is located. The needle tip is pointed cephalad by tilting the needle 60 degrees caudad. Radio-opaque material 0.5 mL is injected into the cervical plexus fascial sheath under image intensification. The local anaesthetic is then injected into the cervical plexus. For surgery, 15–20 mL of local anaesthetic are used. To relieve cervical radiculopathy, 5 mL bupivacaine 0.5 per cent with 40 mg methylprednisolone are used.

PERIPHERAL NERVE BLOCKS IN INFANTS AND CHILDREN

Regional blockade techniques have been developed for children of all ages, including newborns. The distribution and clearance of bupivacaine and lignocaine following several types of regional blockade in babies over 6 months of age resemble those found in adults.[68] Bupivacaine clearance is mildly delayed in newborns.[68] Techniques requiring paraesthesia to be obtained do not succeed in young children because of a lack of cooperation and understanding.[69] Most of these blocks are performed while the child is anaesthetized, making use of a nerve stimulator. With blocks performed when patients are asleep, there may be a greater potential for the intraneural injection of larger volumes of local anaesthetic.

Arm blocks can provide relaxation and analgesia/anaesthesia for fracture reductions and laceration repairs.[70] For brachial plexus block, the axillary approach is the safest and most successful. It can be used in the emergency situation and almost eliminates the risk of pulmonary aspiration.[71] More peripheral blocks, such as those of the median, radial and ulnar nerves, may be performed at the wrist, while the digital nerves may be blocked using a metacarpal approach.

The inguinal paravascular block can be used for lower limb surgery or diagnostic muscle biopsy. Ankle nerve blocks and metatarsal nerve blocks are also used.

Intercostal nerve blocks will provide analgesia in both the chest wall (upper six nerves) and abdomen (lower six nerves) after surgery or trauma. Continuous interpleural local anaesthetic infusions have been used for analgesia after the repair of a coarctation or anterior spinal fusion. Ilio-inguinal and iliohypogastric nerve blocks relieve pain after herniotomy or orchidopexy.[69,70] Blockade of the dorsal nerve of the penis provides analgesia following circumcision, as does topical lignocaine. Wound infiltration with bupivacaine 0.25 per cent, or lignocaine aerosol sprayed into the wound, can be a successful way of providing postoperative analgesia.[69]

Regional anesthesia in children is generally safe. Among 24 409 cases of regional anaesthesia, there were only 23 reported critical incidents, none of which resulted in death or neurological sequelae.[72] Peripheral nerve blockade should be used more widely and, where appropriate, should be used to substitute for central blocks. Wound infiltration and peripheral blocks are most effective for minor inguinal or extremity procedures in which near-complete blockade of the afferent impulses is feasible.[72] For major upper abdominal or thoracic procedures, peripheral blocks provide some analgesia and a reduction in opioid requirement, but they cannot adequately interrupt all the necessary afferent pathways and often require very large doses of local anaesthetics.[72] The duration of peripheral blockade appears shorter in children than in adults.[72] With a fascia lata block, patients with femur fractures or femur osteotomies experience excellent analgesia with full urinary function, and motor and sensory function in the contralateral leg.[72] Continuous peripheral blockade can extend block duration. In infants undergoing coarctation repairs and ductus arteriosus ligations, continuous intercostal blockade reduces analgesic requirements and accelerates tracheal extubation.[72] Between 5 and 10 days of intercostal nerve blockade via percutaneous approaches have been obtained with biodegradable polyester–bupivacaine microspheres.[72]

INTERPLEURAL BLOCK

Interpleural analgesia was first described by Kvalheim and Reiestad in 1984.[52] It involves the placement of a catheter either deep to the internal intercostal membrane but superficial to the pleura, or between the visceral and parietal pleura. Since then, reports involving more than 700 patients have been published on the technique's use in acute and chronic pain.[52]

Technique

Interpleural catheters can be inserted with the patient in the prone, lateral, sitting or supine position.

ANTERIOR APPROACH

In a supine patient, the unilateral arm is abducted 90 degrees or folded above the head. A 16 or 18 gauge Tuohy epidural needle is connected to a three-way tap, and a 5 ml syringe is filled with saline.[73] In the posterior axillary line at the level of T6–8, the skin and periosteum over the selected rib are anaesthetized with local anaesthesia. The needle is placed over the selected rib and angled 45 degrees in a posterior as well as in a cephalad direction. Once the needle is walked off the rib, the introducer is removed, the three-way tap and a well-lubricated 5 ml glass saline-filled syringe (with the plunger removed) are attached, and the needle is slowly advanced. Because of the negative pressure, the meniscus of the saline will drop on entering the interpleural space. The three-way tap is then removed (while occluding the needle with a fingertip), and the interpleural catheter is advanced 5–6 cm into the interpleural space. Additional confirmation of correct catheter placement is that fluid present in the catheter will flow into the chest before the filter is attached.

POSTERIOR APPROACH

The patient can lie prone or on his or her side with the surgical site uppermost. The ipsilateral arm either hangs over the edge of the bed (prone position) or is pulled across the chest (lateral position) to retract the scapula as far anterolaterally as possible. An epidural needle (Tuohy 16 or 18 gauge) is inserted through the 4–9th (usually the 8th) intercostal space about 8–10 cm from the posterior midline.[52] The needle is inserted at an angle of 30–40 degrees to the skin, close to the upper border of the rib. It is walked off the cephalad edge of the rib and advanced about 3 mm. After perforating the posterior intercostal membrane, which is felt as a distinct resistance, the stylet is removed from the needle. A well-lubricated 5 ml glass saline-filled syringe is attached to the needle. As the needle perforates the parietal pleura, the meniscus of the saline will drop. A catheter is then advanced as above.[74] This position can be changed, however, to allow the local anaesthetics to be spread to other areas (e.g. a 30 degree Trendelenburg tilt can be applied if blockade of the upper sympathetic chain is desired).[75]

For ventilated patients, the ventilator should be disconnected before pleural puncture and until the needle is withdrawn from the pleural space. Awake patients are asked to hold their breath at the end of expiration until the pleural space is entered and the needle removed.[52] Aspiration by way of the catheter is attempted to exclude blood vessel or lung puncture. The catheter is then taped to the patient's back.[76] Variations include surgical placement of the catheter at the time of thoracotomy and the insertion of the local anaesthetic solution through the chest drain.[77]

Mechanism of action

There are several possible mechanisms of analgesia.[73] Local anaesthetic crosses the parietal pleura (posteriorly and laterally) to block the intercostal nerves. It also crosses the parietal pleura medially to anaesthetize the lesser (anteriorly) and greater splanchnic nerves, and the sympathetic chain (posteriorly). Sensory nerve endings in the pleurae are topically anaesthetized. Some local anaesthetic may diffuse neuraxially across the dural root sleeve. It is believed that the local anaesthetic solution diffuses from the pleural space through the parietal pleura and innermost intercostal muscles to provide multiple, unilateral intercostal nerve blockade. It provides analgesia but not anaesthesia for surgery. Local anaesthetic solutions in the pleural space may also involve the phrenic nerve, the sympathetic chain and the splanchnic nerve.[20] It remains to be seen whether any local anaesthetic diffuses into the peritoneal cavity, the lung substance or the heart.[20] It has been suggested that lung lymphatic uptake of local anaesthetic may play a role in producing prolonged analgesia.[78]

Indications for use

ACUTE PAIN

The technique has proved to be effective in the management of perioperative pain after unilateral breast surgery, renal surgery, splenectomy, cholecystectomy (with a subcostal approach) and percutaneous biliary drainage.[19] It is less effective for post-thoracotomy pain as the presence of chest drains may remove large quantities of anaesthetic.[20] A bilateral interpleural block has been used for midline upper abdominal surgery.[79]

CHRONIC PAIN

Intrapleural blockade has also been used to treat chronic pain problems. It is effective in treating patients with multiple rib fractures and flail chests, where it may also improve the ventilatory status of these patients.[80,81] With multiple rib fractures, the respiratory function can be dramatically improved, but interpleural blood can dilute the local anaesthetic, and a drain (if present) needs to be clamped for about an hour.[73] It has been used to treat severe, acute and subacute thoracic herpes zoster, chronic thoracic and pancreatic pain, and in complex regional pain syndrome type 1.[82] In cancer pain, this technique has been used to treat pancreatic tumours and tumour invasion of the brachial plexus or vertebral metastases.[20,73,75]

Dose and agents used

Several questions remain unanswered, such as which local anaesthetic is the most appropriate and what the optimal concentration and volume of the drug are.[20,81] Bupivacaine has been the local anaesthetic agent most commonly used for interpleural regional analgesia, but volumes and concentrations have varied. It is usually given in concentrations of 0.25–0.5 per cent. The addition of adrenaline 1:200 000 does not significantly decrease the serum level or increase the duration of blockade.[73,76] The volumes usually used vary from 20 to 60 mL.[77,82] Complete pain relief and peak plasma concentrations are obtained between 15 and 30 minutes, and last between 10 and 15 hours, although long durations of up to 24 hours have been reported after a single injection.[76,77] Continuous interpleural infusions of local anaesthetics have not been reproducibly successful in the early postoperative period.[19]

The effect of interpleural blockade on respiratory function after upper abdominal surgery is controversial, and more detailed studies of respiratory function need to be performed, particularly in relation to diaphragmatic function, which may be impaired.[83] For chronic pain, catheters have been inserted for 5–10 days.[80] Occasionally, a subcutaneous implantable infusion system has been inserted for long-term interpleural analgesia.[84]

Complications

Several serious complications of this technique have been reported, including pneumothorax, pleural effusion and infection.[52] Fortunately, pneumothorax occurs infrequently. The small amount of air that may enter the pleural space during the procedure is probably rapidly absorbed and will not develop into a tension pneumothorax. Intrapulmonary positioning of the catheter and intrathoracic bleeding can also occur. Systemic toxicity reactions such as somnolence, disorientation and convulsions have also been reported.[20] In most studies, the plasma concentrations of bupivacaine reported are sufficiently low that signs of systemic toxicity should not occur.[76] The rate of vascular absorption of local anaesthetics from the pleural space is slower than that following multiple intercostal blockade.[81] Mechanical problems associated with catheter use can also occur.[85] Hypotension and a Horner's syndrome are rarely seen.[73]

Conclusion

The primary advantages of this technique are its simplicity and its ability to provide continuous analgesia, but clear benefits of this technique have not yet been shown.[85] Its efficacy needs to be determined compared with continuous intercostal block, thoracic epidural analgesia and PCA. Controlled studies are required to identify the best drug, its appropriate dosage and the risk-to-benefit ratio of this technique.

INTRAPERITONEAL ANALGESIA

Intraperitoneal analgesia is obtained by instilling local anaesthetic into the peritoneal cavity to reduce perioperative abdominal and pelvic pain.[86] There is an abundance of nociceptors on the visceral and parietal surfaces of the peritoneum yet their contribution to perioperative pain in intra-abdominal and pelvic surgery remains relatively unknown.[86] The post-surgical inflammatory reaction releases histamine, kinins, serotonin and prostaglandins, which may stimulate these receptors. Amide local anaesthetics have potent prolonged anti-inflammatory properties besides their nerve conduction-blocking properties.[86] Pelvic local anaesthetic instillation during laparoscopic sterilization results in a lack of pain during clip application, and a marked reduction in the level of postoperative pain and in the incidence and severity of postoperative shoulder pain.[86] Equipotent dosages of lignocaine and bupivacaine showed no difference in the degree or duration of analgesia.[86] Recommended lignocaine dosages (diluted to 80 mL before peritoneal instillation) are 500 mg for postpartum patients and 1000 mg for non-pregnant patients.[86] Peak plasma concentrations of 2.64 $\mu g/mL$ (for pregnant patients) and 2.3 $\mu g/mL$ (for non-pregnant patients) were shown to be well below toxic levels and were even lower with the addition of 1:200 000 adrenaline.[86] The duration of satisfactory surgical conditions of 45 minutes limits the use of this method as the sole anaesthetic technique in performing diagnostic and laparoscopic procedures. In laparoscopic cholecystectomy, 30 mL bupivacaine 0.5 per cent led to a marked reduction in postoperative pain for 8 hours post-surgery.[86] The instillation of 0.6 mL/kg of bupivacaine 0.375 per cent led to peak plasma concentrations of 0.94 $\mu g/mL$ (± 0.47 $\mu g/mL$), which is straying close to toxic levels.[86] No studies have been reported on the use of the subdiaphragmatic intraperitoneal instillation of lignocaine in laparoscopic cholecystectomy.[86] The intraperitoneal instillation of local anaesthetics does not alter the neuroendocrine response to laparotomy but offers advantages in selective pelvic procedures. It may yet prove to be a valuable adjunct to upper abdominal laparoscopic procedures. Future trials will no doubt clarify the desirability and safety of this practice.

REFERENCES

1. **Bonica, J.J. and Buckley, F.P.** 1990: Regional analgesia with local anesthetics. In Bonica, J.J. (ed.) *The management of pain*, 2nd edn. Philadelphia: Lea & Febiger, 1883–966.
2. **Lamacraft, G., Molloy, A.R. and Cousins, M.J.** 1997: Peripheral nerve blockade and chronic pain management. *Pain Reviews* 4, 122–47.
3. **Wedel, D.J.** 1996: Regional anaesthesia for day case surgery: which blocks? which local anaesthetics? *International Symposium of Regional Anaesthesia*, 9–11 April, Auckland, New Zealand, 82–6.
4. **Mather, L.E.** 1996: Pharmacology of local anaesthetic agents – relevance of chemical properties. *International Symposium of Regional Anaesthesia*, 9–11 April, Auckland, New Zealand, 23–6.
5. **Strichartz, G.** 1996: Target: peripheral nerve. *International Symposium of Regional Anaesthesia*, 9–11 April, Auckland, New Zealand, 16–18.
6. **Strichartz, G.** 1996: Physiology and pharmacology of regional blockade. *International Symposium of Regional Anaesthesia Daily News* 2, 1–2.
7. **Strichartz, G.** 1996: A breadth of local anaesthetic actions: from molecules to man. *150 years on – a selection of papers presented at the 11th World Congress of Anaesthesiologists*. Rosebery, NSW: Bridge Printery, 103–7.
8. **Tucker, G.T.** 1996: Chirality and its relevance to local anaesthetics. *150 years on – a selection of papers presented at the 11th World Congress of Anaesthesiologists*. Rosebery, NSW: Bridge Printery, 97–101.
9. **Charlton, J.E.** 1996: Are other therapies preferable? *International Symposium of Regional Anaesthesia*, 9–11 April, Auckland, New Zealand, 131–4.
10. **Hogan, Q.H. and Abram, S.E.** 1997: Neural blockade for diagnosis and prognosis. *Anesthesiology* **86**(1), 216–41.
11. **Setyna, N.F. and Berde, C.B.** 1995: Diagnostic nerve blocks: caveats and pitfalls in interpretation. *IASP Newsletter* (May/Jun), 3–5.
12. **Raja, S.N.** 1997: Nerve blocks in the evaluation of chronic pain. *Anesthesiology* **86**, 4–6.
13. **Zuccherelli, L.** 1998: Peripheral nerve stimulation and nerve blocks. *Hospital Supplies* (Mar), 18–30.
14. **Gunn, C.G.** 1996: *Treatment of chronic pain: intramuscular stimulation for myofascial pain of radiculopathic origin* 2nd edn. Edinburgh: Churchill Livingstone, 1–165.
15. **Murphy, T.M.** 1990: Chronic pain. In Miller R.D. (ed.) *Anesthesia*, 3rd edn. New York: Churchill Livingstone, 1927–50.
16. **Dessein, P.H., Shipton, E.A. and Cloete, A.** 1997: Fibromyalgia as a syndrome of neuroendocrine deficiency: a hypothetical model with therapeutic implications. *Pain Reviews* 4, 79–88.
17. **Raj, P.P.** 1988: Prognostic and therapeutic local anesthetic blockade. In Cousins, M.J. and Bridenbaugh, P.O. (eds) *Neural blockade*, 2nd edn. Philadelphia: J.B. Lippincott, 899–933.
18. **Dahl, J.B. and Frederiksen, H.J.** 1995: Wound infiltration for operative and postoperative analgesia. *Current Opinion in Anaesthesiology* 8, 435–40.
19. **Shipton, E.A.** 1992: Postoperative pain – an update. *South African Journal of Surgery* 30(1), 2–5.
20. **Raj, P.P.** 1991: Regional techniques for postoperative analgesia. *McGill University Annual Review Course in Anaesthesia* (May), 311–21.
21. **MacHolmes, C.** 1996: Intravenous regional anaesthesia. *International Symposium of Regional Anaesthesia*, 9–11 April, Auckland, New Zealand, 112–15.
22. **Lilienfeld, D. and Payne, K.** 1997: Intravenous regional anaesthesia of the forearm using pethidine alone and with lignocaine. *South African Journal of Anaesthesiology and Analgesia* 3(2), 22–6.
23. **Ehrlich, I.K., Lerman, J., Sikich, N. and MacPherson, B.** 1992: Efficacy of EMLA cream for venipuncture in children. *Anesthesia and Analgesia* 74, 582.
24. **Inada, T., Uesugi, F., Kawachi, S. and Inada, K.** 1997: Lidocaine tape relieves pain due to needle insertion during stellate ganglion block. *Canadian Journal of Anaesthesia* 44(3), 259–62.
25. **Rowbotham, M.C., Davies, P.S., Verkempinck, C., and Galer, B.S.** 1996: Lidocaine patch: double-blind controlled study of a new method for post-herpetic neuralgia. *Pain* **65**, 39–44.

26. **Nicodemus, H.F., Ferrer, M.J.R., Cristobal, V.C. and De Castro, L.R.** 1991: Bilateral infraorbital block with 0.05% bupivacaine in children. *Anesthesiology* 75(3A), A690.

27. **Trankina, M.F.** 1991: Infrapatellar nerve block for chronic pain following diagnostic knee arthroscopy. *Anesthesiology* 75(3A), A738.

28. **Heard, S.O., Edwards, W.T., Ferrari, D.** *et al.* 1992: Analgesic effect of intra-articular bupivacaine or morphine after arthroscopic knee surgery: a randomised, prospective double-blind study. *Anesthesia and Analgesia* 74, 822–6.

29. **Heard, S.O., Edwards, W.T., Ferrari, D., Hanna, D. and Willock, M.M.** 1991: Efficacy of intra-articular morphine or bupivacaine following arthroscopic knee surgery. *Anesthesiology* 75(3A), A670.

30. **Stav, A., Sternberg, A., Landau, M., Ovadia, L. and Weksler, N.** 1992: Intra-articular injection of a proliferant for pain relief in patients with rheumatoid arthritis – preliminary results. *The Pain Clinic* 5(2), 83–9.

31. **Gilliland, B.C.** 1990: Arthritis and periarthritic disorders. In Bonica, J.J. (ed.) *The management of pain*, 2nd edn. Philadelphia: Lea & Febiger, 329–51.

32. **Chan, V.W.S., Chung, F., Cheng, D.C.H., Seyone, C., Chung, A. and Kirby, T.J.** 1991: Analgesic and pulmonary effects of continuous intercostal nerve block following thoracotomy. *Canadian Journal of Anaesthesia* 38(6), 733–9.

33. **Thompson, G.E. and Moore, D.C.** 1988: Celiac plexus, intercostal, and minor peripheral blockade. In Cousins, M.J. and Bridenbaugh PO (eds) *Neural blockade*, 2nd edn. Philadelphia: J.B. Lippincott, 503–30.

34. **Scott, D.B.** 1989: *Introduction to regional anaesthesia.* Norwalk: Appleton & Lange, 1–96.

35. **Shulman, M., Waren, W., Nath, H. and Ivankovich, A.** 1996: Intercostal nerve block with a 5% butamben suspension for the treatment of post-thoracotomy syndrome. *International Symposium of Regional Anaesthesia*, 9–11 April, Auckland, New Zealand, 269.

36. **Ritchie, E.D., Tong, D., Chung, F., Norris, A.M., Miniaci, A. and Vairavanathan, S.D.** 1997: Suprascapular nerve block for postoperative pain relief in arthroscopic shoulder surgery: a new modality? *Anesthesia and Analgesia* 84, 1306–12.

37. **Nash, T.P.** 1990: Facet joints – intra-articular steroids or nerve block? *The Pain Clinic* 3(2), 77–82.

38. **Marks, R.C., Houston, T. and Thulbourne, T.** 1992: Facet joint injection and facet nerve block: a randomised comparison in 86 patients with chronic low back pain. *Pain* 49, 325–8.

39. **Bogduk, N.** 1988: Back pain – zygapophysial blocks and epidural steroids. In Cousins, M.J. and Bridenbaugh, P.O. (eds). *Neural blockade*, 2nd edn. Philadelphia: J.B. Lippincott, 935–54.

40. **Wurm, W.H.** 1992: Role of diagnostic and therapeutic nerve blocks in the management of pain. In Aronoff, G.M. (ed.) *Evaluation and treatment of chronic pain*, 2nd edn. Baltimore: Williams & Wilkins, 218–28.

41. **Purcell-Jones, G., Pither, C.E. and Justins, D.M.** 1989: Paravertebral somatic nerve block: a clinical, radiographic, and computed tomographic study in chronic pain patients. *Anesthesia and Analgesia* 68, 32–9.

42. **Winnie, A.P.** 1991: Regional anesthesia of the extremities. *American Society of Anesthesiologists' Annual Refresher Course Lectures* 19, 233–51.

43. **Philip, B.K.** 1992: Regional anaesthesia for ambulatory surgery. *Canadian Journal of Anaesthesia* 39(5), R3–R6.

44. **Durrani, Z. and Winnie, A.P.** 1992: Diagnostic and therapeutic brachial plexus block for reflex sympathetic dystrophy unresponsive to stellate ganglion block. *Anesthesia and Analgesia* 74, S77.

45. **Hickey, R., Rowley, C.L., Candido, K.D., Ramamurthy, S. and Winnie, A.P.** 1991: A comparative study of 0.25% ropivacaine and 0.25% bupivacaine for brachial plexus anesthesia. *Anesthesiology* 75(3A), A711.

46. **Eledjam, J.J., Deschodt, J., Viel, E.J.** *et al.* 1991: Brachial plexus block with bupivacaine: effects of added alpha-adrenergic agonists: comparison between clonidine and epinephrine. *Canadian Journal of Anaesthesia* 38(7), 870–5.

47. **Gaumann, D.M., Brunet, P.C. and Jirounek, P.** 1992: Clonidine enhances the effects of lidocaine on C-fiber action potential. *Anesthesia and Analgesia* 74, 719–25.

48. **Gaumann, D.M., Forster, A., Griessen, M.** *et al.* 1992: Comparison between the admixture of clonidine or epinephrine to lidocaine in axillary plexus block. *Anesthesia and Analgesia* 74, S107.

49. **Singelyn, F.J., Muller, G. and Gouverneur, J.M.** 1991: Adding fentanyl and clonidine to mepivacaine results in a rapid onset and prolonged anesthesia and analgesia after brachial plexus blockade. *Anesthesiology* 75(3A), A653.

50. **Kayser, V., Gobeaux, D., Lombard, M.C., Guilbaud, G. and Besson, J.M.** 1990: Potent and long-lasting antinociceptive effects after injection of low doses of a mu-opioid receptor agonist, fentanyl, into the brachial plexus sheath of the rat. *Pain* 42, 215–25.

51. **Stan, T.C.** 1996: Longer acting axillary blocks by the addition of methylprednisolone. *International Symposium of Regional Anaesthesia*, 9–11 April, Auckland, New Zealand, 270.

52. **Finucane, B.T.** 1991: Regional anaesthesia – complications and technique. *Canadian Journal of Anaesthesia* 38(4), R3–R10.

53. **Selander, D.G.** 1996: Brachial plexus anaesthesia. *International Symposium of Regional Anaesthesia*, 9–11 April, Auckland, New Zealand, 108–11.

54. **Marino, G., Valoti, O., Liguori, S., Ferri, F. and Rossi, M.** 1996: Another infraclavicular approach to the brachial plexus, please. *International Symposium of Regional Anaesthesia*, 9–11 April, Auckland, New Zealand, 208–9.

55. **Grossi, P., Foggioni, M., Porcheddu, A. and Coluccia,**

R. 1996: Respiratory effects of the infraclavicular brachial plexus block. *International Symposium of Regional Anaesthesia*, 9–11 April, Auckland, New Zealand 186–7.

56. **Raath, R.P.** 1997: Interscalene brachial plexus block. *South African Journal of Anaesthesiology and Analgesia* 3(3), 22–4.

57. **Bosenberg, A.T.** 1996: Supraclavicular brachial block in children using a nerve stimulator. *International Symposium of Regional Anaesthesia*, 9–11 April, Auckland, New Zealand, 163.

58. **Pham-Dang, C., Gunst, J.P., Gouin, F.** *et al*. 1997: A novel supraclavicular approach to brachial plexus block. *Anesthesia and Analgesia* 85, 111–16.

59. **Shantha, T.R.** 1996: Brachial plexus block: a new method. *International Symposium of Regional Anaesthesia*, 9–11 April, Auckland, New Zealand, 221–2.

60. **Bouaziz, H., Narchi, P., Mercier, F.J.** *et al*. 1997: Comparison between conventional axillary block and a new approach at midhumeral level. *Anesthesia and Analgesia* 84, 1058–62.

61. **Marino, G., Rossi, M., Fruga, F., Valoti, O. and Ferri, F.** 1996: Lateral approach to the sciatic nerve. *International Symposium of Regional Anaesthesia*, 9–11 April, Auckland, New Zealand, 209.

62. **Benzon, H.T., Kim, C., Benzon, H.P.** *et al*. 1997: Correlation between evoked motor response of the sciatic nerve and sensory blockade. *Anesthesiology* 87, 547–52.

63. **Vloka, J.D., Hadzic, A., Lesser, J.B.** *et al*. 1997: A common epineural sheath for the nerves in the popliteal fossa and its possible implications for sciatic nerve block. *Anesthesia and Analgesia* 84, 387–90.

64. **Singelyn, F.J., Aye, F. and Gouverneur, J.M.** 1997: Continuous popliteal sciatic nerve block: an original technique to provide postoperative analgesia after foot surgery. *Anesthesia and Analgesia* 84, 383–6.

65. **Beeton, A.G.** 1998: Selected anaesthetic blocks. *Specialist Medicine* XIX (3), 16–18.

66. **Tissot, S., Frering, B., Gagnieu, M.C., Vallon, J.J. and Motin, J.** 1997: Plasma concentrations of lidicaine and bupivacaine after cervical plexus block for carotid surgery. *Anesthesia and Analgesia* 84, 1377–9.

67. **Shantha, T.R.** 1996: Cervical plexus block: a new method. *International Symposium of Regional Anaesthesia*, 9–11 April, Auckland, New Zealand, 222–3.

68. **Sethna, N.F. and Berde, C.B.** 1989: Paediatric regional anaesthesia. In Gregory, G. (ed.) *Paediatric anaesthesia*. Edinburgh: Churchill Livingstone, 674–8.

69. **Lloyd-Thomas, A.R.** 1990: Pain management in paediatric patients. *British Journal of Anesthesia* 64, 85–104.

70. **Broadman, L.** 1990: Regional anesthesia for pediatric patients. *American Society of Anesthesiologists Annual Refresher Course Lectures* 264, 1–7.

71. **Tryba, M., Haensch, K. and Zenz, M.** 1991: Axillary brachial plexus block for emergency procedures in young children. *Anesthesiology* 75 (3A), A757.

72. **Berde, C.** 1996: Regional anesthesia in children: what have we learned? *Anesthesia and Analgesia* 83, 897–900.

73. **Potgieter, D.** 1998: Three useful blocks. *Specialist Medicine* XX (3), 8–15.

74. **Scott, P.V.** 1991: Interpleural regional analgesia: detection of the interpleural space by saline infusion. *British Journal of Anaesthesia* 66, 131–3.

75. **Dionne, C.** 1992: Tumour invasion of the brachial plexus: management of pain with intrapleural analgesia. *Canadian Journal of Anaesthesia* 39(5), 520–1.

76. **Covino, B.G.** 1990: Comparative efficacy of regional analgesia and patient controlled analgesia. *International Anesthesia Research Society Review Course Lectures*, 29–33.

77. **Bridenbaugh, P.O.** 1992: Postoperative pain relief: does the technique matter? *International Anesthesia Research Society Review Course Lectures*, 35–8.

78. **Suresh, V., Johnston, R.V., Traber, D.L., Traber, L.D. and Arens, J.F.** 1991: Pharmacokinetics of interpleural bupivacaine in plasma and lung lymph. *Anesthesiology* 75(3A), A756.

79. **Lee, E.D. and Ben-David, B.** 1991: Bilateral intrapleural block for midline upper abdominal surgery. *Canadian Journal of Anaesthesia* 38, 683–4.

80. **Reiestad, F., McIlvaine, W.B., Kvalheim, L., Haraldstad, P. and Pettersen, B.** 1989: Successful treatment of chronic pancreatitis pain with interpleural analgesia. *Canadian Journal of Anaesthesia* 36(6), 713–18.

81. **Covino, B.G.** 1991: New techniques in regional anesthesia. *International Anesthesia Research Society Review Course Lectures*, 1–6.

82. **Stromskag, K.E., Minor, B.G. and Lindeberg, A.** 1991: Comparison of 40 ml of 0.25% intrapleural bupivacaine with epinephrine with 20 ml of 0.5% intrapleural bupivacaine with epinephrine after cholecystectomy. *Anesthesia and Analgesia* 73, 397–400.

83. **Lee, A., Boon, D., Bagshaw, P. and Kempthorne, P.** 1990: A randomised double-blind study of interpleural analgesia after cholecystectomy. *Anaesthesia* 46, 1028–31.

84. **Levine, C.V. and Levin, B.H.** 1992: Long-term interpleural analgesia using a subcutaneous implantable infusion system. *Canadian Journal of Anaesthesia* 39(4), 408.

85. **Sandler, A.N.** 1992: Update on postoperative pain management. *Canadian Journal of Anaesthesia* 39(5), R53–R56.

86. **Starbuck, N.M.** 1999: Intraperitoneal analgesia. *South African Journal of Anaesthesiology and Analgesia* 5(1), 30–1.

LOCAL ANAESTHETICS IN CENTRAL NEURAL BLOCKADE

Local anaesthesia was first discovered in 1884, and the first spinal anaesthetic was performed in 1898.[1] Regional anaesthesia/analgesia may be defined as 'the administration of analgesic agents in close proximity to the peripheral neural structure or to the central neuraxis'.[2] Central neural blockade can be divided into intrathecal and epidural (cervical, thoracic, lumbar and caudal). Expertise at performing central neural blockade and proper patient selection are necessary if potential complications are to be anticipated and avoided. Central neural blockade with local anaesthetics can be used perioperatively, in labour and in chronic pain.

Patient selection

Patients may qualify for a combined central neural block/general anaesthetic technique or a central neural block on its own. Central neural blockade is being increasingly used for ambulatory (day case) surgery patients.[3] Absolute contraindications to central neural blockade include patient refusal, infection at the site of injection and full anticoagulation. There are numerous relative contraindications, including psychiatric and communicative disorders, neurological disease and cardiac disease.[1] It seems prudent to avoid intrathecal or epidural anaesthesia in untreated patients with overt evidence of sepsis, although a spontaneous meningitis or epidural abscess cannot be differentiated from a procedure-related one.[4]

With anticoagulation, the major concern is the development of intrathecal and epidural bleeding, producing spinal cord or cauda equina compression and paresis.[5] Whether central neural blockade should be performed in patients who are partially anticoagulated or in those who will be subsequently anticoagulated is still hotly debated.[1] Several factors that have anecdotally been associated with epidural haematoma formation include the timing of the anticoagulant dose, having a postoperative indwelling catheter, the concurrent use of antiplatelet agents and spinal puncture from 'catheter manipulation' during times of anticoagulant activity.[6] Other risk factors include being female, a history of a bleeding abnormality and increased age.[7] It is suggested that the use of anticoagulant prophylaxis for venothrombo-embolism does not totally contraindicate central neural blockade. The management of patients undergoing central neural blockade who are receiving antiplatelet therapy remains an area of disagreement. More studies are needed to confirm the safety of performing central neural blockade on patients on current aspirin therapy. Unfortunately, there are no tests that reliably predict platelet function. The skin bleeding time, with its limitations, is the test usually used as an adjunct to clinical factors to assess platelet function. It has, however, been advocated that spinal or epidural anaesthesia can be performed on patients on current antiplatelet therapy without performing a bleeding time, assuming that no additional anticoagulants or coagulation defects are present.[6]

It is essential to make a balanced assessment of the particular risks. Some guidelines are as follows:[6,8]

1. Full anticoagulation with warfarin or heparin, and thrombolytic therapy with streptokinase, should contraindicate central neural blockade until its effects have been reversed. However, the risk of spinal haematoma was, in one study, not enhanced in patients receiving low-dose warfarin at a prothrombin time 1.3–1.5 times normal.[7] Preoperative treatment with oral anticoagulants must be discontinued at least 3 days before the insertion of an epidural catheter. Immediately before catheter placement, coagulation parameters must be determined.[9] An appropriate period should be allowed between epidural catheter placement and heparinization so that any possible puncture-associated bleeding has had the opportunity to cease.[9] For practical reasons, the epidural catheter is best placed the evening before surgery. Before epidural catheter removal, coagulation parameters must be within the normal range.[9]

2. With patients on low molecular weight subcutaneous heparin therapy, the procedure (including removal of the epidural catheter) should be performed at least 1 hour before or 12 hours after the last dose.

3. With patients on unfractionated heparin, the procedure (including removal of the epidural catheter) should be performed at least 1 hour before or 4–6 hours after the most recent dose.

4. With patients on aspirin therapy, ideally 10 days should have lapsed since the last dose, but risks and benefits should be assessed. (Aspirin can be continued up to the day of surgery if no contraindications exist but should be stopped 5 days before surgery if the patient is to be anticoagulated as well.) Bleeding time and physical examination may be helpful in assessing individual risk.

5. With regard to postoperative anticoagulant therapy, the heparin infusion should be stopped 1–2 hours before catheter removal. If the patient is on subcutaneous heparin, the catheter should be removed about an hour before a dose is due. If warfarin is to be given, the catheter should be removed well before the drug becomes effective.

6. In patients with thrombocytopaenia, risks and potential benefits for platelets should be individualized and bleeding times used to help assess platelet function.

7. In addition, for the use of thoracic epidural anaesthesia in coronary bypass surgery, the following is recommended. The intraoperative activated clotting time should not exceed 600–700 seconds; unobstructed venous drainage from the caval veins during cardiopulmonary bypass is mandatory to prevent epidural venous bleeding; after cardiopulmonary bypass, the prebypass activated clotting time should be reached by protamine administration, and other clotting disorders (thrombocytopaenia) should be treated appropriately.[9]

Patient preparation

Patient preparation should be the same as for general anaesthesia, including a history, a physical examination and minimal laboratory testing.[3] All the necessary equipment required to administer a general anaesthetic or to carry out resuscitation must be immediately available.

Supplementary medications can be given to relieve fear and anxiety, and to improve patient compliance. Anxiolytics and hypnotics used include diazepam, midazolam and propofol. Opioids include alfentanil, fentanyl, sufentanil, butorphanol and nalbuphine. The administration of anaesthetic gases (e.g. nitrous oxide) and vapours at subanaesthetic concentrations can also provide analgesia and sedation to supplement regional analgesia. Supplemental oxygen is appropriate whenever sedation is given.[5] Verbal reassurance and music through headphones are also effective supplements.[3]

Monitoring

Appropriate continuous ECG and pulse rate monitoring, as well as regular blood pressure recording, should be undertaken. Pulse oximetry is a useful guard against overgenerous sedation.[5] The direct carbon dioxide monitoring of ventilation is often possible when the catheter is connected to the nasal prongs or a face mask is used to provide supplemental oxygen.[3] Verbal assessment of mental function remains essential.

Complications

These are associated with the local anaesthetics themselves, the physiological changes caused by the blocks and the insertion of needles. Catheters should always be placed close to the appropriate dermatomal level in order to minimize complications. Motor block can occur with increased concentrations of local anaesthetic (e.g. lignocaine 2 per cent, bupivacaine 0.75 per cent or ropivacaine 0.75 per cent) or with certain local anaesthetics (e.g. etidocaine).

LOCAL ANAESTHETIC TOXICITY

Allergic reactions

These are rare and are usually associated with the ester compounds.[1] Cross-reactivity is not known, so patients allergic to one class of local anaesthetic may be treated with another. Treatment is the same as for any anaphylactic reaction.

Idiosyncratic reaction

This is an unusual response (vasovagal attacks and hysteria) defying predictable side-effects.

Local effects

These are the effects on local tissue (nerve and muscle) sometimes attributed to antioxidants, preservative agents or both.[10] Local toxicity is directly related to concentration, and high concentrations of all local anaesthetics are associated with neurotoxicity. Data from animal models suggest that lignocaine may be concentration-dependently more neurotoxic than other currently used local anaesthetics.[7] In central neural blockade, lignocaine 5 per cent and tetracaine 0.5 per cent are able to damage nerves incurably.[10] The addition of dextrose 7.5 per cent only increases toxicity. Transient radicular irritation can occur after an uneventful single injection of intrathecal anaesthesia with hyperbaric 5 per cent lignocaine.[7] Isobaric 0.5 per cent lignocaine has been found to be a safe alternative in outpatient gynaecological surgery.[7] The maldistribution of local anaesthetics within the intrathecal space has led to excessive concentrations, which have been implicated in neurotoxicity and the cauda equina syndrome after continuous spinal anaesthesia with microcatheters in adults.[7] It is noteworthy that sacral-to-cephalad hyperbaric dye ratios were significantly higher for smaller intrathecal catheters.[7] The direction of the needle tip and the speed of injection might also be involved in the observed absence of mixing between injected drugs and spinal fluid.[10] Not more than 2 per cent lignocaine solutions for spinal anaesthesia should be used, even if only a single injection is given.[10]

Local anaesthetics at supratherapeutic concentrations are able to impair mitochondrial respiration.[10] Bupivacaine appears to be more myotoxic than lignocaine.[10] The lowest effective concentrations should always be employed.[5] Intravenous chloroprocaine can cause venous thrombosis,[1] and epidural chloroprocaine has been associated with back pain.[3]

Systemic effects

An incidence of ± 0.2 per cent occurs following epidural blockade.[11] Systemic effects occur following accidental intravascular injection or after the injection of excessive quantities of local anaesthetic into the correct tissue plane.[1] The symptoms and signs include perioral numbness, dizziness, tingling, auditory and visual disturbances, twitching, seizures and, finally, CNS depression with coma, respiratory and cardiac depression, arrest and death. In anaesthetized patients, the first signs of toxicity are frequently cardiovascular.[12] Although the incidence of serious complications following local anaesthetic techniques in children is very low, adding adrenaline (1:200 000) to the local anaesthetic solution provides an early warning marker (ECG T-wave elevation) that may be used as a signal to discontinue the administration of local anaesthetic.[12] Most toxic reactions are self-limiting as plasma levels rapidly decrease as a result of redistribution.

Lignocaine is used as an antiarrhythmic agent, whereas bupivacaine may induce rare but life-threatening accidents when rapidly and massively injected intravenously, and mepivacaine has intermediate properties.[10] At toxic concentrations, bupivacaine alters cardiac function by decreasing the myocardial contractile force and creating arrhythmias, high-degree blocks, major QRS widening, and ventricular tachycardia related to re-entry phenomenon.

Bupivacaine rapidly enters and blocks the sodium channels of cardiac cells. It then accumulates, depressing the maximum conduction velocity (V_{max}) and interfering with cardiac conduction. Re-entrant arrhythmias occur, which may be fatal.[1] Other mechanisms include the blockade of transient and delayed potassium channels, blockade of the calcium channels, the inhibition of cyclic AMP and complex interrelationships with mitochondrial respiration.[10] At the intracellular pH of 6.90–7.10, bupivacaine is distributed inside the phospholipid bilayer in its ionized form rather than the usual un-ionized base. This favours the development of use-dependent or phasic blockade with receptor dissociation slower than association.[10] S(–) bupivacaine is less cardiotoxic than R(+) bupivacaine but has a lower clearance rate.[10] (The toxicity of ropivacaine is discussed in Chapter 16.)

In the case of systemic toxicity, rapid aggressive treatment is important. An airway must be established, ventilation maintained and seizures controlled (with diazepam, midazolam or propofol). The circulation must be evaluated. If vasodilattion and hypotension occur, treatment includes fluid loading with Ringer's lactate solution and the administration of phenylephrine (0.1 μg/kg per minute). Life-threatening ventricular arrhythmias can be treated with phenytoin (5 mg/kg intravenously).[12,13] Bretylium (5 mg/kg intravenously) may also be helpful to treat recalcitrant arrhythmias induced by bupivacaine.[1] Noradrenaline is not the drug of choice in treating bupivacaine-induced asystole as adrenaline may be ineffective and its arrhythmogenic effect may be detrimental in restoring sinus rhythm and cardiac output.[12] For bupivacaine, as long as coronary blood flow is maintained (by cardiac massage), wash-out is possible, and it does not appear necessary to add any 'displacing drug'.

The prevention of systemic toxicity is based on choosing appropriate dosages and drugs, and detecting intravascular injections. Test-dosing continues to be controversial. Adrenaline 15 μg produces an increase in heart rate of approximately 20 beats per minute in normal subjects when injected intravenously. Unreliable responses occur in beta-blocked patients, in the elderly and in those under anaesthesia, who may have a reduced sensitivity to catecholamines.[5] The heart rate changes are easy to miss in the patient in labour because of the heart rate variability already associated with labour.[14] There is also no guarantee that the catheter will not subsequently migrate into a blood vessel or the dura. Test-dosing using air with Doppler monitoring, or just using plain local anaesthetics, has also been suggested.[14] Every dose of local anaesthetic given should be regarded as a test dose and the patient closely observed. Most complications in children are associated with the excessive dosing of local anaesthetics (or opioids).[12] The dose of bupivacaine should therefore be limited to no more than 0.4–0.5 mg/kg per hour, and neuraxial opioids limited to their recommended doses.[12]

Diluting or using a less potent drug will reduce the potential toxicity. Prilocaine and chloroprocaine are rapidly cleared from the plasma and may provide a greater margin of safety.[5] Epidural anaesthesia has a high potential for systemic absorption. Local anaesthetics should always be administered slowly using small quantities (3–5 mL) at a time. However, the haemodynamic effects of epidural anesthesia with local anaesthetics at non-toxic concentrations are almost exclusively the result of sympathetic blockade rather than a direct effect on the myocardium.[10]

To summarize, the following guidelines are necessary to avoid complications:[15]

- Use a test dose and slow injection, even with a small volume of local anaesthetic in an infant.
- If cardiac arrest occurs as the result of bupivacaine toxicity, continue cardiac resuscitation because as long as coronary blood flow is maintained, wash-out is possible.
- Avoid high local anaesthetic concentrations intrathecally, especially with lignocaine.
- The neurotoxic potential of any drug used intrathecally should be carefully considered.
- Avoid antiplatelet therapy for 1 week and low molecular weight heparin for 24 hours before performing epidural or intrathecal anaesthesia.
- Use a nerve stimulator during the performance of peripheral blocks, especially in paediatrics.

PHYSIOLOGICAL EFFECTS OF CENTRAL NEURAL BLOCKADE

Cardiovascular effects

In addition to the direct effect of absorbed local anaesthetic and adrenaline, there is the indirect effect of sympathetic blockade. Hypotension (up to 38 per cent) is one of the most consistent complications reported.[16]

Total spinal anaesthesia may occur when local anaesthetic is injected close to the central neuraxis, either by accidental direct injection into the intrathecal space, by injection into the dural cuff region or by intraneural injection.[1] An overdose with an intrathecal injection (or inappropriate positioning) may also lead to total spinal anaesthesia. This is characterized by flaccidity, apnoea, unconsciousness and circulatory collapse. Treatment includes ventilation and circulatory support. An unexpectedly widespread sensory and sympathetic block occurring after a delayed onset (of 10 minutes or more) and a negative aspiration test after a lumbar epidural may point to a subdural block.[17]

Moderate sympathetic blockade can reduce peripheral resistance and venous return. This may be poorly tolerated in the presence of myocardial ischaemia, acute hypovolaemia and valvular heart disease (mitral or aortic stenosis).[5] A 30 per cent decline in systolic blood pressure is usually associated with a decrease in cardiac output and should be treated. With high sympathetic blockade, sudden bradycardia and cardiac arrest can also occur.[5] In the absence of sympathetic tone, cardiac massage may produce little cerebral blood flow, and adrenaline needs to be given early on.[18]

Respiratory effects

High intrathecal or epidural blockade may interfere with abdominal or chest wall muscle function and may compromise the ability to cough and to clear the airway.

NEEDLE INSERTION

Nerve injury

Such sequelae range from transient, localized disorders of nerve function and loss of control of the urinary and rectal sphincters, through to permanent paraplegia.[18] The incidence of permanent neurological sequelae is extremely low.[1] Transient neurological injury is uncommon, its incidence ranging from 0.1 per cent after epidural blockade to 0.8 per cent after intrathecal blockade.[11] Its aetiology includes trauma, chemical damage, infection, ischaemia and compression.

To limit nerve injury, small-gauge needles should be used wherever possible. Gentleness, precision and careful manual control are essential. Any injection should be discontinued if the patient complains of pain. The use of microvoltage nerve stimulators to locate needle tips is strongly encouraged.

Haematoma formation

This very rare (occurring in only 1 in 190 000 epidurals) but potentially catastrophic complication has been discussed above.[19] Coagulopathies or anticoagulant therapy (e.g. full heparinization) are the predominant risk factors, whereas low-dose heparin thromboprophylaxis or NSAID treatment is rarely associated with spinal bleeding complications.[19] Ankylosing spondylitis has been identified as a risk factor.[19] As dural penetration leads to some degree of bleeding, epidural haematomas might be reduced by the paramedian approach.[20] Haematomas have been known to occur spontaneously.

Medication errors

Injection of the wrong solution may have serious consequences. Overdose or injection into the wrong site may also occur.

OTHER COMPLICATIONS

Post-dural puncture headaches and backache

This is one of the most consistent complaints following central neural blockade. Young, usually female, ambulatory patients seem to be most at risk, the highest incidence occurring in obstetric practice.[21] A history of migraine and pregnancy-induced hypertension represents a significant risk factor.[7] A major aetiological determinant is the size of the needle used. A meta-analysis has confirmed that postdural puncture headaches are significantly reduced when a rounded bevel and a smaller-gauge needle are used.[22] An incidence of 37 per cent has been reported with 18 gauge needles, whereas this decreases to 0.33 per cent with 26 gauge needles.[23,24]. Pencil-point needles are superior to Quincke-type cutting needles in lowering the incidence, even if the former are larger in size.[7] By using smaller gauge needles, the incidence in ambulatory outpatients patients can be reduced to approximately 5.2 per cent.[25] The smallest possible needle should thus be used and only one puncture hole made in the dura. The bevel of a non-cutting needle should be aligned so that it splits the dural fibres longitudinally.

Other factors influencing the incidence of headache include the angle of approach of the needle point.[1] Adequate hydration and the avoidance of Valsalva manoeuvres are also important.[3] Post-dural puncture headache should be differentiated from postpartum headache occurring in the absence of a wet tap. Post-dural puncture headache occurred in 9.6 per cent of patients receiving continuous spinal anaesthesia via 28 gauge microcatheters.[26]

The onset of headache is usually delayed for at least 24 hours. Most are mild and spontaneously resolve (two thirds within one week).[22] Confining patients to bed does not prevent post-dural puncture headache. Conservative therapy consists of rest, hydration (especially with caffeinated beverages), caffeine and analgesics.[3] For the few cases that do not resolve, an epidural blood patch can be performed. For patients over 40 years of age, this should be required 0.5 per cent of the time.[22]

Intrathecal anaesthesia with a 24 gauge Sprotte needle reduced the incidence of back pain (from 30 per cent with an epidural 18 gauge Tuohy needle) to 11 per cent.[7] Intrathecal anaesthesia with a 29 gauge cutting needle increased postoperative back pain fourfold compared with a 26 gauge cutting needle because of increased difficulties associated with small needles.[7]

Catheter techniques

Problems that may occur with catheters include threading difficulties, kinking, occlusion, migration (intravascularly or to dura, lung or spinal cord), knotting, infection, nerve trauma, haemorrhage and breakage.[1,27] Epidural catheters may cause a low incidence of nerve injury (minimized by the use of a microvoltage nerve stimulator for needle tip location) and dural penetration.[12] Non-styletted epidural catheter tip construction and stiffness may be critical features in causing paraesthesia during catheter placement, and subtle neurotrauma resulting in unilateral radiculopathy.[7] In the paediatric population, there are no reports of residual neurological sequelae from indwelling epidural catheters.[12]

Infectious complications after neuraxial anaesthesia are extremely rare events.[7] However, the bacterial culture of spinal catheter tips after 96 or more hours indwelling time revealed significant colony formation, which may assume importance in immunocompromised patients.[7] The infection rate associated with epidural catheters in children is extremely low (0.04–0.5 per cent).[12] Epidural abscesses are usually treated by laminectomy or percutaneous drainage via epidural needles and catheters.[7] However, catheter removal is essential if a patient is septic and the source of the infection is unclear. Leakage around the catheter is frequently the cause of premature discontinuation of epidural infusions.[12]

Nausea, vomiting and urinary retention

Nausea and vomiting may be caused by the haemodynamic changes, the medications used or the surgery. Urinary retention is a common complication of central neural blockade.

Blocks

EPIDURAL BLOCK

Of all the techniques available for postoperative pain relief, none provides greater versatility than epidural blockade with a catheter technique (Figures 9.1–9.3). Analgesia can be provided from the upper chest to the toes. The catheter can be used to extend the block during the postoperative period. The anatomy of the lumbar epidural space on CT examination is complex, showing divisions and transverse connective tissue planes. This might be responsible for failure of drugs to act satisfactorily and the failure of correct positioning of epidural catheters.[20] Epidural block is increasingly becoming a part of the anaesthetic technique. With epidural block, the onset of anaesthesia can be slow but can be hastened using chloroprocaine.

Postoperative epidural analgesia with local

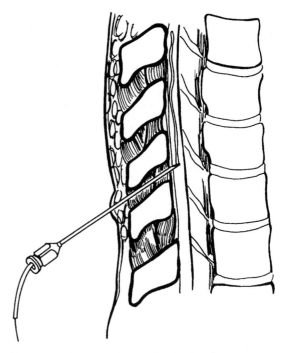

Figure 9.1 Insertion of an epidural catheter.

anaesthetics can be carried out with on-demand bolus injections (e.g. 5–10 mL of 0.25–0.5 per cent bupivacaine every 1–2 hours), timed-bolus injections or continuous infusions (15–20 mg per hour of 0.125–0.25 per cent bupivacaine).[28] The use of continuous local anaesthetic infusions makes it possible to achieve improved analgesia with lower doses. Thoracic, lumbar and caudal epidural catheters permit continuous epidural analgesia for 2–3 days postoperatively. A continuous infusion using a low-dose local anaesthetic–opioid combination can also be used to provide excellent postoperative analgesia.[28] Lumbar epidural block has been extensively used in paediatric practice. A 19 gauge needle with a 23 gauge catheter is very satisfactory for children weighing less than 10 kg.[29]

The effect on the rapidity and onset of epidural blockade of adjusting the pH of local anaesthetic solutions by adding sodium bicarbonate has been tested.[28] Is pH adjustment beneficial? There is still considerable disagreement over this. A recent study concluded that the alkalinization of bupivacaine of 0.5 per cent offered no improvement in the onset of epidural blockade.[30]

CAUDAL BLOCK

Caudal anaesthesia (see Figure 9.2) is probably the most common regional anaesthetic technique for

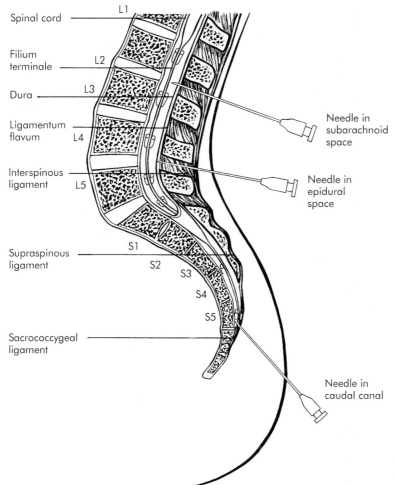

Spinal cord

Filium terminale

Dura

Ligamentum flavum

Interspinous ligament

Supraspinous ligament

Sacrococcygeal ligament

L1
L2
L3
L4
L5
S1
S2
S3
S4
S5

Needle in subarachnoid space

Needle in epidural space

Needle in caudal canal

Figure 9.2 Blocks: epidural, intrathecal and caudal. See text for details.

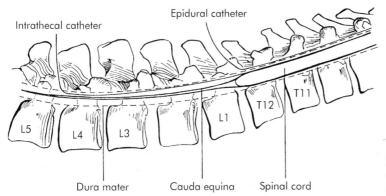

Intrathecal catheter

Epidural catheter

L5 L4 L3

Dura mater

Cauda equina

Spinal cord

L1 T12 T11

Figure 9.3 Techniques of drug delivery via epidural or intrathecal catheters.

surgery below the umbilicus and for postoperative analgesia in children. In children, it is safe and easy to perform, gives reliable results and is applicable to children of all ages.[29] For upper abdominal surgery, an 18 gauge epidural catheter can be passed via the sacral hiatus to the T7–8 vertebrae.[29]

INTRATHECAL BLOCK

Intrathecal anaesthesia (see Figures 9.2 and 9.3 above) is the simplest and most reliable of the regional techniques.[22] It is easy to perform, rapid in onset and highly effective. The most important clinical features are the height (level) and duration of sensory analgesia. The four most important physical characteristics of spinal anaesthetics are the density, the dose, the concentration and the volume of anaesthetic solution injected.[31] Studies reporting the influence of baricity on the spread of spinal anaesthesia have shown variable results.[31] Baricity matters most at the moment of injection. Solutions are made hyperbaric by the addition of glucose in concentrations of between 5 and 8 per cent. The restricted spread following the administration of a 0.83 per cent glucose-containing bupivacaine solution reduces the amount of sympathetic blockade, thereby reducing the chance to develop hypotension.[31] The density of the plain solution of 0.5 per cent bupivacaine is slightly hyperbaric at room temperature, and slightly hypobaric at body temperature.[31] The distribution of hyperbaric anaesthetic solution in the CSF is affected by gravity and influenced by the patient's position during and after intrathecal injection. The fixation time of a hyperbaric solution may take at least 60 minutes.[31] Once a hyperbaric local anaesthetic solution has been injected, placing the patient in a head-down position is not recommended, especially if a high block has already been achieved. If an isobaric solution is injected, the epicentre of local anaesthetic concentration in the CSF remains at the site of the injection regardless of the position of the patient during and after injection.[31] Thus non-isobaric solutions should be used carefully as positional changes extend the sensory block at any time, with potential haemodynamic consequences.[31] Truly isobaric solutions are safe and reliable.

For ambulatory surgery, the agent most commonly used is lignocaine (either hyperbaric 5 per cent or isobaric 2 per cent). For longer action, agents such as bupivacaine (0.5–0.75 per cent) and tetracaine are used.[3] Intrathecal bupivacaine is used in high-risk infants as analgesia persists for several hours after the return of motor function.[29] The intrathecal movement of drugs has been related to many factors, including dose, volume of the drug, baricity and posture.[32]

Use in labour and delivery

Continuous lumbar epidural anaesthesia is the most popular choice for analgesia during labour and delivery.[14] It has an excellent maternal–fetal safety record. Prehydration with a crystalloid solution (500–1000 mL) is necessary if there are no contraindications (pre-eclampsia or heart disease). Plain lignocaine 1.5 per cent or plain bupivacaine 0.25 per cent in a 5 mL dose can be given with the patient on his or her side. After catheter placement and taping, the patient can be turned to the other side and another 5 mL injected.[14] A continuous infusion of plain bupivacaine 0.125 per cent can be started at a rate of 10 mL per hour. Monitoring the level of block and adjustment of the infusion rate may be required.

Hypotension (a 25–30 per cent decrease in systolic blood pressure) is the most common side-effect. Treatment includes position alteration (left uterine displacement or the trendelenberg position), intravenous fluids and ephedrine (5–15 mg).[14]

Physiological advantages of central neural blockade for surgery

Regional anaesthesia can be given before the onset of surgical stimulation and can be extended postoperatively. Neural blockade may actually suppress the spinal cord changes that potentiate pain and predispose to persistent painful sequelae.[33] The impact of the postoperative fatigue syndrome may also be reduced.[33] Regional anaesthesia also has a regional action that may limit its systemic side-effects. It thus has many advantages.[34]

CARDIOVASCULAR SYSTEM

Many studies show that the use of a major nerve conduction block will usually decrease all the classical determinants of myocardial oxygen consumption.[34] This creates a potentially favourable environment for a reduction in myocardial morbidity following myocardial ischaemia or abnormal increases in left ventricular filling pressure (congestive cardiac failure).[34] Catheters provide continuous analgesia postoperatively, when patients are at greatest risk of developing cardiovascular morbidity.

A significant reduction in thrombotic complications occurs with epidural anaesthesia compared with general anaesthesia by sympathetic blockade, and by the local anaesthetic drugs modifying the changes in coagulation induced by surgery.[35] Blood viscosity may be reduced because of redistribution of the fluids associated with sympathetic blockade or from haemodilution as a result of intravenous fluid administration.[36] In vascular surgery, blood flow may be improved.[2]

RESPIRATORY SYSTEM

Central neural blockade can improve diaphragmatic function and thus help to improve postoperative pulmonary function.[34] This can, in some settings, reduce the incidence of postoperative pulmonary complications. Epidural analgesia can reduce the duration of postoperative mechanical ventilation.[34]

NEUROENDOCRINE/METABOLIC RESPONSE TO SURGERY

The usual postoperative increases in catecholamines (and adrenergic tone), cortisol and antidiuretic hormone excretion result in protein catabolism, hypertension, tachycardia, immune suppression and impaired renal excretory function.[34] The use of regional anaesthesia, especially postoperative regional analgesia, results in some measure of control of these responses. There is also an improvement in non-specific assays of immunocompetence, such as the lectin stimulation of lymphocytes, as well as a detectable improvement in more specific assays of immunocompetence, such as natural killer cell cytotoxicity.[34]

SURGICAL BLOOD LOSS

Several studies have shown a reduction in intraoperative blood loss with the use of regional anaesthesia.[34]

PAIN CONTROL

Regional analgesic techniques (especially with catheters) have the potential to bring a marked improvement in postoperative pain control.

GASTROINTESTINAL FUNCTION

The use of regional anaesthesia can result in an earlier return of gastrointestinal function.

SPINAL OPIOIDS IN CENTRAL NEURAL BLOCKADE

The use of spinal opioids (a generic term for epidural and intrathecal) opioids[37] has grown rapidly since their first application in 1979. The aim of using neuraxial opioids is to achieve as good an analgesia as with systemic dosing and to do it with appreciably smaller doses, systemic concentrations and risks of systemic side-effects.[37] Besides postoperative analgesia, spinal opioids are used for labour analgesia, cancer pain, trauma analgesia and some chronic benign pain conditions. Delivery methods include intermittent bolus injection, continuous infusion alone or patient-controlled techniques. Virtually all the known opioids in clinical practice have been used, including the agonist–antagonist compounds.[38]

The unique feature of neuraxial opioid analgesia is the lack of sensory, sympathetic or motor block, which allows patients to ambulate without the risk of orthostatic hypotension or motor incoordination usually associated with neuraxial local anaesthetics or hypotension associated with parenterally administered opioids.[39] The advantages of neuraxial opioids are particularly beneficial in high-risk patients undergoing major surgery, those with compromised pulmonary or cardiovascular function, and grossly obese or elderly patients.[39] In high-risk surgical patients, these techniques are not only associated with better analgesia, but also possibly with improved postoperative outcome.[40]

In terms of analgesia and the restoration of postoperative pulmonary function following abdominal or thoracic surgery, the technique has been found to be superior to alternative methods such as the intermittent intramuscular injection of opioids, PCA with intravenous opioids, intercostal block and epidural block with local anaesthetics.[39] Intrathecal morphine analgesia appears to be superior to a parenteral analgesic–sedative combination in the intensive care patient with multiple injuries, in whom frequent monitoring of the level of consciousness is important.[39] There is no conclusive evidence that neuraxial opioids provide analgesia of a better quality than that provided by parenteral opioids.[39]

The use of opioids administered spinally has the potential of producing greater morbidity than seen with those given by conventional routes.[41] They do, however, produce a pain relief whose quality and duration are greater than those of conventional routes.

Mode of action

New techniques have been used to investigate the epidural space. These include endoscopy, CT scanning, MRI and cryomicrotime sectioning.[42] Apart from passing out of the intervertebral foraminae, there are three possible paths for opioids injected epidurally: vascular absorption (via the rich epidural plexus of veins, the blood vessels around the dorsal nerve root and the plexus of the vena vertebralis interna), absorption into the local tissues (especially nerve epidural fat) and traversing the dura to gain access to the CSF.[43,44] Before reaching the spinal cord, opioids must first cross a hydrophilic zone (the extracellular and intracellular fluids) and then a hydrophobic zone (the cell membrane lipids of the arachnoid membrane).[40] The proportion of opioid absorbed systemically follows the kinetic principles of systemic absorption (e.g. lipid solubility). Some drugs (depending on the maximum molecular radius, the charge distribution and the dissociation constant) will diffuse across the dura into the CSF.[4] Unionized opioids are lipid soluble and pharmacokinetically mobile across lipid membranes yet pharmacologically inactive.[44] The charged, ionized moiety is pharmacologically active but pharmacokinetically immobile.[44] The arachnoid mater is probably the main barrier for opioid drugs.[44] The more lipid soluble the opioid, the faster its passage through membranes and the more rapid its clearance.[44] Depending on the degree of lipid solubility, opioids can attach themselves to endogenous opioid receptors in the substantia gelatinosa (Rexed's laminae II–III) of the dorsal horn of the spinal cord. The unbound opioids will circulate within the CSF and either move to non-active tissues or bind to opioid receptors at a more distant site.[45] Lipophilic opioids (with high octanol:buffer partition coefficients) dissolve and cross the lipophilic arachnoid mater easily but the hydrophobic region with difficulty.[40] Drugs (alfentanil, hydromorphone and pethidine, with greater meningeal permeability coefficients) with intermediate lipophilicity move more readily between the lipid and aqueous zones. Opioids (fentanyl and sufentanil) with high octanol:buffer coefficients move more easily to the intravascular compartment than to the intrathecal compartment.[40] (The optimal octanol:buffer distribution coefficient resulting in maximal meningeal permeability lies between 129

[for alfentanil] and 560 [for bupivacaine]).[40] Thus, spinal cord opioid concentrations after epidural administration are the result of a net difference between the rate of uptake and the distribution to the vascular and intrathecal spaces.[40] Lipophilic opioids (sufentanil and fentanyl) will cross the dura rapidly but also tend to retrace their path into the epidural space.[46] Hydrophilic opioids (morphine) cross the dura poorly but tend to stay in the intrathecal (or subarachnoid) space once there. The extensive spread of an epidural opioid may occur with epidural obstruction (a herniated disc or a space-occupying lesion), caval obstruction and distended peridural veins, inadvertent dural puncture and subdural injection.[44]

Detachment from the opioid receptors is dependent on receptor affinity and lipophilicity. Systemic absorption from the epidural space enables lipophilicity to influence the drug's ability to cross the blood–brain barrier and attach to the supraspinal opioid receptors. Supraspinal regions modulate the transmission or integration of nociceptive messages and/or activating brain stem descending pathways that act on the signal transmission of nociceptive messages.[44] The physiochemical characteristics of each opioid administered epidurally confer a unique profile of analgesia and side-effects. To compensate for systemic absorption and epidural fat sequestration, epidural opioid doses need to be 10–16 times greater than those required for intrathecal administration as no more than 5 per cent of the epidural dose of any opioid is ever likely to reach the CSF.[44]

The principles underlying the systemic kinetic differences between opioids are circumvented by direct intrathecal application.[41] For intrathecal opioids, lipophilicity bears an inverse relationship to potency as the ionized (hydrophilic) part of the drug is the active part at the receptor site.[44] In the CSF, with a limited volume of distribution, since the drug is directly applied to the intrathecal space, morphine is found to be more potent than fentanyl.[44] CSF proteins (3–5 per cent of those in blood) insignificantly influence CSF pharmacokinetics.[44] The rostral migration of opioids in the CSF can occur,[37] depending on the hydrophilicity of the opioid administered. Rostral flow within the CSF to the fourth ventricle and respiratory centre can result in delayed respiratory depression. The mechanism of bulk movement of the CSF in a cranial direction remains unclear, but changes in intra-abdominal and intrathoracic pressure, and the head-down position, are important.[44] Other undesirable side-effects (pruritus, urinary retention, nausea and vomiting) associated with spinal opioid therapy may also be caused by migration to distant sites.[36] The distribution of opioid throughout the CSF can, however, provide widespread analgesia by binding to the receptors in the dorsal horn at multiple levels.

Low-dose plasma opioid concentrations measured after small epidural opioid doses suggest a spinal site of action of analgesia, whereas larger doses of epidural opioids result in systemic absorption, which contributes to supraspinal analgesia.[47] Analgesia is thus produced by a combination of spinal and supraspinal effects; this may be a necessary combination for adequate analgesia. The clinical effects of each opioid are manifested by the ratio of their systemic to their spinal effects. The degree of opioid-sparing via the epidural route is largely dependent on the solubility of the drug.[48]

The epidural-to-intravenous potency ratio is the ratio of epidural and intravenous hourly requirements. For morphine, this value is 9.3, for fentanyl 3.1, for tramadol 2.5, for pethidine 2.4, for alfentanil 2, for buprenorphine 1.5, for sufentanil 1.3, and for methadone 1.2.[44]

Disparities between intravenous and intrathecal potencies can occur. Systemic potency ratios (e.g. of methadone and pethidine) can be poor guides to their spinal effectiveness.[49] (These differences between systemic and spinal dosing have not been applied in determining equi-analgesic doses).[41] The equi-analgesic doses of lipophilic opioids given intrathecally are much higher than was previously realised.[41] Doses similar to systemic doses must be administered to achieve analgesia.

Recent evidence has shown that lipophilic opioids (pethidine, fentanyl and sufentanil) spread rostrally in the CSF, reaching the cisternal CSF in 10–30 minutes.[37,50] High concentrations of lumbar CSF lipophilic opioid may favour redistribution within the intrathecal space by mass diffusion, causing severe delayed respiratory depression.[37,50] This is in addition to the early respiratory depression caused by their rapid systemic absorption.

During intrathecal infusion, the main pharmacokinetic factors involved are diffusion from the drug into the spinal cord and subsequent uptake by blood capillaries draining the cord.[51] Passage through the dura into the epidural space also takes place. Finally, the drug is transported to the cisterna magna and other CSF fluid compartments.[51] The potency of intrathecally administered opioids is inversely related to their lipid solubility.[51]

Binding affinity is defined as the ratio of rate constants for dissociation and association of the drug with the receptor, which determines the concentration of drug required for a specified degree of receptor occupancy. Morphine's binding affinity is 3–4 times that of alfentanil, 60 times that of pethidine, and more than 300 times that of tramadol.[44]

The ideal opioid

No inherently ideal opioid has yet emerged. The ideal spinal opioid should be hydrophilic, have a high affinity for the opioid receptors, require occupation of the small percentage of receptors needed to provide analgesia, have a long duration of analgesia, be free of side-effects and not spread rostrally to the fourth ventricle in the CSF to cause delayed respiratory depression.[46]

Clinical outcome

The neuraxial opioid effects of blunting the neuroendocrine response produce lower protein metabolism and immunodepression.[52] This may result in less infection and less postoperative fatigue. Most studies have shown improved pulmonary function when epidurally administered opioids were used for pain control.[52] Epidural opioids blunt the activation of the sympathoadrenal system, implicated in causing postoperative tachycardia, hypertension, myocardial ischaemia and negative cardiac outcome.[53] With postoperative epidural opioid analgesia, patients are discharged from hospital earlier.[52] Patient satisfaction remains high with this technique. In critically ill and severely compromised patients, there is a real advantage in postoperative outcome with epidural opioids.[52,53]

Compared with the conventional intramuscular route, a significantly earlier recovery of peak expiratory flow rate, fewer pulmonary complications (atelectasis and parenchymal infiltrates) and a shorter hospital stay were seen in patients undergoing thoracic or upper abdominal surgery receiving epidural morphine.[39] In high-risk patients undergoing major abdominal, thoracic or vascular surgery and receiving epidural block and postoperative epidural local anaesthetics and/or opioids, there was decreased postoperative morbidity (fewer cardiorespiratory complications and a lesser stress response) and mortality, as well as improved outcome (shorter hospital stays and lower costs), compared with those receiving general anaesthesia and postoperative parenteral opioids.[39] PCEA opioids in vasculopaths undergoing aortic bypass surgery significantly reduced thrombotic, infectious and cardiovascular complications.[39] In high-risk major surgical patients, epidural analgesia using local anaesthetics and/or opioids is the method of choice and is cost-effective. In a 17-nation survey, most anaesthetists believed that neuraxial opioids (especially morphine) positively affected postoperative outcome.[39]

A recent randomized study assessed the effects of perioperative analgesia with intravenous morphine versus those with epidural morphine, bupivacaine or both after colon surgery.[54] Clinical outcome improvements were seen in both a quicker fulfilment of discharge criteria and a lower cost of hospital stay in patients receiving epidural bupivacaine, either alone or with morphine.[54] This study highlights the importance of an ordered, multimodal recovery pathway designed to control factors other than analgesia that might alter gastrointestinal function.[54] Following coronary artery bypass surgery, thoracic epidural anaesthesia leads to a reduced frequency of perioperative myocardial ischaemia and infarction, and an improvement in pulmonary function, enhancing earlier recovery.[9]

Choice of opioid

Two questions need to be asked before any spinal opioid is used: first, what is its equi-analgesic dose compared with conventional parenteral routes?;[41] and second, what are its side-effects at this dose? There are large interindividual differences in the level and record, of opioid achieved and the degree of analgesia obtained.[37] There are massive differences in CSF concentration between the parenteral, intrathecal and epidural route.[55] Thus, choosing the right dose is as important as choosing the right opioid.[37] Disparities between intravenous and intrathecal potencies can occur. Systemic potency ratios (e.g. of methadone and pethidine) can be poor guides to their spinal effectiveness.[37]

Preservative-free morphine, with its hydrophilicity, remains the prototypical agent. This characteristic allows morphine to travel cephalad by passive CSF flow to provide analgesia at sites distant to its placement. Neuraxial morphine clearly reduces dose, improves pain relief and may decrease serious morbidity and mortality in high-risk surgical patients compared with standard parenteral administration.[56] In contrast, the neuraxial administration of lipid-soluble opioids (alfentanil, sufentanil, fentanyl and butorphanol) has generally failed to demonstrate these benefits.[56] The intrathecal route offers certain availability of the drug in the CSF. Studies with intrathecal injections tend to show a ceiling effect above which only the side-effects increase with increasing dose.[57] A better spinal localization of opioid ensures the resulting segmental analgesia with smaller doses.

Comparisons of epidural versus intravenous lipid-soluble opioids (alfentanil, sufentanil, fentanyl and butorphanol) have uniformly shown no significant differences in analgesic power or side-effects between the two routes of administration.[37] The equianalgesic doses of lipophilic opioids given spinally are much higher than was previously realised.[37] Doses similar to systemic doses need to be given to achieve analgesia, so that the benefit in terms of a dose reduction is also lost.[37] Lipid-soluble opioids tend to be cleared more rapidly from the CSF and generally exert more localized effects.[37] The spinal application of the lipid soluble opioids offers no guarantee against respiratory depression,[37] the latency of which is consistent with that of the systemic effects. Highly lipid-soluble opioids have a rapid onset of action (5–15 minutes).[37] They have a relatively short duration of action (2–4 hours). Thus, in general, highly lipid-soluble opioids should preferably not be given epidurally as the sole agents for postoperative analgesia.[56]

Techniques of delivery (Figure 9.3)

EPIDURAL

Intermittent opioid administration can be either on a pre-timed, on demand (prn) or flexible basis. Because of a large interpatient variation in the analgesic half-life, pre-timed injections can result in a small percentage of patients with inadequate pain relief and a small percentage with possible drug accumulation and side-effects.[46] Injecting on a flexible basis, however, will allow for interpatient variability and result in superior analgesia.

The use of continuous infusions avoids having to give large doses of spinal opioid at any one time.[57] Low-volume infusion rates help to localize the opioid to the desired spinal segments. Concentration in the CSF and plasma ought to be more stable, and adverse effects ought to develop gradually. With low-dose constant epidural infusions, catheters can migrate into the intrathecal space or an epidural vessel.[28] With penetration of the dura, 2 hours or more is required for a significant motor block to develop.[28] The consequence of an intravascular injection would not be a toxic reaction but a gradual loss of analgesia. The use of continuous epidural infusions thus needs careful observation and re-evaluation by a physician at least every 2 hours.

Continuous infusions prevent the regression of analgesia by keeping patients in a steady-state condition of continuous analgesia. They are particularly well suited to the lipophilic agents (fentanyl) and/or local anaesthetics.[46] Epidural infusions are at present more feasible than intrathecal ones because of the availability of suitable catheters. Microcatheters are now available for intrathecal intermittent injections or continuous infusion but are costly.

For epidural opioids, PCA is effective in adjusting the dose to individual requirements.[57] The disadvantage of the use of morphine via this route is its delayed onset of action.[46]

INTRATHECAL

Intrathecal opioid administration has the advantages of simplicity, reliability and low dose requirements, resulting in patients being less sedated, more cooperative and more mobile.[39] There is convincing evidence that morphine doses below 0.5 mg provide excellent postoperative analgesia.[39] The high CSF opioid concentrations obtained raise the spectre of toxicity. Preservative-free morphine and fentanyl have, however, been approved for intrathecal use. Animal spinal cord and toxicity studies with sufentanil have shown conflicting results.[46] For surgery, where postoperative pain would not be expected to be prolonged, single-dose administration (with the local anaesthetic) can be very effective. There is no comparative evidence for the advantages and disadvantages of epidural and intrathecal catheters.[41] There are, however, a few controlled trials on the use of intrathecal opioids in postoperative pain.[55] The intrathecal route offers certain availability of the drug in the CSF compared with the epidural route.

The technique's limited popularity compared with that of the epidural route may be due to unreliable catheter technology, the risk of post-dural puncture headache, delayed respiratory depression and spinal neurotoxicity.

Types of opioid used

For the doses employed, see Table 9.1.[46]

Table 9.1 Postoperative spinal opioid doses[37]

	Systemic dose	Epidural dose	Intrathecal dose	Epidural infusion rate
Morphine	5–10 mg	2-5 mg	0.2–0.5 mg	0.5 mg/hr
Pethidine	50–100 mg	30–50 mg	10–20 mg	10–15 mg/hr
Methadone	5–10 mg	3–6 mg	N/A	0.5 mg/hr
Fentanyl	100–150 μg	25–100 μg	2.5–25 μg	25–50 μg/hr
Sufentanil	10–25 μg	2.5–10 μg	2.5–10 μg	2.5–10 μg/hr

HYDROPHILIC OPIOIDS

Morphine Sulphate

Morphine has low lipophilicity. Epidurally (2–5 mg), it penetrates the dura poorly (only 3.6 per cent).[55] The onset of analgesia is delayed for up to 30–60 minutes.[38] The peak effect is usually not seen before 90–120 minutes, and analgesia lasts 8–20 hours.[38] CSF concentrations are about 25 times those of plasma.[44] When an epidural catheter is in place, it is possible to repeat doses or provide a constant infusion (0.2–0.6 mg morphine/hr) with frequent monitoring by nurses.[58] Catheter placement along the vertebral column does not affect the production of analgesia with morphine, although the onset of analgesia can be prolonged in segments some distance from the catheter site. The clinical advantages of using continuous epidural morphine infusions (0.5–1 mg per hour) over intermittent boluses are a more complete quality of analgesia and a lower risk of respiratory depression (1 in 5000 versus 1 in 100 respectively).[40,48] The long duration of action is due to the low systemic concentration and metabolism, and high receptor affinity, with a low epidural-to-systemic dose requirement ratio.[55] In children, epidural morphine should be limited to bolus doses of no more than 0.05 mg/kg and infusions of no more than 5 μg/kg per hour, and systemic opioids should be avoided.[12]

Intrathecal administration requires very small doses (0.2–0.5 mg) with minimal systemic absorption.[38] Intense postoperative analgesia is produced for 8–24 hours.[37] For lower abdominal and lower extremity surgery, the maximum intrathecal morphine dose should not exceed 0.3 mg.[51] For upper abdominal surgery and thoracotomies, the maximum intrathetcal dose should not exceed 0.5 mg.[51] The intrathecal injection of morphine eliminates the impact of systemic and lipid uptake, thus permitting a more precise administration of small doses. When pain is situated in high thoracic or cervical dermatomes, it is advisable to multiply by a factor of 4–5 when infusing intrathecal morphine at lumbar level.[51] Morphine is more likely to migrate rostrally, with the possibility of delayed respiratory depression. Even low doses of intrathecal morphine (0.3 per cent in doses from 0.2 to 0.8 mg), especially in high-risk patients, may be associated with delayed respiratory depression.[39,51]

LIPOPHILIC OPIOIDS

Pethidine

Pethidine, which has some local anaesthetic properties, may be slightly more effective epidurally than intravenously, yet doses are only reduced by 25 per cent with epidural injection, compared with 75 per cent with morphine.[56] The mean onset time is 5–20 minutes.[44] Peak CSF levels occur after 15–30 minutes, and the drug disappears from the CSF four times faster than morphine.[44] When given intrathecally, its inherent local anaesthetic properties are sufficient to provide sensory anaesthesia in some patients and surgical analgesia in most.[37] Intrathecal pethidine 1 mg/kg has been successfully used for elective caesarean sections, providing postoperative analgesia as well.[59]

Fentanyl

Epidural fentanyl (with a high octanol:buffer coefficient) undergoes preferential vascular absorption rather than meningeal penetration.[40] It has a very rapid onset of action (5–15 minutes), which makes it useful in patients acutely experiencing unacceptable pain.[28] Its duration is short because of rapid disassociation and it usually requires a continuous infusion.

Doses similar to systemic requirements are necessary to achieve analgesia, and catheter placement close to the segments where analgesia is desired is important.[38] Systemic uptake is high, and if continuous infusions are used, plasma concentrations may be identical to those found when the drug is given intravenously to produce similar degrees of analgesia.[38] There are no clinical advantages of administering fentanyl epidurally (regardless of the catheter insertion site) compared with the intravenous route, although after prolonged infusion the epidural space may act as a depot, and epidural requirements may be reduced by 25 per cent when delivered through the lumbar epidural space, and by 40–50 per cent when delivered through the thoracic epidural space.[40,47,48]

The duration of action of epidural opioids does not correlate with their rank of lipophilicity because of differences in receptor affinity and dissociation, and clearance.[44] The analgesic effect of most lipophilic opioids is predominantly through systemic uptake (the result of the drug being redistributed through the plasma to supraspinal levels) rather than spinal mechanisms.[39] There is no clinical advantage of epidural lipophilic opioid administration (fentanyl, alfentanil, sufentanil, pethidine, buprenorphine, butorphanol and methadone) over intravenous administration for analgesia following major surgery.[39] Dosage requirements and the quality of analgesia are similar whether these are administered intravenously or epidurally.[39] Regardless of the mechanism of action, epidural lipophilic

opioid administration may offer no clinical advantages over the intravenous route.[40] The relatively low peak concentration of lipophilic opioids compared with that of hydrophilic morphine results from the fact that even though they do cross more readily into the systemic circulation, their rapid systemic distribution from the plasma to the body distribution compartments prevents their concentrations from rising parallel with their rapid systemic uptake.[44] The more lipophilic the opioid, the higher the distribution volume and the more rapid the clearance rate.[44]

Sufentanil

The characteristics of the lipid-soluble fentanyl are magnified in sufentanil. Doses usually given systemically are necessary and may even be exceeded. Sufentanil has a higher lipid solubility, mu receptor affinity and analgesic potency than fentanyl.[37] Its theoretical advantage is its strong affinity for the mu receptor, where it has to occupy fewer than 30 per cent of the receptors to provide analgesia.[46] Thus, sufentanil's higher intrinsic efficacy is related to its ability to exert an analgesic effect with a lower fractional receptor occupancy (than morphine).[40] Epidural sufentanil yields the best results in patients with chronic opioid use greater than 250 mg per day, who have developed opioid tolerance from decoupling of the opioid receptors from the inhibitory G proteins.[40] Intravenous and epidural sufentanil are, however, almost similar in both quality of analgesia and plasma levels.[37,40] Intrathecal sufentanil provides rapid and effective analgesia for 1–2 hours.[39] Sufentanil concentrations are localized near the site of epidural administration, with higher concentrations in the CSF than in the plasma, supporting a spinal site of action.[47] Sensory and autonomic alterations, and limb rigidity, may occasionally occur following intrathecal sufentanil.[39]

Alfentanil

The lipophilicity of alfentanil lies between that of morphine and that of hydromorphone.[40] Because its coefficient of meningeal permeability is in the optimal range, the rapid intravascular absorption phase seen with other lipophilic opioids (with high peak plasma levels) does not occur.[40] The reason for its short duration of action (30–90 minutes) despite ideal physicochemical characteristics is unknown.[40] Receptor dissociation and CSF clearance are faster for alfentanil than for fentanyl.[44] There is thus no advantage of the epidural over the intravenous route. The dose required for subcutaneous PCA for postoperative analgesia is almost double that required via the epidural route.[48] The addition of hydroxypropyl-beta-cyclodextrin to intrathecal sufentanil prolongs its spinal action and reduces its supraspinal actions.[51]

Tramadol

The epidural injection of 100 mg tramadol hydrochloride in patients undergoing abdominal surgery gives good pain relief for over 9 hours without the danger of delayed respiratory depression seen with epidural morphine.[60,61]

Hydromorphone

Hydromorphone has a lipid solubility greater than that of morphine but less than that of fentanyl.[40] It has a faster onset but shorter duration of action than morphine.[40] From a pharmacokinetic point of view, it appears very similar to morphine. A ratio of 5:1 between morphine and hydromorphone has been used for bolus administration, and a ratio of 3:1 is recommended for continuous infusions.[40] The dose required systemically is approximately double that required for epidural postoperative pain relief.[48]

Diamorphine

Diamorphine has a moderate dural permeability (*in vitro*) but it is more lipophilic than morphine. It has a faster onset of action than morphine, with an early contribution from systemic uptake, leaving the CSF more rapidly and leaving less drug available for cephalad spread.[51,55] The duration of action is less than that of morphine (8–11 hours), with a 1:1 epidural-to-systemic dose requirement ratio.

Buprenorphine

Buprenorphine has poor dural permeability (*in vitro*), with very high lipophilicity and high receptor affinity but limited activity (being a partial agonist). Its action is probably a result of its significant uptake, especially if higher doses of buprenorphine (0.3 mg or above) are used.[55] Nevertheless, it has been found as effective as morphine, with fewer side-effects.[55] Its slow dissociation from opioid receptors increases its duration despite its high lipophilicity.[44] Similar postoperative surveillance for respiratory depression is necessary, especially if higher doses of buprenorphine are used.

Methadone

Methadone is a very poor neuraxial opioid.[46] Intrathecally, it is 18 times more potent than morphine.[62] The long half-life seen with systemic administration is not observed with spinal injec-

tion. Its lipid solubility does not enable it to provide prolonged spinal analgesia.

Neurotoxicity

Prolonged epidural morphine usage has revealed no apparent neurotoxicity.[39] Although neurotoxic data are not available for pethidine and fentanyl, no neurological complications have been reported with their use.[39] In sheep studies, it has been shown that large doses of sufentanil and butorphanol that are safe epidurally result in histopathological cord changes with intrathecal use.[39]

There is no firm evidence that neuraxial opioids on their own provide analgesia superior to that provided via other routes of administration. Disadvantages of spinal opioids include incomplete analgesia and a large interpatient variability in response. The risk-to-benefit ratio for neuraxial opioids needs to be defined and compared with conventional routes.

Side-effects

Opioid antagonists (naloxone 0.04 mg intravenously or naltrexone 50 mg orally) are used for pruritus, nausea, urinary retention and somnolence.[51] Mixed opioid agonist–antagonists (nalbuphine 5–10 mg intravenously or butorphanol 1–2 mg intravenously) are also used for pruritus, nausea, urinary retention and somnolence. Symptomatic treatments for nausea include droperidol intravenous 0.5–1.0 mg, transdermal scopolamine, and intravenous metoclopramide 10 mg.[51] For pruritus, diphenhydramine 12.5–25.0 mg intravenously or propofol 10 mg intravenously can be used.[51]

RESPIRATORY DEPRESSION

The most important and potentially fatal complication of opioid usage is respiratory depression. Early respiratory depression is associated with many opioid techniques, but with neuraxial morphine it may be considerably delayed (e.g. for 6–18 hours after injection) as morphine-laden CSF reaches the medullary depression centres by diffusion and bulk flow.[39] With morphine, this has an incidence of 0.1–0.5 per cent.[63] The risk of delayed respiratory depression is most serious in postoperative and post-traumatic pain but is nearly non-existent in chronic pain treatment with opioids.[44] Even highly lipid-soluble opioids may still cause delayed respiratory depression but in a less predictable manner than morphine.[37,40] Rostral spread via the CSF and by direct transit in the epidural veins may be significant.[39] Also, because systemic concentrations of sufentanil and fentanyl after repeated epidural administration are no different from those after intravenous administration, the risk of respiratory depression is at least equal to the systemic administration of the drug.[48] Intermediately lipid-soluble opioids (alfentanil and hydromorphone) have limited spread within the CSF, with some opioid-sparing effects (so that smaller doses are given), thereby lowering the risk of respiratory depression.[48] Early respiratory depression with epidural morphine may occur within 1 hour, but the same may happen within minutes if lipophilic opioids are used.[39] Late-onset respiratory depression is potentially more dangerous since it may occur unexpectedly some hours after the injection of the opioid. It is slow and progressive in onset. A healthy obstetric population is not a high-risk group for respiratory depression as the respiratory changes in pregnancy confer protection against opioid-induced hypopnoea.[39] Overall, the incidence of respiratory depression is rare, however (occuring in approximately 0.33 per cent of cases).[63]

Spinal opioid-induced respiratory depression is unpredictable. It may be associated with any of the currently available opioids.[39] All patients receiving spinal opioids must be monitored for respiratory depression for 12 hours after every morphine injection (or infusion discontinuation), or for 4–6 hours after lipophilic opioid administration (or infusion discontinuation).[39]

An incidence of 0.09 per cent has been found for respiratory depression associated with the epidural route but this is surely an underestimate.[64] It occurs early on (within 1 hour, but usually between 20 and 45 minutes) after injection. It results from epidural venous systemic uptake and redistribution to the respiratory centre. It may also follow direct venous injection or a spinal tap. Delayed respiratory depression occurs for reasons similar to those for intrathecal opioids.

Respiratory depression associated with the intrathecal route occurs with an incidence of approximately 0.36 per cent.[64] It most commonly occurs 3–6 hours after injection, but may be seen up to 24 hours after injection. Rostral CSF spread of a hydrophillic drug (e.g. morphine) to the respiratory centre occurs.

Multiple factors increase the risk of delayed respiratory depression:[39,43,55]

- the adjuvant use of CNS depressant drugs;
- the concomitant systemic use of opioids and/or sedatives;

- the posture – nursing in a supine position post-injection.
- high opioid doses and rapid injection;
- intrathecal opioids;
- thoracic epidurals;
- increased intrathoracic pressure (coughing and intermittent positive pressure ventilation);
- intermittent positive pressure ventilation, as increasing the pH in the CSF increases the diffusible fraction;
- raised intra-abdominal pressure, encouraging cephalad spread of the opioid;
- a lack of tolerance to opioids (acute versus chronic pain) in the opioid-naive patient;
- increasing age and respiratory disease;
- greatly altered transfer pharmacokinetics of opioid from the epidural to the intrathecal space occurs if a dural puncture occurs during the placement of an epidural catheter and the initial dose should be reduced by a factor of 10;
- high-risk patients;
- the use of water-soluble opioids.

Drug-related factors include:[55]

- intrathecal morphine;
- being a water-soluble opioid;
- having a high diffusible fraction.

The risk of delayed respiratory depression increases many-fold if a concomitant dose of systemic opioid is given.[46] Systemic opioids should never be given while a spinal opioid technique is being used. REM sleep recovers with rebound from a suppression produced by opioids on the first one or two days after major surgery. REM sleep is associated with an increased likelihood of obstructive sleep apnoea and desaturation.[57]

NAUSEA AND VOMITING

The incidence varies from 17 to 34 per cent for morphine.[46] The time of onset coincides with the rostral migration of the drug, being 4–6 hours.[44] The lipid-soluble opioids have a decreased incidence of nausea and vomiting. The incidence following intrathecal opioids is very high, but it appears to be lower epidurally, the incidence increasing with chronic use. Naloxone does not seem consistently to ameliorate nausea and vomiting. Transdermal scopolamine can reduce nausea and vomiting.

URINARY RETENTION

Urinary retention from a reduction in detrusor muscle contraction may necessitate catheterization in 15–50 per cent of patients.[46,65] It may be less with the more lipid-soluble agents. A relaxation of the detrusor muscle and an increase in bladder capacity have been implicated. Treatment with intravenous naloxone (0.4–0.8 mg) is often unsuccessful, and catheterization may be necessary.[44]

PRURITUS

This can be localized or diffuse. The incidence is high with mu receptor agonists (morphine, diamorphine, pethidine and fentanyl), and low with kappa receptor agonists (butorphanol).[39] Pregnant patients appear to be more at risk.[39] The overall incidence varies from 11 to 24 per cent for epidural opioids and up to 46 per cent after intrathecal opioids.[46,55] Pruritus appears 2–3 hours after opioid injection, its duration being shorter than that of the analgesia.[44] Diphenhydramine reduces a localized reaction. Propofol 10 mg reduces pruritus by direct depression of the spinal neurone systems implicated in its production, possibly by blocking the release of excitatory amino acids.[47] Naloxone (2–4 μg/kg per hour) is equally effective in refractory cases.

RECURRENT HERPES SIMPLEX INFECTIONS

Epidural opioids (especially morphine with pruritus) are associated with an increased incidence of recurrent herpes simplex infections in obstetric patients.[39,46] The reason for this association has been questioned. Up to 845 of previously herpes simplex-infected pregnant women have peripartum recurrences whether or not neuraxial opioids are used.[39]

SPINAL HAEMATOMA

For a discussion of spinal haematoma, see 'Local anaesthetics in central neural blockade', above.

MAJOR NEUROLOGICAL DAMAGE

The possibility of permanent neurological damage is always a cause for concern. Permanent neurological sequelae are fortunately rare (see above).[43] Preparations containing preservatives should not be used.

EFFECTS IN CHRONIC USE, AND TOLERANCE

The major problems encountered in acute pain are pruritus, urinary retention and respiratory depression. In chronic pain, however, these are not problematic,[41] as previous opioid exposure seems to minimize their incidence.

In the treatment of chronic pain, tolerance to spinal opioids can instead be seen.[62] This especially occurs when an infusion at higher than the necessary dose is administered. The duration of receptor occupation is very important for the development of tolerance.[44] Tolerance is reported for all the pharmacological actions of morphine except for miosis and constipation.[44] It is a reversible process as, following prolonged application, removal of the drug from the receptor results in restitution of the sensitivity to opioids. There is a cross-tolerance for most of the opioid agonists.[44] No cross-tolerance exists between the different classes of agonist (e.g. between mu and delta agonists).[44]

Monitoring

No consensus of opinion exists regarding the duration, technique or level of monitoring, or on whether these patients should be nursed in general wards or specialized care units.[39] Unfortunately, a respiratory monitor that can be used on a general ward and that is both reliable for and predictive of a respiratory event has not yet been developed.[46] The combination of respiratory inductance plethysmography and pulse oximetry has confirmed the insensitivity of clinical counts of the breathing rate.[57] Pulse oximetry is at present the most feasible way of improving the monitoring of opioid-induced ventilatory disturbances, even though a warning from this device is given only once desaturation has occurred. Properly trained nurses relying on the frequent assessment of ventilation or sedation represent the safest currently used means of monitoring respiratory status.[51] There is increasing evidence that neuraxial opioids are safe for use on surgical wards if the patients are of American Society of Anesthesiologists' (ASA) patient risk classification 1–2, if the personnel are trained, with preprinted guidelines for potential emergencies available; if patient selection and opioid dosing are appropriate; and if respiratory rate and sedation level are checked hourly.[39]

SOME GENERAL PRINCIPLES

A strict protocol needs to be observed by nursing, anaesthetic and surgical staff for the management of these patients. The production of a special chart will facilitate management.

1. Analgesia, respiratory rate and depth, and sedation, should be monitored hourly.[66] With morphine, this monitoring should continue for 24 hours after the bolus dose or after the infusion has been stopped. With the lipid-soluble opioids (fentanyl and sufentanil), this monitoring should continue for at least 4–6 hours after the last bolus dose or after the infusion has been stopped. Blood pressure and pulse rate should also be assessed frequently.

2. Naloxone and oxygen must be easily available if respiratory embarrassment occurs. A bolus of naloxone can initially be given, followed by an infusion (2–5 μg/kg per hour) since its half-life is much shorter than that of the opioids.[46] It must be titrated to effect. Oral naltrexone has also been used.[67] Nalmefene (0.5–2.0 mg) results in a prolongation of the antagonistic effect.[39] Hypotension should be managed by the use of fluids, ephedrine and tipping the bed.

3. All equipment should be regularly checked.

4. No systemic opioids must be administered at the same time.

5. Documentation of what has been done for each patient and standing orders to provide guidelines for all potential emergencies should be available. Adequate communication channels are essential.[55] The nurses must know which doctor to call in an emergency or if there is inadequate pain control.

6. Regular teaching and discussion on the management of pain should be undertaken.

There is a need for prospective studies to determine the safety aspects of intrathecal versus epidural opioids.

Use of spinal opioids for labour and delivery

Challenges include providing pain relief that is safe for mother and baby with preservation of the normal progress of labour and delivery. An absence in changes in autonomic and motor function, in combination with low maternal and fetal drug levels, is highly desirable for the parturient. Intrathecal opioids are particularly attractive for obstetric pain relief as they do not influence progress in labour.[51] Variability in pain relief in the second stage (from a differential effect of opioids on the A delta and C fibre input) may necessitate further anaesthetic intervention.[51]

OPIOID USED

Morphine

Epidural morphine used as a sole agent has yielded poor results.[68] Its average time of onset is 20–45 minutes. Intrathecal morphine (0.5–2.0 mg) produces adequate analgesia in the majority of parturients, with an onset time of 15–60 minutes and an average duration of 6 hours.[55] A high incidence of side-effects occurs, including pruritus, nausea and vomiting, and urinary retention in approximately 50 per cent of patients.[51] Morphine has no advantage over bupivacaine.

Pethidine

The duration of epidural pethidine is short, and its analgesia is unpredictable.[46] In a dose-response study of epidural pethidine for analgesia after caesarean section, 25 mg was found to be the most effective dose in terms of onset and duration.[69] Doses above this only increased side-effects such as nausea and dizziness.[69] Because of its local anaesthetic and autonomic actions, intrathecal pethidine 10 mg is more reliable than intrathecal fentanyl 10 μg or intrathecal sufentanil 5 μg when nearing the second stage of labour.[51] Intrathecal pethidine is being increasingly used for surgery and in patients with allergies to local anaesthetics.[69] Its mechanism in spinal anaesthesia is unknown.

Fentanyl

Epidural fentanyl on its own is ineffective, its use being reserved principally for perineal pain that is unrelieved by bupivacaine. The combination of intrathecal fentanyl (25 μg) and morphine (0.25 mg) has been used with some success during labour.[14] Fentanyl achieves a rapid onset of analgesia, while morphine gives a greater duration of action. Epidural fentanyl is frequently used before delivery to augment regional anaesthesia despite concerns over its placental transfer.[69] Intrathecal fentanyl 25–50 μg results in pain relief of 30–120 minutes' duration, which might be less profound compared with that of sufentanil 10 μg.[51]

Sufentanil

Epidural sufentanil (10–50 μg) can provide satisfactory analgesia.[14] Intrathecal sufentanil 10 μg results in profound but short (1–2 hours) analgesia.[51] When analgesia was requested in labouring parturients (with a cervical dilatation of 7 cm or more), intrathecal sufentanil 10 μg with bupivacaine 2.5 mg resulted in rapid onset and excellent analgesia lasting approximately 130 minutes, allowing most women to deliver vaginally.[69]

Alfentanil

Alfentanil has been looked at in initial studies, but there is little solid information on it.[14]

It thus appears that epidural opioids on their own confer no benefit over local anaesthetics. Intrathecal morphine is effective, but the incidence of unwanted side-effects restricts its use.

MATERNAL SIDE-EFFECTS

Pruritus is the most common maternal side-effect. Conflicting results on the effectiveness of nalbuphine or naloxone treatments have been reported.[69] In labouring parturients, high sensory block has been noticed 10–25 minutes after intrathecal sufentanil 10 µg.[69] Somnolence and respiratory depression have also been reported after intrathecal sufentanil.[69] Suggested mechanisms for the decrease in blood pressure after intrathecal fentanyl and sufentanil administration include a direct action on spinal mu receptors or a decrease in the level of endogenous catecholamines.[69] Epidural opioids delaying gastric emptying in labouring parturients is controversial.[69] Studies are needed to determine whether bupivacaine/ropivacaine concentrations less than 0.125 per cent in a continuous epidural infusion increase maternal ambulation, the ability to micturate and more effective pushing without inducing delayed gastric emptying. Episodes of hypoxaemia occur in healthy women during labour and may be compounded by neuraxial opioids.[69]

FETAL SIDE-EFFECTS

The placental transfer of maternally administered fentanyl, alfentanil and sufentanil is rapid, whether it is given by intravenous (5 minutes), epidural (over 15 minutes) or intrathecal bolus (15 minutes) injections.[69] Controversy exists over whether epidural analgesia is associated with fetal heart rate changes.[69] Even when fetal heart rate changes are significant, no difference in neonatal outcome (Apgar score and umbilical cord gases) has been observed.[69]

Mixtures of opioids

The potential use of opioid mixtures to enhance analgesia has not yet been fully evaluated. Because of the slow onset of morphine and morphine-induced side-effects, the combined administration of morphine with the more lipid-soluble opioids (fentanyl and sufentanil) improves the analgesic profile by decreasing the onset time while lessening the morphine-induced side-effects.[51] The short duration of the highly lipid-soluble opioids can be overcome by the use of intrathecal combinations of fentanyl and morphine, or by the use of a continuous intrathecal fentanyl infusion.[51] Preliminary observations suggest a more rapid onset and a prolonged duration by combining spinal morphine with spinal fentanyl or sufentanil.[70] The epidural combination of fentanyl 50 µg or sufentanil 25 µg with morphine 2 mg improves early postoperative analgesia, lowers the incidence of adverse effects and gives postoperative analgesia for about 20 hours.[71, 72] In labour, adding intrathecal fentanyl 5 µg to morphine 0.25 mg (or diamorphine 2.5 mg) provides analgesia within 5 minutes instead of 45–60 minutes.[72] However, 50 per cent of parturients were shown to develop nausea, vomiting or pruritus, which is unacceptable.[72] The combination of epidural butorphanol 3 mg with morphine 4 mg does not significantly increase respiratory depression or affect sedation or the duration of analgesia, but it does lower the incidence of pruritus and nausea.[73] Epidural butorphanol 3 mg, nalbuphine 10 mg and oral naltrexone 6 mg have been added to epidural morphine to prevent mu opioid side-effects without introducing additional risks such as sedation (butorphanol) or the reversal of analgesia (naltrexone).[73] The incidence of epidural morphine-induced pruritus is reduced with epidural butorphanol.[47]

Conclusion

The risk-to-benefit ratio for spinal opioids needs to be defined and compared with that for conventional routes.[55] There is conflicting evidence on whether they are definitely superior to optimally administered parenteral opioids, especially PCA, although many studies show an analgesia whose quality and duration are greater than those achieved by opioids given by conventional routes.[62] In addition, some studies have shown decreased morbidity, a shorter hospital stay and lowered costs in patients receiving epidural opioids.[46] The modern use of neuraxial opioids has come a long way since their first application in 1979. Recent advances offer anaesthetists and surgeons an exciting challenge to vastly improve the acute pain care of patients under their control.

CLINICAL USE OF CENTRAL NEURAL BLOCK COMBINATIONS

The optimal concentrations and doses of different combinations have not yet been determined. Analgesic effects have been demonstrated following the neuraxial administration of non-opioid drugs such as clonidine, somatostatin, octreotide, ketamine, calcitonin, midazolam and droperidol.[39] Balanced neuraxial analgesia, using a combination of low doses of drugs with separate but synergistic mechanisms, may produce the best results.

Clinical use

WITH ADRENALINE

Lipid-soluble opioids may, however, be combined epidurally with adrenaline (25–50 μg per hour), which restricts systemic absorption and may also enhance analgesia by a direct α_2-adrenergic action on the spinal cord.[56] In labour, adding adrenaline 0.2 mg to intrathecal sufentanil 10 mg may slightly prolong analgesia but lead to an increase in nausea.[37,74]

WITH LOCAL ANAESTHETICS

General surgery

Both basic research and human studies evaluating labour pain and postoperative pain have demonstrated synergistic effects between local anaesthetics (bupivacaine/ropivacaine and lignocaine) and opioids (morphine and fentanyl).[40,70] Combinations result in a reduction in the dose of agents needed, the maintenance or enhancement of the degree of pain relief and a minimization of the risk of unwanted side-effects.[40] This is known as multimodal or balanced analgesia. Even if an extremely low concentration of local anaesthetic is added to the opioid, the quality of analgesia may be far superior.[39] Is the combination an additive or a synergistic effect? The isobologram may help in part in determining the answer.[75] However, a gain in safety from opioid-sparing may be partly illusory if pain is itself a counterbalance for opioid-induced respiratory depression.[76] Studies of epidural opioid alone versus epidural opioid plus local anaesthetic at low infusion rates show that pronounced analgesia is achieved with the combination therapy when pain

is assessed during function.[70] Factors influencing the effective rate of epidural opioid infusion include the site and type of surgery, the type of pain, the choice of opioid and its loading dose, the volume of the injectate, the concentration of the local anaesthetic, the siting of the catheter tip and individual characteristics influencing the pharmacodynamics and pharmacokinetics of the given opioid.[39]

Insertion of the epidural catheter should be at the mid-dermatomal level of the incision when local anaesthetics are used. With thoracic epidural analgesia for upper abdominal surgery, a combination of bupivacaine at approximately 10 mg per hour and morphine at 0.2 mg per hour (after an initial loading dose of 1–2 mg morphine depending on age), or bupivacaine at a rate of around 10 mg per hour and fentanyl of 50–80 μg per hour, seems to be appropriate.[70] The thoracic administration of lipophilic opioids with local anaesthetics (bupivacaine/ropivacaine and sufentanil) may reduce the risk of side-effects through reduced plasma concentrations and result in tailoring to the level of nociceptive input into the spinal cord.[77] However, the risk of respiratory depression is significant if the patient is more than 70 years old or if sedating drugs are also given.[77] Thoracic epidural anaesthesia with low-dose sufentanil/local anaesthetics and with general anaesthesia results in an improved haemodynamic stability before and after coronary bypass surgery, reducing the release of noradrenaline and adrenaline, and facilitating 'fast-track' recovery after cardiac surgery.[77] Thoracic epidural anaesthesia provides favourable effects on the coronary circulation and on myocardial performance.[78] The possible sites of action of the local anaesthetic drugs include the nerve trunks in the paravertebral space, the dorsal root ganglia, the dorsal and ventral spinal roots, the spinal cord itself and the brain.[42] For coronary artery bypass grafting or lung surgery, the epidural catheter is inserted at the T1–2 level, for pulmonary surgery at the T3–4 level, and for upper abdominal surgery at the T7–8 level.[78] In coronary artery bypass grafting, bupivacaine 0.375 per cent with sufentanil 5 μg/mL in a dose of 0.05 mL/cm body length is used.[78] A continuous infusion of bupivacaine 0.125 per cent and sufentanil 1 μg/mL at a rate of 6–12 mL per hour, can be used.[78] For lung surgery, if morphine is used, a epidural loading dose of 1 mg followed by a continuous epidural infusion of morphine 0.2 mg in bupivacaine 0.75 per cent at an infusion rate of 0.8 mL per hour, can be used.[78] For upper abdominal surgery, both regimens can be used.[78] A continuous thoracic epidural infusion of local anaesthetics and opioids provided segmental analgesia with favourable haemodynamics and excellent postoperative pain relief.[78]

During lumbar epidural analgesia, less local anaesthetic (bupivacaine 2.5–5.0 mg per hour) has to be used because of the risk of motor block and orthostatic hypotension.[37] It has been suggested that, in both PCEA and continuous epidural infusion, the concentration of bupivacaine should be between 0.06 and 0.12 per cent in order to limit the volume requirements and preserve improved pain relief during coughing and mobilization.[75]

By administering smaller doses of epidural opioids, the incidence of side-effects may be less than that experienced via the intravenous route.[40] However, properly conducted dose-ranging studies have not been performed in humans to determine the ideal equimolar ratios between opioids and local anaesthetics. The isobolographic method for rigorously defining how drugs interact has not been used in human studies evaluating combinations of local anaesthetics and opioids for epidural analgesia. The epidural administration of small doses of lipophilic opioids in combination with local anaesthetics may offer significant clinical advantages over the systemic administration of opioids alone.[40] Dose-ranging studies will be necessary to determine the ideal concentrations of opioids and local anaesthetics, as well as the ratio of the two drugs to obtain optimal analgesia with a minimal incidence of side-effects. It remains to be seen whether the benefits of local anaesthetics (the maintenance of gastrointestinal motility and the prevention of thromboembolic disease) are still preserved when using extremely low doses.[75]

For postoperative analgesia in children, a caudal bupivacaine–morphine mixture has been successfully used.[79] The dosing of morphine should be reduced by at least 50% for infants less than 6 months of age.[80] The addition of diamorphine 1 mg to intrathecal 0.5% bupivacaine offers a significant improvement in analgesia in patients undergoing lower limb surgery.[29]

Labour

Interest has focused on the ideal dose and combination of drugs to produce excellent analgesia without motor blockade. In labour, most patients' pain is successfully relieved with a loading dose of 10–15 mL bupivacaine/ropivacaine 0.04–0.25 per cent and fentanyl 50 μg or sufentanil 5 μg, followed by an infusion of bupivacaine/ropivacaine 0.04–0.0625 per cent and fentanyl 1.5–2.5 μg/mL or sufentanil

0.10–0.25 μg/mL at a rate of 10–15 mL per hour.[81–83] This provides excellent analgesia in the first two stages of labour with minimal maternal motor weakness, no detrimental effects on uterine or umbilical arterial flow, and no loss of beat-to-beat heart rate variability.[72] The optimum combination having an opioid-sparing synergistic effect has yet to be established.[39]

Interest in the use of intrathecal anaesthesia has been revived because of the Sprotte needle (with a conical tip), which may reduce the incidence of post-dural puncture headache to less than 1 per cent.[14] The Whitacre needle (also with a conical tip) is also associated with a small incidence of post-dural puncture headache.[84] The addition of intrathecal bupivacaine 2.5 mg to sufentanil 10 μg may significantly prolong analgesia compared with sufentanil 10 μg alone.[75] Sufentanil has a dual effect – binding to the dorsal horn and a weak local anaesthetic effect.[75]

Caesarean section

For caesarean section, the addition of fentanyl 100 μg or sufentanil 20 μg to epidural 0.5 per cent bupivacaine/ropivacaine with adrenaline gives improved intra-operative anaesthesia and longer postoperative analgesia, with minimal maternal side-effects and no adverse neonatal effects.[20] This can be followed by the regimen recommended for labour in the period of postoperative analgesia. Intrathecal fentanyl 6.25 μg or sufentanil 1.0 μg mixed with hyperbaric bupivacaine 15 mg prolongs postoperative analgesia to 4 hours, with few side-effects.[72] Adding adrenaline increases nausea and may prolong motor block. The use of intrathecal morphine 0.1 mg with 0.75 per cent bupivacaine prolongs pain relief for 18–27 hours, with minor side-effects (e.g. pruritus).[37,44]

Additional dose–response studies are needed to define the most effective dose and combination of agents that will provide effective analgesia with an acceptable incidence of side-effects.

WITH α_2-ADRENERGIC AGONISTS

Although most clinical data suggest that combinations of α_2-adrenergic agonists and opioids result in only additive effects, it nevertheless appears that the co-administration of these agents does permit reduced doses of opioid with the maintenance of excellent analgesia.[47] The balance between analgesia and side-effects (sedation, bradycardia, hypotension and dry mouth) appears better after epidural than intravenous administration of these drugs.[85] The addition of the α_2-adrenergic agonist clonidine to epidural combination regimens of local anaesthetic and opioid will increase analgesic power, but the infusion rates studied so far (19–25 μg per hour) have resulted in hypotension, which is exaggerated in hypertensive patients and thoracic neuraxial administration.[39,70] Lower clonidine infusion rates still need to be studied.[70] It has been shown that analgesia and serum levels are similar whether clonidine (2 μg/kg) is administered systemically or intramuscularly, suggesting a systemic effect.[39] However, bolus doses of epidural clonidine 30 μg have been added to the combination of bupivacaine 12.5 μg, adrenaline 25 μg and sufentanil 10 μg during the first stage of labour to provide good analgesia, and appear to be safe for both mother and child.[83] Epidural clonidine in the dose range 3–10 μg/kg may prolong postoperative analgesia by 4–7 hours when added to local anaesthetics.[39]

WITH NSAIDs

NSAIDs have considerable opioid-sparing effects and may be useful in lessening opioid side-effects.[58] Fixed-dose combination therapy should enhance the analgesic potency that is necessary in moderate or major abdominal surgery.[70] After caesarean section, the combination of intramuscular diclofenac (75 mg) and low-dose epidural morphine (3 mg) provides analgesia superior to that given by either drug alone.[86] So far, no NSAID has proved superior regarding efficacy or side-effects, and the choice of preparation may therefore depend on other factors, such as duration and site of administration (intravenous, via suppositories, orally or as a cream).[70] A combination of epidural morphine 1–2 mg or intrathecal morphine 0.1–0.2 mg and PCA ketorolac may offer additive analgesia while minimizing spinal opioid side-effects.[37,87]

KETAMINE

Ketamine binds to opioid receptors, interacts with 5-HT systems and has a regional intravenous local anaesthetic action.[39] Epidural ketamine 4–30 mg has been used for lower abdominal surgery with an onset of 20 minutes and a duration of 3–4 hours.[39] The addition of caudal ketamine 0.5 mg/kg to bupivacaine for postoperative analgesia in children significantly improved both the quality and the duration of analgesia.[39] The adverse effects include sedation, blurred vision, tachycardia, hypertension and hallucinations.[39]

Various combinations of local anaesthetics,

opioids and α_2-adrenergic agonists are discussed in Chapter 6.

Technical advances

PATIENT-CONTROLLED EPIDURAL ANALGESIA

To reduce the side-effects, minimum effective analgesic doses should be given; PCEA achieves this. It has proved very successful for the lipid-soluble opioids with the catheter site closest to the spinal dermatomes for which analgesia is required.[48] The loading dose for fentanyl is 50–100 μg, with a maintenance dose of 10–20 μg. For sufentanil, the loading dose is 10–15 μg and the maintenance dose 5–10 μg; and with alfentanil, a loading dose of 500–1000 μg and a maintenance dose of 150–300 μg are given.[48] PCEA with a low-dose, adjustable, continuous infusion avoids fluctuations in pain control and frequent dosing.[48] Intermediate lipid-soluble opioids (alfentanil, pethidine and hydromorphone) hold the greatest promise of effective analgesia with limited risk of respiratory depression as a low continuous infusion combined with small maintenance doses via PCEA.[48] PCEA with opioids lowers pain scores in post-laminectomy, post-thoracotomy and caesarean section patients compared with intravenous PCA with opioids.[85] A number of PCEA studies have shown additional support for a spinal rather than a systemic effect of the 'continuous' supply of lipophilic opioids.[88]

PCEA has proved a viable alternative to continuous epidural techniques with a significant reduction in total dose requirement to achieve a similar level of analgesia (e.g. by 20–25 per cent with the combination of bupivacaine and fentanyl).[39,89,90] Patients receiving epidural injections of local anaesthetics combined with opioids have a more rapid onset of analgesia and a more long-lasting and profound labour pain relief than do patients receiving either drug alone.[39] During the first stage of labour, PCEA has proved to be safe and effective alternative for mother and neonate to continuous infusion epidural analgesia when using an infusion of 0.125 per cent bupivacaine with adrenaline 1:400 000 and fentanyl 2.5 μg/mL with boluses ranging from 2 to 6 mL and lock-out times of 10–30 minutes.[91] PCEA lowers the consumption of bupivacaine and fentanyl compared with continuous infusion epidural analgesia.[91] Post-caesarean section, sufentanil offers no advantages over fentanyl when used for PCEA. Patients received 16 mL per hour of 0.01 per cent bupivacaine and adrenaline $0.5\,\mu g/mL$ with fentanyl $2\,\mu g/mL$ or sufentanil $0.8\,\mu g/mL$.[92] Boluses of 3 mL could be self-administered as desired every 15 minutes. With PCEA following major orthopaedic surgery, fentanyl and bupivacaine have been found to be additive in their analgesic actions, resulting in decreased requirements of each.[93] Using alfentanil in major abdominal surgery, PCEA was found to be no more effective than intravenous PCA, and it was associated with the same incidence of oxyhaemoglobin desaturation.[94] Also after abdominal surgery, PCEA using fentanyl (a $25\,\mu g$ bolus with a lock-out time of 15 minutes) caused less oxyhaemoglobin desaturation than continuous infusion epidural analgesia with fentanyl.[95] However, the advantage of continuous epidural infusion techniques is the continuous and more effective analgesia it provides. Continuous infusion epidural analgesia with bupivacaine and morphine reduces the incidence of postoperative myocardial ischaemia and subsequent infarction in patients undergoing upper abdominal surgery compared with intravenous PCA with morphine.[85]

There remains a lack of randomized studies to identify the best lipophilic opioid, the most appropriate dose regimens for PCEA after different types of surgery, and the cost–benefit ratio of this technique.[39]

MICROCATHETERS

Continuous intrathecal anaesthesia, using microcatheters (28 and 32 gauge) in the intrathecal space, provides a route of administration for a low-dose combination of drugs with additive or synergistic effects (e.g. local anaesthetics, opioids and α_2-adrenergic agonists). These catheters keep the risk of postdural puncture headache to a minimum.[27] Continuous intrathecal analgesia may result in fewer haemodynamic effects than continuous epidural analgesia.[96] They could prove beneficial, especially in high-risk patients, by providing excellent analgesia while causing minimal changes in blood pressure and no motor blockade. For postthoracotomy pain, an intrathecal fentanyl infusion (at $0.26\,\mu g/kg$ per hour) using 32 gauge catheters provides rapid intense analgesia.[97] These catheters await the development of pumps that can produce sufficient pressure to deliver a continuous infusion of drugs. The risk of infection with such use needs further evaluation. At present, the break strength of intrathecal microcatheters is one third to one half of that found for a typical epidural catheter.[98] Cauda equina syndromes have, however, been reported in

association with intrathecal microcatheters and local anaesthetics.[99] However, small spinal catheters do not seem to play an important role despite the previous reports of 1992.[15] Cauda equina syndromes have not been reported in infants or in obstetric patients, despite the use of microcatheters in these patients.[12,51]

Combined epidural–spinal techniques provide the speed and reliability of spinal anaesthesia as well as the advantages of a continuous catheter technique.[28] This gives rapid-onset analgesia with greater flexibility in providing high-quality anaesthesia both during and after surgery. A dual 18 or 22 gauge epidural–spinal needle allows the passage of a 29 gauge spinal needle, which allows for the administration of an intrathecal dose of an opioid (e.g. morphine) at the same time as an epidural catheter is inserted.[28] The use of pencil-point needles (24–26 gauge) has resulted in a very low incidence of post-dural puncture headache, and these may yet become more popular than 29 gauge needle.[28]

For caesarean sections, using a combined spinal–epidural needle technique, an intense sensory and motor blockade may be obtained with the intrathecal local anaesthetic injection. This may be supplemented in the postoperative period by further injection of the drug through the epidural catheter.[56] Instead of an intrathecal local anaesthetic injection, a lipid-soluble opioid (e.g. sufentanil $10\,\mu g$) can be injected for a rapid onset of analgesia.[56,100] A double-catheter, single-interspace, combined spinal–epidural technique has recently been described.[101]

THE FUTURE

The liposomal encapsulation of opioids permits the delivery of relatively large concentrations of a drug in a form that is sequestrated and slowly released into the local biophase. In the rat model, liposomal encapsulation prolongs sufentanil spinal analgesia without decreasing the intensity of the analgesia.[37,102] With liposomal encapsulation, it may be possible in future to produce selective spinal analgesia with the phenylpiperidine-derived opioids, which lasts as long as morphine analgesia but avoids the side-effects associated with rostral spread. In the rat model, the neuraxial use of NSAIDs (ketorolac) and opioids (morphine) has shown significant analgesic synergy.[103,104] Human studies to show the efficacy of neuraxial NSAIDs in reducing neuraxial opioid doses still need to be undertaken.[103,104]

Epidural infusions of bupivacaine and pethidine, in contrast to infusions of bupivacaine and fentanyl, slow the regression of sensory anaesthesia and the development of pain.[105] Future studies should attempt to define the effect of lipid solubility, dose–response relationships and additional anaesthetic properties on the rate of regression of sensory anaesthesia during continuous epidural infusions of local anaesthetics and opioids. In a recent study, epidural fentanyl 4 μg/kg was more effective when given before incision compared with 15 minutes after incision in thoracic surgery.[106] Effective pre-emptive analgesia with neuraxial opioids still needs to be researched. The calcium channel blockers (nifedipine) could in future be used to enhance and prolong postoperative pain relief from neuraxial opioids (morphine).[107] The spinal combination of NMDA antagonists with spinal opioids is being researched in animal models. Intrathecal MK 801 with morphine has been used to abolish hyperaesthesia evoked by carrageenin injury in the rat paw.[107]

SPINAL OPIOIDS IN CHRONIC PAIN CONDITIONS

Opioids can be given by the high-morbidity spinal route in chronic pain when they have failed by conventional routes.[62] This presumes that the failure is based on the drug not reaching the receptors in the CNS. The pain must also be opioid sensitive. Opioids are least effective against neuropathic pain and intermittent somatic pain.

The WHO analgesic regimen is effective in over 80 per cent of cancer patients with severe pain.[108] It begins with simple non-steroidal analgesics and progresses upwards to high-dose opioids, usually by the oral or sublingual route. Between 15 and 20 per cent of patients can nevertheless still suffer severe pain towards the end of their lives despite earlier obtaining effective pain relief from the WHO analgesic regimen.[108] Various options, including continuous subcutaneous infusions of opioids, neurodestructive procedures and spinal opioids can now be used.

Another possible reason to switch to spinal opioids is where tolerance to systemically administered opioids has developed or where they caused pronounced side-effects.[109,110] It is still, however, not clear exactly which patients should receive spinal opioids. Tolerance is difficult to distinguish from increasing dose needs because of disease progression.[111] The suspicion remains that spinal opioids can produce a better quality of analgesia with fewer side-effects than conventional routes, but this is unproven.[62] A false diagnosis of tolerance is frequent in chronic opioid treatment.[44] Dural thickening and fibrotic action after the prolonged use of an epidural catheter can affect dural kinetics.[44] Pseudotolerance caused by dural thickening may be reversed by an injection of a corticosteroid and lignocaine solution epidurally.[44]

The use of spinal opioids in chronic benign pain is a controversial issue. This form of treatment is adopted only when all appropriate therapies have failed.[112]

With morphine, a simple method of converting from the conventional route is to try 1 per cent of the total daily dose as the daily intrathecal dose, and 10 per cent as the epidural dose. Initially, the intrathecal dose may be given once daily and the epidural dose twice daily.[62] The doses may then be increased as the disease or tachyphylaxis develops. An opioid withdrawal syndrome can occur in patients receiving high oral doses of morphine when they convert to spinal opioids.[113]

Technique

In most cases, the epidural route is chosen, although the intrathecal route is also used.[55] The catheter can be connected up to a system allowing the intermittent or continuous infusion of opioid. PCA can also be used. Many systems are in use. They range from a conventional epidural catheter (e.g. the Port-A-Cath), a disposable infusion device (e.g. the Infusor) and a simple subcutaneous reservoir, to an implanted programmable continuous-flow pump reservoir (see Chapter 7).[55] Catheters made up of nylon probably satisfy the requirements for long-term intrathecal catheterization better than those made up of other conventional methods (polyurethane, polyethylene or silicone elastomer).[114]

The main indication for the long-term intrathecal infusion of opioids is in cancer pain not amenable to oral analgesics, including morphine. Only a few studies have dealt with patients receiving intrathecal opioids for chronic non-cancer pain.[44] The feasibility of long-term intrathecal administration has been markedly improved by the introduction of an intrathecal infusion technique. An intrathecal catheter is tunnelled subcutaneously to the anterior thoracic region and connected to an infusion pump implanted subcutaneously in the infraclavicular region.[51] Two types of pump can be used: a gas-operated constant flow pump or a battery-powered pump with a variable flow rate.[51] The latter was programmable by an external device. Other options were the connection of a tunnelled catheter to a subcutaneous access port linked to an external pump or joining the catheter directly to the portable pump.[51] In cancer patients, this method compares favourably with implanted pumps in term of feasibility, complication rate and cost-effectiveness.[51] A retrospective analysis of 51 patients with cancer pain treated with a continuous intrathecal morphine infusion through a tunnelled percutaneous catheter showed adequate pain relief with an acceptable risk-to-benefit ratio.[88] Bupivacaine was added because of insufficient pain relief in 17 of these patients. The effects of the long-term intrathecal co-administration of local anaesthetics await further prospective evaluation. Intrathecal analgesia does, however, remain a viable therapeutic option for cancer pain syndromes refractory to the WHO guidelines for pharmacological tailoring.[115]

In children, a small group require epidural or intrathecal infusions of local anaesthetics/opioids, or neurolytic blockade, beyond that envisaged by the WHO protocol, to achieve adequate analgesia.[116] Indications for this intervention include limiting opioid side-effects, opioid-resistant neuropathic pain, malignant pleural effusion drainage and interpleural chemotherapy.[116] For children under 10 years of age, 20 gauge polyethylene unstyletted catheters via 18 gauge Tuohy needles, both epidurally and intrathecally, with subcutaneous tunnelling have been used.[115]

With recent advances in technology and techniques, many of these patients can be cared for at home (by visiting nurses) or on a outpatient basis. The use of ambulatory PCA devices for home care is an exciting development. Whether one delivery system produces more effective analgesia remains to be determined in controlled trials.[109]

For cancer pain, epidural catheters with tunnelling have been left in place for up to 862 days.[116] Externalized tunnelled silicone rubber catheters have been left in place for up to 1460 days.[116]

Patients with chronic non-malignant pain also deserve 'pain-free' holidays. Temporary epidural infusions of local anaesthetics/opioids (bupivacaine/fentanyl) have been used in 605 ambulatory patients with severe lumbalgia for up to 112 days.[117] Disposable fixed flow rate pumps, propelled by a latex balloon (Home Pump), or the Pain Pump, propelled by a spring, were used satisfactorily with infusion rates of 0.5–2.0 mL per hour.[117] The drugs placed in the pumps varied depending on the prior medications taken by the patient and the intensity of the pain. They usually included bupivacaine 0.25 per cent (90 mL), fentanyl 50 μg/mL (8–10 mL) and droperidol 2.5 mg/mL (2 mL). Daily telephone contact was made with the patient. There were no cardiorespiratory complications, infections occurring in only 0.3% of patients.[117]

There is little comparative evidence to recommend infusion rather than bolus administration. With epidural morphine, both seem to provide an equivalent extent of pain relief.[41] There seems, however, to be a more rapid dose escalation if an infusion is used.[108] An intrathecal infusion may have distinct advantages over an epidural bolus or epidural infusions.[109]

Problems

A wide interpatient variation in dose requirements can occur.[112] Tolerance can occur (especially with infusions) but is readily overcome by increasing the dose.[41, 108] Use has been made of intrathecal DADLE, clonidine, somatostatin and calcitonin to overcome tolerance.[113] Problems encountered with opioids via epidural catheters include pain on injection, occlusion, leak, catheter dislocation, inadvertent intrathecal placement and infection.[112,113] The infection rate is claimed to be lower with catheter tunnelling or implantable intrathecal catheter systems.[62] The advantages of implanting injection reservoirs or systems remains to be seen.[62] When a system should be implanted also remains controversial.

With intrathecal morphine in the lumbar area, pain relief can often be obtained in the cervical dermatomes.[112] Intraventricular morphine is effective for pain in the face and head, but its usefulness may be limited by CSF leakage and catheter maintenance.[62,112]

Toxicity

The high CSF opioid concentrations obtained raise the spectre of toxicity with chronic administration.[41] None, however, has been found in prolonged animal or human (as well as post mortem) studies, even with the long-term infusion of low-dose intrathecal bupivacaine.[41,115] Neuropathological findings after long-term intrathecal infusions of morphine, bupivacaine and their combination seem discrete (e.g. nerve fibre degeneration and fibrosis) and are not related to the duration or to cumulative doses of the intrathecal treatment.[114]

Combinations

For patients who fail to respond to systemic and epidural opioids, especially those with neuropathic pain (e.g. nerve root invasion), low-dose morphine–bupivacaine (0.125 per cent) infusions have been successfully used in the long term.[110] Concern over toxicity and adaption to sympathetic blockade seems unwarranted as little or no sympathetic or sensorimotor impairment occurs with bupivacaine (below 0.25 per cent).[110] An absence of CNS toxicity occurs even at plasma levels considered to be toxic. The mechanism for this tolerance is unknown.

Conclusion

It remains to be seen whether central neural blockade with opioids for chronic pain relief has fewer complications than ablative pain relief procedures. However, in properly selected patients, this method offers an effective alternative for pain relief.

NEUROLYTIC AGENTS IN CENTRAL NEURAL BLOCKADE

With the advent of neuraxial opioids, the role of epidural and intrathecal neurolytic blockade has become unclear.[118] Neurolytic blockade is still one of the most effective methods for the relief of severe intractable pain below the neck.[119] These procedures are, however, best suited to patients whose weakness, debility or short life expectancy makes them unsuitable candidates for neurosurgery.[120] Its major drawback is its limited duration of pain relief, of 2 weeks to more than a year (with an average of 2–4 months), after which sensation and pain return.[121] Thus, the reluctance to use these blocks for the non-terminal cancer patient or for non-cancer pain is certainly justified.

Agents used

Neurolytics, such as alcohol, phenol and chlorocresol, are also used (Figure 9.4). With alcohol, a concentration of 95 per cent will reliably lyse

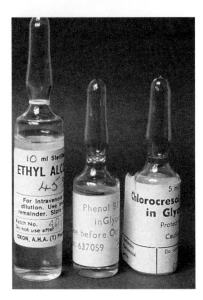

Figure 9.4   Neurolytic agents in central neural blockade – ampoules of alcohol, phenol and chlorocresol.

sympathetic, sensory and motor components.[118] Phenol has an initial local anaesthetic effect, which decreases after 24 hours to reveal its neurolytic effect.[120] It has been reported to spare motor function at a concentration of 3 per cent. In the epidural space, solutions of phenol are the agents of choice. Phenol can be combined with glycerine (7 per cent) to limit its spread.[122] X-ray contrast medium can be added. For intrathecal neurolysis, all the neurolytic agents can be used, each having its own particular indication.[122]

Mechanism of action

Neural destructive effects include a loss of cellular fatty elements, the precipitation of protein, separation of the myelin sheath from the axon and oedema of the axon, and fibrosis (making neural regeneration more difficult).[118]

Patient selection

Patients should have localized pain. Diagnostic nerve blocks should always precede the use of neurolytic agents to assess the effects. Patients must play an active part in the decision to proceed with the neurolysis. They and their families must understand the possible complications and the 'temporary' nature of the procedure.[120] Existing neurological deficits must be documented.

Complications of neurolytic blockade

With neurolytic blocks, there is the inability to control precisely the spread of destructive agents. Post-injection neuritis can occur. In the intrathecal space, neurolytics should be deposited as peripherally as possible to avoid spillover onto the sacral roots destined for the bladder or rectum.[120] A loss of motor function or the inability to control bowel or bladder function can greatly impair the quality of the remaining life.[123]

Techniques

INTRATHECAL BLOCK

The spinal segment to be blocked must be determined. Dermatome and sclerotome charts as well as anatomy books can be consulted.[118] The patient must be properly positioned for the neurolytic to be placed on the posterior sensory roots, and must lie still.[124] X-ray imaging intensification should be used. Alcohol is hypobaric so the painful aspect must be in the superior position. Alcohol is also painful to inject. Following the injection of alcohol, the patient is rotated forward by 45 degrees, allowing the alcohol to rise in the intrathecal compartment to invest the sensory roots.[122] The formulations of phenol in glycerine and chlorocresol in glycerine are hyperbaric, and the patient must be placed in the lateral position with the painful segments dependent. After injection, the patient is rotated 45 degrees backwards to allow the sensory roots to be invested.[122] Chlorocresol is more potent and penetrative than phenol.

Small (up to 0.25 ml) discrete aliquots are injected until the desired pain relief and/or dermal analgesia is obtained.[120] The treatment of several segmental levels is accomplished more safely by using needles at each level. The patient's position should be maintained for 20–30 minutes.

Intrathecal neurolytic blocks can be used for cancers involving cranial nerve distribution or for tumours involving somatic nerves lying between the limb plexuses.[120] For severe pelvic or perineal pain, intrathecal neurolytic block can be most rewarding.[125] A saddle block with the patient in a semi-recumbent position is used in perineal pain. Bilateral blocks in this area are associated with the attendant higher risk of bladder dysfunction.

EPIDURAL BLOCK

The epidural neurolytic route carries less morbidity than the intrathecal route but takes longer. Phenol (5–10 per cent) in contrast medium is used. The volume is determined by the volume of local anaesthetic necessary to perform a diagnostic block successfully.[118] It is particularly useful for bilateral pain and is not associated with major motor blockade.[123] An epidural catheter can also be inserted near the nerve root(s) involved and phenol injected daily over a few days.[124] This technique is useful for isolated bony secondaries.

CORTICOSTEROIDS IN CENTRAL NEURAL BLOCKADE

One of the earliest reports of the use of epidural steroids was published by Lievre in 1957.[126] Overall, the literature on epidural corticosteroids for back pain indicates that there has been widespread endorsement of the procedure over the past 33 years.[127] Most of the literature on caudal and lumbar epidural steroids comprises uncontrolled trials. Unfortunately, very few controlled studies on the efficacy of epidural corticosteroid injections have been published, and recent reviews have questioned the validity of these studies.[123,128,129] The two controlled caudal epidural studies were unable to demonstrate convincing statistical benefits because of their small size.[127] Of the five controlled trials of lumbar epidural corticosteroids, two have been supportive and three unfavourable.[127] The literature on cervical epidural corticosteroids is only anecdotal in quality.[127] There have been few reports on the use of epidural corticosteroids in complaints other than lumbar or sacral nerve root problems.[127]

There is no indication of what constitutes a 'standard' epidural injection.[127] Different authors have reported the use of different corticosteroids in different doses and with a variety of different adjunctive agents, such as normal saline and local anaesthetics of differing concentrations and volumes.[127]

The chief apparent effect is to reduce pain. Most patients may receive relief for a matter of weeks to up to 3 months, only a small proportion obtaining longer-lasting relief.[127] A review of the literature found that immediate pain relief varied from 25 to 89 per cent of cases and reported success rates from 35 to 86 per cent at review between 6 weeks and 5 years.[129] In a recent study, patients with sciatica followed up at 1 month were significantly better after a single epidural injection of corticosteroid with local anaesthetic than after local anaesthetic alone.[130]

Mechanism of action

The beneficial effects of corticosteroids in central neural blockade are thought to be provided by a localized anti-inflammatory effect (see Chapter 6), the inflammation initiated by either mechanical or chemical insults to the nerve root being reduced.[123] Oedema around the nerve roots is related to pressure caused by stenotic intervertebral foramina, osteophytes or the prolapse of an intervertebral disc.[131] The evidence for this belief is, at best, circumstantial.[127] A local anaesthetic-like action has also been suggested.[127]

Side-effects

The most common side-effects are related to the technical aspects of the procedures (e.g. dural puncture), as, for example, in the exacerbation of pain (related to the injectate volume) in about 1 per cent of lumbar steroid injections.[127] Rarely, fluid retention, hypercorticism and allergy are attributed to the corticosteroid agent injected. Animal and human studies have shown no deleterious effects on neural tissue from methylprednisolone or triamcinolone *per se*.[127] However, many of the constituents of commercially available preparations that might be used as epidural corticosteroids contain ingredients that have been shown, directly or by inference, to exert deleterious effects on nerve tissue or the meninges if injected intrathecally.[127] Multiple intrathecal corticosteroid injections appear to be associated with an increased risk of complications (e.g. aseptic meningitis), and this technique has all but disappeared from practice.[123,127,132]

Route of administration

Corticosteroids have been injected into the epidural space by either the lumbar or caudal route exclusively, or by both concurrently.[129] The cervical epidural application comprises a relatively new route of treatment.[131]

Indications

Indications for corticosteroid administration include those patients with lumbosacral radicular pain who have corresponding sensory change.[132] The shorter the symptomatology the better as long-standing symptoms are less likely to benefit from

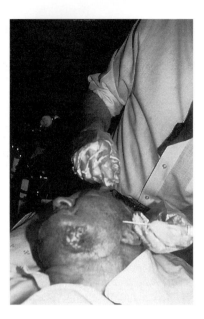

Figure 9.5   Placement of a corticosteroid around the mandibular nerve in a patient with carcinoma of the floor of the mouth.

epidural corticosteroids.[123] Other indications include patients with chronic low back pain or postural low back pain with radiculoid features.[132] The technique is also indicated in patients with metastatic cancer in whom tumour infiltration of the nerve roots causes radicular pain[132] (Figure 9.5). Cervical epidural corticosteroids have recently been used in the treatment of chronic resistant cervicobrachialgia.[131] The indications for the optimal use of epidural corticosteroids remain unresolved.

Agents used

These should be placed as close as possible to the level of nerve root irritation. In lumbar epidurals, the typical formulation has been methylprednisolone (50–100 mg) in 5–10 mL diluent (saline or weak local anaesthetic).[120, 127] For caudal epidurals, the typical formulation has been methylprednisolone 80 mg in 10–30 mL local anaesthetic.[127] The pharmaceutical vehicle in which methylprednisolone is formulated includes polyethylene glycol, which may have the potential of damaging neural tissue.[133] For this reason, intrathecal injection is not recommended. Preparations commonly used for epidural injection contain only 3 per cent polyethylene glycol, which is further diluted by the saline or local anaesthetic.[133] Triamcinolone diacetate 50 mg has also been used.[120]

Number of injections

The literature gives little guidance on the number of times that epidural corticosteroids may safely be given without provoking systemic toxic effects.[133] Reassessment should be carried out 1–2 weeks after initial treatment.[123] If symptoms have improved but some pain is still present, the injection should be repeated. A third block can be performed 1–2 weeks later if some symptoms persist. There is no point in repeating the injections if the first epidural is unhelpful.

Technique

It is important that the offending nerve root be identified and the epidural performed at the appropriate level.[118]

LUMBAR EPIDURAL CORTICOSTEROID INJECTION

The patient is placed in the lateral position with the affected side down. The epidural space is then located. Many patients experience transient exacerbation of their radicular pain as the needle enters the epidural space or on injection of the test dose (after negative aspiration).[132] The local anaesthetic (or saline) and the corticosteroid are then injected. The patient is kept in the lateral position for 10–15 minutes. A reduction in the pain level, decreased sensation in the affected dermatome and an improvement in straight leg raising provide evidence of having reached the affected root.[118]

CERVICAL EPIDURAL CORTICOSTEROID INJECTION

The patient is seated with the neck flexed. Injections are performed at the C5–6 or C6–7 interspace.[131] The needle is inserted in the midline at a 45 degree angle to the skin in a superior direction. The epidural space is identified.[132] After negative aspiration and a test dose, the local anaesthetic (or saline) and corticosteroid are injected. For the next 20 minutes, the patient can be placed in the lateral position with the involved side down, or lie supine in a Trendelenberg position of 45 degrees if more bilateral diffuse involvement of the nerve roots has occurred. Pain relief and improvement in the range of motion are then evaluated.

Conclusion

Despite the enthusiasm that has been shown for epidural corticosteroids, there are no data stem-ming from controlled trials, let alone double-blind controlled trials, that unreservedly vindicate their use. At best, two controlled trials of caudal epidural corticosteroids approach statistical significance, and one controlled study vindicates the use of lumbar epidural corticosteroids plus local anaesthetic in the treatment of patients with lumbar radicular pain, but the latter is incompatible with another similar study of comparable size.[127]

REFERENCES

1. **Finucane, B.T.** 1991: Regional anaesthesia: complications and techniques. *Canadian Journal of Anaesthesia* **38**(4), R3–R10.
2. **Bridenbaugh, P.O.** 1990: Regional anesthesia – advantages and disadvantages. *International Anesthesia Research Society Review Course Lectures*, 24–8.
3. **Philip, B.K.** 1992: Regional anesthesia for ambulatory surgery. *Canadian Journal of Anaesthesia* **39**(5), R3–R6.
4. **Chesnut, D.H.** 1992: Spinal anesthesia and the febrile patient. *Anesthesiology* **76**, 667–9.
5. **Mulroy, M.F.** 1992: Complications of regional anesthesia. *International Anesthesia Research Society Review Course Lectures*, 45–9.
6. **Bullingham, A. and Priestly, M.** 1997: Anaesthetic management of patients being treated with anticoagulants. *Current Opinion in Anaesthesiology* **10**, 234–9.
7. **Schneider, M.C. and Hampl, K.F.** 1995: Complications of epidural and spinal anaesthesia in adults. *Current Opinion in Anaesthesiology* **8**, 414–19.
8. **Wildsmith, J.A.W. and McClure, J.H.** 1991: Anticoagulant drugs and central nerve blockade. *Anaesthesia* **63**, 613–14.
9. **Rolf, N. and Mollhoff, T.** 1997: Epidural anaesthesia for patients undergoing coronary artery bypass grafting. *Current Opinion in Anaesthesiology* **10**, 17–20.
10. **Mazoit, J.X. and Cao. L.S.** 1995: Local anaesthetic toxicity. *Current Opinion in Anaesthesiology* **8**, 409–13.
11. **Massey Dawkins, C.J.** 1969: An analysis of the complications of extradural and caudal block. *Anaesthesia* **24**, 554–63.
12. **Badgwell, J.M. and McLeod, M.M.** 1995: Complications of epidural and spinal anaesthesia in children. *Current Opinion in Anaesthesiology* **8**, 420–5.
13. **Feldman, H.S., Arthur, G.R., Pitkanen, M., Hurley, R., Doucette, A.M. and Covino, B.G.** 1991: Treatment of acute systemic toxicity after the rapid intravenous injection of ropivacaine and bupivacaine in the conscious dog. *Anesthesia and Analgesia* **73**, 373–84.
14. **Hughes, S.C.** 1992: Analgesia methods during labour and delivery. *Canadian Journal of Anaesthesia* **39**(5), R18–R23.
15. **Ecoffey, C.** 1995: Regional anaesthesia. *Current Opinion in Anaesthesiology* **8**, 407–8.

16. **Moore, D.C. and Bridenbaugh, D.L.** 1966: Spinal (subarachnoid) block. *Journal of the American Medical Association* **195**, 123–8.

17. **Calder, T.M. and Harris, A.P.** 1992: Subdural block during attempted caudal epidural analgesia for labour. *Anesthesiology* **76**, 316–18.

18. **Wildsmith, J.A.W. and Lee, J.A.** 1989: Neurological sequelae of spinal anaesthesia. *British Journal of Anaesthesia* **63**(5), 505–7.

19. **Wulf, H.** 1996: Epidural anaesthesia and spinal haematoma. *Canadian Journal of Anaesthesia* **43**(12), 1260–71.

20. **Kaufman, L.** 1991: Pain. In Kaufman, L. (ed.) *Anaesthesia Review 8*. Edinburgh: Churchill Livingstone, 231–53.

21. **Wildsmith, J.A.W. and McClure, J.H.** 1988: Aspects of spinal anaesthesia. In Kaufman, L. (ed.) *Anaesthesia Review 5*. Edinburgh: Churchill Livingstone, 269–85.

22. **Mulroy, M.F.** 1996: Which needles by which approach? *International Symposium of Regional Anaesthesia*, 9–11 April, Auckland, New Zealand, 35–8.

23. **Carbaat, P.A.T. and Van Crevel, H.** 1981: Lumbar puncture headache: a controlled study on the preventative effect of 24 hours bed rest. *Lancet* **2**, 1133–5.

24. **Myers, L. and Rosenberg, M.** 1962: The use of the 26 gauge spinal needle – a survey. *Anesthesia and Analgesia* **41**, 509–15.

25. **Mulroy, M.F., Neal, J.M., Bridenbaugh, L.D. and Plamen, B.** 1989: Is post-spinal headache more frequent to outpatients? *Regional Anesthesia* **45**(2S), 2.

26. **Horlocker, T.T., McGregor, D.G., Matsushige, D.K. et al.** 1997: Neurologic complications of 603 continuous spinal anesthetics using macrocatheter and microcatheter techniques. *Anesthesia and Analgesia* **84**, 1063–70.

27. **Beeton, A.G. and Shipton, E.A.** 1991: Continuous spinal anaesthesia with microcatheters. *South African Medical Journal* **80**, 309.

28. **Shipton, E.A.** 1992: Postoperative pain – an update. *South African Journal of Surgery* **30**(1), 2–5.

29. **Lloyd-Thomas, A.R.** 1990: Pain management in paediatric patients. *British Journal of Anaesthesia* **64**, 85–104.

30. **Verborgh, C., Claeys, M.A. and Camu, F.** 1991: Onset of epidural blockade after plain or alkalinised 0.5% bupivacaine. *Anesthesia and Analgesia* **73**, 401–4.

31. **Veering, B.** 1996: Does solution baricity matter? *International Symposium of Regional Anaesthesia*, 9–11 April, Auckland, New Zealand, 39–43.

32. **Nicol, M.E. and Holdcroft, A.** 1992: Density of intrathecal agents. *British Journal of Anaesthesia* **68**, 60–3.

33. **Justins, D.M. and Richardson, P.H.** 1991: Clinical management of acute pain. *British Medical Bulletin* **47**(3), 561–83.

34. **Yeager, M.P.** 1991: The role of regional anesthesia in improving surgical outcome. *International Anesthesia Research Society Review Course Lectures*, 122–9.

35. **Wildsmith, J.A.W.** 1989: Developments in local anaesthetic drugs and techniques for pain relief. *British Journal of Anaesthesia* **63**, 159–64.

36. **Odoom, J.A. Bovill, J.G. Hardeman, M.R., Oosting, J. and Zuurmond, W.W.A.** 1992: Effects of epidural and spinal anaesthesia on blood rheology. *Anesthesia and Analgesia* **74**, 835–40.

37. **Shipton, E.A.** 1996: Modern use of neuraxial opioids in acute pain. *South African Journal of Surgery* **34**(4), 180–5.

38. **Sandler, A.N.** 1992: Update on postoperative pain management. *Canadian Journal of Anaesthesia* **39**(5), R53–R56.

39. **Rawal, N.** 1996: Opioids and nonopioids – efficacy, safety and cost-benefit. *Pain Reviews* **3**, 31–62.

40. **De Leon-Casasola, O.A. and Lema, M.J.** 1996: Postoperative epidural opioid analgesia: what are the choices? *Anesthesia and Analgesia* **83**, 867–75.

41. **McQuay, H.J.** 1991: Opioid clinical pharmacology and routes of administration. *British Medical Bulletin* **47**(3), 703–17.

42. **Cousins, M.J.** 1996: Advances in thoracic epidural block: anatomical concepts. *International Symposium of Regional Anaesthesia*, 9–11 April, Auckland, New Zealand, 64–7.

43. **Morgan, M.** 1989: The rational use of intrathecal and extradural opioids. *British Journal of Anaesthesia* **63**, 165–88.

44. **Tawfik, M.O.** 1994: Mode of action of intraspinal opioids. *Pain Reviews* **1**, 275–94.

45. **Brose, W.G., Tanelian, D.L., Brodsky, J.B., Mark, J.B.D. and Cousins, M.J.** 1991: CSF and blood pharmacokinetics of hydromorphone and morphine following lumbar epidural administration. *Pain* **45**, 11–15.

46. **Rauck, R.L.** 1991: Epidural and spinal narcotics. *American Society of Anesthesiologists' Annual Refresher Lectures* **274**, 1–7.

47. **Brown, D.V. and McCarthy, R.J.** 1995: Opioids and other analgesics. *Current Opinion in Anaesthesiology* **8**, 337–41.

48. **Glass, P.S. and Grichnick, K.P.** 1995: The role of opioids for epidural analgesia. *Current Opinion in Anaesthesiology* **8**, 283–6.

49. **Dickenson, A.H., Sullivan, A.F. and McQuay, H.J.** 1990: Intrathecal etorphine, fentanyl, and buprenorphine on spinal nociceptive neurones in the rat. *Pain* **42**, 227–4.

50. **Stevens, R.A., Petty, R.H., Hill, H.F. et al.** Redistribution of sufentanil to cerebrospinal fluid and systemic circulation after epidural administration in dogs. *Anesthesia and Analgesia* **76**, 323–7.

51. **Crul, B.J., Van Dongen, R.T. and Snijdelaar, D.G.** 1994: Intrathecal opioids. *Pain Reviews* **1**, 295–307.

52. **De Leon-Casasola, O.A. and Lema, M.J.** 1992: Spinal opioid analgesia: influence on clinical outcome. In Sinatra, R.S., Hord, A.L., Ginsberg, B. and Preble, L.M. (eds) *Acute pain: mechanisms and management*. St Louis: Mosby-Year Book, 293–303.

53. **Beattie, W.S., Buckley, D.N. and Forrest, J.B.** 1993:

Epidural morphine reduces the risk of postoperative myocardial ischaemia in patients with cardiac risk factors. *Canadian Journal of Anaesthesia* **40**(6), 532–41.

54. **Moore, J.M. and Spencer, S.L.** 1997: How can postoperative outcome be improved? *Current Opinion in Anaesthesiology* **10**, 163–6.

55. **Green, D.W.** 1992: The clinical use of spinal opioids. In Kaufman, L. (ed.) *Anaesthesia Review 9*. Edinburgh: Churchill Livingstone, 80–111.

56. **Eisenach, J.C.** 1993: Epidural and spinal narcotics. *American Society of Anesthesiologists Annual Refresher Course Lectures* **135**, 1–7.

57. **Black, A.M.S. and Alexander, J.I.** 1991: Analgesia for postoperative pain. In Atkinson, R.S. and Adams, A.P. (eds) *Recent Advances in Anaesthesia and Analgesia 17*. Edinburgh: Churchill Livingstone, 119–35.

58. **Moote, C.** 1993: Techniques for post-op pain management in the adult. *Canadian Journal of Anaesthesia* **40**(5), R19-R24.

59. **Kafle, S.K.** 1993: Intrathecal meperidine for elective caesarean section: a comparison with lidocaine. *Canadian Journal of Anaesthesia* **40**(8), 718–21.

60. **Delilkan, A.E. and Vijayan, R.** 1993: Epidural tramadol for postoperative pain relief. *Anaesthesia* **48**, 328–31.

61. **Baraka, A., Jabbour, S., Ghabash, M., Nader, A., Khoury, G. and Sibai, A.** 1993: A comparison of epidural tramadol and epidural morphine for postoperative analgesia. *Canadian Journal of Anaesthesia* **40**(4), 308–13.

62. **McQuay, H.J.** 1989: Opioids in chronic pain. *British Journal of Anaesthesia* **63**, 213–26.

63. **Shipton, E.A.** 1994: Control of perioperative pain after abdominal operation. *South African Journal of Continuing Medical Education* **12**, 549–62.

64. **Rawal, N., Arner, S., Gustafsson, L.L. and Allvin, R.** 1987: Present state of extradural and intrathecal opioid analgesia in Sweden: a nationwide follow-up survey. *British Journal of Anaesthesia* **59**, 791–9.

65. **Shipton, E.A. and van der Merwe, C.A.** 1993: Perioperatiewe pynsorg – die nuutste. *South African Journal of Continuing Medical Education* **11**(3), 459–68.

66. **McQuay, H.J.** 1992: Spinal opioids. *South African Society of Anaesthetists Refresher Course Lectures*, 11–13.

67. **Norris, M.C., Leighton, B.L. and De Simone, C.A.** 1989: Naltrexone and subarachnoid morphine following cesarean section. *Anesthesiology* **71**, A873.

68. **Finster, M. and Westrich, D.J.** 1991: Newer trends in obstetric pain relief. *International Anesthesia Research Society Review Course Lectures*, 30–4.

69. **Grange, C.S. and Douglas, M.J.** 1997: Epidural and intrathecal narcotics in obstetrics. *Current Opinion in Anaesthesiology* **10**, 199–202.

70. **Kehlet, H. and Dahl, J.B.** 1993: The value of multimodal or balanced analgesia in postoperative pain treatment. *Anesthesia and Analgesia* **77**, 1048–56.

71. **Schnider, S.M.** 1993: Epidural opioids and local anesthetics for pain management in obstetrics. *American Society of Anesthesiologists' Annual Refresher Course Lectures* **233**, 1–7.

72. **Wittels, B., Glosten, B., Faure, E.A.M.** *et al.* 1993: Opioid antagonist adjuncts to epidural morphine for postcesarean analgesia: maternal outcomes. *Anesthesia and Analgesia* **77**, 925–32.

73. **Camann, W.R., Minzter, B.H., Denney, R.A. and Datta, S.** 1993: Intrathecal sufentanil for labor analgesia. *Anesthesiology* **78**, 870–4.

74. **Grieco, W.M., Norris, M.C., Leighton, B.L.** *et al.* 1993: Intrathecal sufentanil labor analgesia: the effects of adding morphine or epinephrine. *Anesthesia and Analgesia* **77**, 1149–54.

75. **Vercauteren, M.P.** 1995: Current status of perispinal local anaesthetic–opioid combinations in acute pain management. *European Society of Anaesthesiologists' Refresher Course Lectures* RC-22, 103–8.

76. **Fell, D.** 1993: Postoperative analgesia in children. *British Journal of Anaesthesia* **70**, 4–5.

77. **Brodner, G.** 1997: Pain management in patients undergoing thoracic surgery. *Current Opinion in Anaesthesiology* **10**, 54–9.

78. **Gielen, M.** 1996: Thoracic epidural anaesthesia (TEA): effects and applications. *International Symposium of Regional Anaesthesia*, 9–11 April, Auckland, New Zealand, 68–70.

79. **Berde, C.** 1993: Acute postoperative pain management in children. *American Society of Anesthesiologists' Annual Refresher Course Lectures* **136**, 1–7.

80. **Abuzaid, H., Prys-Roberts, C., Wilkins, D.G. and Terry, D.M.S.** 1993: The influence of diamorphine on spinal anaesthesia induced with isobaric 0.5% bupivacaine. *Anaesthesia* **48**, 492–5.

81. **Russell, R. and Reynolds, F.** 1993: Epidural infusions for nulliparous women in labour. *Anaesthesia* **48**, 856–61.

82. **Yee, I., Carstoniu, J., Halpern, S. and Pittini, R.** 1993: A comparison of two doses of epidural fentanyl during caesarean section. *Canadian Journal of Anaesthesia* **40**(8), 722–5.

83. **Le Polain, B., De Kock, M., Scholtes, J.L. and Van Lierde, M.** 1993: Clonidine combined with sufentanil and bupivacaine with adrenaline for obstetric analgesia. *British Journal of Anaesthesia* **71**, 657–60.

84. **Kestin, I.G.** 1991: Spinal anaesthesia in obstetrics. *British Journal of Anaesthesia* **66**, 596–607.

85. **Peacock, J. and Dale, S.** 1996: Patient-controlled analgesia. *Current Opinion in Anaesthesiology* **9**, 313–17.

86. **Sun, H.-L., Wu, C.-C., Lin, M.-S. and Chang, C.-F.** 1993: Effects of epidural morphine and intramuscular diclofenac combination in postcesarean analgesia: a dose-range study. *Anesthesia and Analgesia* **76**, 284–8.

87. **Turner, J.L., Sibert, K.S. and Sinatra, R.S.** 1992: Epidural and spinal analgesia in the post-cesarean delivery patient. In Sinatra, R.S., Hord, A.H., Ginsberg, B. and Preble, L.M. (eds) *Acute pain: mechanisms and management*. St Louis: Mosby Yearbook, 269–78.

88. **Van Dongen, R.T.M., Crul, B.J.P. and De Bock, M.** 1995: Long-term intrathecal infusion of morphine

and morphine/bupivacaine mixtures in the treatment of cancer pain: a retrospective analysis of 51 cases. *Pain* **55**, 119–23.

89. **Gambling, D.R., Huber, C.J., Berkowitz, J.** *et al*. 1993: Patient-controlled epidural analgesia in labour: varying bolus dose and lockout interval. *Canadian Journal of Anaesthesia* **40**(3), 211–17.

90. **Curry, P.D., Pacsoo, C. and Heap, D.G.** 1994: Patient-controlled analgesia in obstetric anaesthetic practice. *Pain* **57**, 125–8.

91. **Cohen, S., Amar, D., Pantuck, C.B.** *et al*. 1993: Post-cesarean delivery epidural patient-controlled analgesia. *Anesthesiology* **78**, 486–91.

92. **Cooper, D.W. and Turner, G.** 1993: Patient-controlled extradural analgesia to compare bupivacaine, fentanyl and bupivacaine with fentanyl in the treatment of postoperative pain. *British Journal of Anaesthesia* **70**, 503–7.

93. **Chauvin, N., Hongnat, J.M., Mourgeon, E., Lebrault, C., Bellenfant, F. and Alfonsi, P.** 1993: Equivalents of postoperative analgesia with patient-controlled intravenous or epidural alfentanil. *Anesthesia and Analgesia* **76**, 1251–8.

94. **Owen, H., Kluger, M.T., Ilsley, A.H., Baldwin, A.M., Fronsko, R.R.L. and Plummer, J.L.** 1993: The effect of fentanyl administered epidurally by patient-controlled analgesia, continuous infusion, or a combined technique of oxyhaemoglobin saturation after abdominal surgery. *Anaesthesia* **48**, 20–5.

95. **Klimscha, W., Weinstabl, C., Ilias, W.** *et al*. 1993: Continuous spinal anesthesia with a microcatheter and low-dose bupivacaine decreases the hemodynamic effects of centroneuraxis blocks in elderly patients. *Anesthesia and Analgesia* **77**, 275–80.

96. **Guinard, J.-P., Chiolero, R., Mavrocordatos, P. and Carpenter, R.L.** 1993: Prolonged intrathecal fentanyl analgesia via 32-gauge catheters after thoracotomy. *Anesthesia and Analgesia* **77**, 936–41.

97. **Stacey, R.G.W., Watt, S., Kadim, M.Y. and Morgan, B.M.** 1993: Single space combined spinal–extradural technique for analgesia in labour. *British Journal of Anaesthesia* **71**, 499–502.

98. **Ley, S.J. and Jones, B.R.** 1991: Strength of continuous spinal catheters. *Anesthesia and Analgesia* **73**, 394–6.

99. **Rigler, M.G., Drasner, K., Krejcie, T.C.** *et al*. 1991: Cauda equina syndrome after continuous spinal anesthetics. *Anesthesia and Analgesia* **72**, 275–81.

100. **Vercauteren, M.P., Geernaert, K., Vandeput, D.M. and Adriaensen, H.** 1993: Combined continuous spinal–epidural anaesthesia with a single interspace, double-catheter technique. *Anaesthesia* **48**, 1002–4.

101. **Eisenach, J.C.** 1993: Aspirin, the miracle drug: spinally, too? *Anesthesiology* **79**, 211–13.

102. **Shipton, E.A.** 1994: Technological advances in regional anaesthesia. *South African Medical Journal* **84**, 128–9.

103. **Malmberg, A.B. and Yaksh, T.L.** 1993: Pharmacology of the spinal action of ketorolac, morphine, ST-91, U50488H, and L-PIA on the formalin test and an isobolographic analysis of the NSAID interaction. *Anesthesiology* **79**, 270–81.

104. **Ferrante, F.M., Fanciullo, G.J., Grichnik, K.P., Vaisman, J., Sacks, G.M. and Concepcion, M.** 1993: Regression of sensory anesthesia during continuous epidural infusions of bupivacaine and opioid for total knee replacement. *Anesthesia and Analgesia* **77**, 1179–84.

105. **Katz, J., Kavanagh, B.P., Sandler, A.N.** *et al*. 1992: Pre-emptive analgesia: clinical evidence of neuroplasticity contributing to postoperative pain. *Anesthesiology* **77**, 439–46.

106. **Pereira, I.T., Prado, W.A. and Dos Reis, M.P.** 1993: Enhancement of the epidural morphine-induced analgesia by systemic nifedipine. *Pain* **53**, 341–55.

107. **Yamamoto, T., Shimoyama, N. and Mizuguchi, T.** 1993: The effects of morphine, MK-801, an NMDA antagonist, and CP-96345, an NK1 antagonist on the hyperesthesia evoked by carrageenin injection in the rat paw. *Anesthesiology* **78**, 124–33.

108. **Gourlay, G.K., Plummer, J.L., Cherry, D.A.** *et al*. 1991: Comparison of intermittent bolus with continuous infusion of epidural morphine in the treatment of severe cancer pain. *Pain* **47**, 135–40.

109. **Follet, K.A., Hitchon, P.W., Piper, J., Kumar, V., Clamon, G. and Jones, M.P.** 1992: Response of intractable pain to continuous intrathecal morphine: A retrospective study. *Pain* **49**, 21–5.

110. **Du Pen, S.L., Kharasch, E.D., Williams, A.** *et al*. 1992: Chronic epidural bupivacaine-opioid infusion in intractable cancer pain. *Pain* **49**, 293–300.

111. **Hogan, Q., Haddox, J.D., Abram, S., Weissman, D., Taylor, M.L. and Janjan, N.** 1991: Epidural opiates and local anaesthetics for the management of cancer pain. *Pain* **46**, 271–9.

112. **Plummer, J.L., Cherry, D.A., Cousins, M.J., Gourlay, G.K., Onley, M.M. and Evans, K.H.A.** 1991: Long-term spinal administration of morphine in cancer and non-cancer pain: a retrospective study. *Pain* **44**, 215–20.

113. **Erdine, S. and Aldemir, T.** 1991: Long term results of peridural morphine in 225 patients. *Pain* **45**, 155–9.

114. **Sjoberg, M., Karlsson, P.A., Nordborg, C.** *et al*. 1992: Neuropathological findings after long-term intrathecal infusion of morphine and bupivacaine for pain treatment in cancer patients. *Anesthesiology* **76**, 173–86.

115. **Krames, E.S.** 1993: The chronic intraspinal use of opioid and local anaesthetic mixtures for the relief of intractable pain: when all else fails! *Pain* **55**, 1–4.

116. **Collins, J.J., Grier, H.E., Sethna, N.F.** *et al*. 1996: Regional anesthesia for pain associated with terminal pediatric malignancy. *Pain* **65**, 63–9.

117. **Aldrete, J.A.** 1996: Temporary epidural infusions in ambulatory patients with severe lumbalgia. *Pain Reviews* **3**, 1–13.

118. **Abram, S.E.** 1990: Techniques for some commonly used nerve blocks. In Abram, S.E. (ed.) *The pain clinic manual*. Philadelphia: J.B. Lippincott, 334–49.

119. **Raj, P.P.** 1990: Management of chronic pain. *American Society of Anesthesiologists' Annual Refresher Course Lectures* **133**, 1–7.
120. **Murphy, T.M.** 1990: Chronic pain. In Miller, R.D. (ed.) *Anesthesia*, 3rd edn. New York: Churchill Livingstone, 1927–50.
121. **Charlton, J.E.** 1989: Common pain syndromes and their management. *Canadian Journal of Anaesthesia* **36**(3), S9–S12.
122. **Budd, K.** 1989: The pain clinic – chronic pain. In Nunn, J.F., Utting, J.E. and Brown, B.R. (eds) *General anaesthesia*, 5th edn. London: Butterworths, 1349–69.
123. **Abram, S.E.** 1989: Pain – acute and chronic. In Barash, P.G., Cullen, B.F. and Stoelting, R.K. (eds) *Clinical anesthesia*. Philadelphia: J.B. Lippincott, 1427–54.
124. **Shipton, E.A.** 1990: The management of intractable pain. *Hospital Medicine* (Aug), 30–4.
125. **McQuay, H.J.** 1989: Common conditions in the pain clinic and their management. In Nimmo, W.S. and Smith, G. (eds) *Anaesthesia*. Oxford: Blackwell Scientific Publications, 1198–215.
126. **Lievre, J.A., Block-Michael, H. and Attali, P.** 1957: L'injection transsacree. Etude clinique et radiologique. *Bulletin du Societé Medicale* **73**, 1110.
127. **Salisbury, J.** 1994: *Epidural use of steroids in the management of back pain*. National Health and Medical Research Council (Australia), 1–76.
128. **Benzon, H.T.** 1986: Epidural steroid injections for low back pain and lumbosacral radiculography. *Pain* **24**, 277–95.
129. **Bogduk, N.** 1988: Zygapophysial blocks and epidural steroids. In Cousins, M.J. and Bridenbaugh, P.O. *Neural blockade*, 2nd edn. Philadelphia: J.B. Lippincott, 935–4.
130. **Rodgers, P., Nash, T., Schiller, D. and Norman, J.** 1992: Epidural steroids for sciatica. *The Pain Clinic* **5**(2), 67–72.
131. **Stav, A., Ovadia, L., Landau, M., Wekler, N. and Berman, M.** 1991: Epidural steroid injection in the treatment of lumbar and cervical pain syndromes: a preliminary retrospective comparison. *The Pain Clinic* **4**(2), 95–102.
132. **Rowlingson, J.C.** 1991: Management of chronic pain. *American Society of Anesthesiologists' Annual Refresher Course Lectures* **113**, 1–7.
133. **Williams, K.N., Jackowski, A. and Evans, P.J.D.** 1990: Epidural haematoma requiring surgical decompression following repeated cervical epidural steroid injections for chronic pain. *Pain* **42**, 197–9.

10

COMPLEX REGIONAL PAIN SYNDROMES AND THE SYMPATHETIC NERVOUS SYSTEM

The nomenclature complex regional pain syndromes (CRPS) replaces that of reflex sympathetic dystrophy and causalgia as the generic, clinical non-mechanistic classification of disorders thought to invoke common neuropathic and clinical features in these groups of patients.[1] These disorders are usually consequent to injury, manifesting with pain and sensory changes that are disproportionate in intensity, distribution and duration to the underlying pathology. Additional features of motor, autonomic, trophic and psychological dysfunctions make up a CRPS diagnostic constellation. CRPS is not a 'thing' but a group of entities that present with somewhat similar clinical presentations and are therefore often lumped together for the sake of clinical unity. CRPS is not limited to limb injuries but may develop with visceral diseases (from intra-abdominal sympathetic involvement), CNS lesions, soft tissue lesions, amputation syndromes (e.g. mastectomy) and back pain.[2] Sympathetically maintained pain is a frequent but variable component of these syndromes as the sympathetic and somatosensory pathways are no longer functionally extinct.[2]

DEFINITIONS

Complex regional pain syndrome type 1

The International Association for the Study of Pain has agreed on four diagnostic criteria for reflex sympathetic dystrophy (now to be called CRPS 1), the last three of which must be present to confirm the diagnosis:[3]

1. the presence of an initiating noxious event or a cause of immobilization;
2. continuing pain, allodynia or hyperalgesia with pain disproportionate to any inciting event;
3. evidence at some time of oedema, changes in skin blood flow or abnormal sudomotor activity in the region of the pain;
4. that this diagnosis is excluded by the existence of conditions that would otherwise account for the degree of pain and dysfunction.

CRPS 1 may develop as a consequence of trauma affecting the limbs, with or without an obvious nerve lesion.[4] It may also develop after visceral disease and CNS lesions or, rarely, without an obvious antecedent event. Precipitants include blunt trauma (e.g. sprains), fractures, lacerations, crush injuries, amputations and burns, surgery, repetitive microtrauma and a variety of disease states (myocardial infarction, neurological diseases and infection and vascular disease).[5] No major injury occurs.

The syndrome consists of pain and related sensory abnormalities, abnormal blood flow and sweating abnormalities, as well as abnormalities in the motor system. The syndrome often results in disuse and presents with a continuous diffuse (often burning) limb pain and various sensory (hyperpathia, allodynia and autonomic) changes. Changes in the structure of both superficial and deep tissues occur (trophic changes). Yet in chronic CRPS type 1, efferent nerve fibres are histologically unaffected, and in afferent fibres, only C fibres show histopathological abnormalities.[6] Skeletal muscles showed a variety of histopathological findings similar to the abnormalities found in the muscles of diabetics.[6]

Complex regional pain syndrome type 2

The International Association for the Study of Pain has defined three criteria for causalgia (now to be called CRPS 2), all of which must be present to confirm the diagnosis:[7]

1. the presence of continuous pain, allodynia or hyperalgesia after nerve injury, not necessarily limited to the distribution of the injured nerve;
2. evidence at some time of oedema, changes in skin blood flow or abnormal sudomotor activity in the region of the pain;
3. that this diagnosis is excluded by the existence of conditions that would otherwise account for the degree of pain and dysfunction.

Particular note should be taken of the similarities between the diagnostic criteria for CRPS 1 and CRPS 2. Most cases of CRPS 2 occur after gunshot wounds, most of which are proximal to the knee or elbow. The great majority of cases are related to injuries, usually partial transections of the medial cord of the brachial plexus, median nerve or sciatic nerve.[5] A recent study to assess the diagnostic criteria of the International Association for the Study of Pain for CRPS suggests that CRPS decision rules may lead to overdiagnosis of the disorder.[8] The addition of trophic tissue changes, range of motion changes and a 'burning' quality to the pain did not improve diagnostic accuracy, but the addition of motor neglect signs did.[8]

Sympathetically maintained pain

One of the motivations for adopting the new terminology was the realization that a sympathetic inclusion or exclusion, as a clinical response to blocks, occurs as a feature of some neuropathic pains but is not the basis of their pathophysiology.[1] That aspect of pain which can be relieved by a local anaesthetic block of the sympathetic ganglia that serve the painful area, or by pharmacotherapy, is termed sympathetically maintained pain.[9] It is pain that is maintained by sympathetic efferent innervation or by neurochemicals or circulating catecholamines.[2,10] Sympathetically maintained pain may be a feature of several types of painful disorder. However, in a given situation, a patient may have a pain syndrome wherein part of the pain is sympathetically maintained pain and another part is sympathetically independent pain. In other words, patients may have both sympathetically maintained pain and sympathetically independent pain. In addition, sympathetically maintained pain is variable over time such that, at one observation, a given patient may have pain that is wholly or partially sympathetically maintained, but at another, usually later, time, the pain may be entirely sympathetically independent.[10]

Sympathetically maintained pain may and may not be present in a patient with CRPS.[11] Sympathetically maintained pain can be present in patients with painful neuropathies associated with connective tissue disorders, acute shingles, post-herpetic neuralgia, painful metabolic neuropathy, traumatic nerve injury and soft tissue injury.[12] It may be a mechanism for the production of pain in a number of these disorders, yet it may also exist independently.[9] Patients have typical spontaneous pain and allodynia but no obvious disturbance of blood flow, no obvious trophic changes and only discrete motor disturbances.[13] They are more likely to have a hyperalgesia to cold stimuli and to show improvement with sympathetic blockade.[4]

In sympathetically independent pain, the factors that maintain the central state of hyperexcitability may be diverse. These may include maintaining nociceptor input in normal nociceptive afferent fibres as a result of factors, such as traction on the periosteum, muscle, vasculature and epineurium, that may arise from trauma or surgery. Another source of ongoing nociceptor input may be regenerating nerve sprouts in an end-bulb neuroma or a neuroma-in-continuity.[14]

CRPS have strict inclusion criteria, but the presence or absence of sympathetically maintained pain is not one of them.[11]

INCIDENCE

There is relatively little information available regarding the overall incidence of CRPS 1 and 2 in the general population. A predominance of CRPS 1 patients occurs between the ages of 40 and 60, few cases occurring in patients under 30 or over 70.[15,16] No obvious sex-related differences have occurred as CRPS is most often precipitated by peripheral trauma (crushing injuries, lacerations, fractures, sprains, burns or surgery) to soft tissue or nerve complexes.[17] The incidence is 1–2 per cet after various fractures, raging from 2 to 5 per cent after peripheral nerve injury, and from 7 to 35 per cent in prospective studies of Colles' fractures.[18] In one prospective study of Colles' fractures, 54 per cent of patients had one or more features of CRPS 2 weeks after removal of the plaster cast.[2] It occurs in 5 per cent of patients after myocardial infarction, with local cold injury and after revascularization of an ischaemic extremity.[18] In 10–26 per cent of cases, no precipitating factor can be found.[18]

The overall incidence in a pain clinic population has been estimated at 6–11 per cent.[19] The overall incidence of CRPS 2 appears to be approximately 4 per cent.[20] When seen in children (peaking at 9–13 years), it appears to be more common in females (4:1), involves the lower limb most frequently and is often diagnosed late.[2,21] Cases have occurred in children as young as 3 years of age. There is no worthwhile evidence to substantiate the claim that psychological factors or certain personality traits predispose to the development of CRPS 1.[21] Few progress to atrophic changes or osteoporosis, and the resumption of weight-bearing should occur as soon as possible.[2] Sympathetic blocks for analgesia have a role in children, to allow physiotherapy and mobilization, although their timing is debatable.[2]

ANIMAL BEHAVIOUR MODEL

Several features of chronic inflammation and nerve damage can be reproduced in experimental animal models to help to understand the mechanisms that underlie the pain and cutaneous disorders in patients with CRPS and other neuropathic disorders, and to examine the validity of new therapeutic approaches.[22] Disturbances in the peripheral nervous system after peripheral nerve injury (e.g. from axotomies or tight, partially tight or loose ligatures) cause perivascular sympathetic fibres to sprout into and surround the dorsal root ganglion, or to sprout to the neuroma. Denervated blood vessels in the periphery lose their sympathetic innervation, which is limited to the segment of the vessel in the affected area.[22] The principal generative site of abnormal activity in sensory neurones is the cell body within the dorsal root ganglion, explaining why the inhibition of peripheral fibre excitability provides only mild or temporary relief.[22] In general, the animal models for sympathetically maintained pain suggest the involvement of α-adrenergic receptors.[12]

MECHANISM OF SYMPATHETICALLY MAINTAINED PAIN

The pathogenesis of CRPS has been speculated as being either a disease process of either peripheral nerves, peripheral soft tissue the spinal cord (Figure 10.1).[17] The pathophysiology of CRPS has not yet been full elucidated, with suggested coupling between sympathetic and somatosensory pathways at central and peripheral sites.[2] Several theories have been proposed but none proven. This is clearly a complex syndrome without a simple pathophysiological explanation, although both direct and indirect methods of excitation of nociceptors by noradrenaline have been proposed.[2] Nerve injury and soft tissue injury may lead to sensitization of nociceptors to adrenergic agents.[12] Different classes of events that may induce CRPS indicate that peripheral (neural and non-neural) and central mechanisms are involved.[23] The crucial pathophysiological process triggered by nerve

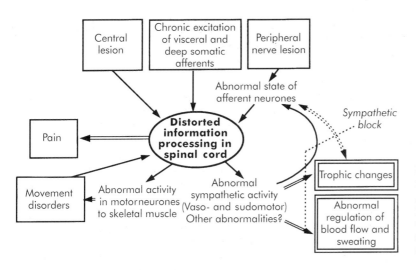

Figure 10.1 Some postulated neural mechanisms for the generation of complex regional pain syndromes following central lesions, the chronic stimulation of visceral afferents and peripheral nerve lesions.

injury is an increase in neuronal excitability, which most probably results from the remodelling of membrane electrical properties.[24] C polymodal nociceptors activate and sensitize dorsal horn WDR neurones, which then respond to activity in large-diameter A mechanoreceptors, which are activated by light touch.[2] In sympathetically maintained pain, A mechanoreceptor activity is maintained by sympathetic efferent action in the absence of cutaneous simulation.[2] Subcutaneous local anaesthetic injection, cooling of the receptor field and the intravenous injection of the alpha-blocker phentolamine abolishes the sympathetic activation of WDR neurones.[2]

Sympathetic efferent fibres travelling with somatosensory afferent fibres account for sympathetically maintained pain. As a result of injury, nociceptors upregulate the expression of α_1-adrenergic receptors.[9] These are activated by the release of noradrenaline in the local tissues, and pain develops.[12] There is thus a coupling between the α_1-adrenergic receptor function and the activation of the pain signalling system, resulting in central sensitization. New evidence suggests that central mediation may be via the NMDA receptors.[25] Input from low-threshold mechanoreceptors leads to pain. In sympathetically maintained pain, the efferent activity in the sympathetic nervous system acquires the capacity to activate C polymodal nociceptors and may thus be directly activated by noradrenaline.[2,9] The ongoing activity in the nociceptor also maintains the central signalling neurones in a sensitized state.[14] Also, following nerve damage, noradrenaline perivascular axons have been shown to sprout into the dorsal ganglion and form basket-like structures around large-diameter sensory

neurones, allowing sympathetic stimulation to repetitively activate sensory neurones.[2]

There may, however, be two possible locations of the action of noradrenaline in the same axon: one in the periphery and the other in the dorsal root ganglion. It is possible that, during the time course of the disease, the location of the origin of abnormal ectopic impulses shifts in the same fibres from the periphery to the dorsal root ganglion.[26] Thus, cutaneous noradrenaline application can aggravate the pain in some but not all sympathetically maintained pain patients.[27] The noradrenaline reaction can change over time (as can the pain-relieving effects of sympatholytic therapy).[27]

Noradrenaline may also act indirectly via prostaglandin release, which stimulates the nociceptor.[2] Under pathological conditions, the noradrenaline released from sympathetic postganglionic neurones can stimulate prostaglandin release.[2] CRPS with patchy osteoporosis may have two components: neuropathic pain (including severe spontaneous pain or persistent mechanical allodynia) and prolonged regional inflammation, the early phase of which might be indicated by the positive inflammatory symptoms of pain (tenderness), heat, swelling and loss of function, and their alleviation by corticosteroids.[28] Inflammation *per se* may therefore play a part in the development of CRPS 1. Immunoglobulin G labelled with indium-111 is concentrated in the affected extremity, proving an increased microvascular permeability for high molecular weight proteins, an important characteristic of inflammation.[18,29] Thus sympathetically maintained pain could be postulated to occur if inflammation persisted or the C nociceptor responsiveness to noradrenaline did not disappear with healing.[2]

GENETIC PREDISPOSITION

In CRPS 1, a two-fold increase in A3, B7 and DR2(15) MHC antigens was found to be associated with poor treatment outcomes, reflecting a possible genetic diasthesis.[30] Caucasians show a higher incidence of CRPS in some series.[2]

DIFFERENTIAL DIAGNOSIS

For a hot, red painful extremity, the differential diagnosis includes local pathology (sprain and fracture), septic arthritis, cellulitis and allergy.[2] Vascular insufficiency (Raynaud's disease, thrombosis and thromboangiitis obliterans) or disuse may result in a cold, blue atrophic limb.[2]

CLINICAL COURSE

Regardless of the cause or location of the precipitating event, the symptoms almost always appear in the distal part of an extremity.[31] They spread independently of both the source and the site of the precipitating event, presenting with a stocking and glove anatomical distribution. Three stages of progression traditionally occur, although the value of staging is questionable as the duration of the first two stages is variable and it is not possible to predict who will progress to the third atrophic stage, even when prolonged limb disuse increases atrophic changes.[2,32]

Stage I (acute phase)

This phase, which may last from days to months, is often missed. Burning pain, tenderness and local muscle spasm occur at the site of the injury. The limb may be warm, red and dry, or cool and pale. This condition responds rapidly to treatment.[20] Sympathetic hypoactivity occurs with rapid nail and hair growth, and heat intolerance.

Stage II (dystrophic phase)

Pain can remain unchanged, increase or decrease. Sympathetic hyperactivity now occurs. Local brawny oedema is often the first notable change in the skin, with gradual thickening and coarsening of the skin over a time course of days to a few weeks. Abnormal sympathetic activity induces increased vasoconstriction on the post-capillary side compared with the precapillary side, leading to the oedema.[33] Changes distal to the site of injury are seen. Muscle shortening and stiffening of the local and then the regional joints takes place. The affected limb is cold and moist,[20] and may be pale or cyanotic. Patchy osteoporosis occurs.[28] The response to treatment is attenuated. Symptoms may persist for many months.

Stage III (atrophic phase)

The pain (usually aching) now becomes constant. The skin thus loses its normal wrinkles and becomes smooth and tight. The hair coarsens, and the nails become thickened and brittle. The capsules of the joint shrink, the movements of such joints being painful.[34] The muscles atrophy. The affected limb is cold, damp and almost immobile. Diffuse osteoporosis occurs. Psychological abnormalities may be present.[20] Treatment is unlikely to help, and the changes may be permanent.[20]

Recurrences

Many aspects of the bilateral presentation or recurrence of CRPS 1 are unknown.[35] However, recurrent CPRS episodes have been reported to occur in 10–30 per cent of patients, and migratory symptoms involving multiple extremities have also been reported.[2] In a series of 1183 patients, the incidence of recurrence was 1.8 per cent per patient per year.[35] Young patients in whom a CRPS 1 started with a cold skin temperature have the highest chances of experiencing a recurrence. Recurrences can be found in one or more limbs other than the first limb. Most recurrences are spontaneous and present with few signs and symptoms.[35] Very rarely do amputations for pain result in relief.[2]

DIAGNOSIS OF SYMPATHETICALLY MAINTAINED PAIN

The diagnosis of sympathetically maintained pain can be complex, based on clinical symptoms and signs supplemented by carefully performed and interpreted tests, as there are few data on the sensitivity and specificity of these tests.[2,11] No single test has adequate sensitivity and specificity to distinguish conclusively between sympathetically maintained pain and sympathetically independent pain.[2] There is no definitive way to diagnose sympathetically maintained pain on the basis of signs, symptoms or clinical history. In particular, signs that may be inferred to represent increased sympathetic activity in the painful area do not denote the presence of sympathetically maintained pain. Sympathetically maintained pain may be suspected in a patient who has otherwise unexplained pain, and pain in one of the extremities or the face. The presence of cooling hyperalgesia is a sensitive but non-specific marker for sympathetically maintained pain.[12] (Only approximately 50 per cent of patients with sympathetically independent pain have cooling hyperalgesia.[12])

The diagnosis of sympathetically maintained pain may be substantiated by the intravenous infusion of the non-specific α-adrenergic blocking agent phentolamine (which is conducive to the avoidance of placebo blocking effects).[36] Pain relief from phentolamine shows that the direct blockade of afferent fibres is likely not to be responsible for the relief of pain as phentolamine has no direct effect on somatic function.

CLINICAL FINDINGS OF CRPS 1 AND 2

Because of the diffuse nature, the differences in pain intensity and clinical features, and a variable onset time of these clinical features, this syndrome may be missed.[20] Patients should be graded according to the intensity of their presenting sensory, autonomic and motor changes as being mild, moderate or severe.

History

Trauma may precede the onset. Pain is usually continuous and burning, felt initially in the distal part of the limb but later spreading diffusely to involve the limb girdle. It can be exacerbated by exposure to cold, anxiety and light touch.

Physical findings[20,31,37]

Pain

The pain is disproportional in distribution, severity and duration to that expected from the inciting event.[2] An initial burning distal pain becomes diffuse and aching, fluctuating in intensity.[2] This may be accompanied by hyperalgesia to thermal stimulation, joint movement, light touch and deep pressure. Hypoaesthesia or hyperaesthesia, and allodynia to cold and mechanical stimuli, may occur.

Autonomic deregulation

Vasomotor and sudomotor control are substantially altered in CRPS.[38,39] Alterations in blood flow occur, and the skin may feel warm (early CRPS 1) or cold and be pale. It may have a reddened or cyanosed appearance. In the acute stage, vasomotor control is decreased in the affected limb, whereas sudomotor function is enhanced.[38] Later, hyperhydrosis or hypohydrosis may be present. Oedema of the extremity may occur in fewer than 50 per cent of patients. This may be because of increased filtration pressure (from sympathetic vasoconstriction of the post-capillary venules exceeding precapillary arterio-constriction) or neuropeptide release (from sympathetic post-ganglionic neurones or primary afferent nociceptors).[2] Increased or decreased sweating can occur with side-to-side asymmetry between the affected and non-affected limbs.[2]

Motor dysfunction

Reduced joint movement, reduced muscle strength and tremor may be apparent but are not essential criteria for CRPS.[2] Patients attempt to protect their hyperalgesic limb by limiting its range of movement.

Trophic changes

The skin may appear smooth and shiny, with muscle wasting. Changes in the hair (coarse hair) and nail growth patterns (thickening) may occur. Joint stiffness from trophic changes and/or functional motor disturbances may be apparent.[2] Osteoporosis is a non-specific sign, occurring in a small percentage of cases.

Psychological reactive disturbances

Stressful life events are more common in CRPS patients.[40] There is no evidence that a particular psychological profile predisposes to CRPS.[2] As symptoms are disproportionate to the injury, maladaptive behaviours may be misinterpreted as psychopathology.[2] Anxiety, depression and hopelessness, in common with other chronic pain patients, may occur. Behavioural responses are especially important with CRPS as immobilization and limb overprotection exacerbates demineralization, vasomotor changes, trophic changes and oedema.[2]

DIAGNOSTIC TESTS FOR CRPS 1 AND 2[20,37]

AUTONOMIC

Autonomic dysfunction can be detected by changes in skin temperature (thermography and thermometry).[2] Bilateral symmetrical multidigital temperature measures using surface thermistors or thermography show consistent discrepancies (cooler or warmer) on the affected side. In the ice cold stress challenge test, both extremities (the involved and the uninvolved) are cooled to 5°C and then warmed up again. The clinician then looks at all the digits to determine what the blood flow (even capillary flow) is in that extremity, in terms of both temperature and laser flow Doppler studies.[25] The thermal grill may be a useful tool in understanding CRPS.[41] Touching cool elements with the affected CRPS hand produces an intense burning sensation (cold allodynia), whereas touching warm elements produces a pleasant warm sensation.[41] In CRPS patients, the intravenous administration of sodium amytal, a medium-acting barbiturate, tended to warm many of their limbs as a result of central changes in thermoregulatory control.[42] Stress infrared thermography has been found to be a sensitive and specific indicator of CRPS 1.[43]

SENSORY

There are lowered thresholds to pinprick, light touch and cold.

MOTOR

A reduced measure of strength as well as decreased active and passive range of motion occur.

LOCAL ANAESTHETIC BLOCKADE RESPONSE

Sympathetic block with local anaesthetic usually abolishes the diffuse burning pain and allodynia,

raises the skin temperature to 35–36°C and abolishes the vasoconstrictor response to cold stimulation. However, sympathetic blockade is not always reliable and specific for sympathetic pain as local anaesthetic can spread to nearby somatic nerves in which sensory fibres run. The systemic load of local anaesthetic in the paravertebral space may independently evoke pain relief.[9] It is difficult to obviate placebo effects. Invasive sympathetic blocks may be associated with a high expectation of pain relief, and the number of placebo responders can vary markedly from zero to 100 per cent, usually being about 30 per cent.[2] False negatives may occur if the local anaesthetic fails to reach the targeted ganglia. Damaged primary afferents generate spontaneous ectopic impulses, which are highly sensitive to the low doses of local anaesthetic that may be obtained from systemic absorption.[44] False-positive results may indicate the spread of local anaesthetic to the somatic fibres.[2] Additionally, sensory fibres from deep somatic elements may be blocked as they traverse the sympathetic rami and chain.[2] Large local anaesthetic doses may contribute to systemic analgesia, while low lignocaine concentrations have a selective action on nociceptive transmission in the spinal cord.[2]

BONE SCAN

Non-specific changes may occur with imaging, partly because of disuse.[2] Long bone periarticular osteoporosis and diffuse small bone osteoporosis may be seen on plain X-rays.[2] Three-phase (flow, pool and static phase) scanning shows distinctive patterns of increased flow, pooling and delay in the affected limb.[2] MRI can show skin thickening or thinning and soft tissue oedema.[2] There may be a poor correlation between clinical staging, bone scanning and thermography in staging CRPS 1.[45]

INTRAVENOUS REGIONAL BLOCKADE WITH GUANETHIDINE

Guanethidine absorbed into the sympathetic nerve terminal causes initial noradrenaline release before persistent noradrenaline depletion for a couple of days.[2] A negative test does not exclude sympathetic–afferent coupling proximal to the cuff (spinal cord).[2] Burning during intravenous injection from noradrenaline release has been suggested to indicate sympathetically maintained pain.[2]

INTRAVENOUS PHENTOLAMINE

A new diagnostic test using phentolamine has been developed.[46,47] Systemic α-adrenergic blockers have been found to decrease the pain and hyperalgesia associated with sympathetically maintained pain without affecting sympathetically independent pain. The patient is placed in the supine position. ECG and blood pressure monitoring are mandatory. An intravenous line is established (screened off from the patient), and a baseline pain level is established via sensory testing (using a visual analogue scale [stimulus independent], a soft hairbrush, blunt pressure or a tuning fork [mechanical test] and a drop of acetone or ethyl chloride [cold test]).[9] The patient receives a bolus of Ringer's solution (300–500 mL) followed by 2 mL/kg per hour throughout the test. Sensory testing takes place every 5 minutes for at least 30 minutes or until a stable pain level is achieved. If the pain level decreases substantially, the patient may be a placebo responder and phentolamine is not given. Propranolol (up to 2 mg) is slowly titrated intravenously. Phentolamine (1 mg/kg) is then slowly infused over 10 minutes with the patient blinded in order to block α-adrenoreceptor function adequately. A lower dose is given in children. Sensory testing is repeated every 5 minutes during the infusion and for 30 minutes afterwards.[9] This test allows sympathetically maintained pain to be assessed anywhere in the body, avoids false-positive results from somatic nerve blockade and allows blinded placebo controlled infusions to be administered.[2] Because of minor potassium channel blockade and direct smooth muscle relaxation by phentolamine, the specificity of this test has been questioned.[2] The analgesic response to intravenous phentolamine has been shown to be predictive of pain reduction following subsequent sympathetic blocks.[2]

NON-SPECIFIC CONFIRMATORY TESTS

These include radiographic densitometry testing for osteopaenia, water displacement plethysmography for measures of swelling, tests of sudomotor function such as skin conductivity or potentials, quantitative sweat testing (e.g. ninhydrin or starch iodide) and plain X-rays (for patchy demineralization of the bones). An objective measure of the interruption of sympathetic function is the skin potential response, which can be monitored using a ECG lead on the palm and the dorsum of the hand to show the potential difference, which is altered by sweat gland activity.[10]

OTHERS

Vasomotor tone can be determined by measuring skin blood flow with laser Doppler flow meters and skin temperatures by infrared thermometry. Resting and evoked sweat output can be measured by the quantitative sudomotor axon reflex test.[48]

THERAPY OF SYMPATHETICALLY MAINTAINED PAIN

Sympatholysis remains the mainstay of treatment for sympathetically maintained pain.[11] Some patients have sustained relief from one or more sympathetic ganglion blocks (with local anaesthetic).[11] Local anaesthetic sympathetic ganglion blockade inhibits the release of noradrenaline from the sympathetic terminals, and the central sensitization is reversed such that low-threshold mechanoreceptors no longer produce activity in the central pain-signalling neurones.[9] Systemic phentolamine may be just as useful.[49] Others require sustained sympatholysis, which may be achieved by continuous epidural infusions of low concentrations of local anaesthetic, by oral agents (phenoxybenzamine and prazosin), by transdermal clonidine (which relieves the pain by inhibiting noradrenaline release in the affected skin) or by neuroablative sympatholysis (neurolytic, radiofrequency or surgical).[9,11,36]

The roles of neurolytic and surgical sympathectomy are not clear.[2] Surgical sympathectomy can dramatically relieve sympathetically maintained pain, but often only minimal or short-term improvements are achieved, especially if a diagnostic delay occurs.[2] A recent study of long-term outcome after surgical sympathectomy showed that 100 per cent of patients who underwent sympathectomy within 12 months of injury, 69.2 per cent of those who had sympathectomies within 24 months of injury and only 44.4 per cent of patients who were treated by surgical sympathectomy after 24 months of injury obtained permanent symptom relief.[50] Patient age, sex and occupation, the site and type of injury, the presence of trophic changes and the duration of follow-up were not significantly related ($P > 0.05$) to surgical outcome.[50] It has been suggested that neuroablative procedures should be reserved for CRPS type 2 after conservative management has failed (C.J. Glynn, 1997, personal communication). Also, treatment failures reflect an inadequacy of diagnosis or a lack of knowledge of sympathetic denervation. For example, failure to remove the thoracic T2 and T3 ganglia will result in a lack of denervation of the hand.[12] Some patients require contralateral sympathectomy as well. Endoscopic surgery using radiofrequency techniques can be safe and effective in about a third of patients.[2,12]

Surgeons may occasionally be involved with the placement of percutaneous catheters, the release of muscle or joint contractures and the pinning of contracted joints.[51]

MANAGEMENT OF CRPS

Early recognition and treatment are associated with the best chance of a successful outcome in patients with CRPS.[2] There are very few controlled studies for any of the therapeutic modalities used in CRPS *per se*, and a void of detailed outcome measures.[1] Few blinded randomized studies of different treatment modalities have been performed so treatment is based on clinical experience and symptom control.[52] A critical review of controlled clinical trials for CRPS showed long-term analgesic effectiveness with corticosteroids.[53] There was limited support for the long-term effectiveness of topical dimethylsuphoxide, epidural clonidine and intravenous regional ganglion blockade with bretylium and ketanserin.[53] Topical capsaicin showed a significant analgesic effect.[53] Intranasal calcitonin, intravenous phentolamine, and intravenous regional ganglion blockade with guanethidine, reserpine, droperidol and atropine were ineffective.[53] Patients with sympathetic pain who were not repeatedly treated with sympathetic blocks were followed up for 10 years.[54] Their sensory abnormalities remained fairly constant, with allodynia to both cooling and heat persisting. A failure rate of some 40 per cent of patients to achieve lasting benefit from the management of CRPS has prompted a new algorithm to advance management.[1,55] One recent longitudinal study of CRPS in 1348 patients revealed that 96 per cent of the study subjects still suffered some pain and disability regardless of the duration of the disease or the course of treatment.[17]

The central theme is functional restoration with a coordinated progressive approach that introduces each of the treatment modalities in an individual way with extreme flexibility to achieve both remission and rehabilitation.[55] The underlying principles are motivation, mobilization and desensitization facilitated by the relief of pain, as well as the use of pharmacological and interventional procedures to treat signs and symptoms.[55] Self-management techniques are emphasized, and functional rehabilitation is the key to success of this algorithm.[55] There is no specific treatment that will successfully relieve the pain of CRPS types 1 and 2 in all patients. Reactivation with specific exercise therapy and stimulation to re-establish function is an essential goal for CRPS therapy.[1,55] The various modalities used, including analgesia by pharmacological means or by regional anaesthesia or the use of neuromodulation, behavioural management and the qualitatively different approaches that are unique to the management of children with CRPS, are provided to facilitate functional improvement in a stepwise but methodical manner.[55] These patients usually require multimodal therapy to provide adequate analgesia in order to use the affected limb normally. The management of biosocial factors is critical to achieving a successful outcome.[55] Psychotherapy helps patients to cope, comply and continue.[11] Priorities of care are pain relief, functional restoration, the treatment of psychological co-morbidity, patient motivation and compliance with therapy, and the avoidance of known precipitating nociceptive triggers.[1] Treatments should not advance to surgical procedures until all other options have been tried to their limits.[1] Clinical features and the response to blocks or trials of treatment may help to reveal the extent to which the pain is composed of true nociceptive stimuli, sympathetically maintained pain or central pain. More specific targeted treatments can then be applied.

Treatment of the precipitating injury

Treatment must include adequate management of the precipitating injury to minimize ongoing nociceptive stimulation from traumatized tissue, inflammation or infection.[2] Possibilities include debridement, fracture reduction, the repair of torn tendons, muscles, ligaments or nerves, and the treatment of any infection. In the animal model, the pre-emptive use of local anaesthetic delayed the development of autotomy after peripheral nerve section by several weeks.[56] Use should therefore be made of regional anaesthetic techniques wherever possible when treating the precipitating injury.[57]

Analgesic interventions

SYMPATHETIC BLOCKS

These are carried out if sympathetic pain is suspected in order to diagnose the site of the pain and the contribution (if any) of the sympathetic nervous system.[20] Before the block is performed, a baseline history and examination are recorded. False-positive (e.g. blockade of adjacent somatic nerve fibres or a placebo response) and false-negative responses can occur, and the therapeutic result may outlast the block.[58] A successful block is followed by subjective and functional improvement. The effect of the block should be assessed in comparison to the baseline examination, and objective evidence that the block is working should be obtained.

Intravenous regional block

There is animal and clinical evidence that tourniquet occlusion itself is capable of producing pain relief from A beta fibre blockade, irrespective of the additional action of systemic lignocaine on sodium channels, or of NMDA and spinal-mediated wind down or a placebo response.[1] This poses a question on the continued use of intravenous regional local blocks.

Guanethidine. This produces a blocking effect on sympathetic nerve endings by uncoupling pharmacological mechanisms associated with release of noradrenaline, adenosine triphosphate and neuropeptide Y, all of which can affect the tone of vascular smooth muscle.[59] It may last for up to 3 days, sometimes longer (Figure 10.2).[20] Uniform pressure is applied to the limb for 20 minutes. This pressure must exceed the systolic pressure by a minimum of 50 mm and 100 mm in the upper and lower limb respectively. The initial dose should be limited to 10 mg because of the marked release of noradrenaline giving vasoconstriction on first use. In subsequent blocks (within 3–5 days), there is less release of noradrenaline, and the dose of guanethidine can be increased. It should not exceed 30 mg in any single block or 150 mg in any course of treatment.[59] The dose of guanethidine is adjusted according to the size of limb and the physical status of the patient. Saline diluent 25 mL are used in the arm and 50 mL in the thigh. Postural hypotension may occur.

Two recent studies have shown no benefit of intravenous regional guanethidine over placebo ischaemic arm blocks in the treatment of CRPS.[60,61] Yet a recent study claimed that some patients diagnosed 17–26 years ago still had long-lasting pain

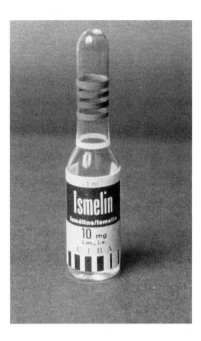

Figure 10.2 Ampoule of guanethidine (Ismelin®) for intravenous regional sympathetic nerve blockade.

relief after intravenous regional guanethidine blockade.[62] However, randomized controlled trials have not supported the use of guanethidine in 'reflex sympathetic dystrophies.'[63] Patients in all groups reported less than 30 per cent of the maximum possible pain relief during the first week after the injections, and on only two occasions (one saline and one low-dose guanethidine) was relief reported for longer than a week.[63] There was also no evidence of a dose response for guanethidine.[63]

Bretylium. Bretylium 2 mg/kg in 30–50 mL normal saline or 0.5 per cent lignocaine can be given using a similar tourniquet technique (Figure 10.3).[32] A well-designed study showed the combination of bretylium with lignocaine to be more effective than lignocaine alone in patients with a previous positive improvement after sympathetic nerve blockade.[64]

Clonidine. No reported difference in pain intensity was found with intravenous regional sympathetic blockade with clonidine despite the sympathetic blockade being effective.[65]

Ketorolac. Ketorolac 60 mg has been found to have some beneficial effects in CRPS patients because of the reduction of prostaglandin release and interfer-

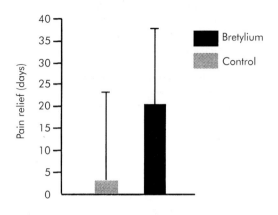

Figure 10.3 Twelve patients with CRPS type 1 received two control treatments (with 0.5 per cent lignocaine) and two treatments (with 0.5 per cent lignocaine + bretylium 1.5 mg/kg) in a randomized double-blind fashion. A standard intravenous regional technique was used. Bretylium + lignocaine provided more than 30 per cent pain relief for a mean of 20 (± 17.5) days, whereas lignocaine alone provided relief for only 2.7 (± 3.7) days.

ence with the vasoconstriction produced by thromboxane.[2]

Others[59]. Other drugs are also available:

- ketanserin, a selective serotonin type 2 receptor antagonist, which, in double-blind trials, resulted in greater pain reduction than the control treatment;[2]
- lysine acetylsalicylate (to block prostaglandins);
- naftidrofuryl (to block bradykinin);
- methylprednisolone 80 mg in 30–50 mL 0.5 per cent lignocaine;[32]
- labetolol (a mixed alpha- and beta-receptor blocking drug);
- reserpine, hydrallazine and thymoxamine.

Local anaesthetic sympathetic block

Early sympathetic blockade has been advocated in adults, although its efficacy has been difficult to determine because of limitations in the current literature, and natural resolution or placebo response cannot be discounted (as there are no controlled trials).[2] Of 500 patients treated with sympathetic blocks and reviewed after 3 years, 46 per cent received satisfactory pain relief.[66] If sympathectomy (whether local anaesthetic ganglion blockade or intravenous regional blockade) fails to produce the desired pain relief, continuous sensorineural blocking techniques such as epidural infusion (with local

anaesthetic) can be tried. This combines sensory and sympathetic blockade.[67]

Stellate (cervicothoracic) ganglion block. Classical approaches to the stellate ganglia are found in many standard text books.[68,69] Anterior paratracheal as well as lateral, anterolateral, superior and posterior approaches have all been described. An anterior paratracheal approach is most commonly used, the needle being placed on the anterior tubercle of the 6th cervical vertebra (C6) on the involved side[70] (Figures 10.4 and 10.5). Another approach has the needle angled more medially to make contact with the body of the vertebra rather than the transverse process.[71] This decreases the possibility of vertebral artery puncture or pneumothorax. The blockade of all sympathetic fibres to the upper arm may not be achieved with a stellate ganglion block at C6, and a paravertebral upper thoracic block or interpleural administration in a head-down position has been advocated.[2]

The regional anatomy predicts the potential complications of placement of the needle, and the patient must be carefully monitored. An aspiration test, the use of a prior test dose of local anaesthetic and the use of an isolated needle are recommended.[72] If placed properly, 5 mL local anaesthetic will block the stellate ganglion.[14] This will not reliably block all the fibres from the upper extremities, since contributions from T2 and T3 may be present. A volume of 10 mL local anaesthetic (lignocaine) is injected slowly after re-aspiration to provide an adequate block to the arm, even in patients with

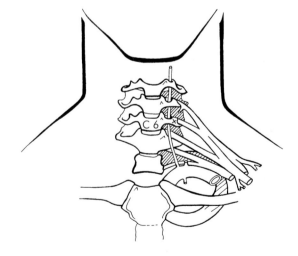

Figure 10.4 Stellate ganglion block. The C6 paratracheal technique. Note the point of contact (X) and the vertebral artery passing behind the C6 anterior tubercle.

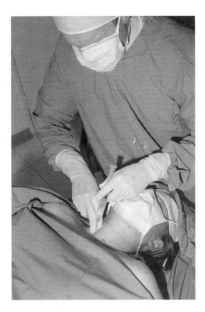

Figure 10.5 Stellate ganglion block in a patient with CRPS type 1 of the upper limb.

anomalous Kuntz nerves.[14,70] A continuous technique has been described in which a thin radio-opaque catheter is introduced under X-ray control using the paratracheal technique.[73] If blockade is being performed for sympathetically mediated viscera (including the heart), 15–20 mL of solution should be administered. A similar approach with the needle directed more caudally towards the lateral mass of C7 at its lower level or T1 near the neck of the first rib is advised for cases requiring sympathetic blockade of the arm.[74]

Horner's syndrome may be present without complete sympathetic denervation of the upper limb (which may receive a sympathetic supply down to T9).[70] An observation of increased venous prominence and warming and dryness of the extremity, along with an attenuation of the skin potential or skin conductance response, is indicative of successful upper extremity sympathetic blockade. Complications include a temporary hoarseness and feeling of a lump in the throat (recurrent laryngeal nerve block), a haematoma, phrenic nerve and brachial plexus blockade, intrathecal and epidural spread, pneumothorax and convulsions from injection into the vertebral artery.

Neurolytic blockade has been successfully used in the management of sympathetic pain. A percutaneous paratracheal approach is made under X-ray control and, following the injection of 0.5 mL contrast medium, phenol 0.5 mL 5 per cent in glycerine or water is instilled.[75] Methyl prednisolone 40 mg and 1–2 mL local anaesthetic may be added.[73] Again, the arm may partially escape, and in these cases an injection of the sympathetic chain at T2 and T3 can be used as a supplement. Because of the proximity of the pleura and the somatic nerves, this technique is not commonly practised.[73] Phenol allows nerve regeneration to occur over time because the concentrations used by most practitioners are too low. When volumes containing 1 g or more (10 mL of 10 per cent solution) are used, phenol can be quite toxic if injected intravascularly, leading to confusion and arrhythmias.[74] Its advantages are a lack of pain on injection, and ready compatibility and enhanced solubility with most commercial iodinated contrast media. Absolute ethyl alcohol is very safe and effective in the destruction of nerve tissue but is painful on injection and incompatible with most commercial iodinated contrast media.[74] Thermocoagulation provides an alternative form of neural destruction, one limited by the radius of effect from each needle placement, such that repeated procedures are often required.[74] Morphine injected around the stellate ganglion does not modulate the sympathetic nervous system nor does it provide pain relief.[76]

Paravertebral thoracic sympathetic block. Permanent selective sympathectomy of the arm is more reliably attained with a posterior approach, injecting alongside the dorsal quadrant of the vertebral bodies just ventral to the heads of the ribs at T2 and T3 levels.[74] Dorsal thoracic approaches with CT imaging offer more benefit when neuroablative sympathectomy is performed, given the lower risks of serious complications.[74] An alternative technique is radiofrequency neurolysis under fluoroscopic control.[74]

Lumbar sympathetic block. There are several variations of the technique, using X-ray control, depending on whether the lumbar sympathetic chain is invested with local anaesthetic or neurolytic on the anterolateral aspect of the body of one, two or three lumbar vertebrae.[75] The patient is placed either on their side or prone (see Figure 10.6). Needle insertion should be 8–10 cm from the midline. Some specialists prefer to avoid the transverse process so that the needle proceeds directly to the lateral aspect of the vertebral body (see Figure 10.6).[69] Safe, reliable, lasting and effective sympathetic blocks are readily obtained by a single injection technique at L3 paravertebrally, or by a double needle technique at the L3 and L4 levels.[74] When a bilateral procedure is

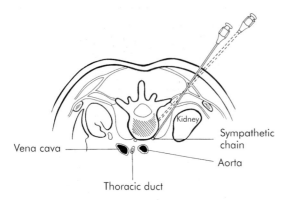

Figure 10.6 Lumbar sympathetic block. Note the initial and final needle positions. See text for details.

required, this can be obtained by a single injection placed in the sagittal plane in a compartment between the vertebral bodies and the great vessels.[74]

A single injection technique uses the tip of the twelfth rib to act as a marker for needle insertion 2–3 cm below and medial to that point (see Figures 10.7–10.11). This allows easy access to the L3 vertebral body and placement next to the sympathetic chain. This technique provides a good spread over two or three segments with volumes of 10–15 mL of local anaesthetic solution. It is vitally important to aspirate to ensure that neither blood nor CSF is present and check that there is no resistance to injection, as it is to inject slowly. The use of contrast medium mixed with local anaesthetic under X-ray control will increase the safety of the technique.[69] For continuous blockade, a catheter can be passed through the needle. Under CT guidance, percutaneous lumbar sympathetic plexus catheter placement is easily performed, achieves short-term pain relief in the majority of patients and generally proves effective in the long-term pain relief of CRPS patients.[77]

The observation of venous prominence, warmth of the ipsilateral extremity, attenuation of the skin potential or skin conductance response and a drop in blood pressure indicate successful sympathetic blockade.[78] Complications include perforation of the kidney or ureter, anaesthesia of the genitofemoral nerve, perforation of an intervertebral disc and subarachnoid block.[78] Perforation of the great vessels is also a possibility.

A neurolytic block can be used where pain relief with serial blockade using local anaesthetic is not prolonged. For a neurolytic block, aqueous phenol solution is the agent of choice.[75] A contrast agent

Case study

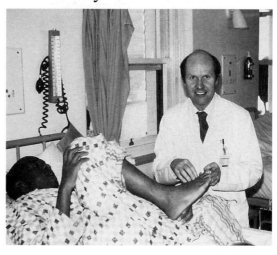

Figure 10.7 Mr AS is a 28 year old man who complained of severe pain over the L_5-S_1 dermatomes of his right leg. He had been shot in his right buttock. He had been placed on intramuscular pethidine for 6 weeks with no relief of his pain and could not walk.

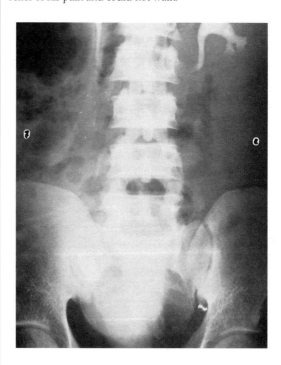

Figure 10.8 When referred to the Pain Relief and Research Unit at the University of Witwatersrand, an x-ray revealed a bullet fragment at the greater sciatic notch. A diagnosis of CRPS type 2 was made.

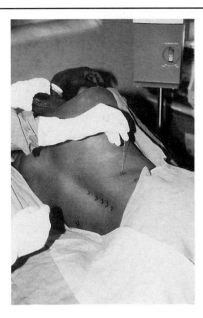

Figure 10.9 A lumbar sympathectomy was performed at L$_3$.

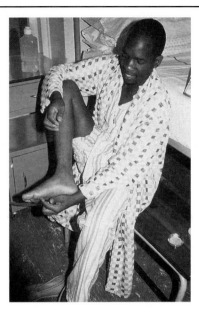

Figure 10.11 The pain decreased. The pethidine was stopped. He received aggressive physiotherapy and was soon able to walk around, and was discharged.

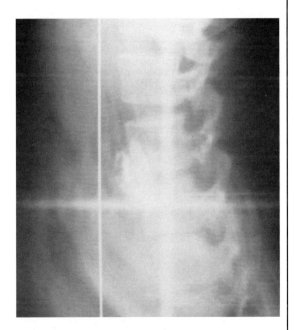

Figure 10.10 Contrast dye was used to confirm the correct placement of the needle.

should first be used to determine linear spread. Saline 0.5 mL should be injected before removing each needle to prevent the needles depositing neurolytic solution on the somatic nerve roots during removal. If segmental somatic nerve neuritis does occur, it can be treated with oral anticonvulsants or with a local injection of bupivacaine and methylprednisolone.[75]

Coeliac plexus block. Blockade of the coeliac plexus will interrupt the sympathetic and afferent pathways that traverse it. It has been shown to be an effective method for the relief of upper abdominal pain. In combination with lumbar sympathetic blockade, it has been used in treating painful disorders of the abdomen and the leg, including CRPS type 2.[79] It is now primarily reserved for the treatment of pain caused by malignancy of the upper abdominal viscera and for chronic pancreatitis.

The classical technique for percutaneous injection of the coeliac plexus involves the bilateral placement of needles just anterior to the body of L1 and posterior to the aorta and diaphragmatic crura, with the patient in the prone position.[80] X-ray control is used and contrast injected. Correct placement is indicated by a layering-out of the contrast in a narrow line along the anterior aspect of the vertebral column. For diagnostic and therapeutic blocks with local anaesthetic, 20 mL of 1 per cent lignocaine with 1:200 000 adrenaline is used on each side. For destructive blocks, 5–10 mL of 1 per cent lignocaine are injected bilaterally to document abdominal pain relief and lack of somatic blockade, and to mitigate against the pain induced by the alcohol that will follow. Twenty-five millilitres of 50 per cent alcohol in saline are then injected through each needle.[76] If 100 per cent alcohol is used, 20 mL of the solution consisting of equal parts of alcohol 100 per cent and bupivacaine 0.5 per cent are injected on each side.[65] The needles are purged with 1 mL saline before removal.

Techniques have recently been described making use of CT scanning or ultrasound to position the needle accurately. The CT scan calculates the distance from the point of entry at the skin to the coeliac artery, the angle of needle entry and the depth.[81]

The transaortic approach, using CT with the patient prone, results in more anterior positioning of the needle tip so that it lies anterior to the diaphragmatic crura. The needle is introduced at a distance of 4 ± 1 cm from the left of the midline, the tip being positioned over the posterior wall of the aorta at the level of the coeliac trunk.[82] The aorta is then perforated and the needle driven across it. There is now less tendency for the injected solution to spread posteriorly to the paravertebral nerve roots or sympathetic chain, minimizing the risk of orthostatic hypotension or paresis (if a neurolytic is used).[82]

In the transcrural technique, the needles are introduced at a distance of 6 ± 1 cm from both sides of the midline at a 45 degree angle to the table top until the L1 vertebral body is contacted.[82] The needle is then withdrawn until the tip lies antero-laterally to the aorta and caudally to the diaphragm at the level of the coeliac trunk.

Recent studies describe the percutaneous approach to the coeliac plexus guided by CT or ultrasound with the patient in the supine position. The point of entry is situated in the upper abdominal wall, 1–2 cm below and to the left of the xiphoid process and perpendicular to the skin. The coeliac trunk and the abdominal aorta are then localized with CT or ultrasound, and the needle tip is positioned over the coeliac plexus in the upper pre-aortic area according to the angle of needle entry and the depth, which is calculated by CT or ultrasound.[82] The advantage of this approach is that it allows the patient to remain supine. The spread obtained covers the coeliac plexus without involving the retrocrural region and the psoas compartment (containing the sympathetic chain and lumbar plexus), thus reducing the risk of neurological complications. When compared with CT, ultrasound is quicker and more economical, avoids radiation and does not require a contrast medium: it may prove the future method of choice.[82] CT does, however, provide a better quality image than ultrasound.

Possible complications include pain on injection of alcohol and pain at the site of injection. Orthostatic hypotension is common during the first 48 hours.[78] Increased peristalsis may also occur. Other possible complications include subarachnoid injection, retroperitoneal haematoma and neuralgias of the lower thoracic and lumbar somatic nerves (especially L1), as well as visceral perforation and pneumothorax. Paraplegia is a very rare complication.[78,79]

A recent study using four different percutaneous anterior and posterior approaches to the coeliac plexus was undertaken in patients with chronic pancreatic pain from pancreatitis or carcinoma.[82] All the approaches were effective in treating chronic pancreatic pain, with no significant difference in the analgesia obtained. Patients with pancreatic carcinoma did, however, respond better than those with chronic pancreatitis. Generally speaking, subsequent blocks do not seem to achieve the same degree of success as the original one, especially in patients with chronic pancreatitis.[79] An epidural catheter can also be inserted into the region of the coeliac plexus for continuous infusion.[79]

Splanchnic nerve blocks. An excellent alternative procedure to coeliac plexus blockade is the ablation of the afferent supply to the plexus, namely the greater and lesser splanchnic nerves.[75] The lateral body of T12 is traversed by the nerves, and they can be blocked above the diaphragm at the upper border of T12 with a technique similar to the classical coeliac plexus approach. Needles are placed from either side so that the tips lie on the anterolateral surface of the body of T12.[69] One millilitre of contrast is injected to check that a linear spread has been obtained, on the anteroposterior and lateral views, along the anterolateral aspects of the vertebral bodies immediately above the diaphragm. Local anaesthetic can be injected for a diagnostic block.

For neurolysis, 5 mL of 7 per cent aqueous phenol is instilled through each needle.[75] This procedure is more comfortable for the patient, requires a lower volume of drug and does not result in the same degree of hypotension as does coeliac plexus blockade.[75] If ethyl alcohol is used, at least 21 mL or more of ethyl alcohol 75 per cent need to be injected into each needle.[83] The needles must be kept as close as possible to the vertebral body in order to avoid a pneumothorax.

Interpleural local anaesthesia. Patients with CRPS 1 in the upper limb can be treated with local anaesthetic (0.5 per cent bupivacaine with adrenaline 1:200 000) via an interpleural catheter inserted through the fourth intercostal space.[84] The patient is positioned in the lateral decubitus position with the affected side up and the head down 20 degrees. The local anaesthetic is slowly injected into the pleural space and diffuses through the medial surface of the parietal pleura to block the cervical portion of the sympathetic chain, including the stellate ganglion.[84] The catheter can be left *in situ* (for up to 5 days), and top-up doses can be given.[84]

REGIONAL LOCAL ANAESTHETIC BLOCK

Anecdotal reports attest to the value of somatic in addition to sympathetic blockade in the management of advanced CRPS 1 as pain may be arising from somatic sources.[67] Patients unresponsive to intermittent sympathetic blockade may benefit from continuous local anaesthetic blockade for several days to obtain analgesia and assess the passive range of movement.[2] Continuous sympathetic blockade can be obtained by a catheter in the vicinity of the sympathetic chain.[25] Infraclavicular catheters over the brachial plexus may be a better way of providing sympathetic blockade to the upper extremity than are stellate ganglion blocks, and lumbar paravertebral catheters have been used to provide prolonged lumbar sympathetic blockade.[2,25] Dilute concentrations of local anaesthetics should be used to minimize motor block.[2]

EPIDURAL OR INTRATHECAL BLOCK

This was discussed in Chapter 9. In resistant cases with established central sensitization, treatment at a spinal cord level is often required to provide analgesia and to facilitate physiotherapy.[2] Epidural catheter infusions using local anaesthetics, opioids and α_2-adrenergic agonists (and maybe NMDA antagonists such as ketamine) as combinations may be the optimal therapy for CRPS. Catheters can be placed in the cervical, thoracic and lumbar epidural spaces. The careful monitoring of patients with cervical epidural infusions is essential.[2] Following the continuous epidural administration of a very low dose of ketamine (25 μg/kg per hour) for 10 days, complete pain relief was obtained in a patient with CRPS type 2 without any side-effects.[85]

Implantable pumps with intrathecal catheters have made possible the long-term administration of intrathecal drugs.[2] Intrathecal morphine as well as local anaesthetic has benefited intractable CRPS patients.[2,86]

CLONIDINE

When applied to limbs with CRPS, transdermal clonidine, by reducing noradrenaline release at presynaptic α_2-adrenergic receptors, decreases pain/hyperalgesia in the areas of application.[2] There is no consistent evidence for the use of oral clonidine in CRPS.[2] Neuraxially administered α_2-adrenergic agonists diminish pain in CRPS by reducing the sympathetic nervous system activity and decreasing the transmission of pain information at the level of the spinal cord.[87] Epidural clonidine (300 and 700 μg) significantly reduced pain in extremely recalcitrant CRPS 1 patients, offering hope for such cases.[87] Some of these patients then obtained sustained analgesia on epidural infusions of clonidine (10–50 μg per hour) for a mean duration of 43 days.[87] Smaller bolus doses of epidural clonidine, followed by infusions of 20–30 μg per hour for 5–7 days, have been used.[2] When recurrent or prolonged treatment was required, a subcutaneous portal and tunnelled epidural catheter was inserted for the patient to self-administer clonidine until the symptoms resolved.[2]

Post-sympathectomy neuralgia

This occurs 5–10 days after a surgical or chemical sympathectomy, its incidence ranging from 30 to 50 per cent.[88,89] Classically, it consists of an aching discomfort in the dermatomal distribution immediately proximal to that of the sympathetic denervation. The aetiology of the pain remains obscure.[88] It usually resolves spontaneously over 2–10 weeks.[88] It was recently proposed to be a complex neuropathic and central deafferentation/reafferentation syndrome dependent on the transection of paraspinal somatic and visceral afferents within the sympathetic trunk, the cell death of many axotomized afferent neurones and the persistent sensitization of spinal neurones by painful conditions prior to sympathectomy. Viscerogenic convergence, collateral afferent sprouting and sympathetically maintained pain mechanisms seem important in the development of this syndrome.[89] It is rare in the absence of prior pain.[89]

Physical and exercise treatment

The overriding principle is the restoration of function, increasing the range of movement in the painful area to recover function, promoting circulation and increasing the level of bone mineralization, thereby minimizing the effects of disuse.[2] Much of the physiotherapy literature is, however, without outcome audit.[1] Once adequate pain relief has been achieved, it is most important that regular physiotherapy should be instituted (a case of 'use it frequently or lose it'). Aggressive mobilization and exercises with heavy weights should be avoided so as not to exacerbate the complaint. Physiotherapeutic rehabilitation is dealt with more specifically in Chapter 15.

Desensitization

If it is not painful, gentle self-stimulation with contrast temperature baths, gentle squeezing, massage and gentle rhythmical movements is effective. TENS has been used with varying efficacy, successfully treating sympathetically maintained pain in both adults and children.[20] However, other reports indicate an exacerbation of pain with TENS.[32] Electroacupuncture has been used in the treatment of sympathetic pain, showing an improvement in 70 per cent of the patients treated with intensive physiotherapy.[90] Double-blind studies and larger patient numbers are needed to establish the validity of TENS and electroacupuncture in the treatment of CRPS.

Reactivation

On the hour, every hour, self-exercising with low-tension pulleys, light stress loading and ball compression provides somatic afferent stimulation, increases function and decreases swelling. Hand therapy is often the backbone of a treatment programme in CRPS.[91] Scrub and carry movements are often used for upper limb involvement.[2]

Flexibility and strengthening

Under adequate analgesia, the patient then slowly begins to walk, swim or dance as improvement allows. In patients with lower limb involvement, weight-bearing is particularly important.[2]

Ergonomics, aerobics and functional rehabilitation

Normalization of use, gait retraining, work hardening and therapeutic recreation can be valuable extensions of physiotherapy skills.

Implanted peripheral nerve stimulators

Destructive surgical procedures seem of little use in the management of sympathetic pain. Chronic electrical stimulation (either epidurally or centrally) may have a better chance of success, but there is a tendency for patients to escape from control despite the continued efficient operation of their stimulating device over time.[20,92] In CRPS, an 80 per cent success of dorsal column stimulation (in 79 cases) has been reported, but with neurological complications in four of the patients.[93] CRPS patients may have greater vascular reactivity and be more susceptible to spinal artery spasm.[2] A recent trial in 36 patients with advanced CRPS treated with spinal cord stimulation, peripheral nerve stimulation or a combination of both showed pain relief averaging 53 per cent after 3 years.[94]

In recent years, peripheral nerve stimulators have been implanted for the treatment of CRPS 1.[95] The concept is a non-electrode that circumferentially goes around and then sits under a nerve, applying stimulation to it.[96] The technique involves surgically exposing a peripheral nerve and placing that electrode under or next to the nerve, with the electrode tail coming out. Testing should occur over a 2–4-day period. Finally, the tail is internalized with a permanent extension wire to an implanted generator. The technique is identical in both technique and hardware to spinal cord stimulation.[96] The surgical technique used creates a barrier between the nerve and the electrode by covering the electrode with a thin fibrous membrane from intramuscular septa.[95] Nerves used include the median, ulnar, saphenous and tibial nerves. Temporary stimulation is evaluated for a few days. If the result is satisfactory, a permanent programmable stimulating battery pack is implanted.

A rapid reversal of hyperhidrosis, vasoconstriction and allodynia should occur.[95] More long-term follow-up of this modality of treatment is needed. In patients with peripheral nerve symptoms, this technique may be more effective than spinal cord stimulation.[96] In CRPS 1 stage III patients, analysis has shown a long term 67–70 per cent success rate with peripheral nerve stimulation.[96]

Psychotherapy

Patients should be supported to take an active role in their rehabilitation. After the building of a good doctor–patient relationship, the emotional component of the pain and disability needs to be discussed with patients and, if necessary, treated.[97] Patients are anxious, unhappy, frustrated and angry about their pain and disability. They need to be made aware that pain and disability are not the same thing. Other associated features of CRPS are fear avoidance behaviours, an externalized locus of control, somatization, sleeplessness, depression and passiveness.[1] Specific psychological interventions include relaxation training (with relatively good outcomes in 70 per cent of patients), biofeedback and cognitive behavioural management (with some benefit in more than 50 per cent of children) to break the pattern of disuse and the fear of pain.[1,2] Coping strategies can be taught in individual or group sessions. Patients need to understand their condition. Resolution of the vascular changes of CRPS 1 after electroconvulsive therapy raises questions of the possible cerebral contributions of CRPS type 1.[98]

Oral drugs

Differences in the mechanisms of CRPS conditions have meant that clinical trials of these drugs have met with limited success. Few oral drugs are supported by large controlled trials.[2] Short-term heavy opioid dosing may allow the introduction of other therapies.[1] The agents that have been used include the following.[20,99]

α-Adrenergic blockers

Phenoxybenzamine (a post-synaptic α_1- and pre-synaptic α_2-blocker) and prazosin (a selective α_1-blocker) have both been used. In early CRPS, 92 per cent of patients in one series were cured by phenoxybenzamine and/or nifedipine without physiotherapy.[100]

β-Adrenergic blockers

Propranolol has also been used. It possibly acts by blocking the prejunctional β_2-receptor, which will release noradrenaline if stimulated.[20]

Calcium channel blockers

Sympathomimetic amines depend on calcium flux for their action.[20] α-Adrenergic stimulation (with noradrenaline) produces peripheral vasoconstriction secondary to increased calcium entry and mobilization in vascular smooth muscle cells. Calcium channel blockers such as nifedipine have been used.[100] In chronic CRPS, 40 per cent of patients in one series were cured using nifedipine and/or phenoxybenzamine without physiotherapy.[100]

NSAIDs and corticosteroids

Both NSAIDs and, particularly, corticosteroids (e.g. prednisolone) have been successfully used in the management of CRPS. Their actions on central neuronal excitability are often overlooked. They should be used in early care with extensive oedema and joint involvement.[1] In early CRPS 1, they probably decrease plasma extravasation by stabilizing basement membranes. In early CRPS 1, oral steroids can be given at high doses for 3 days and then tapered off over 7–10 days.[32]

Topical capsaicin

Topical capsaicin, the pungent principle of red pepper, has been successfully used in CRPS 1 to reduce local burning, hyperaemia and thermal hyperalgesia.[70] It is particularly effective where thermal hyperalgesia is present. It acts by desensitizing the C fibre nociceptors.[101,102]

Others

A variety of secondary analgesics have been used with success in anecdotal cases and uncontrolled trials. These include the psychoactive agents (tricyclics), membrane-stabilizing drugs (gabapentin and mexilitene), calcitonin and D-phenylalanine.[1,99]

CONCLUSION

Validated scientific facts in the areas of the pathophysiology and treatment of CRPS are lacking, with many hypotheses remaining to be confirmed or modified.[2] The treatment of CRPS emphasizes regaining function by seeking movement and self-generated activation. Factors initiating sympathetically maintained pain remain unclear.[2] Early multimodal intervention is required to reduce pain and autonomic dysfunction, and allow early mobilization.[2] Ongoing functional and pain assessments reduce the secondary effect of disuse.[2] Future drug development includes adenosine, NMDA antagonists (ketamine and magnesium infusions) and cholinergic stimulation.[1] Finally, among a battery of candidates currently emerging in animal models for potential use in CRPS, selective ion channel modulators (particularly subtype-selective potassium channel openers and sodium channel blockers), growth factors and enzyme inhibitors are the most promising.[22,103] Furthermore, the development of NO synthetase inhibitor compounds, or low molecular weight analogues of neural growth factor, may help in unravelling the complexity of the CRPSs and their relationship to the sympathetic nervous system.[11] It remains to be seen whether aggressive early analgesia and/or activation can prevent long-term neuropathic CRPS pain.

REFERENCES

1. **Boas, R.A.** 1996: Treatment guidelines for complex regional pain syndromes. *Refresher Course on Complex Regional Pain Syndromes, 8th World Congress on Pain,* Vancouver, Canada, 1–17.
2. **Walker, S.M. and Cousins, M.J.** 1997: Complex regional pain syndromes: including 'reflex sympathetic dystrophy' and 'causalgia'. *Anaesthesia and Intensive Care* **25**, 113–25.
3. **Merskey, H. and Bogduk, N.** 1994: *Classification of chronic pain.* Seattle: IASP Press, vol. 2, 41–2.
4. **McMahon, S.B.** 1991: Mechanisms of sympathetic pain. *British Medical Bulletin* **47**(3), 584–600.
5. **Bonica, J.J.** 1953: *The management of pain.* Philadelphia: Lea & Febiger, 948.
6. **Van der Laan, L., Ter Laak, H.J., Gabreels-Festen, A. and Goris, R.J.** 1998: Complex regional pain syndrome type 1 (RSD): pathology of skeletal muscle and peripheral nerve. *Neurology* **51**(1), 20–5.
7. **Merskey, H. and Bodduk, N.** 1994: *Classification of chronic pain.* Seattle: IASP Press, vol. 2, 210–12.
8. **Galer, B.S., Bruehl, S. and Harden, R.N.** 1998: IASP diagnostic criteria for complex regional pain syndrome: a preliminary empirical validation study: International Association for the Study of Pain. *Clinical Journal of Pain* **14**(1), 48–54.
9. **Campbell, J.N.** 1996: Complex regional pain syndrome and the sympathetic nervous system. In Campbell, J.N. (ed.) *Pain 1996 – an updated review.* Seattle: IASP Press, 89–96.
10. **Haddox, J.D.** 1996: A call for clarity. In Campbell, J.N. (ed.) *Pain 1996 – an updated review.* Seattle IASP Press, 97–9.
11. **Shipton, E.A. and Hopley, L.A.** 1996: Complex regional pain syndromes and the sympathetic nervous system. *South African Journal of Anaesthesiology and Analgesia* **2**(3), 1.
12. **Campbell, J.N., Raja, S.N., Selig, D.K., Beltzberg, A.J. and Meyer, R.A.** 1994: Diagnosis and management of sympathetically maintained pain. In Fields, H.L. and Liebeskind, J.C. (eds) *Progress in pain research and management.* Seattle: IASP Press, vol. 1, 85–100.
13. **Wilson, P.R.** 1990: Sympathetically maintained pain – principles of diagnosis and therapy. In Stanton-Hicks, M., Janig, J. and Boas, R.A. (eds) *Reflex sympathetic dystrophy.* Boston: Kluwer, 25–8.
14. **Raj, P.P.** 1995: Sympathetic blocks. *Pain and the Sympathetic Nervous System: Special Interest Group Newsletter* (Summer), 5–8.
15. **Kleinest, H.E., Cole, W.M., Wayne, L. et al.** 1973: Post traumatic sympathetic dystrophy. *Orthopedic Clinics of North America* **4**, 917–27.
16. **Pak, T.J., Martin, G.M., Magnes, J.L. et al.** 1970: Reflex sympathetic dystrophy. *Minneapolis Medicine* **53**, 507–12.
17. **Aprile, A.E.** 1998: Complex regional pain syndrome. *AANA Journal* **65**(6), 557–60.
18. **Veldman, P.H.J.M., Reynen, H.M., Arntz, I.E. and Goris, R.J.A.** 1998: Signs and symptoms of reflex sympathetic dystrophy: prospective study of 829 patients. *Lancet* **342**, 1012–16.
19. **Abram, S.E.** 1990: Reflex sympathetic dystrophy: incidence and epidemiology. In Stanton-Hicks, M., Janig, W. and Boas, R.A. (eds) *Reflex sympathetic dystrophy.* Boston: Kluwer, 9–15.
20. **Charlton, J.E.** 1991: Management of sympathetic pain. *British Medical Bulletin* **47**(3), 601–18.
21. **Lynch, M.E.** 1992: Psychological aspects of reflex sympathetic dystrophy: a review of the adult and paediatric literature. *Pain* **49**, 337–47.
22. **Babbedge, R., Dray, A. and Urban, L.** 1995: Complex regional pain syndromes (CRPS): mechanisms and therapy from experimental models. *Pain Reviews* **2**, 298–309.
23. **Janig, W.** 1990: Pathobiology of reflex sympathetic dystrophy: some general considerations. In Stanton-Hicks, M., Janig, J. and Boas, R.A. (eds) *Reflex sympathetic dystrophy.* Boston: Kluwer, 41–54.
24. **Kelly, J.F.** 1994: Sixth International Congress Meets. *Pain and the Sympathetic Nervous System: Special Interest Group Newsletter* (Winter), 1.
25. **Rauck, R. and Salem, W.** 1994: Techniques and treatment modalities for reflex sympathetic dystrophy. *Pain and the Sympathetic Nervous System: Special Interest Group Newsletter* (Winter), 2–3.
26. **Wall, P.D.** 1995: Noradrenaline-evoked pain in neuralgia. *Pain* **63**, 1–2.
27. **Torebojk, E., Wahren, L., Wallin, G., Hallin, R. and Koltzenburg, M.** 1995: Noradrenaline-evoked pain in neuralgia. *Pain* **63**, 11–20.
28. **Moriwaki, K., Yuge, O., Tanaka, H., Sasaki, H., Izumi, H. and Kaneko, K.** 1997: Neuropathic pain and prolonged regional inflammation as two distinct symptomalogical components in complex regional pain syndrome with patchy osteoporosis. *Pain* **72** (1–2), 277–82.
29. **Oyen, W.J.G., Arntz, I.E., Claessens, R.A.M.J., Van der Meer, J.W.M., Corstens, F.H.M. and Goris, R.J.A.** 1993: Reflex sympathetic dystrophy of the hand: an excessive inflammatory response? *Pain* **55**, 151–7.
30. **Mailis, A. and Wade, J.** 1994: Profile of Caucasian

women with possible genetic predisposition to reflex sympathetic dystrophy: a pilot study. *Clinical Journal of Pain* **10**, 210–17.

31. **Blumberg, H., Griesser, H.J. and Hornyak, M.E.** 1990: Mechanisms and role of peripheral blood flow dysregulation in pain sensation and edema in RSD. In Stanton-Hicks, M., Janig, W. and Boas, R.A. (eds) *Reflex sympathetic dystrophy*. Boston: Kluwer, 81–95.

32. **Kettler, R.E.** 1990: Sympathetically maintained pain. In Abram, S.E. (ed.) *The pain clinic manual*. Philadelphia: J.B. Lippincott, 121–33.

33. **Blumberg, H., Hoffmann, V., Mohadjer, M. and Scheremet, R.** 1994: Clinical phenomenology and mechanisms of reflex sympathetic dystrophy: emphasis on edema. In Gebhart, G.F., Hammond, D.L. and Jensen, T.S. (eds) *Progress in pain research and management*. Seattle: IASP Press, vol. 2, 455–81.

34. **De Takats, G.** 1992: Reflex dystrophy of the extremities. *The Pain Clinic* **5**, 41–54.

35. **Veldman, P.H.J.M. and Goris, R.J.A.** 1996: Multiple reflex sympathetic dystrophy: which patients are at risk for developing a recurrence of reflex sympathetic dystrophy in the same or another limb? *Pain* **64**, 463–6.

36. **Shipton, E.A.** 1995: Sympathetic pain – an update. *Modern Medicine* (Jun), 79–81.

37. **Abram, S.E., Blumberg H., Boas, R.A.** *et al*. 1990: Proposed definition of reflex sympathetic dystrophy. In Stanton-Hicks, M., Janig, W., Boas, R.A. (eds), *Reflex sympathetic dystrophy*. Boston: Kluwer, 206–8.

38. **Birklein, F., Riedl, B., Claus, D. and Neundorfer, B.** 1998: Pattern of autonomic dysfunction in time course of complex regional pain syndrome. *Clinical Autonomic Research* **8**(2), 79–85.

39. **Birklein, F., Rield, B., Neundorfer, B. and Handwerker, H.O.** 1998: Sympathetic pattern in patients with complex regional pain syndrome. *Pain* **75**(1), 93–100.

40. **Geertzen, J.H., de Bruijn-Kofman, A.T., de Bruijn, H.P., van der Wiel, H.B. and Dijkstra, P.U.** 1998: Stressful life events and psychological dysfunction in complex regional pain syndrome type I. *Clinical Journal of Pain* **14**(2), 143–7.

41. **Heavner, J.E., Calvillo, O. and Racz, G.B.** 1998: Thermal grill illusion and complex regional pain syndrome type I (reflex sympathetic dystrophy). *Regional Anesthesia* **22**(3), 257–9.

42. **Mailis, A., Plaper, P., Ashby, P., Shoichet, R. and Roe, S.** 1997: Effect of intravenous sodium amytal on cutaneous limb temperatures and sympathetic skin responses in normal subjects and pain patients with and without complex regional pain syndromes (type I and II). Part I. *Pain* **70**(1), 59–68.

43. **Gulevich, S.J., Conwell, T.D., Lane, J.** *et al*. 1997: Stress infrared telethermography is useful in the diagnosis of complex regional pain syndrome, type I (formerly reflex sympathetic dystrophy). *Clinical Journal of Pain* **13**(1), 50–9.

44. **Fields, H.L.** 1992: Editorial. *Pain* **49**, 161–2.

45. **Raj, P.P. and Kelly, J.F.** 1994: Multidisciplinary man-

agement of reflex sympathetic dystrophy. *Pain and the Sympathetic Nervous System: Special Interest Group Newsletter* (Winter), 4–6.

46. **Raja, S.N., Treede, R.D., Tewes, P.A., Davis, K.D., Lim, C. and Campbell, J.N.** 1991: A new diagnostic test for sympathetically maintained pain: systemic phentolamine administration. *Anesthesiology* **71**, A732.

47. **Raja, S.N., Meyer, R.A. and Campbell, J.N.** 1992: Intravenous phentolamine: a placebo-controlled diagnostic test for sympathetically maintained pain. *PSNS – A Publication on Pain and the Sympathetic Nervous System* (Spring), 2–3.

48. **Wilson, R.** 1994: Laboratory findings in reflex sympathetic dystrophy: a preliminary report. *Clinical Journal of Pain* **10**, 235–9.

49. **Dellemijn, P.L., Fields, H.L., Allen, R.R., McKay, W.R. and Rowbotham, M.C.** 1994: The interpretation of pain relief and sensory changes following sympathetic blockade. *Brain* **117**, 1475–87.

50. **Schwartzman, R.J., Liu, J.E., Smullens, S.N., Hyslop, T. and Tahmoush, A.J.** 1997: Long-term outcome following sympathectomy for complex regional pain syndrome type I (RSD). *Journal of Neurological Science* **150**(2), 149–52.

51. **Cooney, W.P.** 1997: Somatic versus sympathetic mediated chronic limb pain. Experience and treatment options. *Hand Clinics* **13**(3), 355–61.

52. **Johnson, P.W. and Carpenter, R.L.** 1990: Temporary increase in leg pain resulting from lumbar sympathetic blockade. *Pain* **42**, 201–3.

53. **Kingery, W.S.** 1997: A critical review of controlled trials for peripheral neuropathic pain and complex regional pain syndromes. *Pain* **73**(2), 123–39.

54. **Wahren, L.K. and Torebjörk, E.** 1992: Quantative sensory tests in patients with neuralgia 11 to 25 years after injury. *Pain* **48**, 237–44.

55. **Stanton-Hicks, M., Baron, R., Boas, R.** *et al*. 1998: Complex regional pain syndromes: guidelines for therapy. *Clinical Journal of Pain* **14**(2), 155–66.

56. **McQuay, H.** 1992: Pre-emptive analgesia. *British Journal of Anaesthesia* **69**(1), 1–3.

57. **McQuay, H.J., Carroll, D. and Moore, R.A.** 1988: Postoperative orthopaedic pain – the effect of opiate premedications and local anaesthetic blocks. *Pain* **33**, 291–6.

58. **Charlton, J.E.** 1986: Current views on the use of nerve blocking in the relief of chronic pain: In Swerdlow, M. (ed.) *The therapy of pain*. Lancaster: MTP Press, 133–64.

59. **Hannington-Kiff, J.G.** 1990: Intravenous regional sympathetic blocks. In Stanton-Hicks, M., Janig, W. and Boas, R.A. (eds) *Reflex sympathetic dystrophy*. Boston: Kluwer, 113–24.

60. **Jahad, A.R., Carroll, D., Glynn, C.J. and McQuay, H.J.** 1995: Intravenous regional sympathetic blockade for pain relief in reflex sympathetic dystrophy: a systematic review and a randomised double-blind crossover study. *Journal of Pain and Symptom Management* **10**, 13–20.

61. **Ramamurthy, S. and Hoffmann, J.** 1995: Intravenous regional guanethidine in the treatment of reflex sympathetic dystrophy/causalgia: a randomised double-blind study. *Anesthesia and Analgesia* **81**, 718–23.

62. **Wahren, L.K., Gordh, T. and Torebjork, E.** 1995: Effects of regional intravenous guanethidine in patients with neuralgia in the hand: a follow-up study over a decade. *Pain* **62**, 379–85.

63. **McQuay, H.J. and Moore, R.A.** 1998: *An evidence-based resource for pain relief.* Oxford: Oxford University Press 27, 212–15.

64. **Hord, A.H., Rooks, M.D., Stephens, B.O., Rogers, H.G. and Fleming, L.L.** 1992: Intravenous regional bretylium and lidocaine for the treatment of reflex sympathetic dystrophy: a randomised double-blind study. *Anesthesia and Analgesia* **74**, 818–21.

65. **Glynn, C.J. and Jones, P.C.** 1990: An investigation of the role of clonidine in the treatment of reflex sympathetic dystrophy. In Stanton-Hicks, M., Janig, W. and Boas, R.A. (eds) *Reflex sympathetic dystrophy.* Massachusetts: Kluwer, 187–96.

66. **Koizen, F.** 1992: Reflex sympathetic dystrophy syndrome: a review. *Clinical and Experimental Rheumatology* **10**, 401–9.

67. **Cicala, R.S., Jones, J.W. and Westbrook, L.L.** 1990: Causalgic pain responding to epidural but not to sympathetic block. *Anesthesia and Analgesia* **70**, 218–19.

68. **Scott, D.B.** 1989: *Techniques of regional anaesthesia.* Norwalk: Appleton & Lange, 206–9.

69. **Lofstrom, J.B. and Cousins, M.J.** 1988: Sympathetic neural blockade of upper and lower extremity. In Cousins, M.J. and Bridenbaugh, P.O. (eds) *Neural blockade in clinical anesthesia and management of pain,* 2nd edn. Philadelphia: J.B. Lippincott, 461–500.

70. **Rowlingson, J.C.** 1991: Management of chronic pain. *American Society of Anesthesiologists' 42nd Annual Refresher Course Lectures* **113**, 1–7.

71. **Racz, G.B.** 1989: *Techniques of neurolysis.* Boston: Kluwer, 234–9.

72. **Winnie, A.P.** 1969: An immobile needle for nerve blocks. *Anesthesiology* **31**, 577–8.

73. **Linson, M.A., Leffert, R. and Todd, D.P.** 1983: The treatment of upper extremity reflex sympathetic dystrophy with prolonged continuous stellate ganglion blockade. *Journal of Hand Surgery* **18**, 153.

74. **Boas, R.A.** 1996: Sympathetic blocks – practical pointers. *International Symposium on Regional Anaesthesia,* April, Auckland, New Zealand, 104–7.

75. **Budd, K.** 1989: The pain clinic – chronic pain. In Nunn, J.F., Utting, J.E. and Brown, B.R. (eds) *General anaesthesia,* 5th edn. London: Butterworth, 1349–69.

76. **Glynn, C. and Casale, R.** 1993: Morphine injected around the stellate ganglion does not modulate the sympathetic nervous system, nor does it provide pain relief. *Pain* **53**, 33–7.

77. **Wechsler, R.J., Frank, E.D., Halpern, E.H., Nazarian, L.N., Jalali, S. and Ratner, E.R.** 1998: Percutaneous lumbar sympathetic plexus catheter placement for short- and long-term pain relief: CT techniques and results. *Journal of Computer Assisted Tomography* **22**(4), 518–23.

78. **Abram, S.E.** 1990: Techniques for some commonly used blocks. In Abram, S.E. (ed.) *The pain clinic manual.* Philadelphia: J.B. Lippincott, 334–49.

79. **Cousins, M.J., Dwyer, B. and Gibb, D.** 1988: Chronic pain and neurolytic neural blockade: In Cousins, M.J. and Bridenbaugh, P.O. (eds) *Neural blockade in clinical anesthesia and management of pain,* 2nd edn. Philadelphia: J.B. Lippincott, 1053–84.

80. **Abram, S.E.** 1989: Pain – acute and chronic. In Barash, P.G., Cullen, B.F. and Stoelting, R.K. (eds) *Clinical anesthesia.* Philadelphia: J.B. Lippincott, 1427–54.

81. **Petriccione Di Vadi, P. and Wedley, J.R.** 1990: The use of coeliac plexus block in abdominal cancer pain: a review. *Pain Clinic* **3**(4), 223–7.

82. **Montero-Matamala, A., Aguilar-Sanchez, J.L. and Vidal-Lopez, F.** 1992: Percutaneous anterior and posterior approach to the coeliac plexus: a comparative study using four different techniques. *The Pain Clinic* **5**(1), 21–8.

83. **Ogawa, S., Suzuki, H., Yazaki, S., Saito, H., Saeki, S. and Kato, J.** 1991: A clinical study of volumes and concentrations of ethyl alcohol for splanchnic nerve block. *The Pain Clinic* **4**(1), 37–41.

84. **Reiestad, F., McIlvaine, W.B., Kvalheim, L., Stokke, T. and Pettersen, B.** 1989: Interpleural analgesia in treatment of upper extremity reflex sympathetic dystrophy. *Anesthesia and Analgesia* **69**, 671–3.

85. **Takahashi, H., Miyazaki, M., Nanbu, T., Yanagida, H. and Morita, S.** 1998: The NMDA-receptor antagonist ketamine abolishes neuropathic pain after epidural administration in a clinical case. *Pain* **75**(2–3), 391–4.

86. **Becker, W.J., Ablett, D.P., Harris, C.J. and Dold, O.N.** 1995: Long term treatment of intractable reflex sympathetic dystrophy with intrathecal morphine. *Canadian Journal of Neurological Science* **22**, 153–9.

87. **Rauck, R.L.** 1995: Reflex sympathetic dystrophy – effect of epidural clonidine. *Pain and the Sympathetic Nervous System: Special Interest Group Newsletter* (Summer), 2–3.

88. **Campbell, J.N.** 1990: An unusual presentation of the post sympathectomy syndrome. *The Pain Clinic* **3**(4), 243–5.

89. **Kramis, R.C., Roberts, W.J. and Gillette, R.G.** 1996: Post-sympathectomy neuralgia: hypotheses on peripheral and central neuronal mechanisms. *Pain* **64**, 1–9.

90. **Chan, C.S. and Chow, S.P.** 1981: Electroacupuncture in the treatment of post-traumatic sympathetic dystrophy. *British Journal of Anaesthesia* **53**, 899–902.

91. **Bengston, K.** 1997: Physical modalities for complex regional pain syndrome. *Hand Clinics* **13**(3), 443–54.

92. **Tasker, R.P.** 1990: Reflex sympathetic dystrophy – neurosurgical approaches. In Stanton-Hicks, M., Janig, W. and Boas, R.A. (eds) *Reflex sympathetic dystrophy.* Boston: Kluwer, 125–34.

93. **Law, J.D.** 1993: Spinal cord stimulation for intractable pain due to reflex sympathetic dystrophy. *CNI Review,* 17–22.

94. **Calvillo, O., Racz, G., Didie, J. and Smith, K.** 1998: Neuroaugmentation in the treatment of complex regional pain syndrome of the upper extremity. *Acta Orthopaedica Belgica* **64**(1), 57–63.

95. **Racz, G.B., Lewis, B., Heavner, J.E. and Scott, J.** 1990: Peripheral nerve stimulator implant for treatment of RSD. In Stanton-Hicks, M., Janig, W. and Boas, R.A. (eds) *Reflex sympathetic dystrophy.* Boston: Kluwer, 135–41.

96. **Hassenbusch, S.** 1994: Interventional techniques. *Pain and the Sympathetic Nervous System: Special Interest Group Newsletter* (Winter), 3–4.

97. **Glynn, C.** 1995: Complex regional pain syndrome, reflex sympathetic dystrophy, and complex regional pain syndrome type II, causalgia. *Pain Reviews* **2**, 292–7.

98. **King, J.H. and Nuss, S.** 1993: Reflex sympathetic dystrophy treated by electroconvulsive therapy: intractable pain, depression, and bilateral electrode electroconvulsive therapy. *Pain* **55**, 393–6.

99. **Charlton, J.E.** 1990: Reflex sympathetic dystrophy: non-invasive methods of treatment. In Stanton-Hicks, M., Janig, W. and Boas, R.A. (eds) *Reflex sympathetic dystrophy.* Boston: Kluwer, 151–64.

100. **Miuzelaar, J.P., Kleyer, M., Hertogs, I.A. and De Lange, D.C.** 1997: Complex regional pain syndrome (reflex sympathetic dystrophy and causalgia): management with the calcium channel blocker nifedipine and/or the alpha-sympathetic blocker phenoxybenzamine in 59 patients. *Clinical Neurology and Neurosurgery* **99**(1), 26–30.

101. **Cheshire, W.P. and Snyder, C.R.** 1990: Topical capsaicin in reflex sympathetic dystrophy. *Pain* **42**, 307–11.

102. **Dubner, R.** 1991: Topical capsaicin therapy for neuropathic pain. *Pain* **147**, 247–8.

103. **Shipton, E.A.** 1996: New concepts in pain management. *South African Journal of Anaesthesiology and Analgesia* **2**(1), 4–8.

INTERVENTIONAL THERAPY

INTRODUCTION

The basic premise of any interventional technique should be to choose the one with the simplest and least hazardous intervention, that is associated with the highest likelihood of achieving desirable results.[1] When contemplating an interventional technique, the risk to benefit ratio must be considered. While arguments for using neurolytic procedures by any of the three techniques outlined are well established for pain of malignant origin, indications for their use in non-malignant states are becoming clearer, and the results of carefully selected indications more than justify their retention in the pain armamentarium.[2] Patient selection and timing of neural destruction for pain relief are based on the exhaustion of the more conservative modalities, a lack of available, clinically superior options, and the availability of a capable physician and support systems after the procedure.[3] It is only after these modalities have proved unsatisfactory, either because of inadequate pain control or complications from the therapy itself (nausea, constipation, sedation), that neurolysis should be considered.[4] Patient selection and education is therefore essential, as there are limitations, complications, and side-effects that patients must accept prior to initiating interventional therapy.[4] A full knowledge of the possible consequences of long-term neuronal blockade is essential before such steps are taken, especially if the result is irreversible.[5] Permanent damage to nerves can lead to unpleasant sequelae. The risk of the destruction of motor nerves, mixed nerves, or sphincter innerva-tion (resulting in incontinence or bowel dysfunction) must always be considered when using permanent neurolytic agents.[1] Damage to nerve tissue can also lead to central nervous system changes later to be evidenced as a neurological pain syndrome. However, after informed consent, the patient may be willing to accept loss of function, especially if some pre-existing organ dysfunction exists and the pain is severe.[1] Consideration for neurolytic intervention in cancer pain is indicated when the pain symptoms cannot be controlled adequately with medications and other conservative therapy, and when life expectancy is limited (from 6 to 18 months).[4] Nevertheless, procedures may be performed during the last days of life, if warranted by unrelieved pain or suffering, or in those patients who are extremely ill and weak.[4] Yet early invasive pain treatment may allow cancer pain patients an improved quality of life without pain, unnecessary sedation, and side-effects.[1] For successful outcome, excellent anatomical knowledge and technical precision are necessary.[2] The introduction of cryotherapy and radiofrequency have improved the safety and specificity of neurolysis.

The purpose of performing a diagnostic nerve block in the management of chronic pain is to determine pain pathways and pain mechanisms, and to serve as a prognostic block for interventional procedures.[6] Diagnostic blocks include paravertebral, intercostal, trigeminal and facet nerve blocks, local infiltration, sympathetic blockade, and neuraxial blockade (Figure 11.1).[7,8] There are diagnostic, prognostic, therapeutic and prophylactic indications for nerve blocks (see Chapter 8).

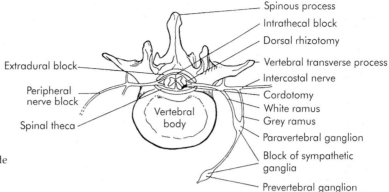

Figure 11.1 Sites for neural blockade (using local anaesthetics or neurolytic agents).

THERAPEUTIC INTERVENTIONS

If a patient might benefit from nerve blocks, therapeutic nerve blocks are undertaken. These include the addition of corticosteroids (methyl prednisolone), or guanethidine for sympathetic blocks for more lasting pain relief.[5] If diagnostic blocks confirm the likelihood that nerve pathways can be interrupted more permanently, then several ways exist of intervening and producing a long-term effect. Physical therapy can either be destructive or stimulatory.[9] Neuroablation can be done with chemical neurolysis, cryotherapy (cold), radiofrequency (heat) or surgery.[9] When a patient is pain-free after neuroablation, opioids should not be stopped abruptly, lest a withdrawal syndrome be provoked.[3] Neurostimulation can be external or internal.

LOCAL ANAESTHETICS

Chemically, local anaesthetics exist in two forms, that of the amino-esters and that of the amino-amides. They can also be classified based on their clinical properties:[10]

- low potency with short duration (e.g. procaine, 2-chloroprocaine);
- intermediate potency with intermediate duration (e.g. lignocaine, mepivacaine, prilocaine);
- high potency with long duration (e.g. bupivacaine, tetracaine, etidocaine).

Bicarbonation and carbonation of local anaesthetics

Local anaesthetics are supplied at a low pH to prolong shelflife.[10] The addition of bicarbonate increases the pH of these solutions and the percentage of uncharged forms. These diffuse through the nerve membrane, hastening the onset of block (see Chapter 8).

When carbon dioxide is mixed with local anaesthetics under pressure, it rapidly diffuses through the nerve membrane and decreases the axoplasmic pH.[10] This increases the intracellular concentration of charged forms of local anaesthetic, which is important for receptor binding and ultimate neural blockade, thus supposedly hastening onset of block.

Toxicity

There is not a great difference in toxicity between equipotent doses of most local anaesthetics. The systemic toxicity of local anaesthetics depends on:[11]

- the dose;
- the site of injection – vascular sites lead to rapid absorption;
- the drugs used – when large doses are required, it is best to use drugs of lowest toxicity (e.g. prilocaine, mepivacaine, chloroprocaine and procaine);
- the speed of injection – when high dosage is required, injections of small aliquots over several minutes reduces toxicity;
- the addition of adrenaline (also noradrenaline, phenylephrine) – the local vasoconstriction caused slows absorption and decreases the maximum plasma concentrations of most local anaesthetics between 20 per cent and 50 per cent.

Dosage

In regional anaesthesia, maximum dosage recommendations are confused and without scientific foundation. The commonest cause of toxicity is accidental intravenous bolus injection. A maximum recommended dose of any local anaesthetic given in this way will still cause overt toxicity with convulsions.[11] The maximum plasma concentrations following absorption depend primarily on the site of injection. An intercostal block, for example, produces more than three times the maximum plasma concentration of lignocaine than is seen after local infiltration.[12] If it is assumed that toxic symptoms occur at a plasma lignocaine concentration of 5 μg/ml, this would be achieved by giving approximately 300 mg intercostally, 500 mg epidurally, 600 mg in the brachial plexus region and 1000 mg subcutaneously.[12] The addition of adrenaline 1/200 000 decreases the maximum plasma concentration of lignocaine by 50 per cent after subcutaneous infiltration but by only 20–30 per cent after intercostal, epidural or brachial plexus blocks. It also decreases the maximum plasma concentration of bupivacaine significantly less than that of lignocaine. The maximum recommended dose should thus be adjusted for each site of injection, as well as for the presence or absence of adrenaline.

The maximum recommended dose of plain lignocaine is 200 mg in the UK and 300 mg in the USA. The maximum recommended dose of an adrenaline-containing lignocaine solution is 500 mg. The former dose is too small (e.g. for brachial plexus blocks, epidural blocks), and the latter assumes that adrenaline allows a 150 per cent dosage increase, for which there is no evidence.[12] It has therefore been suggested that the maximum recommended dose of plain lignocaine should be doubled to 400 mg.[11] The maximum recommended dose of bupivacaine is 150 mg. Bupivacaine is at least four times more potent and toxic than lignocaine, yet the maximum recommended dose of lignocaine is only 1.3–2 times greater than that of bupivacaine.[12] The present situation regarding maximum recommended doses for local anaesthetic agents is thus unsatisfactory (Tables 11.1 and 11.2).

Table 11.1 Comparative potencies of local anaesthetics (%)[11]

Lignocaine	0.5	1	1.5	2	
Mepivacaine	0.5	1	1.5	2	
Prilocaine	0.5	1	1.5	2	
Bupivacaine	0.125	0.25	0.375	0.5	0.75
Etidocaine	0.25	0.5	0.75	1	1.5
Chloroprocaine	0.5	1	1.5	2	3
Procaine	1	2			

Table 11.2 Concentrations of local anaesthetics commonly used for anaesthesia (lower concentrations are generally used for analgesia alone)

	Topical (%)	Peripheral (%)	Spinal (%)	Epidural (%)
Lignocaine	4–10 (0.25–0.5 for intravenous regional	0.5–1.5	5.0	1.5–2.0
Bupivacaine	–	0.25–0.5	0.5–0.75	0.5–0.75
Ropivacaine	–	0.25–0.5	–	0.5–1.0
Mepivacaine	–	1.0–1.5	–	2.0
Tetracaine	–	–	0.5–1.0	–
Chloroprocaine	–	1.0–3.0	–	3.0
Etidocaine	–	–	–	1.0–1.5 (not for analgesia)

CRYOANALGESIA

The principle of using extreme cold to produce insensibility to pain has been known and used for centuries. Its clinical application to produce analgesia, however, was not introduced until 1976 when Lloyd, Barnard and Glynn coined the term 'cryoanalgesia' to describe the destruction of peripheral nerves by extreme cold for the relief of pain that required somatic blockade[13] (Figure 11.2).

Apparatus and technique

Image intensification is a valuable addition to probe location especially in the vertebral areas.[14] The cryoprobe consists of a fine needle probe with a built-in thermocouple (to confirm the temperature achieved at the tip) and an electrical connection to the tip (for nerve stimulation). The temperature

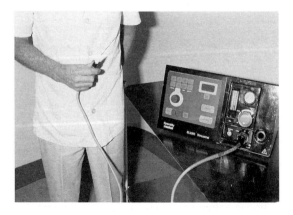

Figure 11.2 Cryotherapy. The Spembly-Lloyd cryoprobe machine.

drop at the end of the probe is generated by allowing nitrous oxide or carbon dioxide to expand through a small orifice using the Joule–Thompson effect.[15,16] This effect occurs when a gas under pressure is ejected through a nossle.[14] As the gas expands, it cools. The probe temperature falls to $-70°$ C in the distal 5 mm to form a 2–4 mm ice ball which freezes the nerve. With percutaneous insertion the lesion is made using two, 2-minute freeze cycles separated by a 1-minute warming period, which is likely to increase the destructive effect.[17] A larger 14-gauge gas expansion cryoprobe will create a freeze zone lesion of approximately 6–8 mm in diameter.[1] An exposed nerve may be picked up on the tip of the probe at surgery. With percutaneous insertion, the skin and subcutaneous tissues are anaesthetized with local anaesthetic. A large intravenous cannula can be used to create a tract through the tissue through which the probe is inserted.

Most modern cryoprobes allow for stimulation for appropriate location of motor and sensory nerves. Accurate location of the probe tip to the nerve can be achieved using the stimulatory mode where maximum twitch response with minimum current indicates that the tip is lying adjacent to the nerve.[16,17] With purely sensory nerves, a tingling sensation or pain occurs along the nerve on stimulation. The probe should only be withdrawn when fully thawed to prevent adherence to and tearing of surrounding tissue. The patient should be warned about the resulting numbness in the area supplied by the nerve. This usually wears off after several weeks.

Mechanism of action

There is Wallerian degeneration with axonal disintegration and break up of the myelin sheaths, but with minimal disruption of the endoneurium, the basal lamina and other connective tissue.[18] The nerve will subsequently regenerate. The resultant conduction block produces analgesia lasting usually from days to weeks but occasionally up to 6 months.[1] Less fibrous tissue may be produced than with other forms of peripheral nerve destruction. The incidence of post-lesion neuralgia is less with this technique.[15]

Advantages

The advantages of this technique are its simplicity, low cost, and reversibility of the lesion and any of its side-effects.[16] There may be a transient, mild neuritis but there is no reported neuroma formation after this form of neurolysis.[1]

Disadvantages

A large (e.g. 14 gauge) intravenous cannula should always be used to provide a sheath for the percutaneous insertion of the cryoprobe. This prevents freezing of the skin and tissue superficial to the probe tip.[18] Somatic block should be carried out lateral to the paravertebral muscles if possible to avoid spinal cord or 'feeder' artery involvement.[18] Cryoanalgesia should not be used on mixed nerves with a large motor component as it can result in paralysis of the muscles supplied by that nerve.[15] Side-effects are, however, usually limited to pain at the insertion site and occasionally to neuritic pain along the course of the nerve. If this does not resolve, a mixture of local anaesthetic and corticosteroid is injected at the site of the cryolesion, or the patient placed on antidepressant–anticonvulsant combination therapy.

Results

The duration of pain relief is dependent on the completeness of the nerve destruction, making it important to position the ice ball correctly.[18] The duration of this block will only last days to weeks, as opposed to several weeks or months with radiofrequency thermocoagulation (RFTC), phenol or alcohol.[1] The median duration of pain relief varies from about 2 days to about 6 months, but usually with a minimum of about 3 weeks.[15,18]

Indications

Cryoanalgesia is thus put to best use in relieving postoperative and post-traumatic chest pain, and to improving medium-term pain relief in chronic pain syndromes.[17] There is no absolute contraindication to cryoanalgesia except for patient refusal. However, for technical reasons, mainly the size of the probe that is used, cryotherapy is limited to certain neural structures.[2]

ACUTE PAIN

Cryoanalgesia has been used to produce very prolonged analgesia, particularly during thoracotomy, when the probe can be applied to the intercostal nerves under direct vision.[19] It does not, however, block visceral pain and the prolonged numbness may worry the patient. An external approach to the intercostal nerves can be used for analgesia for fractured ribs.[18]

CHRONIC PAIN

Intercostal cryoanalgesia can be used to treat patients with various chronic chest pain syndromes (e.g. post-thoracotomy scar pain and post-herpetic neuralgia).[17] Cryoanalgesia of the branches of the trigeminal nerve (e.g. infraorbital, mental) has been used to treat different types of facial pain, such as trigeminal neuralgia, post-herpetic neuralgia and atypical facial pain. Cryoanalgesia of the branches of the trigeminal nerve has been used to treat the pain from head and neck cancer.[18] These include the supraorbital, supratrochlear, infraorbital, mental and lingual branches as well as the main divisions (e.g. mandibular, maxillary). The tonsillar bed can be frozen twice for 2 minutes in patients suffering from glossopharyngeal neuralgia[14] (radiofrequency lesioning can also be used). To treat occipital neuralgia, cryoanalgesia of the greater occipital nerve has been used. Cervical nerve root involvement has also been treated with cryoanalgesia.

For low back pain, percutaneous facet nerve cryoanalgesia of the medial branch of the zygapophyseal joint has been used.[2] To treat coccydynia, cryoanalgesia of S5 and coccygeal nerves can be performed.[18] For perineal pain, insertion of the cryoprobe through the sacral hiatus up to the level of the 4th sacral foramen can give good analgesia over the dorsal surface of the scrotum, perineum and the anus.[14]

Cryotherapy may be used for other peripheral nerves such as the ilioinguinal, hypogastric and genitofemoral nerves.[2] Various peripheral nerve entrapment syndromes can be treated by cryoanalgesia. The cryoprobe can also be used for tumour debulking, resulting in greater patient comfort.[9] It may be used for certain neuropathic pains, such as those arising from large neuromas (e.g. the sciatic and femoral nerves in an amputee).[2]

Using the cryoprobe, central lesions can be produced in the anterior pituitary. This technique can be used instead of alcohol in patients with disseminated malignancy, especially in bone, with pain unresponsive to routine therapy.[20] This method has also been used in the treatment of non-cancer pain.[21]

PERCUTANEOUS RADIOFREQUENCY THERMOCOAGULATION (RFTC)

Radiofrequency current can be used for producing therapeutic heat lesions in the peripheral or central

nervous systems. RFTC can be applied at the first sensory neurone level to many somatosensory nerves, including divisions of the trigeminal nerve, the gasserian ganglion, peripheral nerve rhizotomies, such as the intercostal, paravertebral, the medial branch of the zygapophyseal (facet) joints and the dorsal root ganglia.[2] These are generally safe and have few neurological deficits.[22] The indications for use in the periphery are similar to those for cryotherapy. Procedures at the second sensory neurone level, such as percutaneous anterolateral cervical cordotomy, do carry a risk of neurological deficits, including bowel and bladder incontinence, and motor weakness.[2,22] RFTC is used in lesions of the sympathetic trunk, particularly the upper thoracic and sympathetic ganglia, for conditions such as hyperhidrosis and complex regional pain syndromes (CRPS); in the lumbar sympathetic trunk, it is used for CRPS and end-stage arteriosclerotic disease with rest pain, sympathetically maintained pain associated with a metabolic polyneuropathy, phantom limb pain, and certain peripheral vascular conditions (Raynaud's and Buerger's disease).[2] Thoracic and lumbar sympathectomies can be performed for visceral pain and for radiation neuritis.[22] Procedures at the third sensory level include stereotactic hypophysectomy, mesencephalic spinothalamic tractotomy, and medial thalamotomy and are infrequently performed but have much greater risks (see Chapter 13).[22] The lesion, however, is likely to be permanent.[16]

Apparatus and technique

In certain chronic, benign pain syndromes, RFTC is only considered after failure of conservative management.[22] In chronic malignant pain syndromes, RFTC may be the first line of treatment. The basic principle of RFTC involves placement of a fine insulated electrode shaft with an uninsulated tip into the nervous tissue.[22] The shaft is connected to an electrical generating source, and the electrical impedance of the surrounding tissue allows current to flow from the generator source into the tissue itself, thereby generating heat. The hottest part of the lesion will be in the tissue adjacent to the electrode tip. RFTC makes use of the percutaneous insertion of a Teflon-coated 20-gauge insulated needle with either a 5- or 10-mm non-insulated tip.[1] The RTFC machine will allow sensory stimulation from 50 to 70 Hz and motor stimulation at 2–5 Hz to ensure proper placement of the needle on the appropriate nerve. Once this is done, the needle tip is heated with a thermocouple electrode. A heat lesion has a central area of total destruction surrounded by a zone that is damaged selectively.[15] At temperatures just above 45°C, lesions are confined to smaller nerve fibres (including A delta and C fibres). For any given electrical current, thermal equilibrium is established in about 60 seconds. The size of the lesion is controlled by maintaining a constant electrode tip temperature for 1–2 minutes.[15] A thermistor or thermocouple in the electrode tip ensures accurate temperature measurement. Typically, the needle tip is heated to 80–90°C for 60–90 seconds, depending on lesion size.[1]

Lesion generators deliver an alternating current with a frequency above 250 kHz.[15] The available generators use 500 kHz[22] (Figure 11.3). A wide power range and fine output resolution gives accurate temperature control. Variables measured include temperature, current, voltage and impedance. Impedance measurement aids in identifying various tissue types. Electrical stimulation facilities are also in-built. To maintain patient cooperation, local anaesthesia or neuroleptanalgesia are used. X-ray control is used to position an insulated cannula close to the target area. The electrode is inserted through the cannula and the position of its tip is determined both radiologically and by electrical stimulation. Controlled lesions are generated via Teflon-coated needles that have active tips of varying sizes to generate lesions of varying sizes.[22] The cannula used for lesioning comes in various lengths and diameters. A water-soluble non-ionic contrast dye is injected into the epidural space or root sleeve to outline the dura and dorsal root ganglion.[22] The thermocouple electrode is inserted through the cannula for stimulation to identify the nerve or the dorsal root ganglion, followed by thermocoagulation. The most common side-effects are neuritic pain and hyperaesthesia in the treated dermatomes, which most often resolve spontaneously.[15]

Advantages of RFTC

When compared to chemical neurolysis, the advantages of RFTC include the following:[1,22]

■ there is minimal risk to the patient, and it can be performed percutaneously on an outpatient basis;
■ there is a decreased incidence of neuritis with relatively few postoperative thromboembolic phenomena;
■ the lesion size is controllable and selective (the size of the needle plus approximately 1 mm radius);

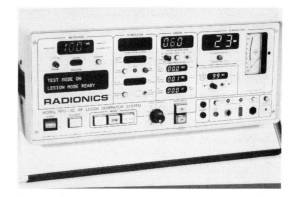

Figure 11.3 Radiofrequency lesioning. The Radionics RFG–3C RF lesion generator.

■ good monitoring of the lesion temperature can be performed with a thermocouple electrode;
■ electrode placement is facilitated with electrical stimulation and impedance monitoring;
■ most RFTC can be performed under monitored anaesthetic care (intravenous sedation with monitoring);
■ during sympathectomies, no profound hypotension occurs, and in lumbar sympathectomies, the incidence of impotence is rare;
■ when properly performed, there is a low incidence of morbidity and mortality, and procedures can be repeated if needed.

Lesions

The goal of RFTC is to relieve pain but to preserve proprioception, touch and motor function. Patients may experience increased pain for days to a few weeks after RFTC.[22] This can be treated with repeated local anaesthetic/corticosteroid infiltration or with oral anticonvulsants.[22]

Dorsal root ganglia lesions are used to treat pain in the distribution of one (or two) nerve roots on the same side. Analgesia is obtained by destroying the cell bodies of the neurones. After a diagnostic local anaesthetic block, a radiofrequency probe is inserted under X-ray control into the appropriate intervertebral foramen. The dorsal root ganglia are situated posteriorly in the intervertebral foramina at the level of a line joining the facet joint spaces (on an anteroposterior view).[15] The nerve root is then outlined by contrast. If the probe tip is correctly placed, electrical stimulation produces paraesthesia in the painful area or reproduces the pain itself. Local anaesthetic is then injected through the probe or intravenous sedation given, and RFTC is performed.[15]

HEAD, NECK, THORACIC, LUMBAR AND SACRAL PAIN

Percutaneous radiofrequency trigeminal gangliolysis (PRTG)

With the patient supine, the foramen ovale is visualized using a C-arm fluoroscope to obtain a sub-mentovertex view.[22,23] An intravenous short-acting induction agent (propofol) is given. A 22-gauge, 100-mm long, Teflon-coated lesioning needle with a 5-mm active tip is advanced (from a point 2.5 cm lateral to the corner of the mouth, aiming towards the medial ipsilateral pupil and a point about 2.5 cm anterior to the tragus of the ipsilateral ear) submucosally to the skull base, until it enters the foramen ovale.[22,23] For the first division, the medial aspect is entered, for the second division, the midpoint, and for the third division, the lateral aspect of the foramen ovale is entered under lateral fluoroscopy.[22,23] CSF is encountered 5–10 mm past the entrance.[23] The stylet is removed and the thermocouple probe inserted.[22] The patient is woken up. An isolated pulse (1 millisecond duration, 100–400 mV, and 50–75 Hz) is used to localize the electrode position by the production of facial paraesthesiae.[23] Motor stimulation ensures that the patient does not have any eye or masseter movement or weakness. The patient is again given propofol and the first lesion is made (90 seconds at 75°C).[23] If necessary, additional lesions can be made until adequate hypaesthesia is obtained. With trigeminal neuralgia, 78–100 per cent of patients have immediate pain relief, and 39–85 per cent will remain in remission.[23] Postoperative paraesthesias occur in 20 per cent of patients, and dyaesthesias in 5.2–24.2 per cent of patients.[23]

Occipital pain

Occipital headache may be relieved by RFTC of the 2nd cervical dorsal nerve root ganglion. A 22-gauge, 100-mm long radiofrequency lesioning needle with a 5-mm active tip is inserted in a lateral position toward the intervertebral foramen of C1 and C2 vertebrae, until it enters the dorsal root ganglion area.[22] This is situated about halfway across the facet line of C1 and C2 vertebrae. An open-mouth fluoroscopic view, and contrast to outline the dura and the dorsal root ganglion confirms correct placement.[22] Propofol is given and the site thermocoagulated.

Neck pain

Radiofrequency lesioning of the 3rd cervical dorsal nerve root ganglion is performed for pain in the ear, the suboccipital, posterior auricular and sub-mandibular areas (e.g. from neck cancer). With oblique fluoroscopy and the patient supine, the radiofrequency cannula (22-gauge, 100 mm long with 5-mm active tip) is advanced in an anteroposterior direction until it enters the midpoint of the facet joint.[22] Injected contrast outlines the dura and the dorsal root ganglion. Motor stimulation (giving posterior auricular and submandibular fasciculations) should be twice the voltage needed for sensory stimulation.[22] Ideally, 0.4–0.8 V at 50 Hz gives paraesthesia, and motor fasciculation is noted at 1.2–1.5 V.[22] Propofol is given and the site thermocoagulated. For pain from the 4th to the 7th cervical nerves, a similar approach is used.[22] A lesion of the 8th cervical nerve dorsal root ganglion is avoided, owing to technical difficulties and the possibility of hand muscle weakness.[22] Cancer pain patients tolerate a higher temperature (67–80°C) and a longer duration of lesioning (about 120 seconds).[22]

Thoracic pain

Thoracic pain (from chest wall, ribs, and pleura) is treated by selective RFTC of the dorsal root ganglia of the corresponding thoracic nerves.[22] The first and second thoracic dorsal root ganglia are thermocoagulated for cancer pain of the upper extremities. A Kirschner wire (0.062 inches in diameter) is introduced percutaneously through a 12-gauge cannula until it contacts the infrapedicle area of the corresponding vertebra through which a drill hole is made.[22] Under lateral fluoroscopy, the wire is guided into the intervertebral foramen and removed, whilst a 20-gauge, 15-cm long radiofrequency lesioning needle with a 5-mm active tip is introduced. Dye is injected to outline the dura and the dorsal root ganglion before RFTC is performed.

Stereotactic percutaneous thermocoagulation of the upper thoracic sympathetic T2 and T3 ganglia (if lung and visceral pleura are involved, and for head, neck, upper extremity and upper chest pain) avoids the major surgical complications associated with open surgical sympathectomy.[22] A positive diagnostic stellate ganglion block with local anaesthetic is first performed. With the patient prone, a 20-gauge, 15-cm long radiofrequency lesioning needle with a 10-mm active tip is inserted under local anaesthesia and intravenous sedation, and under fluoroscopy, slightly obliquely to the mid- to antero-lateral aspect of T2 and T3 vertebral bodies.[22] Two lesions (at 80°C for 120 seconds) a few millimetres apart are made in the sympathetic chain cephalad, next to the midpoint, and on the caudad aspect of each vertebral body.[22] Pneumothorax occurs in 5–10 per cent of cases, but usually resolves sponta-neously.[22] Rarely, post-sympathectomy neuralgia occurs, but disappears in 4–6 weeks[22]. Sympathetic pain involving the lower chest area is treated in a similar manner in the lower thoracic sympathetic chain.[22]

Abdominal pain

Pain from the lower abdominal viscera (descending and sigmoid colon, rectum, uterus, ovaries and fal-lopian tubes) is amenable to stereotactic lumbar sympathectomy after a positive diagnostic lumbar sympathetic ganglion blockade with local anaes-thetic.[22] With the patient prone over a lower abdominal wedge, a 20-gauge, 15-cm long radiofre-quency lesioning needle with a 10-mm active tip is inserted (under local anaesthesia and mild intra-venous sedation, and under oblique fluoroscopy) on to the anterolateral aspect of the 2nd through to 5th vertebral bodies.[22] Dye is injected to outline the sympathetic chain. Electrical stimulation excludes proximity to somatic nerves. Two lesions (at 80°C for 120 seconds) a few millimetres apart are made in each sympathetic ganglion.[22]

Pelvic pain responds to RFTC of the hypogastric plexus (in conjunction with a lumbar sympathec-tomy).[22] Two Teflon-coated needles (20-gauge, 15-cm long with a 10-mm active tip) are inserted on either side about 1 cm anterior to the anterior bor-der of the 5th lumbar or 1st sacral vertebral body.[22] Dye outlines the hypogastric plexus, followed by RFTC at 80°C for 120 seconds.

Lumbar pain

For pain involving the lumbar dermatomes or less, a needle is aimed inferior to the superior pedicle, under oblique fluoroscopy, and enters the interver-tebral foramen at the same level as the medial pedi-cle border.[22] On lateral fluoroscopy, the needle tip should ideally be situated in the posterior third of the intervertebral foramen. Injected dye shows the dura, the dorsal root ganglion and the nerve root sleeve.[22] Paraesthesia should be obtained at about 0.5–0.8 V and motor stimulation of the ganglion at about 1.2–1.5 V.[22]

At the 5th lumbar vertebra (L5) and the sacral ver-tebrae (S1–S5) below, burr holes have to be drilled to access the root ganglia.[15] A Kirschner wire (0.062 inches in diameter) is introduced percutaneously through a 12-gauge cannula until it contacts the dorsal aspect of the 5th vertebral body (just below the pedicle), through which a drill hole is made until the wire enters the dorsal aspect of the inter-vertebral foramen.[22] The wire is replaced with a 20-

gauge, 15-cm long, Teflon-coated radiofrequency lesioning needle with a 5-mm active tip. Dye is injected to make the dura and dorsal ganglion visi-ble.[22] Motor and sensory thresholds are determined by stimulation. The dorsal aspect of the dorsal root ganglion is then thermocoagulated.

Sacral pain

The same technique as for the 5th lumbar nerve dorsal root ganglion applies for the RFTC of the sacral ganglia, where a burr hole is made through the dorsal layer of the sacrum.[22] The dorsal root ganglion of S1 is midway between the S1 foramen and the superior border of the sacral bone.[22] The dorsal root ganglion of S2 is midway between S1 and S2 foramina. The dorsal root ganglion of S3 is situated on the upper border of the S2 sacral fora-men, and that of S4 and S5 is situated at the level of the S2 sacral foramen.[22] Pain from pelvic malig-nancy usually involves the S3 and S4 nerves. The coccygeal nerve is approached through the sacro-coccygeal hiatus, is outlined with dye, and then thermocoagulated.[22]

POSTERIOR PRIMARY RAMUS LESION

The medial branch of the posterior primary ramus provides branches to the facet joints. Facet joint pain occurs in the posterior ramus distribution as well as in part or all of the anterior primary ramus distribution. After a prognostic local anaesthetic block, the radiofrequency probe can be inserted at the cephalad or caudad end of the joint to lesion the nerve supply to both aspects.[15] Alternatively, the probe can be inserted in the groove at the base of the transverse process in which the nerve runs before supplying the joint. The lesion is then made using a temperature of 80–90°C for 60–160 sec-onds.[15]

CORDOTOMY

For a discussion of percutaneous cervical cordo-tomy, see Chapter 13.

NEUROLYTIC AGENTS

There have never been clear guidelines for neu-rolytic blocks in terms of indications or outcome, and well-controlled studies are lacking.[24] Reliable permanent pain relief cannot be produced because of axonal regeneration, the development of deafferentation pain or both.[25] Neurolytic blocks are best suited for patients whose weakness, debility or short life expectancy make them unsuitable candidates for neurosurgery.[24] Great care must be exercised to relieve the pain without producing unwarranted motor or autonomic dysfunction, or producing unintentional damage to non-targeted tissues. These problems can be minimized by careful patient selection (e.g. limited life expectancy, persistent pain unmodified by less invasive measures and amenable to peripheral neurolysis), and attention to technique.[26] Optimal results are obtained by the judicious use of image intensification and CT guidance to verify needle localization, as well as careful aspiration, the use of a nerve stimulator, eliciting paraesthesias and the clearing of the needle of neurolytic before it is withdrawn.[25]

The principal indications for chemical neurolysis are malignancy and non-malignant pain.[2] While in the former case, there may be few absolute contraindications, any argument for using neurolysis in the case of chronic non-malignant pain must be clear, and the indications well established owing to the known side-effects and complications.[2] Specific indications are paraplegic spasticity, peripheral nerve injection for painful neuralgias, sympatholysis of the cervical, thoracic or lumbar sympathetic trunks, visceral nerve blocks of the splanchnic nerves or the coeliac plexus, cranial nerve neurolysis, motor point injections in striated muscle, and on the nerve supply to, or direct intra-articular injections into, specific joints (zygapophyseal, atlanto-occipital, sacroiliac) or their capsules.[2]

Patient selection for this procedure is discussed in Chapter 9.

Mechanism of action

Phenol (5–12 per cent), alcohol (50–95 per cent), and chlorocresol (2–4 per cent) are commonly used neurolytic agents. They produce protein denaturation and extraction of lipid membrane components.[27] Their action is non-selective as to fibre size and type, and they cause necrosis and glia scarring.[27] Neural regeneration can occur as long as the cell body is intact.[24] Nerve sprouting and neuroma formation may take place at the site of the nerve disruption. When the basal lamina around the Schwann cell tube persists, regeneration can occur without painful neuroma formation.[17] This is in contrast to surgical section of the nerve.

Agents used

PHENOL

In low concentrations, phenol has a local anaesthetic effect and selectively blocks small fibres while sparing motor function. However, when the time of exposure and the concentrations are adequate, the action is non-selective as to fibre size or type.[27,28] It acts by protein denaturation.[4] Clinically, an initial local anaesthetic effect (warmth and numbness) gives way to chronic denervation.[4] Phenol is clinically used in a concentration from 5 to 12 per cent. It is a clear and colourless acid with a pungent odour.[4] It is unstable at room temperature, hyperbaric relative to CSF and poorly soluble in water.[4] It is highly soluble in glycerine, which can be added to limit spread and localize tissue fixation.[28] The combination is heavier than cerebral spinal fluid and for intrathecal work can be directed appropriately to prevent loss of anterior horn function. Radio-opaque contrast medium can also be added for neuraxial work. Phenol is most destructive in an aqueous medium and less so in glycerine. Various concentrations of phenol have been prepared with saline, water, glycerine and different contrast dyes[4]. Concentrations below 6 per cent may be mixed with water or saline; above this, phenol must be mixed with glycerine or contrast dyes to prevent precipitation owing to its low solubility.[1] It is so viscous that it is difficult to inject in needles smaller than a 20-gauge. It binds more readily to tissues and diffuses less than alcohol.[1] It does not readily pass through the dura, the dural sleeve or the nerve roots, thereby exhibiting selective neurolysis.[1] Shelf life exceeds 1 year when preparations are refrigerated and not exposed to light.[4]

After injecting, a biphasic action is observed, characterized by an initial local anaesthetic effect producing subjective warmth and numbness that gives way to chronic denervation. Phenol is quicker in action than alcohol. It is not as effective at destroying the nerve cell body, and is thus less predictable is its spread and effect; its block also tends to be of shorter duration.[15] Phenol is less likely to produce a chemical neuritis than alcohol. The neurolytic potency of 5 per cent phenol is equivalent to 40 per cent alcohol.[4]

The adult toxic dose of 8–15 g is never approached in clinical practice.[15] Inadvertent intravascular injection may lead to convulsions, and circulatory and respiratory collapse.[15,29] A dose of 66 mg has been suggested as the maximum amount that should be injected in one bolus.[30] The injection site may be tender for a few days and influenza-like symptoms may be experienced for 48 hours.[15] Skin ulceration can occur if phenol is injected too superficially.[28] If motor function is inadvertently affected by phenol, it is more likely to be restored than if it had occurred with alcohol.[15] Topical phenol for chemical face peels is associated with cardiac dysrhythmias in up to 30 per cent of adults.[26] Sites of use in order of preference are epidurally, paravertebrally, on peripheral nerve roots, intrathecally and on cranial nerves.[4]

ETHYL ALCOHOL

This is the most reliable agent for the production of peripheral neurolysis but, because of its non-selective action, it can cause serious damage to neurological tissue remote from the injection site.[31] Because of its high diffusibility and solubility, large volumes are needed to produce adequate neurolysis, resulting in less precise lesions.[1] The neurolytic action is thought to occur through a dehydration action on the nerve tissue, with the extraction of cholesterol, phospholipids and cerebrosides, and the precipitation of mucoproteins.[4] It is clear and colourless (usually in 1 ml ampoules), and stable at room temperature, but readily absorbs water on exposure to air.[4] It can be injected readily through small-bore needles.[4] Owing to its hypobaric nature (specific gravity 0.805 compared to CSF which is 1.005), it floats upwards and special positioning for intrathecal work is required. A concentration of 95 per cent will reliably lyse sympathetic, sensory and motor components.[24] There is great discrepancy on the differential efficacy at concentrations of less than 80 per cent.[28] A concentration of 50 per cent seems reliable for coeliac plexus block. Denervation and pain relief may accrue over a few days post-injection.[4]

With ethyl alcohol (unlike phenol), post-injection neuritis is common (up to 10 per cent on peripheral nerves), caused by the incomplete destruction of somatic nerves and subsequent regeneration (e.g. intercostal spillage following paravertebral block of the thoracic sympathetics).[1,28] Alcohol irritates the tissues and can cause pain, burning and local tenderness.[15] Local reaction seems to be less common in cranial nerves than in other peripheral nerves.[4] In peripheral neurolysis, absolute ethyl alcohol has been shown to have a lower incidence of generalized side-effects than phenol, as there is no hepatic or cardiac toxicity at commonly used doses.[4] It causes significant pain on injection. A disulfiram-like effect can occur.[1] Accurate injection placement

ensures that the minimum volume is used. Sites of use in order of preference are intrathecally, on the coeliac ganglion, on the lumbar sympathetic chain, on the cranial nerves, paravertebrally, and epidurally (in low concentrations).[4] When injected intrathecally, it is hypobaric and may spread significantly.[1]

CHLOROCRESOL

This has a greater ability to penetrate cancerous tissue surrounding nerve roots than does phenol or alcohol.[15] It is used with glycerine as a 2 per cent solution for epidural work and as a 5 per cent solution for intrathecal work. Immediate sensory changes do not occur, making localization difficult and pain relief is delayed usually for up to 24 hours.[15]

GLYCERINE

Percutaneous retrogasserian glycerol rhizolysis (PRGR) is where glycerine is injected into the cistern of Meckel's cave in patients with trigeminal neuralgia producing long-lasting pain relief.[23] No permanent injury to surrounding structures occurs and there is preservation of facial sensation in most patients.[31] Less disturbance of facial sensation is said to occur with glycerine compared to 0.2–0.3 ml of absolute ethyl alcohol.[15] Glycerine may preferentially affect small myelinated or unmyelinated nerve fibres, and particularly large myelinated fibres, which have been implicated in the genesis of trigeminal neuralgia.[23] Glycerine is not associated with scarring in Meckel's cave.[2] With the patient supine, the foramen ovale is visualized using a C-arm fluoroscope to obtain a submentovertex view.[22,23] An intravenous short-acting induction agent (propofol) is given. A 20-gauge, 100-mm long, spinal needle is advanced (from a point 2.5 cm lateral to the corner of the mouth, aiming towards the medial ipsilateral pupil and a point about 2.5 cm anterior to the tragus of the ipsilateral ear) submucosally to the skull base, until it enters the foramen ovale.[22,23] Under lateral fluoroscopy, the needle is slowly advanced through the ganglion into the cistern.[23] Cerebrospinal fluid (CSF) is encountered 5–10 mm past the entrance.[23] The patient is allowed partially to recover and placed in the sitting position with the orbitomeatal line just past the horizontal, with the neck slightly flexed.[23] Contrast is injected and the cistern is visualized. The contrast is then allowed to flow back out of the needle. Anhydrous glycerol is injected from a 1 ml syringe.[23] The patient is warned about the occurrence of transient facial dysaesthesias. The patient should remain sitting with the head tipped forward slightly for 2 hours.[23] Selective discrimination of the division affected can be achieved by tilting the head into characteristic positions.[23] Within 48 hours, 72–96 per cent of patients experience effective pain relief.[23] Recurrence rate ranges from 18.5–72 per cent over a 3–72 months follow-up period.[23] The most common side-effect is headache. Other complications include paraesthesias, dysaesthesias, anaesthesia dolorosa (0–2 per cent), corneal hypesthesia, keratitis (rarely), masticatory muscle weakness, herpes labialis and haematoma at needle entry site.[23]

Although glycerine has been shown to damage axons and myelin sheaths, it does not appear to have the same degree of neurolytic effects when injected around a peripheral nerve or intrathecally.[32] It has been suggested that substance P and/or calcitonin gene-related peptide are released from the terminals of the trigeminal neuro-vascular system during glycerine injection and lead to an increase in cerebral blood flow.[32] Glycerine 0.5 mL has been found to be useful for inserting into the intravertebral foramina to cover the dorsal root ganglia in segmental pain.[9]

SCLEROSANT SOLUTION

The solution contains phenol 2 per cent, dextrose 20 per cent, glycerine 25 per cent and water up to 100 per cent. It has been used (with local anaesthesia) for injection into strained ligaments and joint capsules for pain relief.[15] Intra-articular injection has been used in patients with destructive arthritis where conservative treatments have failed and in whom surgery is contraindicated.[33] A chemical synovectomy is produced which decreases the involvement of the unmyelinated afferent neurones and the release of neurotransmitters.

OTHERS

Osmotic neurolysis using hypertonic or hypotonic solutions (e.g. saline) intrathecally has been used for transient (up to 3 weeks) blockade of unmyelinated C fibres.[27] Hypertonic saline has been useful for movement-related pain due to spinal neoplasms.[1] Clinical experience shows the safe use of epidural hypertonic saline for prolonged analgesia without motor paralysis or neuritis.[1] Ammonium salts have also been used with some success in an attempt to block small fibres selectively.[27] Butyl amino-benzoate, a non-water-soluble local anaes-

thetic, has been used epidurally to treat patients with advanced malignancies.[27]

Complications (see Chapter 9)

Complications can be avoided by the use of small volumes of agent, fluoroscopic control of contrast mixtures, and attention to detail.[2] The use of careful prognostic local anaesthetic blocks beforehand will prevent the possibility of producing unacceptable anaesthesia, and will help to eliminate the placebo problem.[2]

The complications from peripheral neurolysis have been reported to range from 2 to 28 per cent.[2] The most common is neuritis (up to 10 per cent) of the blocked nerve, followed by anaesthesia dolorosa.[2] Anaesthesia dolorosa is usually not a consequence of a single nerve neurolysis and is caused by imbalances in afferent input. Another complication is agent migration to distant structures.[2] Intercostal paravertebral somatic nerve injection may be associated with neurolytic spread to the dural cuff, CSF and the spinal cord.[2] Complications of thoracic sympathetic neurolysis are pneumothorax, neuraxial injection and peripheral neuritis, whilst genitofemoral neuralgia is the most frequent complication of neurolysis of the lumbar sympathetic trunk.[2] Impotence may be associated with sympathetic neurolysis.[2] Rarer complications encountered include skin sloughing, and prolonged motor paralysis or perineal dysfunction.[24]

Common neuroablative techniques

PERIPHERAL NERVE

To ensure effective analgesia, neural interruption is planned proximal to the source of irritation, and accuracy is essential.[4] Because the sensory distribution of peripheral nerves overlaps, blockade of neighbouring segments is recommended.[4] As many peripheral nerves are of mixed function, a prognostic block with local anaesthetic beforehand is essential to evaluate the concomitant motor deficit.[4]

Entrapment syndrome

The entrapment of a perforating cutaneous nerve in the abdominal wall can be disabling. If surgery is not feasible, then by using a nerve stimulator to locate the optimum position, 2–3 mL of phenol 5 per cent aqueous solution can be injected on to the nerve.[15] This can be repeated. If the pain persists, cryotherapy or radiofrequency lesions can be made.[17]

Intercostal neuralgia

Intercostal neuralgia can be treated with 1 mL of phenol 7 per cent aqueous solution. Adjacent segments need to be blocked as well because of dermatomal overlap. In upper intercostal neurolysis (where the overlying scapula and muscle increase the risk of a pneumothorax), a more proximal paravertebral or intrathecal blockade should be performed.[4,34] Alternatives include cryotherapy or radiofrequency lesioning as discussed above.[18]

Muscle spasm

Blockade of the facial nerve with phenol has been used to treat hemifacial spasm of unknown origin.[18] To relieve spasticity in head-injured patients or in children with cerebral palsy, blocks of motor points with phenol 3–5 per cent in aqueous solution in affected muscles can be used.[26] These points elicit maximal muscle contraction when using a nerve stimulator. Occasionally neurolytic blocks of various peripheral nerves of the arms and legs are performed to restore normal functional position of the limbs.

Neuromas

Patients with intractable pain from neuromas that developed after amputation or other surgery can be treated with neurolytic blockade. Phenol–glycerine (50 mg/1000 mg/mL) can be used, starting with small amounts and repeating, if necessary.[35] Between 8 and 22 months of pain relief can be achieved in this way.[35]

Trans-sacral block

In patients with pain from pelvic or rectal malignancies with intact bowel and bladder function, selective neurolysis of the sacral nerve roots via their dorsal foramina is useful.[4] Successive diagnostic local anaesthetic blocks of individual sacral roots will determine the pain pathways involved.[4] Avoidance of bilateral 2nd and 3rd sacral root blocks is likely to preserve bladder function.[4] Trans-sacral block of the S4 segment with 2 mL of phenol 6 per cent aqueous solution is useful in patients with severe unremitting perineal pain caused by inoperable rectal cancer or following rectal surgery. The coccygeal nerve can also be blocked in the anterior sacrococcygeal ligament using 1 mL of absolute ethyl alcohol.[36] These techniques provide a minimal risk of sphincter disturbance.

Others

Rarely, if local anaesthetic fails, neurolytic solutions may be used for blockade of the obturator nerve and the nerve to quadratus femoris to relieve the pain caused by osteoarthritis of the hip.[18]

NERVE PLEXUS

Brachial plexus

Neurolytic blocks can also be performed for cancer pain involving the brachial plexus (e.g. a Pancoat's tumour). Phenol 5 per cent 15 mL in aqueous solution is injected into the plexus via the interscalene or supraclavicular routes. A catheter can be inserted into the plexus if repeated injections need to be given.[15] This procedure results in loss of sensation and mobility in the arm. If the tumour involves only the lower cords, a percutaneous cervical cordotomy or dorsal root ganglia lesions should be considered.[15] When the pain does not involve the whole extremity, paravertebral or more distal blocks may be considered to preserve maximum function.[4] For cervical plexus pain, 3–5 mL of phenol 5 per cent in aqueous solution can be injected at the level of each cervical transverse process.[18]

Hypogastric plexus

For perineal pain secondary to pelvic malignancy, a neurolytic block (with 5 mL phenol 6 per cent in aqueous solution) of the hypogastric plexus can be carried out using biplanar radiological facilities and after a diagnostic local anaesthetic blockade.[4,37,38] The pelvic organs are innervated by somatic and sympathetic fibres.[4] Unlike neuraxial blocks, this is usually not associated with loss of sphincter tone and paresis of the lower extremities, but injury to sacral nerve fibres or to a hollow viscus (rectum, bladder, ureter) can still occur.[4,37]

CRANIAL NERVES

Phenol is the most common agent used for the branches of these nerves.

Trigeminal

Ablative procedures may be considered in trigeminal neuralgia or in trigeminal pain from inoperable malignant disease.

Peripheral branches. Ablative lesions of the peripheral branches (e.g. supraorbital, maxillary, mandibular nerves) can be achieved at the exit

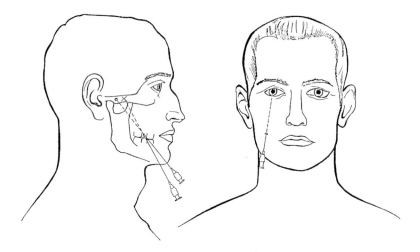

Figure 11.4 Trigeminal ganglion. A skin wheal is raised 3 cm lateral to the angle of the mouth at the level of the upper second molar. A 10 cm (22 gauge) needle is advanced posteromedially and superiorly, with its axis pointing to the midpoint of the zygomatic arch (side view). From the front, the needle axis must point to the pupil. At 6–7.5 cm, the advancing needle contacts the infratemporal plate just anterior to the foramen ovale. A marker is placed 1.25 cm from the skin surface, and the needle is withdrawn into the subcutaneous tissue. It is readvanced with its axis pointing to the articular tubercle (side view). In the front view, its axis points to the pupil. It is advanced until the marker reaches the skin.

foramina of the three divisions of the nerve from the scar using neurolytic chemicals (or cryolesions or radiofrequency lesions).[15] One such example is the treatment of trigeminal neuralgia with pain localized to the distribution of the infraorbital nerve by a maximum of 1 mL phenol 5 per cent aqueous solution. The anaesthesia that may be produced by these lesions may be extremely distressing.

Trigeminal ganglion. Lesions of the ganglion may be induced with either glycerine or radiofrequency current using a similar approach as discussed above (Figure 11.4).

Glossopharyngeal and vagus nerves. For advanced neoplastic progression in head and neck pain, neurolytic blockade of the 9th or 10th cranial nerves or upper cervical nerves (C2 and C3) may be required for complete pain relief.[4,25] Bilateral destruction of the 9th and 10th cranial nerves is not recommended because of potential interference with swallowing mechanisms and protective airway reflexes. Both nerves are blocked at the base of the skull with 2–3 mL of absolute ethyl alcohol, as they exit through the jugular foramen.[18] Extensive radiotherapy to the occiput and the neck makes the paravertebral approach to the cervical nerves difficult.[4] The epidural route should then be used.

NEURAXIAL NEUROLYSIS

Neuraxial neurolysis is discussed more fully in Chapter 9. Its advantages are:

- good results in properly selected cases;
- ease of performance with minimal or no hospitalization;
- duration of pain relief adequate for the preterminal state and suitable for debilitated patients;
- ease of repetition and a low complication rate with proper techniques.[4]

The degree and extent of sensory loss depends on the actual numbers (not types) of fibres destroyed, which is determined by the quantity and concentration of the neurolytic agent used.[4] Chemical rhizolysis can be performed at any level up to the midcervical region. Above this, agent spread to medullary centres carries significant risk of cardiovascular collapse.[4] Controlled studies comparing alcohol and phenol neurolysis are not available. In 58 per cent of patients, good analgesia is obtained with an average duration of 3–4 months.[4] No controlled studies comparing intrathecal with epidural neurolysis have been conducted. The advantages of intrathecal neurolysis over epidural neurolysis are as follows:[4]

- return of CSF verifies correct positioning;

- more precise lesion location (from gravity and posture), and more profound and longer duration of analgesia;
- ease of performance on an out-patient basis.

The main advantage of epidural neurolysis over intrathecal neurolysis is its applicability to pain of a wide distribution or bilateral, with greater control, owing to the ability to re-inject the patient several times over a number of days via the epidural catheter.[1,4] Risks of meningeal irritation, post-dural puncture headaches, and intracranial spread or ventral nerve root spread are also reduced.[4] The major disadvantage of intrathecal neurolysis is the possibility of permanent spinal cord damage with loss of motor, bowel, bladder and sexual functions.[1] Backache is the most common patient complaint after epidural neurolysis.[1] An epidural catheter made from spiral stainless steel coils coated with fluoropolymers has recently been introduced to facilitate radiological localization, aspiration and repositioning.[4]

When pain is related to brachial plexus infiltration (from tumour or fibrosis), neuraxial neurolysis often provides effective analgesia.[4] Chemical rhizotomy is ideal in patients with radicular thoracic or upper abdominal pain.[4] Intercostal muscle paresis may occur. Lumbar intrathecal neurolysis should be planned at the level at which the involved nerve roots exit from the spinal cord (that is between the low thoracic vertebrae).[4] Unilateral perineal and pelvic pain can be treated by placing the patient laterally (with dependency dictated by agent choice), and injecting the agent through a low lumbar puncture.[4] For bilateral pain, the procedure is reversed after a few days.

SYMPATHOLYSIS AND VISCERAL NERVE NEUROLYSIS

The techniques are explained more fully in Chapter 10. The principal indications for sympatholysis are CRPS, end-stage arteriosclerotic disease, sympathetically maintained pain in association with neuralgias, and for metabolic neuropathies (Raynaud's disease, Buerger's disease, the Crest syndrome).[2] For prolonged block of the sympathetic trunk, phenol 6–16 per cent will provide reliable interruption depending on the duration desired.[2] For technical reasons, a smaller concentration (phenol 6–7 per cent) is used for the cervical, stellate or upper thoracic ganglia, primarily to limit any adverse effects on adjacent structures or mixed nerves.[2] Neurolytic stellate ganglion block is hazardous because the cervicothoracic ganglion may be difficult to locate precisely and prevent spread.[4] Characteristic spread of contrast, needle aspiration, evidence of sympathetic local anaesthetic block, injection of 1–2 mL of aqueous phenol 6 per cent, and needle flushing before removal are all recommended.[4] In the lumbar region, phenol 7–16 per cent may be used to provide up to 10 months duration of effect.[2] Lumbar sympatholysis is for pelvic pain of urological, gynaecological or rectal origin, or for lower limb lymphoedema or CRPS.[4] In a small series of patients, complications were not observed after injections of 10 mL of phenol 10 per cent through a single needle positioned in the correct fascial plane near the 2nd lumbar vertebra.[2]

The principal indications for the interruption of the splanchnic or coeliac plexus are for malignancy (involving the pancreas, the distal oesophagus, stomach, liver and bile ducts, small bowel, proximal colon, adrenals and kidneys) and for non-malignant pain such as pancreatitis.[2] There is an immediate incidence of 85–94 per cent good-to-excellent pain relief following neurolytic coeliac plexus blocks (NCPB).[4] Although splanchnic nerve blocks allow for a degree of lateralization, both this and coeliac plexus neurolysis will provide analgesia for up to 10 months.[2,39] To produce optimal results, the following is recommended:[4]

- two needles should be used (the left tip at the junction of the lower and middle thirds of the 1st lumbar vertebra, and the right needle tip 1 cm higher);
- needle insertion is no greater than 7–7.5 cm lateral to corresponding spinal process at the inferior border of the 12th rib;
- radiological (especially CT) guidance is mandatory;
- 25 mL of solution (alcohol) should be injected through each needle;
- insertion depth may exceed that traditionally taught.

PITUITARY ABLATION

Diffuse pain from advanced malignant disease (especially with bone metastases from breast, prostate, and renal tumours) can be treated by pituitary ablation (Figure 11.5). Surgery, ionizing radiation, radioactive implants, alcohol, cryotherapy and radiofrequency lesioning have all been used.[15] All techniques produce pain relief in about 70 per cent of cases for 3–4 months.[15] Pain relief may be rapid and striking, while ascending nociceptive pathways

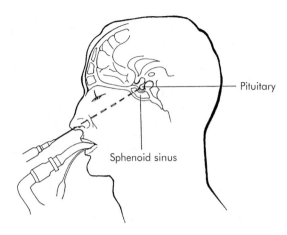

Figure 11.5 Pituitary ablation. Technique for alcohol injection, cryotherapy or radiofrequency lesioning.

remain intact.[3] Pain relief has been reported in about two-thirds of patients, whether or not the primary tumour is hormone-dependent.[3] The mechanisms for this effect are not clearly understood.[40] For chemical, radiofrequency or cryodestruction the probe is passed via the nose through the sphenoid bone into the pituitary fossa under biplanar x-ray control. Transient complications include diabetes insipidus, pupillary dilation, headache and blurring of vision.[18] Rarely, persistent CSF leakage, coma and blindness can occur.[3] The need for hormone replacement varies.

LASERS

Recently, lasers have been used to treat peripheral nerves more precisely without affecting the surrounding tissue.[17] They produce Wallerian degeneration and can be finely controlled and focused. Unfortunately, direct visual access to the nerve is needed.

STIMULATION ANALGESIA

The provision of analgesia by the interventional use of electrical currents is discussed in Chapter 12.

OTHER MODALITIES

Strontium-89 is a systemically injectable radionucleotide for decreasing pain secondary to bone metastases.[1] Seventy-five per cent of patients with metastatic prostrate cancer and more than 50 per cent with metastatic breast cancer obtain satisfactory pain relief.[1]

Percutaneous trigeminal ganglion compression (PTGC) is performed under general anaesthesia for trigeminal neuralgia. A number 14 needle is inserted under fluoroscopic control into the foramen ovale in the manner previously described.[23] A number 14 French Fogarty embolectomy catheter is advanced 15–20 mm into the needle and inflated for 1 minute with contrast to achieve a 'pear shape' in Meckel's cave.[23] This compresses the retrogasserian nerve fibres. Immediate analgesia occurs in 89.9–100 per cent of patients, and the average recurrence time is 4.2–6.5 months.[23] Complications similar to PRGR can occur.[23]

REFERENCES

1. **Arthur, J.M. and Racz, G.B.** 1997: The role of invasive techniques. In Parris, W.C.V. (ed.) *Cancer pain management: principles and practice*. Boston: Butterworth–Heinemann, 215–29.
2. **Stanton-Hicks, M.** 1996: Should we destroy nerves? *International Symposium of Regional Anaesthesia*, Auckland, New Zealand, 9–11 April, 127–30.
3. **Jacox, A., Carr, D.B., Payne, R., Berde, C.B.** *et al.* 1994: *Management of cancer pain*. Rockville: Agency for Health Care Policy and Research Publication, No. 94–0592, vol. 9; 1–257.
4. **Jain, S.** 1997: The role of neurolytic procedures. In Parris, W.C.V. (ed.) *Cancer pain management: principles and practice*. Boston: Butterworth–Heinemann, 231–43.
5. **Wells, J.C.D. and Miles, J.B.** 1991: Pain clinics and pain clinic treatments. *British Medical Bulletin* **47**(3), 762–85.
6. **Abram, S.E.** 1990: Diagnostic and prognostic nerve blocks. In Abram, S.E. (ed.) *The pain clinic manual*. Philadelphia: J.B. Lippincott, 91–3.
7. **North, R.B., Han, M., Zahurak, M. and Kidd, D.H.** 1994: Radiofrequency lumbar facet denervation: analysis of prognostic factors. *Pain* **57**, 77–83.
8. **North, R.B., Kidd, D.H., Zahurak, M. and Piantadosi, S.** 1996: Specificity of diagnostic nerve blocks: a prospective, randomised study of sciatica due to lumbosacral disease. *Pain* **65**, 77–85.
9. **Shipton, E.A.** 1990: The management of intractable pain. *Hospital Medicine* August, 30–4.
10. **Datta, S.** 1991: Pharmacology of local anesthetics. *American Society of Anesthesiologists' Annual Refresher Course Lectures* **276**, 1–5.
11. **Scott, D.B.** 1989: *Introduction to regional anaesthesia*. Norwalk: Appleton and Lange, 1–96.

12. **Scott, D.B.** 1989: Maximum recommended doses of local anaesthetic drugs. *Br J Anaesth* **63**(4), 373–374.

13. **Lloyd, J.W., Barnard, J.D.W. and Glynn, C.J.** 1971: Cryoanalgesia: a new approach to pain relief. *Lancet* **2**, 932.

14. **Raj, P.P.** 1986: Cryoanalgesia. In Raj, P.P., (ed.) *Practical management of pain.* Chicago: Year Book Medical Publishers, 774–82.

15. **Budd, K.** 1989: Ablative nerve blocks and neurosurgical techniques. In Nimmo, W.S. and Smith, G. (eds.) *Anaesthesia.* Oxford: Blackwell Scientific Publications, 1243–64.

16. **Budd, K.** 1989: The pain clinic – chronic pain. In Nunn, J.F., Utting, J.E. and Brown, B.R. (eds.) *General anaesthesia,* 5th edn. London: Butterworths, 1349–69.

17. **Bonica, J.J., Buckley, F.P., Moricca, G. and Murphy, T.M.** 1990: Neurolytic blockade and hypophysectomy. In Bonica, J.J. (ed.) *The management of pain,* 2nd edn. Philadelphia: Lea and Febiger, 1980–2043.

18. **Cousins, M.J., Dwyer, B. and Gibb, D.** 1988: Chronic pain and neurolytic neural blockade. In Cousins, M.J., Bridenbaugh, P.O. (eds.) *Neural blockade,* 2nd edn. Philadelphia: J.B. Lippincott, 1053–84.

19. **Justins, D.M. and Richardson, P.H.** 1991: Clinical management of acute pain. *British Medical Bulletin* **47**(3) 561–83.

20. **Duthie, A.M., Ingham, V., Dell, A.E. and Dennett, J.E.** 1983: Pituitary cryoablation: the results of treatment using a transsphenoidal cryoprobe. *Anaesthesia* **38**, 448.

21. **Budd, K.** 1989: Recent advances in the treatment of chronic pain. *British Journal of Anaesthetics* 1989 **63**, 207–212.

22. **Kantha, S.** 1997: Stereotactic techniques. In Parris, W.C.V. (ed.) *Cancer pain management: principles and practice.* Boston: Butterworth–Heinemann, 181–95.

23. **Burchiel, K.J.** 1996: Pain in neurology and neurosurgery: tic douloureux (trigeminal neuralgia). *Pain 1996 – an updated review.* Seattle: IASP Press, 41–60.

24. **Kettler, R.E.** 1990: Neurolytic nerve blocks for cancer pain. In Abram, S.E. (ed.) *The pain clinic manual.* Philadelphia: J.B. Lippincott, 289–95.

25. **Patt, R.B.** 1992: Control of pain associated with advanced malignancy. In Aronoff, G.M. (ed.) *Evaluation and treatment of chronic pain,* 2nd edn. Baltimore: Williams and Wilkins, 313–39.

26. **Morrison, J.E., Matthews, D., Washington, R., Fennessey, P.V. and Harrison, L.M.** 1991: Phenol motor point blocks in children: plasma concentrations and cardiac dysrhythmias. *Anesthesiology* **75**, 359–62.

27. **Wurm, W.H.** 1992: Role of diagnostic and therapeutic nerve blocks in the management of pain. In Aronoff, G.M. (ed.) *Evaluation and treatment of chronic pain,* 2nd edn. Baltimore: Williams and Wilkins, 218–28.

28. **Raj, P.P. and Denson, D.D.** 1986: Neurolytic agents. In Raj, P.P., (ed.) Practical management of pain. Chicago: *Year Book Medical Publishers,* 557–65.

29. **Brown, D.L. and Rorie, D.K.** 1994: Altered reactivity of isolated segmental lumbar arteries of dogs following exposure to ethanol and phenol. *Pain* **56**, 139–43.

30. **Bryce-Smith, R.** 1966: Local and regional analgesia. *Postgraduate Medical Journal* **41**, 367.

31. **Myers, R.R. and Katz, J.** 1988: Neuropathology of neurolytic and semidestructive agents. In Cousins, M.J. and Bridenbaugh, P.O. (eds.) *Neural Blockade,* 2nd edn. Philadelphia: J.B. Lippincott, 1031–51.

32. **Dingh, Y.R.T., Thurel, C., Serrie, A., Cunin, G. and Seylaz, J.** 1991: Glycerol injection into the trigeminal ganglion provokes a selective increase in human cerebral blood flow. *Pain* **46**, 13–16.

33. **Stav, A., Sternberg, A., Landau, M., Ovadia, L. and Weksler, N.** 1992: Intra-articular injection of a proliferant for pain relief in patients with rheumatoid arthritis: preliminary results. *The pain clinic* **5**(2) 83–9.

34. **Nagaro, T., Amakawa, K., Yamauchi, Y., Tabo, E., Kimura, S. and Arai, T.** 1994: Percutaneous cervical cordotomy and subarachnoid phenol block using fluoroscopy in pain control of costopleural syndrome. *Pain* **58**, 325–30.

35. **Kirvela, O. and Nieminen, S.** 1990: Treatment of painful neuromas with neurolytic blockade. *Pain* **41**, 161–5.

36. **Yamada, K., Ishihara, Y. and Shimada, S.** 1990: The coccygeal nerve block in the anterior sacrococcygeal ligament for intractable perineal pain after operation for rectal cancer. *Pain* **42**, S87.

37. **Khan, Y., Jain, S., Kestenbaum, A. and Shah, N.** 1990: Hypogastric plexus block: a new technique for the treatment of perineal pain. *Pain* **42**, S23.

38. **De Leon-Casasola, O.A., Kent, E. and Lema, M.J.** 1993: Neurolytic superior hypogastric plexus block for chronic pelvic pain associated with cancer. *Pain* **54** 145–51.

39. **Fujita, Y.** 1993: CT-guided neurolytic splanchnic nerve block with alcohol. *Pain* **55**, 363–6.

40. **Blumenkopf, B.** 1997: Neurosurgical approaches. In Parris, W.C.V. (ed.) *Cancer pain management: principles and practice.* Boston: Butterworth–Heinemann, 471–6.

12 STIMULATION ANALGESIA

Neuroaugmentation techniques have been in common use for nearly 30 years.[1] The application of stimulation techniques to alleviate pain is a common phenomenon observed across different cultures.[2] The usefulness of manual and electro-acupuncture for pain relief has been established,[3] and the participation of endogenous opioids and descending pain inhibitory systems in acupuncture analgesia has been demonstrated.[3] Electrical stimulation of the nervous system is a clinically established method of relieving pain arising from damage or disease of the somatosensory pathways.[4] Pain relief from primary afferent neurone stimulation has led to the development of electrical devices that can be used to stimulate different parts of the nervous system.[2]

Electrical nerve stimulation has been shown to be useful in many chronic pain states and deserves wider application.[1] Spinal cord stimulation is an important treatment mode for many patients with a failed back syndrome, for whom stimulation can replace or supplement surgery.[1] Its effective use requires a thorough understanding of the pain states to be treated, an appreciation of the co-morbidities that accompany chronic pain, an infrastructure to support the patient and the physician, and the dedication to lifelong care for the patient with an implant.[1]

Stimulation analgesia can be divided into peripheral and central stimulation. Peripheral nerve stimulation can be very effective in relieving chronic pain, but the number of potential candidates remains small.[1] Brain stimulation has not yet found a clearly defined place in pain management.[1] Most research has been in clinical efficacy, and more basic research into the mechanisms of action is needed to improve efficacy.

Spinal cord stimulators (mainly for neuropathic and ischaemic pain) and brain stimulators (mainly for tremor) are implanted in patients in many European countries.[5] Federal legislation and safeguards are extensive to protect the clinical condition and safety of patients, to meet safety and efficacy requirements in the design and construction of the stimulators and the materials used therein, and to ensure independent checks.[5] Official attitudes towards the indications considered appropriate, and the devices themselves, that are approved for reimbursement also vary widely between countries.[5] The main country outside the European Union where implantation is carried out is Switzerland.[5] Neither peripheral vascular disease nor angina is an approved use in the USA, the major indication there being failed back surgery syndrome for about 66 per cent of patients requiring spinal cord stimulation (a similar situation to that found in Australia).[5,6]

Deep brain stimulation has never been performed in particularly large numbers for pain, and a marked decline in its use for this purpose has been seen in recent years.[5] There has, however, been a growing interest in thalamic stimulation for parkinsonian and essential tremors, and for multiple sclerosis.[5] Nearly all cases of deep brain stimulation are performed in Europe.[5]

In 1996, worldwide sales amounted to approximately 10 100 spinal cord stimulators (including replacement pulse generators) and 1200 deep brain stimulators.[5] In 1997, the global market in neuro-modulation devices was worth more than US$200 million, with an annual growth rate of 15–20 per cent and rising.[5]

PERIPHERAL STIMULATION

Acupuncture

Acupuncture refers to the practice of inserting sharp needles into the body to treat pain and diseases.[7] Classical acupuncture has been practised in China for at least 2500 years. Acupuncture analgesia can be divided into classical acupuncture, Westernized acupuncture, electrical acupuncture and ear acupuncture. The widespread use of these techniques testifies to patient compliance and clinical effectiveness.[8] The reported response rate is, however, not uniform because of stimulation variables, the variations in the pain conditions treated and the inadequacy of placebo controls.[8] Age does not appear to determine the response.[2]

Classical acupuncture

The Chinese believe that life energy (Ch'i) follows specific pathways or meridians in the body upon which the acupuncture points lie.[9] Any pain or disease process can unbalance the circulation of Ch'i. This can be corrected by the insertion (with or without manual rotation) of acupuncture needles into specific points along the meridians near the body surface.[9] Classically, there are 12 bilaterally symmetrical meridians and two non-paired midline control meridians, each representing internal organs.

Westernized acupuncture

The traditional Chinese system involves the use of points that differ from patient to patient, with the possibility of varying them in subsequent sessions. In Westernized acupuncture, standard points are chosen *a priori*. Interestingly, many acupuncture points are close to nerves or to known trigger points.[9] Acupuncture points are sites of low direct current skin resistance and may be identified by using a skin resistance meter.[9]

On the selection of an acupuncture point, a 30 gauge stainless steel needle is inserted deep into the muscle until the patient experiences a tingling, soreness, numbness or heaviness (Teh Ch'i). Acupuncture points can be stimulated by digital pressure (acupressure), electrically and by the use of lasers. Acupuncture analgesia is of slow onset and long duration, and thus an induction period (2–30 minutes) is required for stimulation.[10] This is unlike TENS, in which analgesia begins almost immediately after stimulation.[2] Acupuncture needs to be given on a regular basis and rarely produces a cure.[11] Unlike TENS, however, it is effective in regions distant from the site of stimulation.

Electroacupuncture

With electroacupuncture, electrical stimulation with a pulse generator is applied by needles inserted into the acupuncture points. Electrical stimulation parameters may be defined in terms of frequency, polarity, intensity and waveform characteristics.[2] The insertion of needles means that current can be delivered with depth and precision. Most generators deliver pulsed direct current with a square wave.[9] The frequency, pulse width and voltage can be varied.

Generally, in chronic pain, a low frequency (2–4 Hz), high-intensity stimulation and a long treatment duration are used.[2] In acute pain, the use of low-intensity, high-frequency, short-duration stimulation is preferred.[2] Electroacupuncture (with low-frequency, high-intensity current at distant acupuncture points) and TENS (with high-frequency, low-intensity current applied near surgical sites) results in sufficient pain relief for the skin and fascia; however, pain in the deeper structures still remains.[3] High-intensity, high-frequency electroacupuncture with non-insulated needle electrodes produces more potent analgesic effects than TENS (with different types of surface electrode) in the skin and fascia.[3] High-intensity, high-frequency electroacupuncture with insulated needles gives a significant increase in the pain threshold in muscle and periosteum, demonstrating deep pain relief by the use of insulated needle electrodes and high-frequency, high-intensity current pulses.[3]

Electroacupuncture produces more analgesia than manual acupuncture.[12] Recent results have shown a significant increase in the release of neuropeptides (CGRP, neuropeptide Y and vasoactive intestinal polypeptide) in the saliva of healthy subjects treated with electroacupuncture.[13] The electrical stimulation of acupuncture points with surface electrodes is a relatively new and non-invasive treatment with potential application in the management of patients with peripheral vascular disease.[14]

Ear acupuncture

Ear acupuncture is a specialized form of acupuncture (Figure 12.1). According to the theory of this method, all parts of the body and all the inner organs are reflected on well-localized reflex zones on the auricle of the ear.[15] The entire auricle can be viewed as a representation of an inverted fetus *in utero*. When an organ becomes diseased or painful, the corresponding point on the auricle becomes painful.[15]

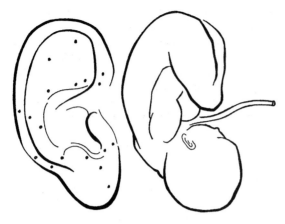

Figure 12.1 Ear acupuncture.

PHYSIOLOGICAL EFFECTS

For acupuncture analgesia, an intact nervous system is required. Local anaesthetic injected into the muscle beneath an acupuncture point prevents the development of analgesia.[10] Acupuncture creates a number of physiological changes. Electroacupuncture has been shown markedly to enhance motor and sensory nerve regeneration.[7] In rats, acupuncture-like sciatic nerve stimulation lowers blood pressure for prolonged periods.[7] Acupuncture can increase temperature and microcirculation, thus promoting the healing of chronic ulceration (probably as a result of the release of vasoactive intestinal peptide).[7] Adrenocorticotrophic hormone is also released by acupuncture. This might be responsible for the effects of acupuncture in treating arthritis and asthma.[7] Stimulation of the sixth point on the pericardial meridian (P6) inhibits emesis in postoperative adult patients.[16] Acupuncture also has an anti-ischaemic effect and has been successfully used in treating severe angina.[15] Stimulation of the median nerve to mimic electroacupuncture diminishes regional myocardial ischaemia triggered by a sympathetically mediated increase in cardiac oxygen demand.[17] The mechanism of this effect is related to the reduction in cardiac oxygen demand secondary to a decreased pressor response.[17]

MECHANISMS OF ACTION

There are a great number of conflicting data on the mode of action of acupuncture and its efficacy.[11] Both psychophysiological and neurophysiological mechanisms for its analgesic effectiveness have been hypothesized. Personality differences are felt to be an important source of variation in response.[18]

It has been shown that acupuncture may have a more pronounced effect on the affective (the unpleasantness) than the sensory component of pain.[19]

With acupuncture, an interaction takes place at different levels of the CNS between impulses from the origin of the pain and afferent impulses from the site of stimulation. Low-frequency, high-intensity acupuncture stimulation is considered to act by stimulating small muscle afferents (type III and A delta fibres) to produce both segmental and suprasegmental inhibition via endorphinergic and serotonergic pathways.[7,11]

In the rat model, electroacupuncture may activate multiple conflicting neuronal circuits that interact and ultimately modulate the analgesic outcome. Low-frequency electroacupuncture appears to be mediated via proenkephalin-derived peptides acting on mu opioid receptors.[8] It is naloxone reversible. High-frequency electroacupuncture appears dynorphinergic and is probably mediated via kappa opioid receptors.[8] Larger doses of naloxone are thus needed to block its analgesic effects. However, on first exposure, opioid antagonists (naloxone and naltrexone) may even potentiate analgesia.[20,21] In the rat model, it has also been found that the arcuate nucleus of the hypothalamus mediates low- but not high-frequency electroacupuncture, and that the central peri-aqueductal grey area is necessary for electroacupuncture analgesia.[22,23] Cross-perfusion experiments have shown transferral of the acupuncture-induced analgesic effect from donor rabbit to recipient rabbit when CSF is transferred.[12] The prevention of electroacupuncture-induced analgesia by naloxone and by antiserum against endorphins suggests that endorphins are involved.[12] In both experimental animal and human studies, both low-frequency (2 Hz) and high-frequency (100 Hz) electroacupuncture selectively induce the release of enkephalins and endorphins.[12] In man, the results of naloxone on acupuncture analgesia following experimentally induced and clinical pain are inconclusive.[19]

PATIENT SELECTION

Acupuncture is used in the treatment of acute and chronic organic pain of musculoskeletal and neurogenic origin. Acupuncture analgesia was first used to provide analgesia for surgery (an appendicectomy) in 1958,[7] but the results of acupuncture in acute perioperative pain relief have generally been disappointing.[9] Patients with post-herpetic neuralgia, diabetic neuropathy, CRPS type 1, osteo- and rheumatoid arthritis, tension headaches, low back and cervical pain syndromes, post-surgical pain syndromes (resistant phantom limb) and temporo-mandibular joint syndromes may be helped by acupuncture when conventional therapy fails.[2,18,24] Patients should be motivated psychologically to help ensure success. Concomitant insomnia, anxiety or depression should first be treated.[2] Caution is advised with acupuncture in pregnancy and in patients with pacemakers. Epileptic patients should lie down and should not be stimulated too vigorously.[2] Aseptic techniques should be observed. Disposable sterile needles prevent complications arising from infectious diseases (e.g. AIDS). Treatments can initially be given biweekly (usually up to a total of six) and then weekly thereafter if the patient responds.

SIDE-EFFECTS

Commonly, hyperaemias occur at the site of needle insertion from the release of histamine-like substances.[2] Lightheadedness and syncope may occur (in fewer than 1 per cent of patients).[2] Patients should therefore lie down during initial therapy. A haematoma may occur at the site of needle insertion. Pneumothorax and damage to the spinal cord have rarely been reported.[9]

EFFICACY

The absence of a standardized methodology of stimulus parameters (frequency, intensity and waveform) makes the analysis of efficacy difficult. With low back pain, however, studies reported a good to excellent response to acupuncture in 72–89 per cent of patients.[2] Real acupuncture seems to be effective in 60–75 per cent of patients, sham acupuncture in 50 per cent of patients and placebo in 30 per cent of patients.[25] Three systematic reviews of acupuncture in chronic non-malignant pain show an effect, but the effect in clinical practice is often short-lived (3 days).[26]

TENS

TENS is simple to use, safe and efficacious, and requires very little preparation time for implementation (even self-implementation). Many clinical studies on the use of TENS for pain relief are poorly conducted and lack any long-term follow-up assessment.[4] It is difficult to come to any clear conclusion, from published work, regarding the parameters of stimulation and pain relief

obtained.[27] In particular, studies investigating the contribution of TENS to post-surgical pain control with adults have reported encouraging results, and TENS has also been found to be useful in treating chronic musculoskeletal pain, angina and procedural pain among adults.[28] For children's procedural pain, such as that from venepuncture, pain intensity is lowest when TENS is used, especially in the higher age groups (above 7 years).[28]

No clear rules therefore exist on optimal frequencies to be used in the treatment of various disorders,[4] and there is an absence of standardized methodology. Up to 70 per cent of chronic pain patients may initially respond well to TENS, but, by the end of the first year, this rate drops to around 30 per cent.[4] One half to three quarters of chronic pain patients who obtain successful analgesia, however, reach over 50 per cent pain relief.[29] With TENS, because pain relief is temporary, stimulation has to be repeated regularly.[30]

MECHANISM OF ACTION

TENS has been found significantly to elevate ice pain threshold in healthy subjects.[31] High-frequency, low-intensity TENS is considered to activate large muscle (type I) and large skin (A beta) fibres (possibly via interneurones with GABA receptors) to produce gating by segmental inhibition.[7] TENS with surface electrodes significantly increases the pain thresholds of skin and fascia but not those of muscle and periosteum.[3] The analgesia is often of rapid onset and short duration, and tolerance can develop from continuous therapy. It seems to be unaffected by naloxone.[8]

There is also evidence that TENS can produce conduction block in C fibres.[32] In rats, however, an increase in CSF dynorphin A (from preprodynorphin) occurs following stimulation, suggesting a dynorphinergic opioid mechanism.[8] Thus, these analgesic effects may be a combination of large-fibre stimulation, nociceptor blockade and an opioid mechanism.

Low-frequency (2–4 Hz), high-intensity stimulus TENS (acupuncture) provides analgesia for certain patients unresponsive to conventional TENS.[32] Like acupuncture, it is considered to act by stimulating small muscle afferents (type III and A delta fibres) to produce both segmental and suprasegmental inhibition via endorphinergic and serotonergic pathways.[7] The analgesia produced has a slow onset and long duration, and can be reversed by naloxone.[8] In rats, an increase in CSF met-enkephalin-arg-phen (from proenkephalin) occurs.[8]

TENS has been shown to be clinically most effective when the frequency is high and the intensity low.[33] It has been found that the application of TENS to somatic receptive fields most commonly reduces the activity of spontaneously firing cells, decreases the activity of noxious stimulus-evoked dorsal horn neurones and more frequently deceases cell activity with high-frequency, low-intensity stimulation variables as opposed to low-frequency, high-intensity ones.[33] This model can be used to glean information about the basic gating mechanisms and to evaluate the numerous variables associated with the application of TENS (e.g. the differential effects of the stimulation modes, the influence of varying the frequency, intensity and pulse duration; the placement of the electrodes; the influence of supraspinal mechanisms; the long duration of stimulation; and the effects on noxious inflammatory somatic and viscerally evoked activity).[33] Non-noxious TENS applied segmentally produces inhibitions of the RIII reflex (a nociceptive flexion reflex elicited by electrical stimulation of the sural nerve at the ankle) only during the 2-minute conditioning period.[34] When given segmentally, noxious TENS produces a facilitatory effect during the 2 minutes of application, followed by significant inhibitory after-effects.[34] Heterotopic noxious TENS administration results in inhibitions of the RIII reflex both during and after the 2-minute conditioning period.[34] The application of noxious piezo-electric current, whether segmentally or heterotopically, produces powerful and long-lasting inhibitory after-effects, underlying the potential use of piezo-electric current in the treatment of pain.[34] In rats, noxious heat-related impulses are attenuated by the presence of specific electrical stimulation, supporting the clinical application of TENS to block pain.[35]

PARAMETERS AND MODES

Stimulators consist of small battery-powered portable units that can be worn undetected under the clothing.[30] Stimulation pulses are delivered to nerve fibres transcutaneously via surface electrodes connected to the stimulator by cables. A thin layer of electrode gel is placed between the electrode and the skin to facilitate contact.[30] The three most common parameters that can be adjusted in TENS units to produce various stimulation modes are the current intensity (amplitude), the pulse width and the rate.[36] Various modes are available:

1. *Conventional mode.* This consists of a low pulse width (75 microseconds), high rate (85 pulses per second) and high-intensity current set to a comfortable tingling paraesthesia without muscle contraction.[36] It is used for acute and chronic pain.

2. *Low-frequency high-intensity stimulation.* This mode consists of a high pulse width (200–220 microseconds), low rate (2–4 pulses per second) and high-intensity of current. Current amplitude is increased to the point of mild discomfort and muscle stimulation.[32] Stimulation is carried out for short periods (5–15 minutes). This is often effective in chronic pain.

3. *Brief intense mode.* This consists of a high pulse width (200–220 microseconds), a high rate (100–150 pulses per second) and a high-intensity current, set to the highest level of pain.[36] It is used for joint pains.

4. *Burst stimulation.* Short bursts of high-frequency stimulation are delivered at 1–2 Hz.[32] Low-intensity current is used for acute superficial pain, while high-intensity current is used for chronic deep pain.[36]

5. *Modulated mode.* Patients unresponsive to the above modes may respond to the modulated mode. Here rate, pulse width and intensity are fluctuated at short (1–2 second) intervals.[36] A recent advance is the use of a randomized frequency and amplitude, which has led to the development of a new generation of stimulators.[29,32]

Patients seem to prefer specific and individualized pulse frequencies and pulse patterns to treat their pain condition.[37] It has been suggested that a speedier reduction in pain occurs with high-frequency as opposed to low-frequency TENS and that patients who present with a longer experience of pain take longer to achieve relief with TENS.[38] It has recently been shown that chronic pain patients prefer modulated stimulation modes (such as frequency modulation and burst) to the conventional constant mode.[4,27] This has emphasized the necessity of offering each patient an initial trial of a range of stimulation modes in order to establish individualized parameters.[4,27]

A sinusoid-waveform TENS stimulus of constant current intensity has the ability to evoke discrete frequency-dependent subjective sensations.[39] This has led to the development of a neurometer to measure current perception thresholds. This can provide a new parameter for the evaluation of chronic pain relief using TENS or electroacupuncture.[40]

SIDE-EFFECTS

TENS has remarkably few physiological side-effects. The only common adverse effect of TENS is skin irritation in about one third of patients, probably due in part to drying out of the electrode gel.[29] Frequently rotating stimulation sites, changing the type of electrode employed and using topical corticosteroids can minimize this problem.[32] Allergic reactions to electrodes, gel or tape are occasionally encountered.[29] The declining response to TENS with time remains a problem.

METHODS OF USE

Educating the patient on the correct electrode placement and the control of settings is critical for effective use.[36] One or more pairs of electrodes are placed on the skin directly over, or in the vicinity of, the pain.[11] The active electrode (the cathode), from which stimulation actually occurs, should normally be placed proximally.[30] Other placement options of electrodes include dermatomes, acupuncture points, trigger points, spinal nerve roots or over a nerve plexus.[36] With pain in an extensive area, two electrode pairs driven by a dual-channel unit can be used.[30]

As continuous mode TENS is that most often used initially, patients are instructed as follows:[37]

- Set all controls (pulse intensity in mA, and frequency) to the minimum settings.
- Increase the pulse intensity to a strong but comfortable level.
- Increase the pulse frequency to the maximum comfortable level.
- Experiment with all the stimulator settings but hunt for the most appropriate one.
- If sufficient pain relief is not obtained, try other modes.

TENS should initially be tried for a minimum of 1 hour to determine its efficacy (improvement or aggravation) and any adverse skin reactions.[29] Most patients treat themselves at home several times daily, each time for 20–60 minutes.[30] Also, in most patients (approximately 80 per cent), pain relief only occurs during stimulation.[30]

CLINICAL USE

The use of TENS has been associated with significant reductions in the use of pain-related medications (NSAIDs, opioids, sedatives, muscle relaxants and corticosteroids) and physical therapy.[41] Cost simulations of medication and physical therapy indicate that, with long-term TENS use, costs can be reduced by up to 55 per cent for medication and up to 69 per cent for physical therapy.[41] In a recent review, 58–72 per cent of chronic pain patients reported an initial positive effect from TENS use, 13–74 per cent reported a continued positive effect at 6 months, and 27–66 per cent of chronic pain patients reported a reduction of pain at 1 year.[41] These TENS-associated improvements, when combined with reduced complications and costs, are important points that clinicians must consider when constructing a treatment plan for chronic pain patients.

Acute pain

In the perioperative situation, immediately after wound closure, sterile adhesive electrodes are applied to the skin on either side of the incision.[42] The wound is dressed, and the electrodes are connected to a stimulator.

There have, however, been few well-controlled studies on the efficacy of TENS in acute postoperative and post-traumatic pain. Although TENS has been successfully used as a adjunct following anal surgery and thoracotomy, it has not been shown to be universally effective in acute pain.[43-45] Controversy also exists over the effect of TENS on opioid requirements.[42] Clearly, TENS is not effective as the sole treatment for moderate or severe pain after surgery.[46] In 15 out of 17 randomized controlled trials on the use of TENS in acute postoperative pain, there was no analgesic benefit over placebo.[47]

Nevertheless, TENS has been widely used as an analgesic adjunct in the management of labour pain.[30] No adverse effects on the fetus or newborn have been detected.[30] However, 10 randomized controlled trials on the use of TENS in labour pain showed that TENS offered no significant effect on pain in labour.[48] A recent application of TENS is the relief of angina when all other methods fail;[49] it seems to have an anti-ischaemic effect, but the mechanism of action is unclear. It may be explained by reduced sympathetic activity since plasma adrenaline and noradrenaline levels drop during TENS.[49]

Chronic pain

Clinicians cannot assume that any particular pain will not respond to TENS as a wide range of chronic pain conditions have been successfully treated using this method.[29] However, when sensory loss is such that there are insufficient large (A beta) cutaneous fibres to stimulate, TENS is of no benefit and may even aggravate the pain.[50,51]

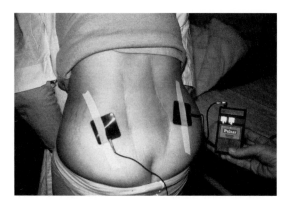

Figure 12.2 Transcutaneous electrical nerve stimulation (TENS) – a patient, suffering from post-laminectomy pain, receiving treatment with a TENS machine.

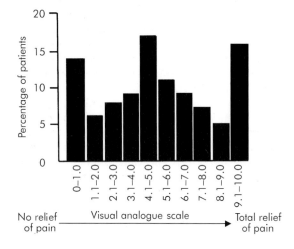

Figure 12.3 Pain relief, using transcutaneous electrical nerve stimulation (TENS) on a long-term basis in 168 chronic pain patients; 47 per cent found that TENS reduced their pain by half or more.

Myofascial pain is particularly responsive to TENS. In cancer pain, TENS appears to be very useful for the accompanying myofascial pain (trigger points) and variably effective for neuropathic pain (Figures 12.2 and 12.3).[32] It is also useful for isolated bony secondaries (spine and rib).[32] TENS can also relieve abdominal discomfort after irradiation.[52]

Other painful conditions treated with TENS include post-herpetic neuralgia (mild), central post-stroke pain, phantom limb and stump pain,

and CRPS type 1.[51,53,54] TENS has been found to be highly effective in the complex treatment of glossalgia.[55]

In chronic lumbar radiculopathy, electrodes are placed over the dermatomal distribution of the affected nerve root.[56] It has been found that TENS is more effective than placebo-TENS in reducing the intensity of chronic low back pain immediately after each treatment session as well as 1 week after the end of the treatment, which confirms that TENS is clinically useful as a short-term analgesic procedure for chronic low back pain rather than as an exclusive or long-term treatment.[57] TENS reduces both the sensory-discriminative and motivational affective components of chronic low back pain in the short term, but much of the reduction in the affective component may be a placebo effect.[57] Because of the additive effect of TENS over a short time, its repetitive use over a short period of time to potentiate this effect has been recommended.[57] In chronic back pain, combined TENS and neuromuscular electrical stimulation therapy has been found to be a more effective analgesic than either given alone.[58]

TRANSCRANIAL TENS

Transcranial TENS (TCES) with high-frequency (166 kHz) intermittent current (100 Hz, Limoge current) has been used in cardiothoracic, general and neurosurgery to reduce opioid requirements and provide longer-lasting postoperative analgesia.[59] In the rat model, the effects of TCES have been found to be centrally mediated, and adding L-tryptophan augments these analgesic effects.[59,60]

GENERAL

With TENS, the onset and offset of analgesia are rapid (within 30 minutes).[61] When post-TENS analgesia occurs, it usually lasts less than 30 minutes.[29] Neither age nor sex has any predictive value for the response to TENS.[29] In chronic pain patients, it has been found that the combination of TENS and vibratory stimulation alleviated pain in more cases than either modality given alone, and it had stronger and more long-lasting analgesic effects.[61,62]

Patients are often loaned a TENS machine to take home. If the technique benefits the patients, they then purchase their own machine. For convenient use in daily life, a cordless mini-TENS has been introduced.[63] Auricular TENS seems effective in relieving pain only when high-intensity TENS is used.[64]

Peripheral nerve stimulation

PERIPHERAL NERVE STIMULATION FOR ANALGESIA

Peripheral nerve stimulation has been successfully to treat pain of neuropathic origin in the upper extremeties, lower extremeties and intercostal nerves.[65,66] Patients with single nerve pathology are the best candidates for peripheral nerve stimulation, but those with multiple lesions have been successfully screened and implanted.[65,66] Clinical syndromes, especially neuropathic conditions, responding favourably to peripheral nerve stimulation, include CRPS types 1 and 2, direct nerve injury (operative, traumatic, entrapment and post-injection) and plexus avulsion injuries.[66] The insertion of electrodes alongside peripheral nerves has been used for the relief of chronic pain, usually resulting from peripheral nerve or nerve root injury (of the upper or lower limbs).[30] Sympathetically maintained pain has also been successfully treated in this way (see Chapter 10).

Clinical selection criteria include:[65,66]

- chronic intractable pain that is resistant to other therapies;
- pain that can be temporarily relieved by a local anaesthetic injection;
- a lack of psychological contraindications or drug dependency and abuse;
- objective evidence of pathology (from selective tissue conductance studies, somatosensory evoked potentials or electromyography);
- pain relief from temporary screening.

The peripheral nerve to be stimulated needs to be exposed surgically. Apparatus implantation is similar to that described under 'Spinal cord stimulation' below. A new approach, using the Resume™ type padded electrode beneath the injured nerve, has resulted in dramatically better success rates (i.e. good pain relief in over 70 per cent of patients during a 10–70 month follow-up).[67] The electrode sites for the upper extremity are usually above the elbow.[67] Sites for the lower extremity are the sole of the foot above and medial to the ankle, and the common peroneal nerve implant above the knee for the top and outside of the calf area.[67] For sciatic nerve stimulation, electrodes have been placed in the upper thigh or close to the sciatic nerve where it exits from the pelvis (this often being used to treat patients suffering from intrasciatic injections of corrosive medications).[67] The electrode placement is carried out as a two-stage procedure under general

anaesthesia proximal to the injury. Firstly, the Resume™ peripheral nerve stimulation electrode is implanted, and the lead wires are externalized for test stimulation.[67] For example, for the median or ulnar nerves, a longitudinal incision is made on the medial aspect of the arm, centred between the elbow and the axilla.[65] A dissection is carried out to the neurovascular bundle to free the nerve and to isolate an area of about 4 cm long for electrode placement.[65] The electrode is placed underneath the nerve with multiple peripheral sutures to hold it in place, and a fascial tissue flap is folded over the electrode to prevent its direct contact with the nerve.[65] Soft tissue is sutured loosely to hold the nerve over the electrode. The lead is brought percutaneously to a small wound in the shoulder area and attached to a temporary connector brought through the skin.[67] The wounds are closed and dressed with transparent dressings. The temporary leads are connected to the battery pack, and the electrical stimulation is adjusted (over the next 3 days) after evaluating the electrode requirements for the best results.[65] If the technique works, the best electrode combination is determined before proceeding to stage two, namely implanting the more expensive (over $5000) permanent stimulating system (Itrel 2 Medtronic™).[65,67]

Complications include infection, bleeding, drug reactions, spinal cord injury, CSF leak, poor analgesia, fibrosis at the stimulator tip and/or motor stimulation.[65,66] Mechanical problems include lead fracture or shearing, perioperative lead movement, extension cable fracture, battery malfunction and transmitter malfunction.[65,66]

PERIPHERAL NERVE STIMULATION IN MUSCLE FUNCTION

Peripheral nerve stimulation is used to restore muscle function after an upper motor neurone type of paralysis.[68] Spectral myography shows that electrical stimulation produces immediate changes in the motor unit by increasing the recruitment number and action potential velocity, and gives a selective recruitment of type II fibres.[69] Functional electrical stimulation for quadriplegic or paraplegic patients consists of direct stimulation of the motor nerves to allow movement in paralysed limbs.[70] Multiple electrodes are implanted on several nerves of the upper or lower extremities. The electrodes are connected to a sophisticated, multiprogrammable pulse generator that fires the electrodes sequentially according to a predetermined programme.[70] This stimulation leads to sequential activation of the muscle groups required to perform a movement. A 16-channel functional electrical stimulation system (for total implantation) has been found to be feasible for short-distance, independent, walker-support walking in paraplegia.[71]

OTHER NERVE STIMULATION ROUTES

Recently, stimulation of the sacral plexus through electrodes percutaneously implanted via the sacral foramina has been described.[72] Electrodes are placed along the plexus in the retroperitoneal area for pain arising from the sacral plexus. Percutaneous electrode placement and stimulation of the gasserian ganglion is used for the treatment of atypical trigeminal neuralgia.[73] In facial pain of central origin (post-stroke), chronic electrical stimulation of the gasserian ganglion can relieve pain in up to 71 per cent of patients.[74] In post-herpetic neuralgia, there is a positive response to percutaneous intermittent intraneural spinal nerve stimulation and intraganglionic gasserian ganglion stimulation using effective low-frequency stimulation.[75] Epidural electrical stimulation of the motor cortex contralateral to the painful area has been successfully employed in patients with facial neuralgia, producing a long-term reduction in facial pain.[76]

For refractory epilepsy, effects comparable to the best regimens of antiepileptic drugs with fewer side-effects are obtained by chronic electrical stimulation of the vagus nerve.[70] The electrode is placed around the vagus nerve in the neck, and the pacemaker is placed in a subcutaneous pocket in the clavicular area.[70]

CENTRAL STIMULATION

Spinal cord stimulation

The first multiprogrammable electronics were introduced in 1980, and totally implantable neural stimulator systems in 1981.[66] In 1988, non-invasive programmable implantable pulse generators with radiofrequency capabilities became available.[66] In the 1990s, the successful adaption of multilead electrode arrays, implantable pulse generators, implantable radiofrequency receivers and objective patient screening methods has led to high success rates.[66]

Spinal cord stimulation has evolved as a reversible, non-destructive, low-morbidity technique for the management of chronic, intractable pain. Despite the extensive use of spinal cord stimulation for the control of various chronic pain conditions, most clinicians previously reported only modest success rates.[77] In a compilation of 15 clinical studies, overall success rates of 66 per cent in the short term (under 1 year) and 52 per cent in the long term were found.[43,78] In a recent nationwide survey in Belgium, it was found that thorough psychiatric screening improved outcome but that work resumption was not necessarily a likely outcome of spinal cord stimulation.[79] In general, the effectiveness of spinal cord stimulation decreases over time.

With modern techniques and appropriate patient selection, sustained success can be achieved in 70–80 per cent of patients.[80] From literature searches, it is clear that evidence on spinal cord stimulation is limited.[81] It is likely to be biased because of the lack of randomization and blinding as it has been conducted by enthusiasts and reporting has been limited.[81] To correct this, randomization, follow-up assessments at uniform times by independent observers, descriptions of clinical and demographic information, the use of valid pain measures and the assessment of multiple outcomes (e.g. back and leg pains, physical functioning, drug use, work status, health care use and quality of life) have been suggested.[81] In general, however, most patients with implanted spinal cord stimulators report at least 50 per cent relief of pain at a 7-year mean follow-up.[82] Overall morbidity has been quite low.[82] Sixty per cent of patients reported that they would go through the same procedure for the same result.[82] In a large study of 171 patients, patients reported using their spinal cord stimulators for on average 11.5 ± 8.1 hours daily, with an average latency before analgesia of 8.3 ± 15.7 minutes and an average duration of analgesia of 2.0 ± 6.6 hours after the spinal cord stimulation had been switched off.[82] Only 68 per cent of patients with pain syndromes of peripheral origin received permanent implants compared with 87 per cent and 90 per cent of those with failed back surgery syndrome and spinal cord injury, respectively.[82] Spinal cord stimulation has been found to be a new and effective way of relieving chronic diabetic neuropathic pain.[83] It is estimated that about 12 000 patients world wide annually are subjected to spinal cord stimulation treatment.[84]

MECHANISM

Spinal cord stimulation most probably works through a spectrum of neurophysiological mechanisms varying from the simple blocking of pain transmission by a direct effect on the spinothalamic tracts, effects on the central sympathetic systems, segmental inhibition via coarse fibre activation and brain stem loops, to thalamocortical mechanisms.[85] The effects of spinal cord stimulation on the inhibitory transmission of nociceptive impulses may be exerted segmentally in the spinal cord, at a supraspinal level or both.[85] The basics include electrical contact with a cathode (negative electrode), which causes excitation of the nervous tissue.[65] The inside of the cell is negatively charged. Thus, the exposure of an external negative charge causes depolarization to a positive potential on the inside of the cell, which therefore causes an action potential and a non-noxious message.[65]

Segmental parts of the gate theory

The gate theory proposes that activity in the A beta fibres should cause the presynaptic inhibition of both A beta and nociceptive A delta fibres,[86] but this does not occur.[86] Yet, there is evidence that spinal cord stimulation has an inhibitory control over the dorsal horn nociceptive neurones (high-threshold, nociceptive-specific spinothalamic tract cells, and WDR lamina V neurones), modulating the perception of pain.[77,80,84,85] The effects on the WDR neurones are partly dependent on GABAergic mechanisms.[84] High-frequency, low-amplitude stimulation silences most dorsal horn cells, including noxious ones.[66] The level of several transmitters/neuromodulators (GABA, substance P, noradrenaline and glycine) increases in the dorsal horn after spinal cord stimulation.[85] The release of GABA and the activation of GABA-B receptors by spinal cord stimulation inhibits the release of the excitatory amino acids (glutamate and aspartate) in the dorsal horn, possibly suppressing nociceptive transmission.[85] Spinal cord stimulation increases the substance P content in the CSF.[84] Spinal cord stimulation in rats with mononeuropathy decreases the extracellular levels of glutamate and aspartate in the dorsal horn concomitant with an increase in GABA release. In neuropathic pain and allodynia, long-term pain relief may be obtained by an influence on dorsal horn humeral transmission and neuromodulators, having secondary effects on the distorted dorsal horn biochemistry after neural damage.[85]

The effect of spinal cord stimulation on neuropathic pain and allodynia may be due to activation of GABAergic and adenosine-dependent mechanisms, inhibiting excitatory amino acid release, which is chronically elevated in such conditions.[84,85,87] Many other mechanisms are probably also active. Both adenosine and the GABA-B agonist

baclofen can be used in 'subclinical' doses to potentiate the effect on spinal cord stimulation in previously unresponsive cases, thereby transforming them into responders.[85]

Supraspinal mechanisms

Long-lasting inhibitory after-effects may be dependent upon the involvement of supraspinal relays. The most obvious evidence for a supraspinal effect of spinal cord stimulation is the fact that paraesthesias are perceived even in phantom limbs.[80] Spinal descending pathways originating in the dorsal column nuclei, terminating deep in the dorsal horn, have recently been described.[84] These may be activated by spinal cord stimulation and play an important role in pain modulation.[84] The inhibition of spinothalamic responses by spinal cord stimulation has been recorded in the human ventrolateral thalamus.[80] Furthermore, evoked potentials in the human somatosensory cortex are reduced by spinal cord stimulation, thus modulating information travelling along the primary somatosensory pathways.[77] Spinal cord stimulation relieves pain after anterolateral cordotomy (which damages the spinothalamic tracts).[80] The electrodes are placed caudal (and contralateral) to the cordotomy lesion, indicating an action of spinal cord stimulation at the thalamic level and/or above.

It has recently been shown that, following spinal cord stimulation, action potentials in A fibres of the dorsal columns drive cells to excite cells in the anterior pretectal nucleus.[84,86] The anterior pretectal nucleus projects to and excites lateral brain stem nuclei and also projects back in the dorsal lateral funiculus, which then sends inhibitory axons to the dorsal horn to inhibit the deep spinothalamic tract cells.[86] This inhibition will reduce the response of these cells to nociceptive A delta or C fibres.[86] The anterior pretectal nucleus is thus an important central relay of the antinociceptive effects of spinal cord stimulation. The analgesic effects of anterior pretectal nucleus cell excitation may also be mediated via rostral projections from this nucleus to areas such as the somatosensory cortex and the intralaminar and posterior thalamic nuclei.[86] Antidromic action potentials descending in the dorsal columns operate the segmental spinal gate, giving rise to brief analgesia.[86] In animals, if spinal cord stimulation is started at the time of nerve section or 3 days before, the start of autotomy is markedly delayed.[84] Spinal cord stimulation applied infrequently and during a limited period of time may induce long-lasting changes of spinal plasticity.[84]

Additional pretectal projections are as follows.[86]

The deep spinothalamic cells project to the thalamus via the anterolateral funiculus. The shallow lamina 1 projection neurones project to the anterior pretectal nucleus and parabrachial nuclei. These project back to the spinal cord via the dorsal lateral funiculus. Noxious stimuli will excite both lamina 1 and deep spinothalamic cells. Lamina 1 cells set up a reverberatory re-excitation of the anterior pretectal nucleus and medullary relays. This reverberatory circuit inhibits the spinothalamic cells to reduce their response to noxious stimuli. Spinal cord stimulation is an effective way of enhancing the activity of this system of neurones.[86]

More basic laboratory research is required on the anti-aversive effects of spinal cord stimulation and deep brain stimulation.[86] Pharmacological methods of enhancing spinal cord stimulation for therapeutic benefit have been suggested.[86] Glutamate mediates transmission to the anterior pretectal nucleus from the dorsal columns. The inhibitory axons descending to the spinal cord from the lateral brain stem are likely to release a catecholamine to act upon the α_2-adrenergic receptors. This suggests that antidepressants inhibiting noradrenaline uptake may be useful potentiators of the descending inhibition.

The effects in motor disorders probably involve different mechanisms. Inhibition at a local level must be responsible for the reduction in muscle spasm seen with spinal cord stimulation below a complete spinal cord transection.[80] The inhibition by spinal cord stimulation of detrusor hyperreflexia and the increase in bladder capacity in patients with multiple sclerosis and other conditions is not understood.[80] In normalizing the micturition reflex, spinal cord stimulation appears to be sympathomimetic.[80] A reduction in the aversive element of pain is particularly apparent in angina pectoris. Many patients report analgesia lasting for 1.5–2.0 hours after switching off the stimulator but often say that they still have pain during stimulation, albeit pain that it is less unpleasant and easier to cope with.[80]

Spinal cord stimulation and the autonomic nervous system

Experimental studies favour the concept that spinal cord stimulation delivered at a low 'clinical' amplitude generally exerts a transitory inhibition of sympathetic activity via a central spinal mechanism.[85] In the treatment of ischaemic pain, the probable effect of spinal cord stimulation is to inhibit sympathetically maintained peripheral vasoconstriction mediated via nicotinic ganglionic receptors and α_1-adrenergic receptors at the neuroeffector junction.[85] Pain relief seems secondary to a re-established balance between oxygen supply and demand. Recent rat studies indicate additional antidromic vasodilatation probably brought about via A delta fibres in the higher part of the velocity spectrum for this fibre group and mediated by CGRP, the mechanism appearing to be NO dependent.[85] There may also be an inhibitory effect on transmission in the spinothalamic pathways, mediated via vagal afferent activation in cervical segments.[85] Spinal cord stimulation releases intracardiac endorphins and lowers systemic catecholamine concentrations.[85] Spinal cord stimulation increases the lower levels of CSF endorphins and serotonin found in chronic pain sufferers as well as increasing transcutaneous oxygen pressures and decreasing transcutaneous carbon dioxide pressures in patients with peripheral vascular disease.[65,66]

One hypothesis suggesting that dysautonomic pain syndromes are in fact mediated by damaged visceral afferents within autonomic nerves suggests potentially exciting explanations for the actions of spinal cord stimulation, possibly involving afferents from blood vessels. Clonidine has been found to inhibit the temporal summation elicited by repeated electrical stimulation and may therefore attenuate spinal cord hyperexcitability.[88] Inhibition of the sympathetic nervous system is more likely with high-frequency, low-amplitude stimulation.[66] Further research on the mechanisms of spinal cord stimulation would enable the indications to be better defined and the outcome to be predicted with a higher degree of reliability than to date.

INDICATIONS

Successful spinal cord stimulation therapy requires careful patient selection, a meticulous implantation technique and comprehensive patient management (including physical therapy).[89] Spinal cord stimulation is most often used in chronic neuropathic pain associated with non-malignant conditions of the trunk or limbs (Figure 12.4).[11,66] These include arachnoiditis, radicular pain with intraspinal fibrosis, spastic torticollis, post-traumatic neuropathic pain (post-amputation and phantom limb pain, coccydynia), peripheral neuropathies (post-herpetic neuralgia and intercostal neuralgia) and CRPS.[11,66,90] Spinal cord stimulation is generally not effective in treating nociceptive pain from nerve irritation (heat, pressure, chemicals and cancer pain) or central deafferentation pain from CNS damage (stroke and

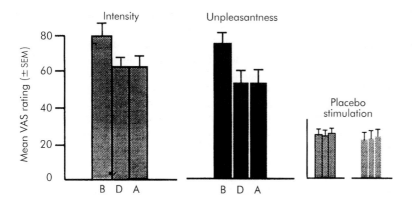

Figure 12.4 Mean visual analogue scale (VAS) ratings given by patients to describe their clinical pain (intensity and unpleasantness) during 30 minute periods before (B), during (D) and after (A) dorsal column stimulation. Placebo stimulation is shown in the inset.

spinal cord injury).[89] The most common condition for which spinal cord stimulation has been applied is chronic low back and sciatic pain (e.g. the failed back surgery syndrome).[91] Many patients with failed back surgery syndrome, particularly those with a neuropathic, deafferentation element, do benefit from spinal cord stimulation.[80] Nociceptive pain (from inflamed facet joints or periosteal irritation) does not respond to spinal cord stimulation.[80] Spinal cord stimulation is occasionally used for spinal cord lesions (where sufficient dorsal column fibres persist).[92] In the failed back surgery syndrome, the success rate overall is not more than 41 per cent in the long term.[93] A prospective, randomized study of spinal cord stimulation versus reoperation in this syndrome found a statistically significant advantage for spinal cord stimulation over reoperation.[94]

With spinal cord stimulation, success is:[80,84]

- almost certain (approaching 90 per cent) in angina and ischaemic limb pain;
- very likely in CRPS types 1 and 2, peripheral nerve lesions, brachial plexus damage, cauda equina damage, nerve root avulsion and amputation stump pain;
- reasonably likely in failed back surgery syndrome (leg pain more than back pain), partial spinal cord lesions, phantom limb pain and postherpetic neuralgia;
- unlikely in nociceptive pain (including that of cancer), thalamic syndromes, vaginal, penile, rectal and perianal pains, other midline pains and intercostal neuralgia;
- very unlikely in facial anaesthesia dolorosa, atypical facial pains, complete cord lesions and abdominal pains.

Spinal cord stimulation does not relieve postoperative wound pain. The clinical efficacy of spinal cord stimulation for each type of pain still needs to be reliably estimated.[91]

The beneficial effects of spinal cord stimulation in peripheral vascular disease are remarkable in terms of pain relief, increased activity, refractory ulcer healing and limb salvage.[70] These effects are mediated via changes in the microcirculation correcting maladaptive processes occurring in the microcirculation distal to major occlusions.[55] The density of perfused capillaries increases significantly during stimulation, and the capillary red cell velocity increases considerably within a day of starting stimulation.[80] Spinal cord stimulation is effective in severe vasospastic disorders (e.g. frostbite), although diabetics respond less well.[80] In critical limb ischaemia, limb salvage rates are increased to 75 per cent at 6 months (in Fontaine grades III and IV), 70–83 per cent at 1 year, 56–64 per cent at 2 years, and 43 per cent at 3 years.[80]

In intractable angina pectoris, considerable relief of pain is achieved in nearly all patients, exercise tolerance is increased, and ST segment depression is reduced.[80] There is a significant reduction in the frequency of angina attacks, increased work capacity, an improved lactate metabolism and a reduction in glyceryl trinitrate intake.[80,95] The suggested mechanism is through an inhibition of sympathetic discharge, resulting from stimulation of the intermediolateral column of the cord, which leads to coronary vasodilatation. It can be concluded that spinal cord stimulation is a treatment modality that is very favourable and strongly recommended in patients in whom no more open surgery or other therapeutic methods can be used.[96] Spinal cord stimulation only interferes with the function of cardiac pacemakers at high voltage.[80]

Spinal cord stimulation has a 'normalizing' effect on the neurogenic bladder.[80] Marked and often sustained improvements in bladder function occur in a high proportion of patients with multiple sclerosis.[80] With spinal cord stimulation, moderate but greatly functional improvement can be achieved in cerebral palsy, dystonia, mild spasmodic torticollis and parkinsonism.[80]

Little work has been done on the effect of high cervical spinal cord stimulation on cerebral blood flow. A significant reversal of cerebral ischaemia, whether resulting from 'fixed' cerebral vascular disease or potentially reversible vasospasm, as seen after subarachnoid bleeding, could be of great benefit.[80] High cervical spinal cord stimulation might even help to reverse coma.

Spinal cord stimulation has efficacy in pain states of neuropathic or ischaemic origins but not in acute pain or pain of nociceptive origin.[97] Spinal cord stimulation is most appropriately used in patients with a unilateral, single focus of pain. It is less effective for bilateral foci of pain and is not at all effective for multiple, multilevel areas of pain.[97]

PATIENT SELECTION

Technical improvements in implanted spinal cord stimulation devices have led to enhanced system reliability and improved clinical results.[82] The assessment of patient suitability is difficult with this expensive technique,[11] but includes pharmacological, psychological and physiological scrutiny.[11] Spinal cord stimulation should be used only after the failure of syndrome-specific conservative therapies.[97] Appropriate selection criteria include the absence of untreated drug habituations, a psychological interview and clearance, a trial of efficacy, a sufficiently long life expectancy and the absence of any surgical contraindications.[79,97] Patients with obvious psychological difficulties, drug abuse or major issues of secondary gain are rejected.[98] Some patients are reconsidered after completing a behavioural programme.[82] However, there is no association between the preoperative use of opioids and benzodiazepines, and the outcome.[82] Spinal cord stimulation should be restricted to patients who have an objective (somatic) basis for their pain complaints and for whom conventional medical, surgical and behavioural therapy has been tried and found to be unsuccessful.[79,98,99] Other relative contraindications include patient aversion to electrical stimulation or an implant, a patient with a demand pacemaker or needing a future MRI, an active and uncontrolled coagulopathy, localized or disseminated infection and a physician's lack of experience with the implantation technique.[66] NSAIDs should be stopped in the weeks before surgery.[6]

Unfortunately, trial stimulation has never proved to be as comprehensive a screening test as was initially hoped, and it might actually be a poor predictor of outcome of permanent spinal cord stimulation.[80] No significant predictors of the outcome of percutaneous stimulation trials, apart from the diagnosis, have been found.[82] Few studies have compared the outcomes in those selected by a trial with those implanted directly without a trial.[80] Trial stimulation relates to 'screening in' potential responders; virtually nothing is known of the technique's effectiveness in 'screening out' potential failures. There is a tendency for the trial electrode (lead) to be left *in situ* and used as permanent electrode in those patients responding positively. Nevertheless, a percutaneous trial remains an important aspect of the procedure.[82] A trial will demonstrate that appropriate paraesthesiae can be achieved in a particular patient, will indicate the optimal placement and will educate the patient with regard to permanent implantation, although it will not predict long-term success.[55] TENS is not a useful predictor of outcome from spinal cord stimulation, and many non-responders to TENS respond to spinal cord stimulation.[80] There is still a need to explain why patients carefully selected for permanent implantation on the basis of pain relief during a temporary trial frequently achieve success rates of little more than 50 per cent.[80] In a small number of patients, spinal cord stimulation may exacerbate their pain.[80] Trial stimulation is now more useful (but still flawed) in multifactorial, 'dirty' diagnostic groupings, particularly the failed back surgery syndrome, which includes a variety of aetiologies and pain mechanisms.[80] Assessments of outcome include pain relief, activity levels and a reduction in medication. Achieving stimulation overlap of the lower back is recognized as technically difficult and may require complex electrode geometries and extensive psychophysical testing.[82] Short-term pain relief is significantly better in females, and a superior outcome is also found in patients with a smaller number of prior operations.[82] There is an association between weakness on the preoperative neurological examination and functional outcome score, and unilateral pain syndromes are not necessarily more easily treatable.[82] Return to work is an important outcome measure.[82] In one study, there was an improvement from 41 per cent working preoperatively to 54 per cent at a mean 7-year follow-up.[82]

In a study over 18 years in 320 patients, an analysis of prognostic factors has revealed a number of significant determinants of outcome, including:[82]

- the importance of achieving a close correspondence of stimulation procedures with the topography of each patient's pain (which has been enhanced by the development of multichannel devices);

- the fact that associations between certain patient characteristics (e.g. axial lower back pain) and outcome are of some value in patient selection.

A temporary monopolar electrode is usually inserted percutaneously as a screening method to demonstrate satisfactory pain relief before the implantation of a permanent system.[98] A superposition of stimulation paraesthesiae upon the topography of a patient's pain has been found to predict the successful relief of pain.[98] Temporary insertion also produces an opportunity to map potential sites for permanent electrode implantation and educates the patient in the technical goals of the procedure.[98]

PSYCHOLOGICAL EVALUATION

To date, no definitive reproducible studies have verified any specific, statistically significant psychological factors, as measured by established psychological tests, to predict the outcome of spinal cord stimulation therapy.[99] There has been little investigation of the psychological characteristics of patients classed as false negatives or screening failures who do not go on to implant or trial.[99] Certainly, major depression or anxiety, active suicidal behaviour, untreated self-harm behaviour and drug dependence are problems susceptible to pretreatment.[6] Exclusion factors include personality disorders, serious cognitive defects and an inability to understand and/or manage the device.[6] However, more time should be devoted to adjunctive therapies (such as psychological pretreatment) to enhance the success rate of spinal cord stimulation. When long-term follow-up psychological test data become available, this may allow a further refinement of patient selection.[82]

INSERTION TECHNIQUE

Over the past two decades, spinal cord stimulation devices and techniques have evolved from single systems, with electrodes requiring laminectomy, into programmable multichannel systems in which electrodes may be placed percutaneously.[82]

Placements are always epidural. The majority are implanted percutaneously in the thoracic spine for lower body and lower limb pain. Relatively few are implanted for upper limb pain. Open, surgical electrode implantation gives superior results in the cervical spine because of the degree of location security.[80] The electrodes must be placed rostral to the upper neurological level of the pain, ipsilaterally for unilateral pain and over the midline of the cord for bilateral pain.[80] To obtain significant pain relief, the spinal cord stimulation-induced paraesthesiae should cover the painful area, yet this does not guarantee success. To stimulate the shoulder, the cathode should be at C2–4, for the whole hand at C5–6, for the anterior thigh at T7–8, for the legs and buttocks at T8–9 and for the foot at T9–10.[80] The low back and perineum remain difficult to target selectively. For angina, the electrodes are placed at T1–2, slightly to the left of the midline.[80] For peripheral vascular disease of the lower limbs (including frostbite), the most successful placements have been at T10–L1 (particularly T10).[80] For vascular disease affecting the upper limbs, C5–T1 has successfully been used.[80] For motor disorders (spasmodic torticollis and dystonia), C2–4 has been the favoured electrode position.[80]

The spinal cord stimulator can be driven either by an external transmitter and radiofrequency coupling, via an internal receiver–transducer, or by a totally intracorporeal, powered pulse generator analogous to a cardiac pacemaker. The advantage of the former is that there is no external apparatus (except for the magnet that switches it on and off).[80] The disadvantages are that the patient has limited control (usually on and off, with a choice of two amplitudes), that telemetric programming is required to change the stimulus parameters, and that battery expiry after a few years requires surgical replacement.[80] The advantages of radiofrequency systems are lower recurring costs and more patient control over the amplitude and other parameters (fine-tuning).

The most popular parameter combination is probably 80–85 cycles per second, a pulse width of 0.20 or 0.21 milliseconds and an amplitude just above the perception threshold.[80] In angina, the parameters are 50–85 cycles per second, a pulse width of 0.2 or 0.21 milliseconds and an amplitude of 3–6 V.[80] For peripheral vascular disease and vasospastic disease, the parameters are 50–120 cycles per second and a pulse width of 0.20 or 0.21 milliseconds.[80] A much higher frequency of 1100–1400 cycles per second with a smaller pulse width of 0.05–0.10 milliseconds has proved effective in extrapyramidal movement disorders and spasticity.[80]

Spinal cord stimulation is applied with low intensity, just suprathreshold for the low-threshold, large fibres conceivably contained in the dorsal columns.[84] Stimulation-evoked paraesthesia should cover or invade the entire painful area. To be effective spinal cord stimulation must be applied continuously for periods of at least 20–30 minutes.[84] It is most effective for ongoing spontaneous pain, especially neuropathic pain of peripheral origin.[84] It generally takes 10–20 minutes before a reduction in pain is perceived, this lasting for 1–3 hours after the cessation of stimulation.[84]

Multicontact electrodes allow for the reconfiguration of the pattern of stimulation to compensate for lead migration or malposition, and they achieve a better coverage of pain sites by paraesthesiae.[100]

Temporary monopolar epidural electrode

Percutaneous insertion of the monopolar electrode (with a remote indifferent skin electrode) into the epidural space is carried out under local anaesthesia with the patient in a sitting or preferably prone position (Figure 12.5).[65] There is no need for sedation.[82] Image intensification is used to place the stimulating

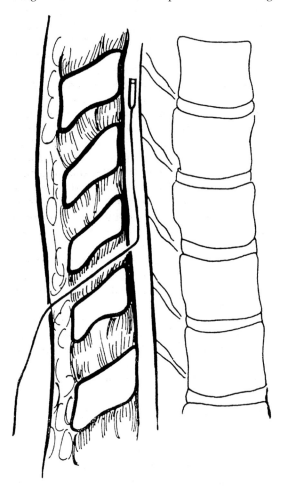

Figure 12.5 Dorsal column stimulation. The epidural electrode and lead have been placed at the mid-thoracic level. This position is generally used for pain relief of the pelvis and legs.

tip at the mid- or lower thoracic level for leg pain or the mid-cervical region for arm pain.[91,92] The electrode tip should be in the midline above the highest painful segment. Once superposition of stimulation paraesthesiae upon the topography of a patient's pain has been achieved, the electrode is fixed to the interspinous ligament and brought out through a paravertebral incision.[91,92] The clinician should be certain that the system to be implanted can withstand changing positions from recumbent to ambulatory and make sure that the paraesthesia coverage does not vary significantly with ambulation.[66] The patient should receive intravenous prophylactic antibiotic cover about 30 minutes before the percutaneous implantation, which is maintained for as long as the percutaneous lead is present and for a brief period subsequent to total system implantation.[66] After a percutaneous test of at least 2–3 days, in which patients have reported at least 50 per cent pain relief with improved activity and analgesic use, a permanent implant can be offered.[82]

Multichannel devices

Permanently implanted multiple electrodes may be inserted percutaneously.[98] Commercially available bipolar systems have been followed by quadripolar systems.[80] The majority of systems used have 4 channels available, but 8- and 16- (dual octapolar) channel systems have recently been introduced. Four channels have proved superior to 2 for both pain syndromes and motor disorders.[80] Local anaesthetic is used as electrode placement can be guided more precisely by patient feedback. Individual electrode placement can be optimized by trial stimulation, by increasing the number of available electrodes or by using an electrode system that allows a wide range of spatial configurations.[80] In future, systems will be capable of varying the amplitude (and other parameters) to individual electrodes independently of others in the array. There is evidence that plate electrodes can deliver successful stimulation in some patients in whom narrower, percutaneous leads have suffered primary or secondary failure.[80] Insulated plate electrodes have technical advantages offsetting the slightly more invasive procedure (laminotomy) necessary to implant them.[101] Yet, for low back pain and leg pain, a 'guarded cathode' or 'split anode' configuration (i.e. a cathode flanked by anodes) performs best.[80] Unwanted dorsal root stimulation can be reduced by decreasing the interelectrode distance (contact separation) and by an awareness of the fact that the threshold for cathodal stimulation is much lower than that for anodal stimulation.[80]

Laminectomies are only performed if placement is technically difficult. The configuration of a central cathode with anodes above and below seems to be preferred by patients.[98] After a trial stimulation period, permanent internalization is performed. The position of the cord can be checked with ultrasound prior to electrode positioning at laminotomy/laminectomy.[80] The electrodes are connected to an inductance coil buried subcutaneously (infraclavicularly, in the lower ventral thoracic wall or in the abdominal wall).[52,91,92] This is usually performed under a general anaesthetic. A radiofrequency coupled power pack is worn outside the body, placed on the skin over this coil, and impulses are generated within the buried system to stimulate the cord.[102] The decision of whether to place an implantable programmable neurological stimulator power source or a radiofrequency receiver with an external transmitter and antennae depends on whether the physics of the implanted system is exceeded during the screening period.[66] If the external power source is guided by an audible signal, problems may be experienced by patients with impaired hearing.[66] Once capable of operating the system, patients are discharged 12–24 hours later.[66]

Fully implantable stimulators are available. These are switched on and off by an external magnet.[91] The implanted battery may be depleted rapidly when used for spinal cord stimulation.[102] Fully implantable stimulators do, however, offer advantages in terms of convenience and patient compliance. A computer-controlled, patient-interactive neural stimulation system has been described.[103]

Patients should not bend, lift, twist or stretch their body for 6–8 weeks following lead placement.[89] They should work with the clinician for 6–8 weeks post-implant to achieve optimal settings and pain relief. Overall, multichannel (quadripolar) systems have a significantly greater clinical reliability than do single channel systems (hazard ratio = 0.45; $P=0.001$).[82] Percutaneously inserted electrode arrays with multichannel systems have the same reliability as did systems with laminectomy electrodes.[82]

COMPLICATIONS

Reviews on complications can be outdated in 5 years as stimulation systems are constantly improving.[6] Superposition of stimulation paraesthesiae upon the topography of a patient's pain is not sufficient for pain relief.[82] Electrode position is critical to achieving a satisfactory overlap of pain by stimulation paraesthesiae, and arrays of multiple electrodes are therefore technically advantageous.[82] Also, numb areas do not respond to spinal cord stimulation.[6] A computer-controlled, patient-interactive system to facilitate the clinical use of these systems is being developed.[82] It is difficult to achieve analgesia in the low lumbar and sacral segments with spinal cord stimulation, as the high current required produces severe paraesthesiae.[32] Complications include electrode migration and dislodgement, infection (1–3 per cent) and equipment failure (lead fracture, insulation failure and current leakage being infrequent).[80] It is difficult to distinguish true electrode migration (infrequent now with anchoring techniques) from malposition.[82] Spinal cord compression (from haematoma, ectopic CSF, electrodes or excess silicon) has rarely occurred.[80] Prolonged, exaggerated postoperative pain localized to the incisions and more diffuse over the back can occur in 5–10 per cent of patients and last several months.[80] The mechanism is unknown but appears clinically to be a fasciitis. Other rare complications include excessive receiver mobility or failure, subcutaneous wound haematomas, hypersensitivity to or skin erosion from the implanted materials, intracranial subdural haematoma (following open implantation in the sitting position) and non-fatal pulmonary embolism.[80] With time, fibrosis under the stimulating electrodes increases the distance between the electrodes and the neural tissue, giving rise to late failures, a steadily progressive phenomenon.[32] Late failure by no means seems to be declining despite technical advances, nor does it account for all cases.[32,80] The extent to which late failure represents true tolerance (rather than a cognitive or perceptive phenomenon) needs to be elucidated.[80] On–off cycling might give better pain relief than continuous stimulation,[80] but the true explanation is unknown.

Recent technical improvements in implanted spinal cord stimulation systems (especially multichannel systems) have led to improvements in clinical results over time (e.g. over 2 years) and decreased the incidence of complications.[98]

COST-SAVING WITH SPINAL CORD STIMULATION

Spinal cord stimulation enjoys several advantages over surgery. It has a low morbidity rate (less than 5 per cent).[100] It has been found in patients who responded positively to spinal cord stimulation therapy that the implantation costs have been offset by the additional back surgery avoided.[100] The annualized costs of spinal cord stimulation complications and maintenance care were also considerably less than the non-surgical chronic care costs for the therapeutic alternative.[100] The reduction in demand for medical care made by failed back surgery syndrome patients over a 5-year period has resulted in savings of more than $3000 for the internally powered system and $7000 for the externally powered system compared with treatment alternatives.[100] It has been found that if a proposed therapy costs $20 000 or more per year and has an efficacy rate of 78 per cent or less, spinal cord stimulation therapy is more cost-effective.[100] Spinal cord stimulation has the potential to reduce direct medical costs, disability costs and other social costs that may justify its cost-effective application in selected patients. One study showed a 22 per cent cost saving with spinal cord stimulation compared with reoperation at 3 years, and that spinal cord stimulation pays for itself after 2 years.[6] In most failed back surgery syndrome patients, spinal cord stimulation has eliminated the need for further back surgery.[100] The improvements in pain with spinal cord stimulation are greater and more sustained than those seen with surgical intervention.[6] Other advantages include testability, reversibility, non-destructiveness, the association with a low complication rate and the ability to address difficult-to-treat neuropathic pain problems.[6]

LONG-TERM FAILURE

In a review of 126 patients followed for an average of 37.8 months initially reporting over 50 per cent pain relief, 20 per cent had discontinued the use of stimulation or requested removal of the system.[78] Reasons for failure were disease progression (in 55 per cent), tolerance (continued appropriate paraesthesiae with loss of pain relief in 41 per cent) and painful hardware (in 4 per cent).[78] An improvement in long-term outcome may be attained by using higher frequencies in cases of tolerance and by exploring the use of more complex arrays and programming to anticipate disease progression.[78] In general, the keys to good outcome in spinal cord stimulation are careful patient selection, meticulous technique, avoiding complications and rigorous follow-up and equipment maintenance.[6]

Deep brain stimulation

Electrical stimulation of the brain offers hope to patients who have failed to respond to other chronic pain treatment techniques. There is considerable evidence, in both basic and clinical studies,

suggesting that deep brain stimulation can modify the activity of nociceptive neurones and that this approach should be a feasible alternative in the treatment of chronic intractable pain.[104] Studies in monkeys suggest that stimulation of the ventroposterolateral nucleus of the thalamus produces inhibition of spinothalamic tract neurones located in the dorsal horn and that this may play a role in pain relief from ventroposterolateral nucleus stimulation.[105] The importance of the medial thalamic nuclei and supraspinal structures (including the cortex) in modulating pain and participating in pain relief has recently received renewed interest. Electrical stimulation of the parabrachial area, including the Kollicker–Fuse nucleus, has been shown to inhibit nociceptor-induced activation of the dorsal horn neurones.[72] Intracerebroventricular self-injection of beta-endorphin as a form of analgesic self-medication occurs in rats in response to intermittent electrical shocks.[106]

SITES USED

The most commonly used deep brain stimulation sites in humans are located in three areas:[104]

- the somatosensory areas of the ventrobasal thalamus (including the ventroposterolateral and ventroposteromedial nuclei);
- the caudal medial thalamic areas (including the periventricular grey matter, central medialis and parafascicularis);
- near the junction of the third ventricle and the sylvian aqueduct (rostral ventral periaqueductal grey/caudal ventral periventricular grey).

MECHANISM OF ACTION

Behavioural animal studies support the clinical findings of analgesia produced by stimulation of the medial areas but not by stimulation of the ventroposterolateral and ventroposteromedial nuclei.[104] Neurophysiological animal studies show evidence for the activation of pain inhibiting pathways by stimulation of these areas.[104] In neither area does there appear to be clear dependence on endogenous opioid pathways for the analgesia.

STIMULATION PARAMETERS

These parameters vary greatly. Stimulation is almost always bipolar, with a wide range of frequencies (2–200 Hz) and pulse widths (0.1–50.0 milliseconds).[104]

INDICATIONS

Dorsal cord stimulation has been used to treat virtually every known chronic pain of both neuropathic and nociceptive origin.[105] As with spinal cord stimulation, a thorough assessment of the likelihood of success has to be made before using this expensive method of treatment.[11] Patients must also be evaluated adequately during the initial trial percutaneous stimulation. Dorsal cord stimulation is reserved for patients who are incapacitated by their pain after a minimum of 6 months from the start of their pain, in whom conventional methods of pain treatment have failed.[105] The pain should have a clearly defined aetiology. Contraindications include patients with a strong psychological component to their pain (e.g. excessive neurotic concerns with bodily functions and disease processes), patients with a prior history of frequent surgically related procedures and patients with chronic undefined pain in the genital, rectal or pelvic areas.[105] It is not necessary to discontinue opioids at the time of electrode implantation.[105]

Nevertheless, somatosensory thalamic stimulation is used for post-traumatic and post-herpetic neuralgias (particularly in the face), sciatica, brachial plexus lesions and central pain caudal to the thalamic relay nuclei (e.g. extensive spinal cord lesions).[91,104] Periventricular and peri-aqueductal grey area stimulation is in turn used for the nociceptive discogenic and arthrogenic components of low back pain.[91]

SURGICAL TECHNIQUE

Peri-aqueductal or periventricular grey area electrodes are placed contralateral to the side of unilateral pain, or an electrode is placed in the non-dominant hemisphere for bilateral pain.[105] The most common combination of electrodes and targets are two electrodes, one in the periventricular grey matter and one in the ventroposterolateral nucleus, located contralateral to the pain.[105] The 'rule' that ventroposterolateral/ventroposteromedial nucleus stimulation is necessary for neuropathic pain and peri-aqueductal/periventricular grey stimulation for nociceptive pain is not clinically valid.[105] Many chronic pain patients (e.g. failed back surgery syndrome patients) present with a combination of both. Somatosensory thalamic or internal capsular stimulation produces effective pain relief contralateral to the electrode placement.[72]

Electrodes are implanted stereotactically under local anaesthesia via a 15 mm burr hole centred anterior to the coronal suture and 15–20 mm lateral to the midline.[72] MRI is used to obtain a mid-sagittal T1-weighted MRI, to locate the anterior and posterior commissures. An axial T1-weighted image at the level of the anterior–posterior commissure plane is then obtained.[105] CT localization can be employed if implanted hardware makes MRI impossible. Intraoperative physiological target localization is essential since the stereotactic coordinates represent only starting points for localization of the physiological targets.[105] Microelectrode recording, microstimulation and macrostimulation are used to identify targets accurately.[105]

The electrode is bipolar and concentric, with an inner fine tungsten rod microelectrode and an outer stainless steel tube insulated except for 0.5 mm around the end nearest the tip of the microelectrode.[105] Microstimulation takes place through the fine electrode recording tip, while macrostimulation takes place though the uninsulated portion of the outer tube. The correct target for pain relief in the somatosensory thalamus is one from which stimulation-induced paraesthesiae encompass the body region where the patient's pain is located.[105] After the stereotactic coordinates of the desired targets have been identified, permanent stimulating electrodes are introduced into the brain at these sites. Percutaneous leads are tunnelled under the scalp and led out under the scalp through the skin a short distance away through small wounds. A postoperative MRI scan confirms correct placement and assesses possible cerebral bleeding.[105] Trial stimulation is begun 24–48 hours after implantation. All possible stimulation combinations (bipolar and monopolar) are explored during the trial stimulation period of 5–7 days.[105] If pain relief ensues, a receiver is implanted subcutaneously in the infraclavicular region. This can be activated via a flat antenna taped to the skin and connected to a transmitter–stimulator (as in spinal cord stimulation).[91] Fully implantable and programmable stimulators can also be used for chronic stimulation, or else the electrodes are removed.[91,105]

COMPLICATIONS

About 20 per cent of patients experience procedural complications, most of which are relatively minor in nature.[105] These include the occasional bleed, a localized tissue reaction, infection (at the receiver, or along the subcutaneous tunnel), electrode displacement, malfunction of the implanted device and tolerance to deep brain stimulation.[91] Electrode implantation more rarely produces a dysaesthesia (in the sensory thalamus) or a slight diplopia (in the periventricular grey region).[91] Only about 4 per cent of complications are permanent (hemiparesis and disorders of extraocular movements), and fewer than 1 per cent of patients are permanently disabled or die.[105]

RESULTS

Of those patients with a permanent implant, 59.0–62.2 per cent experienced long-term pain relief.[105] Nociceptive pain responds better (70 per cent of patients relieved) than neuropathic pain (50 per cent of patients relieved).[105]

CONCLUSION

Detailed information regarding the homologous stimulation sites in man that are appropriate and clinically effective is still needed.[104] Many sites and parameters could also be tested within a single model. Real and placebo stimulation could then be examined in a double-blind manner and measures of clinical and experimental pain applied.[104] MRI and improved neuronal recording should enable more accurate electrode placements. The implantation of two electrodes costs about $60 000.[105] Treatment of the sensory–motor cortex has recently shown promising results in the treatment of some forms of intractable pain.[70]

Magnetic fields

Nociception is influenced by an exposure to magnetic fields.[107] In humans, a significant reduction in pain-related somatosensory-evoked potential amplitudes is observed after exposure to oscillating magnetic fields.[107]

REFERENCES

1. **Long, D.M.** 1998: The current status of electrical stimulation of the nervous system for the relief of chronic pain. *Surgical Neurology* **49** (2), 142–4.
2. **Ng, L.K.Y., Katims, J.J. and Lee, M.H.M.** 1992: Acupuncture: a neuromodulation technique for pain control. In Aronoff, G.M. (ed.) *Evaluation and treatment of chronic pain*. Baltimore: Williams & Wilkins, 291–8.
3. **Ishimaru, K., Kawakita, K. and Sakita, M.** 1995: Analgesic effects induced by TENS and electroacupuncture with different types of stimulating electrodes on deep tissues in human subjects. *Pain* **63**, 181–7.
4. **Tulgar, M., McGlone, F., Bowsher, D. and Miles, J.B.** 1991: Comparative effectiveness of different stimulation modes in relieving pain. Part II: A double-blind controlled long-term clinical trial. *Pain* **47**, 157–62.
5. **Simpson, B.A.** 1998: Neuromodulation in Europe: regulation, variation, and trends. *Pain Reviews* **5**, 124–31.
6. **Burchiel, K.J.** 1998: Spinal cord stimulation. Part 1: Long term efficacy: considerations and outcomes. Part 2. The Sir Sidney Sunderland Lecture: Spinal cord stimulation. In *Highlights from the advanced pain therapy seminar and the Australian Pain Society meeting.* Tasmania: Medtronic, 2–15.
7. **Nash, T.P.** 1992: Development of medicine and stimulation produced analgesia. *The Pain Clinic* **5**(3), 181–5.
8. **Han, J.S., Chen, X.H., Sun, S.L.** *et al.* 1991: Effect of low- and high-frequency TENS on Met-enkephalin-Arg-Phe and dynorphin A immunoreactivity in human lumbar CSF. *Pain* **47**, 295–8.
9. **Charlton, J.E.** 1989: Acupuncture, TENS, hypnosis, and behavioural therapy. In Nimmo, W.S. and Smith, G. (eds) *Anaesthesia*. Oxford: Blackwell Scientific Publications, 1230–42.
10. **Nash, T.P.** 1992: Acupuncture and postoperative vomiting in children. *British Journal of Anaesthesia* **68**, 633.
11. **Wells, J.C.D. and Miles, J.B.** 1991: Pain clinics and pain clinic treatments. *British Medical Bulletin* **47**(3), 762–85.
12. **Ulett, G.A., Han, S. and Han, J.S.** 1998: Electroacupuncture: mechanisms and clinical application. *Biological Psychiatry* **44**(2), 129–38.
13. **Dawidson, I., Angmar-Mansson, B., Blom, M., Theodorsson, E. and Lundeberg, T.** 1998: The influence of sensory stimulation (acupuncture) on the release of neuropeptides in the saliva of healthy subjects. *Life Sciences* **63**(8), 659–74.
14. **Balogun, J.A., Biasci, S. and Han, L.** 1998: The effects of acupuncture, electroneedling and trancutaneous electrical stimulation therapies on peripheral haemodynamic functioning. *Disability and Rehabilitation* **20**(2), 41–8.
15. **Hansson, S.O. and Mannheimer, C.** 1991: Treatment with ear acupuncture in patients with severe angina pectoris. *The Pain Clinic* **4**(1), 53–6.
16. **Dundee, J.W., Ghaly, R.G., Bill, K.M., Chestnutt, W.N., Fitzpatrick, K.T.J. and Lynas, A.G.A.** 1989: Effect of stimulation of the P6 anti-emetic point on postoperative vomiting. *British Journal of Anaesthesia* **63**, 612–18.
17. **Li, P., Pitsillides, K.F., Rendig, S.V., Pan, H.L. and Longhurst, J.C.** 1998: Reversal of reflex-induced myocardial ischaemia by median nerve stimulation: a feline model of electroacupuncture. *Circulation* **97**(12), 1186–94.
18. **Tavola, T., Gala, G., Conte, G. and Invernizzi, G.**

1992: Traditional Chinese acupuncture in tension-type headache: a controlled study. *Pain* **48**, 325–9.

19. **Lundeberg, T., Eriksson, S.V., Lundeberg, S. and Thomas, M.** 1991: Effective acupuncture and naloxone in patients with osteoarthritis pain: a sham acupuncture controlled study. *The Pain Clinic* **4**(3), 155–61.

20. **Bossut, D.F. and Mayer, D.J.** 1991: Electroacupuncture analgesia in rats: naltrexone antagonism is dependent on previous exposure. *Brain Research* **549**(1), 47–51.

21. **Bossut, D.E., Huang, Z.S., Sun, S.L. and Mayer, D.J.** 1991: Electroacupuncture in rats: evidence for naloxone and naltrexone potentiation of analgesia. *Brain Research* **549**(1), 36–46.

22. **Wang, Q.A., Mao, L.M. and Han, J.S.** 1990: The role of periaqueductal grey in mediation of analgesia produced by different frequencies electroacupuncture stimulation in rats. *International Journal of Neuroscience* **53**, 167–72.

23. **Wang, Q.A., Mao, L.M. and Han, J.S.** 1990: The arcuate nucleus of hypothalamus mediates low but not high frequency electro acupuncture analgesia in rats. *Brain Research* **513**(1), 60–6.

24. **Johnson, M.I., Ashton, C.H., Marsh, V.R. and Thompson, J.W.** 1992: Treatment of resistant phantom limb pain by acupuncture: a case report. *The Pain Clinic* **5**(2), 105–12.

25. **Lewith, G.T. and Machin, D.** 1983: On the evaluation of the clinical effects of acupuncture. *Pain* **16**, 111–27.

26. **McQuay, H.J. and Moore, R.A.** 1998: *An evidence-based resource for pain relief.* Oxford: Oxford University Press 23, 195–200.

27. **Tulgar, M., McGlone, F., Bowsher, D. and Miles, J.B.** 1991: Comparative effectiveness of different stimulation modes in relieving pain. Part I: A pilot study. *Pain* **47**, 151–5.

28. **Lander, J. and Fowler-Kerry, S.** 1993: TENS for children's procedural pain. *Pain* **52**, 209–16.

29. **Johnson, M.I., Ashton, C.H. and Thompson, J.W.** 1991: An in-depth study of long-term users of transcutaneous electrical nerve stimulation (TENS). Implications for clinical use of TENS. *Pain* **44**, 221–9.

30. **Sjolund, B.H., Eriksson, M. and Loeser, J.D.** 1990: Transcutaneous and implanted electric stimulation of peripheral nerves. In Bonica, J.J. (eds.) *The management of pain.* Philadelphia: Lea & Febiger, 1852–61.

31. **Johnson, M.I., Ashton, C.H., Bousfield, D.R. and Thompson, J.W.** 1989: Analgesic effects of different frequencies of transcutaneous electrical nerve stimulation on cold-induced pain in normal subjects. *Pain* **39**(2), 231–6.

32. **Abram, S.E.** 1990: Electrical stimulation for cancer pain management. In Abram, S.E. (ed.) *The pain clinic manual.* Philadelphia: J.B. Lippincott, 282–8.

33. **Garrison, D.W. and Foreman, R.D.** 1994: Decreased activity of spontaneous and noxiously evoked dorsal horn cells during transcutaneous electrical nerve stimulation (TENS). *Pain* **58**, 309–15.

34. **Danziger, N., Rozenberg, S., Bourgeois, P., Charpentier, G. and Willer, J.C.** 1998: Depressive effects of segmental and heterotopic application of transcutaneous electrical nerve stimulation and piezo-electric current on lower limb nociceptive flexion reflex in human subjects. *Archives of Physical Medicine and Rehabilitation* **79**(2), 191–200.

35. **Wang, S.F., Chen, Y.W. and Shyu, B.C.** 1997: The supressive effect of electrical stimulation on nociceptive responses in the rat. *Physical Therapy* **77**(8), 839–47.

36. **Yeh, C., Shiell, M., Lamke, J. and Volpe, M.** 1992: Physical therapy: evaluation and treatment of chronic pain. In Aronoff, G.M. (ed.) *Evaluation and treatment of chronic pain.* Baltimore: Williams & Wilkins, 285–90.

37. **Johnson, M.I., Ashton, C.H. and Thompson, J.W.** 1991: The consistency of pulse frequencies and pulse patterns of transcutaneous electrical nerve stimulation used by chronic pain patients. *Pain* **44**, 231–4.

38. **Nash, T.P., Williams, J.D. and Machin, D.** 1990: Tens: does the type of stimulus really matter? *The Pain Clinic* **3**(3), 161–8.

39. **Katims, J.J., Long, D.M. and Ng, L.K.Y.** 1986: Transcutaneous electrical nerve stimulation: frequency and wave form specificity in humans. *Applied Neurophysiology* **49**, 86–91.

40. **Katims, J.J., Naviasky, E., Ng, L.K.Y., Bleecker, M.L. and Rendell, M.** 1986: New screening device for the assessment of peripheral neuropathy. *Journal of Occupational Medicine* **28**(12), 1219–21.

41. **Charbal, C., Fishbain, D., Weaver, M. and Wipperman Heine, L.** 1996: Long-term transcutaneous electrical nerve stimulation (TENS) use: impact on medication and physical therapy utilization and costs. *International Association for the Study of Pain Eighth World Congress*, 18 August, Vancouver, 1–15.

42. **Ready, L.B.** 1990: Acute postoperative pain. In Miller, R.D. (ed.) *Anesthesia.* New York: Churchill Livingstone, 2135–46.

43. **Dai, K.H., Lin, T.H. and Lin, Z.Z.** 1990: Comparative study between transcutaneous nerve stimulation and analgesic in the treatment of postoperative anal pain. *Pain* (suppl. 5), S73.

44. **Miller, K.** 1990: Transcutaneous electrical nerve block technique after thoracotomy. *Pain* (suppl. 5), S232.

45. **Justins, D.M. and Richardson, P.H.** 1991: Clinical management of acute pain. *British Medical Bulletin* **47**(3), 561–83.

46. **Commission on the Provision of Surgical Services.** 1990: *Report of the working party on pain after surgery.* London: Royal College of Surgeons of England/College of Anaesthetists, 1–36.

47. **McQuay, H.J. and Moore, R.A.** 1998: *An evidence-based resource for pain relief.* Oxford: Oxford University Press 20, 172–8.

48. **McQuay, H.J. and Moore, R.A.** 1998: *An evidence-based resource for pain relief.* Oxford: Oxford University Press 21, 179–86.

49. **Mannheimer, C., Emanuelsson, H. and Waagstein, F.** 1990: The effect of transcutaneous electrical nerve stimulation on catecholamine metabolism during pacing induced angina pectoris and the influence of naloxone. *Pain* **41**, 27–34.

50. **Bowsher, D.** 1991: Neurogenic pain syndromes and their management. *British Medical Bulletin* **47**(3), 644–66.

51. **Brusky, J.** 1990: Herpes zoster and postherpetic neuralgia. In Abram, S.E. (ed.) *The Pain Clinic Manual*. Philadelphia: J.B. Lippincott, 127–34.

52. **Shipton, E.A.** 1990: The management of intractable pain. *Hospital Medicine* (Aug), 32–4.

53. **Sweet, W.H. and Poletti, C.E.** 1992: Causalgia and sympathetic dystrophy (Sudeck's atrophy). In Aronoff, G.M. (ed.) *Evaluation and treatment of chronic pain*. Baltimore: Williams & Wilkins, 135–44.

54. **Rodriguez, J.L., de Vera, J.A., Robaina, F.J. and Martin, M.A.** 1990: Transcutaneous electrical nerve stimulation for chronic pains. *Pain* (suppl. 5), S74.

55. **Grechko, V.E. and Borisova, E.G.** 1996: Use of transcutaneous electrical nerve stimulation in the complex treatment of glossalgia. *Neuroscience and Behavioural Physiology* **26**(6), 584–6.

56. **Abram, S.E. and Hebar, R.L.** 1990: Radiculopathy. In Abram, S.E. (ed.) *The Pain Clinic Manual*. Philadelphia: J.B. Lippincott, 105–17.

57. **Marchand, S., Charest, J., Li, J., Chenard, J.R., Lavignolle, B. and Laurencelle, B.** 1993: Is TENS purely a placebo effect? A controlled study on chronic low back pain. *Pain* **54**, 99–106.

58. **Moore, S.R. and Shurman, J.** 1997: Combined neuromuscular electrical stimulation and transcutaneous electrical nerve stimulation for treatment of chronic back pain: a double-blind, repeated measures comparison. *Archives of Physical and Medical Rehabilitation* **78**(1), 55–60.

59. **Stinus, L., Auriacombe, M., Tignol, J., Limoge, A. and Le Moal, M.** 1990: Transcranial electrical stimulation with high frequency intermittent current (Limoge's) potentiates opiate-induced analgesia: blind studies. *Pain* **42**(3), 351–63.

60. **Malin, D.H., Lake, J.R., Hamilton, R.F. and Skilnick, M.H.** 1990: Augmented analgesic effects of L-tryptophan combined with low current transcranial electrostimulation. *Life Sciences* **47**(4), 263–7.

61. **Guieu, R., Tardy-Gervet, M.F. and Roll, J.P.** 1991: Analgesic effects of vibration and transcutaneous electrical nerve stimulation applied separately and simultaneously to patients with chronic pain. *Canadian Journal of Neurological Sciences* **18**(2), 113–19.

62. **Guieu, R., Tardy-Gervet, M.F., Blin, O. and Pouget, J.** 1990: Pain relief achieved by transcutaneous electrical nerve stimulation and/or vibratory nerve stimulation in a case of painful legs and moving toes. *Pain* **42**, 43–8.

63. **Hyodo, M., Toyota, S. and Kawachi, A.** 1990: Cordless mini-TENS – an investigation into its effects in treating shoulder stiffness and other painful disorders. *The Pain Clinic* **3**(2), 103–7.

64. **Johnson, M.I., Hajela, V.K., Ashton, C.H. and Thompson, J.W.** 1991: The effects of auricular transcutaneous electrical nerve stimulation on experimental pain threshold and autonomic function in healthy subjects. *Pain* **46**, 337–42.

65. **Leak, W.D. and Ansel, E.A.** 1996: Neural stimulation: spinal cord and peripheral nerve stimulation. In Raj, P.P. (ed.) *Pain medicine – a comprehensive review*. St Louis: C.V. Mosby, **32**, 327–33.

66. **Raj, P.** 1998: Interventional techniques. In Rawal, N. (ed.) *Management of acute and chronic pain*. London: BMJ Books, 198–219.

67. **Racz, G.B.** 1997: Role of peripheral nerve stimulation for the management of intractable pain. In Jain, S. (ed.) *Current concepts in acute, chronic, and cancer pain management*. New York: World Foundation for Pain Relief and Research, 406–22.

68. **Bhadra, N. and Peckham, P.H.** 1997: Peripheral nerve stimulation for restoration of motor function. *Journal of Clinical Neurophysiology* **14**(5), 378–93.

69. **Montes Molina, R., Tabernero Galan, A. and Martin Garcia, M.S.** 1997: Spectral electromyographic changes during a muscular strengthening training based on electrical stimulation. *Electromyography and Clinical Neurophysiology* **37**(5), 287–95.

70. **Barolat, G.** 1997: Recent advances in neuromodulation and the mechanisms of spinal cord stimulation. In Jain, S. (ed.) *Current concepts in acute, chronic, and cancer pain management*. New York: World Foundation for Pain Relief and Research, 399–402.

71. **Kobetic, R., Triolo, R.J. and Marsolais, E.B.** 1997: Muscle selection and walking performance of multichannel FES systems for ambulation in paraplegia. *IEEE Transactions in Rehabilitation Engineering* **5**(1), 23–9.

72. **Barolat, G.** 1991: Percutaneous retroperitoneal stimulation of the sacral plexus: initial report and technical note. *Stereotactic and Functional Neurosurgery* **56**(4), 250–7.

73. **Steude, U., Kobal, G. and Hamburger, C.H.** 1990: Atypical trigeminal neuralgia: nine years experience with the therapeutic electrostimulation of the gasserian ganglion. *Pain* (suppl. 5), S78.

74. **Taub, E., Munz, M. and Tasker, R.R.** 1997: Chronic electrical stimulation of the gasserian ganglion for the relief of pain in a series of 34 patients. *Journal of Neurosurgery* **86**, 197–202.

75. **Pernak, J.** 1998: Acute herpes zoster and postherpetic neuralgia. *8th World Congress, The Pain Clinic*, 6–10 May, Tenerife, 36–8.

76. **Rainov, N.G., Fels, C., Heidecke, V. and Burrkert, W.** 1997: Epidural electrical stimulation of the motor cortex in patients with facial neuralgia. *Clinical Neurology and Neurosurgery* **99**(3), 205–9.

77. **Marchand, S., Bushnell, M.C., Molina-Negro, P., Martinez, S.N. and Duncan, G.H.** 1991: The effects of

dorsal column stimulation on measures of clinical and experimental pain in man. *Pain* **45**, 249–57.

78. **Oakley, J.C.** 1998: Long-term failure of spinal cord stimulation. *8th World Congress, The Pain Clinic*, 6–10 May, Tenerife, 75.

79. **Kupers, R.C., Van Den Oever, R., Van Houdenhove, B.** *et al*. 1994: Spinal cord stimulation in Belgium: a nation-wide survey on the incidence, indications and therapeutic efficacy by the health insurer. *Pain* **56** 211–16.

80. **Simpson, B.A.** 1994: Spinal cord stimulation. *Pain Reviews* **1**, 199–230.

81. **McQuay, H.J. and Moore, R.A.** 1998: *An evidence-based resource for pain relief.* Oxford: Oxford University Press 28, 219.

82. **North, R.B.** 1997: Spinal cord stimulation for chronic, intractable pain; experience over two decades. In Jain, S. (ed.) *Current concepts in acute, chronic, and cancer pain management.* New York: World Foundation for Pain Relief and Research, 425–42.

83. **Tesfaye, S., Watt, J., Benbow, S.J., Pang, K.A., Miles, J. and MacFarlane, I.A.** 1996: Electrical spinal-cord stimulation for painful diabetic peripheral neuropathy. *Lancet* **348**, 1698–701.

84. **Meyerson, B.A.** 1996: Mechanisms of spinal cord stimulation as pain treatment. In Campbell, J.N. (ed.) *Pain 1996 – an updated review.* Seattle: IASP Press, 207–15.

85. **Linderoth, B.** 1998: Basic physiological mechanisms of spinal cord stimulation in the relief of pain. *8th World Congress, The Pain Clinic*, 6–10 May, Tenerife, 41–2.

86. **Roberts, M.H.T. and Rees, H.** 1994: Physiological basis of spinal cord stimulation. *Pain Reviews* **1**, 184–98.

87. **Cui, J.G., O'Conner, W.T., Ungerstedt, U., Linderoth, B. and Meyerson, B.A.** 1997: Spinal cord stimulation attenuates augmented dorsal release of excitatory amino acids in mononeuropathy via a GABAergic mechanism. *Pain* **73**, 87–95.

88. **Curatolo, M., Petersen-Felix, S., Arendt-Nielsen, L. and Zbinden, A.M.** 1997: Epidural epinephrine and clonidine: segmental analgesia and effects on different pain modalities. *Anesthesiology* **87**(4), 785–94.

89. **Alfano, S., Darwin, J. and Picullel, B.** 1994: *Spinal cord stimulation: patient guidelines for clinicians.* Minnesota: Medtronic, 1–80.

90. **Pallares, J., Pallares, M.J., Fenollosa, P.** *et al*. 1990: Treatment of reflex sympathetic dystrophy of the upper limb by means of spinal cord stimulation. *Pain* (suppl. 5), S78.

91. **Meyerson, B.A.** 1990: Electric stimulation of the spinal cord and brain. In Bonica, J.J. *The management of pain.* Philadelphia: Lea & Febiger, 1862–82.

92. **Tasker, R.R.** 1988: Neurostimulation and percutaneous neural destructive techniques. In Cousins, M.J. and Bridenbaugh, P.O. (eds) *Neural blockade.* Philadelphia: J.B. Lippincott, 1085–117.

93. **De La Porte, C. and Ven De Kelft, E.** 1993: Spinal cord stimulation in failed back surgery syndrome. *Pain* **52**, 55–61.

94. **North, R.B., Kidd, D.H., Lee, M.S. and Piantodosi, S.** 1996: A prospective, randomised study of spinal cord stimulation versus reoperation for failed back surgery syndrome: initial results. In Campbell, J.N. (ed.) *Pain 1996 – an updated review.* Seattle: IASP Press, 453–6.

95. **Romano, M., Zucco, F., Allaria, B. and Grieco, A.** 1998: Epidural spinal cord stimulation in the treatment of refractory angina pectoris. Mechanisms of action, clinical results and current indications. *Guida Italiana Cardiologo* **28**, 71–9.

96. **Augustinsson, L.E.** 1998: Spinal cord stimulation (SCS) in severe angina pectoris. *8th World Congress, The Pain Clinic*, 6–10 May, Tenerife, 35.

97. **Krames, E.S.** 1996: Implantable technologies: when to use spinally administered opioids or spinal cord stimulation: an algorithm for decision-making. In Campbell, J.N. (ed.) *Pain 1996 – an updated review.* Seattle: IASP Press, 201–6.

98. **North, R.B., Ewend, M.G., Lawton, M.T. and Piantadosi, S.** 1991: Spinal cord stimulation for chronic, intractable pain: superiority of 'multi-channel' devices. *Pain* **44**, 119–30.

99. **Doleys, D.M., Klapow, J.C. and Hammer, M.** 1997: Psychological evaluation in spinal cord stimulation therapy. *Pain Reviews* **4**, 189–207.

100. **Kidd, D.H. and North, R.B.** 1996: Spinal cord stimulation: an effective and cost-saving treatment in the management of chronic pain. In Cohen, M.J.M. and Campbell, J.N. (eds) *Pain treatment at a crossroads: a practical and conceptual reappraisal; progress in pain research and management.* Seattle: IASP Press, 173–81.

101. **North, R.B. and Kidd, D.H.** 1998: A prospective, randomised comparison of spinal cord stimulation electrode designs. *8th World Congress, The Pain Clinic*, 6–10 May, Tenerife, 57.

102. **North, R.B.** 1991: Reply to J Devulder. *Pain* **46**, 237.

103. **North, R.B. and Fowler, K.F.** 1987: Computer-controlled, patient-interactive, multichannel, implanted neurological stimulators. *Applied Neurophysiology* **50**, 39–41.

104. **Duncan, G.H., Bushnell, M.C. and Marchand, S.** 1991: Deep brain stimulation: a review of basic research and clinical studies. *Pain* **45**, 49–59.

105. **Young, R.F. and Rinaldi, P.C.** 1994: Brain stimulation for relief of chronic pain. In Wall, P.D. and Melzack, R. (eds) *Textbook of pain.* Edinburgh: Churchill Livingstone, 1225–33.

106. **Dib, B. and Falchi, M.** 1997: Intracerebroventricular self-injection of beta-endorphin by rats in response to intermittent electrical shocks. *International Journal of Clinical Pharmacological Research* **17**(1), 37–46.

107. **Sartucci, F., Bonfiglio, L., Del Seppia, C.** *et al*. 1997: Changes in pain perception and pain-related somatosensory evoked potentials in humans produced by exposure to oscillating magnetic fields. *Brain Research* **769**(2), 362–6.

13 SURGICAL INTERVENTION

INTRODUCTION AND GUIDELINES

There are few clear indications for surgical intervention in chronic pain.[1] In general, the results are often poor following surgical intervention. For these reasons, strict guidelines should be adhered to before surgical intervention is contemplated. An identifiable organic cause of the pain (either neuropathic or nociceptive) should be accurately diagnosed.[2,3] In chronic malignant pain, the patient's prognosis should be taken into account. If patient survival is forecast to be less than 2 months, no ablative procedures should be considered.[3] If patient survival is forecast to be between 2 and 5 months, percutaneous procedures (neurolysis or radiofrequency or cryoprobe lesioning) should be used.[3] Only if a patient's prognosis is of more than 5 months should ablative surgery be considered.[3]

The role of psychological behavioural patterns in patients with chronic pain of non-malignant origin can predispose to surgical failure (see Chapter 14). Compensation and litigation may also influence therapeutic outcome. Conservative therapy as well as other options, such as the use of neuraxial analgesics, cryotherapy, radiofrequency lesioning and neurolysis, should first be explored.[1] Other factors to be considered are both the patient's and family's expectations, patient fitness and the anatomical origin of the pain.[1] It is essential that more than one diagnostic block with local anaesthetic is carried out if any meaningful evaluation is to be obtained.[4] It is important to obtain informed consent from the patient beforehand. Only surgical procedures with a low risk, a low incidence of side-effects and for which there is a good reason to expect satisfactory results should be chosen. With surgery, outcome depends on a myriad of factors.[5] The specificity and sensitivity of the diagnostic tests, the surgeon's knowledge and skill, and the surgical procedure chosen are three variables that non-surgeons may underappreciate.[2,3,5] The task of the pain specialist is to select patients who may benefit from a surgical procedure and select the right surgeon to do the right procedure.[5] Because of the multidimensional nature of pain, surgical intervention should ideally be a multidisciplinary decision between surgeons and pain specialists (for lesion sites, see Figure 13.1).[5]

NERVE REPAIR

Peripheral nerves, when injured, may take one of three gross anatomical forms:[6]

- amputation neuroma;
- neuroma-in-continuity;
- no macroscopically observable abnormality.

Nerve repair may be one of the most important means of preventing neuroma formation from nerve injuries that are clearly neurotmetic and can be repaired acutely or within the first few weeks after injury.[6] For other nerve lesions, in which the completeness or nature of the lesion is uncertain, a

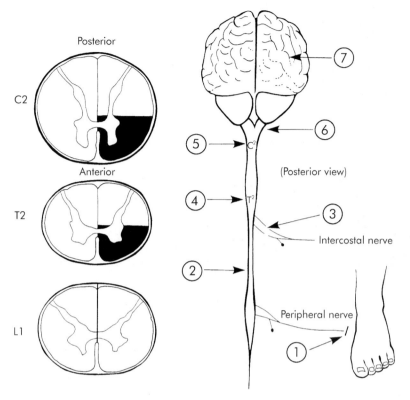

Figure 13.1 Surgical lesion sites.
1, peripheral neurectomy;
2, commissural myelotomy;
3, rhizotomy;
4, thoracic cordotomy;
5, cervical cordotomy;
6, medullary tractotomy;
7, cerebral operations.

waiting period of 2–3 months is appropriate before primary anastomosis or graft repair is attempted.[6] Nerve repair should be viewed as the best option for preventing post-traumatic neuromas in critical nerves. It has been realized that the basic process of axonal regeneration and neuroma formation is inevitable. The carbon dioxide laser scaling of cut nerves has unfortunately shown no difference in neuroma size compared with scalpel transection.[6] Attempts are now made to limit and direct nerve regeneration and to situate the resulting neuroma in a location that will not be subject to repetitive mechanical trauma.[6] When a nerve is placed into muscle tissue, there is less production of connective tissue and little evidence of invasion or regeneration into the surrounding innervated muscle.[6] This is because of the microenviroment of the nerve end, the existing innervation of the surrounding muscle and the lack of neurotropism for sensory fibres.[6] Good results have been reported with nerve implantation into bone marrow, which is not mechanically traumatized and limits neuroma formation.[6]

Innervation tissue can also be transplanted over the painful neuroma in the form of a muscle flap (abductor digiti quinti or pronator quadratus in the upper extremity).[6] Nerve graft techniques can also be used to control neuroma regrowth. This can restore sensorimotor function but may not cure the pain.[6] Free neurovascular tissue islands can also be used, and the free end of an acutely trimmed proximal host nerve can be anastomosed to the graft nerve.[6] A nerve graft can be used to direct the regenerating axons into muscle or another non-neural target. Surgical success with painful neuroma manipulation ranges from 65 to 82 per cent.[6] Many surgical failures are the result of incomplete initial neuronal excision. Seventy-six per cent of patients reoperated for plantar interdigital neuromas have complete or marked pain relief.[6] In the larger mixed nerves of the extremity, resection of the nerve site injury may not be feasible.

When a chronically injured nerve is surgically exposed, it is dissected from the scar in a plane around the external epineurium (external neurolysis) and transposed to a site that is not subject to repetitive mechanical trauma. A swelling in the course of the nerve (neuroma-in-continuity) is frequently found. If there is no resolution of the pain after 3–6 months, internal neurolysis is considered.[6] In this, the external epineurium is microsurgically removed. The scarred internal epineurium is dissected, separating the individual fascicles and taking care not to violate the perineum.[6] This technique is reserved for distal nerves (median and ulnar nerves at the wrist or the posterior tibial nerve in the tarsal tunnel) to improve function of the marginal fascicles and reduce the associated pain. If this fails, distal nerves can be divided into constituent fascicles, and the individual fascicles are then tested, while exposed, for electrophysiological integrity. Conducting segments can be spared, and non-functional fascicles can either be divided and implanted into muscle or grafted on to non-fibrotic distal remnant fascicles, with good success in restoring sensorimotor function.[6] The optimum management strategies for painful neuromas and neuromas-in-continuity are still unknown.

PERIPHERAL NEURECTOMY

There are few (if any) indications for neurectomy. It is performed when a specific peripheral nerve is involved (e.g. by tumour).[2] This has largely been supplanted by neuraxial opioids or lytic nerve blocks. There are several problems that limit the applicability of neurectomy. Because of significant overlap in the distribution of innervation among the peripheral nerves, pain is rarely limited to the zone of a single peripheral nerve.[7] Furthermore, most peripheral nerves are mixed motor and sensory. Disadvantages include motor loss, a loss of all sensory modalities in the skin and joints, neuroma formation (with pain), denervation hypersensitivity or the return of the original pain.[1,8] Properly controlled studies of the efficacy of peripheral neurectomy are rare, and few long-term successes can be anticipated.[8] In cancer pain, multilevel neurectomies for chest wall pain are indicated when a discrete pain-producing lesion involves several intercostal nerves.[9]

Neurectomy may also be effective in alleviating pain originating from a paraspinal tumour involving nerves distal to the neural foramina.[9] Cranial neurectomies have selected indications in neuralgia resulting from cancer.[9] Peripheral nerves resected include the supraorbital, infraorbital and mandibular nerves, the lateral femoral cutaneous nerve and the intercostal nerves.[2,8]

RHIZOTOMIES

Spinal rhizotomies

This is the interruption of the dorsal roots (epidurally or intrathecally) of the spinal nerves within the spinal canal. In patients with malignant and non-malignant disease, it can be performed intrathecally (via a laminectomy) or epidurally (via a laminotomy and medial facetectomy). In the former, the entire dorsal root is sectioned, whereas in the latter, the multiple rootlets are cut.[7] Selective posterior rhizotomy limits the involvement to the venterolateral aspect of the rootlet, where the small fibres are organized.[7] Advantages include the absence of motor blockade and the fact that the procedure results in an area being rendered totally anaesthetic. Spinal rhizotomy is used for well-circumscribed pain.[1] It has proved useful in the management of malignant pain in a restricted or segmental distribution, such as the brachial plexus, the chest wall and the pelvis.[7] Its results, however, are unpredictable and often disappointing as a patient's innervation may not be what would be predicted from anatomy texts because of the alteration in the receptor fields of the dorsal horn neurones.[1,2] For segmentally restricted malignant pain, excision of the sensory ganglia (ganglionectomy) is often performed at the same time.[7] This removes the dorsal root ganglia at multiple levels to catch the few myelinated afferent fibres that enter the ventral horn (up to 20 per cent), but it is not clear whether this improves efficacy.[8] In malignant pain, satisfactory relief may be achieved by sectioning roots invaded by the tumour.[2] Total dorsal rhizotomy of a limb will render it anaesthetic and functionally useless;[8] this may be lessened by sparing one dorsal root.[9] In practice, this procedure is only considered for localized pain in the trunk or abdomen, or, rarely, for an extremity that is functionless preoperatively.[9]

Complications of spinal rhizotomy include infection, bleeding (epidural or intrathecal), trauma and infarction of the spinal cord, CSF fistula and the development of pain in the anaesthetic area.[8] The use of percutaneous rhizotomies using a radiofrequency or cryoprobe, or neurolysis (to place the tip of an infusion catheter at the precise segment within the epidural space under radiographic guidance), is associated with a lower morbidity and should be considered in patients too ill for surgery (see Chapter 11).[2,10]

The peripheral interneural administration of

neurotoxins such as adriamycin results in rapid retrograde axoplasmic transport to the ganglion.[11] This is thought to be useful for selectively inducing permanent lesions in target sensory ganglia. In patients with neuropathic pain, preliminary studies have produced good short-term results,[11] and this method merits further investigation.

Cranial rhizotomies

Rhizotomy of the trigeminal, nervus intermedius and glossopharyngeal nerves has been used for facial or oral pain secondary to malignancy.[8] Local anaesthetic nerve blocks should first be performed as a diagnostic procedure to relieve the pain and to let the patient experience the resulting numbness. A retromastoid craniectomy approach is used to section the trigeminal and glossopharyngeal nerves. If deep ear pain is present, sectioning of the nervus intermedius is also undertaken.[8] Percutaneous rhizotomy using radiofrequency lesioning of the trigeminal and glossopharyngeal nerves has also been described, whereby electrodes are placed in the foramen ovale (gasserian ganglion) or the jugular foramen, or chemical neurolysis is applied at the gasserian ganglion.[8,9] The technique of microvascular decompression of the trigeminal (see below) and glossopharyngeal nerves has largely displaced rhizotomies. A posterior inferior cerebellar artery or an ectatic basilar artery may compress the trigeminal nerve.[2]

DORSAL ROOT ENTRY ZONE LESIONS

The original dorsal root entry zone lesion has been expanded in concept to include deafferentation pain syndromes at all levels of the spinal cord or higher and should be limited to patients failing first-line procedures.[11] The dorsal root entry zone lesion is designed to destroy the first five layers of Rexed in the dorsal root entry zone of the dorsal horn in which lesions are placed in order to destroy the secondary neurones carrying nociceptive and thermal sensation (Figure 13.2).[11,12] It is mainly used in the management of specific types of neuropathic pain (mostly for pain following spinal cord injury), including brachial plexus avulsion pain, severe post-herpetic neuralgia, phantom limb (not stump) pain and post-paraplegia pain, and in patients with diffuse pain that often involves the entire body and limbs below the level of the cord lesion.[3,13–15] Dorsal root entry zone lesions are performed under general anaesthesia and require a laminectomy over each section to be lesioned (eg. C4–T1 laminectomies for brachial plexus avulsion).[16] Dorsal root entry zone lesions of the subnucleus caudalis are used for post-herpetic pain involving the trigeminal nerve and for other severe intractable facial pain.[12]

A 0.25 mm diameter thermocouple temperature-monitoring electrode with a 2 mm long tip is introduced into the spinal cord.[13] Not only are the dorsal root entry zones at each level lesioned, but so also is all the contiguous substantia gelatinosa between

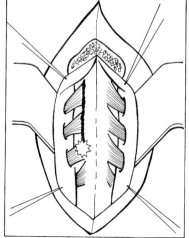
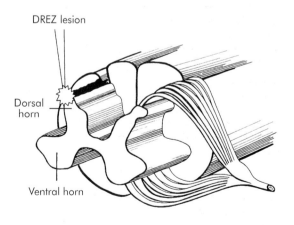

Figure 13.2 Dorsal root entry zone (DREZ) lesions: site of DREZ lesion.

the roots (with lesions 1 mm apart).[13] It is still unclear how many segments above or below the involved level of injury the lesions should be made.[16] Lasers (carbon dioxide and argon) have also been used for faster lesioning of the dorsal root entry zones.[16] The most serious complication of dorsal root entry zone lesioning is ipsilateral motor weakness, in approximately 5 per cent of patients.[12] In avulsion injuries (cervical and conus), pain is relieved in around 70 per cent of patients.[12] In paraplegia, pain has been relieved in 54–90 per cent of patients.[12,16]

Dorsal root entry zone lesions of the subnucleus caudalis have relieved post-herpetic pain involving the trigeminal nerve in over 50 per cent of patients.[16] This method has recently received increasing interest following the use of a computer-assisted dorsal root entry zone microcoagulation technique, which has been claimed to increase the success rate.[15] Indications for nucleus caudalis dorsal root entry zone lesions include post-herpetic neuralgia, anaesthesia dolorosa, malignancy and intractable facial pain secondary to dental procedures, glaucoma, salivary stones, Caldwell–Luc procedures, facial trauma and brain stem vascular lesions.[11] It has recently been applied to deafferentation pain associated with malignancy, with good results.[7] In addition, a trigeminal nucleus caudalis dorsal root entry zone procedure has been developed for pain arising from carcinoma of the orbit.[7] The nucleus caudalis is approached through a suboccipital craniectomy with a cervical laminectomy at C1–3. A modified electrode with a 3 mm long tip (with insulation along the first millimetre) is used for lesioning the subnucleus caudalis as it helps to spare the more superficial spinocerebellar tracts.[13] Lesions are made in the spinal trigeminal tract and the nucleus caudalis from just above the obex to C2 using an angled radiofrequency electrode.[11] Two rows of lesions are made, one above the other, from C2 level to slightly above the obex. Lesions are made by heating the electrode tip to 75°C for 15 seconds.[13] Typically, dorsal root entry zone lesions in the trigeminal nucleus caudalis result in hypoaesthesia over the entire ipsilateral hemiface plus the cornea and invariably the cheeks and anterior tongue. The nuclear afferents for cranial nerves VII, IX and X run along the dorsal aspect of the nucleus caudalis so that strategic inclusion of these can tailor pain therapy from dental or oropharyngeal structures.[11] Post-herpetic neuralgia patients have 67–100 per cent satisfactory pain relief over the long term, while only 50 per cent of patients with trigeminal neuralgia and atypical facial pains have satisfactory pain relief.[11] Care should be taken not to injure the ascending spinocerebellar paths, which would result in ipsilateral ataxia.[11] The nucleus of XI, the crossed pyramidal tract and the dorsal columns are nearby and are attractive targets for a misguided probe.

MAJOR SURGICAL PROCEDURES FOR TRIGEMINAL NEURALGIA

Microvascular decompression

The treatment of trigeminal neuralgia by lesioning the trigeminal ganglion with either glycerine or radiofrequency is discussed in Chapter 11. Microvascular decompression can be used in young patients or in those in whom the additional risk of a craniotomy is outweighed by the benefits of a high probability of long-term palliation of pain with minimal or no sensory loss.[11] It can be used in patients intractable to medical therapy or who are unable to tolerate the drugs (carbamazepine and phenytoin sodium). It is also particularly reserved for those with involvement of the ophthalmic division of the trigeminal nerve, in which radiofrequency lesioning produces a high incidence of ophthalmic complications (e.g. corneal anaesthesia and extraocular palsy).[2,17] Microvascular decompression lasts longer than radiofrequency lesioning and is not associated with numbness or with pain in the numb area, which is found with the latter technique.[17,18]

Frequently, an artery or vein, or less often an arteriovenous malformation or tumour, compresses the trigeminal nerve at its junction with the pons (the root entry zone).[11] The ageing process, with arterial elongation and sagging of the hindbrain, may contribute to venous and arterial compression of the cranial nerves.[19] The most common cause (in approximately 80 per cent) of trigeminal neuralgia is compression at the root entry zone at the brain stem by an arterial branch of the superior cerebellar artery.[2] Pain restricted to the second division is most commonly caused by the blood vessel on the lateral side of the nerve, usually an aberrant trigeminal vein.[19] Pain is occasionally restricted to the first division, being caused by a blood vessel on the caudal side of the nerve.[19]

No methods exist of definitely diagnosing neurovascular compression. A CT or MRI scan should be used to exclude a tumour (meningioma, neurinoma or cholesteatoma) in the cerebellopontine angle, middle fossa or clivus.[2] Multiple sclerosis at the root entry zone may also have to be excluded. Magnetic resonance angiography is a new non-invasive modality that may prove useful in defining vascular relationships at the level of the root entry zone. Under general anaesthesia and with a continuous facial electromyogram and somatosensory evoked potential monitoring, a high lateral retromastoid craniectomy is performed with the patient in the semi-sitting (with a chest Doppler and a right atrial catheter for the detection and treatment of air embolism) or lateral recumbent position.[11] The head is secured by skeletal fixation. Using microsurgical techniques, the dura and then the arachnoid are opened, and the cerebellopontine angle is exposed by retracting the cerebellum medially with a self-retaining retractor.[11,19] Branches of the petrosal vein are coagulated and divided. The porous acusticus is then identified, with the cranial nerves VII and VIII and there arachnoid investment, and they are gently teased away from trigeminal nerve, exposing the arterial or other source of cross-compression, which typically lies at the junction of the nerve and the root entry zone.[11] Brain stem auditory evoked potential monitoring helps to prevent damage to the auditory nerve.[19] The vascular compression is relieved by placing synthetic sponges (e.g. of Teflon felt) between the artery and the nerve.[19] Veins demonstrably indenting or deviating the nerve are coagulated and divided. If no compressive artery is found, the nerve root is partially sectioned.[2] Final haemostasis is assured by the Valsalva manoeuvre, the retractors are removed, and the dura, muscle, fascia and skin are closed.[11]

Morbidity using this technique is low. Important complications, however, include ipsilateral hearing loss (with major permanent hearing loss in up to 8 per cent of cases) from conduction problems by failing to avoid entering the mastoid air cells, and nerve deficit as a result of excessive exposure or retraction.[11] CSF leaks occur in 0–2.8 per cent of patients.[11,19] Transient cranial nerve deficits (e.g. transient diplopia), have an incidence of 4 per cent,[11] while the incidence of facial paresis is 0.4–2.8 per cent.[11] Herpes labialis occurs in 0–50 per cent of cases and is related to intraoperative nerve manipulation.[11] Mortality rates range from zero to 1.4 per cent..[11,19] This technique completely relieves the pain in 80–90 per cent of patients.[19]

Neurovascular compression is found in 70–90 per cent of microvascular decompression of compression.[11] Findings include at the root entry zone 59–76 per cent arterial (usually the superior cerebellar artery), 5–14 per cent venous and 23 per cent mixed arteriovenous in origin, 3.6 per cent tumour, 2 per cent venous angioma, 2 per cent osseous contact and 0.25 per cent each of an aneurysm, an arteriovenous malformation or of no pathology.[11] In 70 per cent of cases, the lateral mesencephalic segment of the superior cerebellar artery near its bifurcation compresses the trigeminal nerve at multiple points on the nerve's medial surface.[11] After microvascular decompression, arterial contact at the root entry zone has a significantly better prognosis than venous or no contact (73 per cent versus 51 per cent cure, respectively).[11] After microvascular decompression, the recurrence rate is 17 per cent for arterial compression, 75 per cent for venous compression and 60 per cent for both.[11] Microvascular decompression arrests trigeminal neuralgia, with gradual fall-out because of recurrences. In long-term follow-up, patients can at no time be considered to be cured.[11] Negative prognostic indicators include advanced neurovascular compression, venous compression, longer symptom duration, a sensory deficit of more than two divisions, prior surgery, and the presence of a permanent pain component or bilateral disease.[11] Those patients without any evidence of compression generally undergo a partial sensory rhizotomy, with satisfactory results in 85 per cent.[11] Although inconsistencies exist, neurovascular compression remains the best explanation for many cases of trigeminal neuralgia, and microvascular decompression still has by far the highest percentage 'cure rate'.[11]

Partial sensory rhizotomy

Partial sensory rhizotomy is currently most commonly used as an alternative to microvascular decompression when no neurovascular impingement is noticed (in 14–21 per cent of cases).[11] However, it often produces a significant, variable sensory deficit and a greater incidence of dysaesthesia and recurrence, which makes microvascular decompression more attractive as an initial procedure. Upon visualization of the root, the lateral two thirds are coagulated with bipolar cautery and then divided close to Meckel's cave, preserving touch sensation on the majority of the face.[11] One half to one third of the nerve is preserved. Alternatively, the classical subtemporal Frazier procedure is performed under general anaesthesia with the patient in skeletal fixation in the sitting position. A vertical incision is made in front of the external auditory meatus superiorly to the zygoma. After a 4 cm craniectomy, an extradural dissection is carried out medially and anteriorly to the foramen spinosum.[11] This is plugged with wax, and the middle meningeal artery is coagulated and divided. Dissection proceeds medially to the foramen ovale, where the third division is identified and the dura dissected from the dura propria and the ganglion proper.[11] The third and the second divisions of the ganglion are exposed, and the trigeminal root is visualized. A dura propria incision posterior to the ganglion is made and the CSF of the cistern encountered. The nerve rootlets are then cut close to the lateral two thirds of the ganglion, sparing the ophthalmic fibres. It is important also to spare the motor root.[11] The dura is closed and the wound closed in layers. It is possible to produce a dissociated sensory loss of pinprick and light touch by sectioning the posterior portion of the root.[11]

Immediate pain relief is obtained in 86–100 per cent of patients, tapering to 50 per cent being pain-free at 5 years.[11] The mortality is similar to that of microvascular decompression (0.8–1.6 per cent).[11] The initial sensory loss is up to 100 per cent, although the eventual sensory loss is variable.[11] Other complications include persistent paraesthesiae (up to 36 per cent of cases), persistent dysaesthesiae (0–8 per cent), anaesthesia dolorosa (0–2.3 per cent), corneal anaesthesia (0–4.6 per cent), keratitis (up to 15 per cent approached subtemporally), cranial nerve injuries (up to 10 per cent), persistent hearing loss (0–3.2 per cent), CSF leak (0–4 per cent), aseptic meningitis (4 per cent) and labial herpes (50–100 per cent).[11] In those patients with vascular contact but no distortion of the trigeminal root entry zone, both partial sensory rhizotomy and microvascular decompression have been advocated.[11]

Medullary trigeminal tractotomy

Destruction of the descending spinal tract of the trigeminal nerve in the dorsal medulla produces analgesia and thermoanalgesia in the distribution of the ipsilateral nerve with the preservation of light touch, the corneal reflex and a modicum of thermal sensibility.[2,11] The afferent impulses and reflexes for mastication and swallowing are intact. The procedure can be performed as an open or percutaneous stereotaxic procedure and can be carried out bilaterally. This is primarily a procedure pain for malignant disease of the head and neck, and can be combined with a nucleotomy and rhizotomy.[11] A

cervical rhizotomy is added in patients with malignant pain in the distribution of cranial nerves V, VII, IX or X. In the open procedure, under general anaesthesia, needle electrodes are inserted into the ipsilateral supraorbital, infraorbital and mental foramina. A second electrode is placed subcutaneously nearby for later bipolar stimulation of each trigeminal division. A similar pair of electrodes is applied to the ipsilateral wrist for median nerve stimulation. The patient is placed prone with skeletal fixation, and, through a ventral suboccipital incision, the arch of C1 and 3 cm of the foramen magnum are opened.[11] The dura is opened in the midline, exposing the medulla and upper cervical cord. Square wave pulses are delivered to each facial electrode and the median electrode. The lateral 'physiological' border of the funiculus cuneatus, followed by the rostral–caudal and medial–lateral boundaries of the descending tract, is identified.[11] Each site is referenced to a common landmark. A radiofrequency electrode is inserted to a depth of 3 mm into the descending tract in the area that has shown the maximal evoked potential from stimulation of the trigeminal division(s) from which the pain originates, and a radiofrequency lesion (60 mA and 30 seconds) is made.[11] The area is resurveyed, and radiofrequency lesions are repeated until the evoked potentials are eliminated. It is preferable to perform a tractotomy after localization by evoked potentials recorded from the brain stem during continuous peripheral trigeminal stimulation.

In trigeminal neuralgia patients, 58 per cent are pain-free and 42 per cent have partial pain relief, a trend that continues after 6 years.[11] Satisfactory pain relief is obtained in 50–85 per cent of patients with malignant pain of the head and neck.[11] Stereotactic trigeminal nucleotomy of the second-order neurones at the oral pole of the nucleus caudalis provides satisfactory pain relief in 76 per cent of patients with deafferentation pain from post-herpetic neuralgia or anaesthesia dolorosa.[11,19] Ipsilateral limb ataxia occurs in 10 per cent of patients and contralateral sensory loss in 14 per cent of patients.[11] Proprioceptive loss in the ipsilateral arm and leg occasionally occur. Although all these side-effects are transient, they can occasionally persist. Keratitis, hemiparesis, facial palsy, masticatory paresis and anaesthesia dolorosa are exceedingly rare.[11]

Conclusion

In trigeminal neuralgia, conservative medical management should always be pursued before resorting to surgery. In young, healthy patients, failing medical therapy, microvascular decompression provides the longest-lasting modality but with a steady attrition rate each year.[11] In patients without clear-cut neurovascular compression, partial sensory rhizotomy offers reliable pain relief, with a fair certainty of eventual recurrence and a higher complication rate.[11] Both microvascular decompression and partial sensory rhizotomy carry a 1 per cent mortality rate.[11] The choice of a percutaneous procedure (see Chapter 11) is a rational choice in both the young and the elderly. They are simple and generally safe to perform. However, none offers more than a median of about 3 years of reasonable pain relief before recurrence.[11] Although more effective for symptomatic trigeminal neuralgia or multiple sclerosis, percutaneous radiofrequency trigeminal gangliolysis results in more dysaesthetic complications than does percutaneous trigeminal ganglion compression or percutaneous retrogasserian glycerol rhizolysis.[11] Tractotomy and dorsal root entry zone lesions have limited application today.

CORDOTOMY

Introduction

A cordotomy occurs when the anterolateral quadrants of the spinal cord (containing the ascending system for pain transmission) are sectioned[2]. It provides a selective loss of pain and temperature perception several segments below and contralateral to the segment at which the lesion is placed.[9] The lesion should be placed much above the pain level because pain and temperature fibres cross the spinal cord within two segments of their entry.[2] The level must also be chosen where anterior horn cells are less important as the cordotomy will damage them. The C2 or T2 levels are usually acceptable. For pain cephalad to the mid-chest, the C2 level is chosen. Cordotomy is indicated for unilateral somatic cancer pain below the level of the mandible that is unresponsive to medication.[2,17] In cancer pain, bilateral cordotomies are generally not performed because of the high risk of respiratory failure (from sleep-induced apnoea), thus essentially eliminating its applicability for widespread metastatic involvement.[2,7] If performed bilaterally, 4–6 weeks must be allowed between procedures, with appropriate pulmonary function tests. For visceral or bilateral pain, bilateral cordotomy may be

required.[9] Cordotomy is occasionally used for chronic benign pain. The closer the pain is to the midline, the greater is the risk of a contralateral pain developing after cordotomy.[2] It is of interest that, in unilateral chronic pain, there is a decrease in blood flow in the contralateral thalamus, which is thought to be a functional effect of the increase in spinothalamic input.[20] This is abolished by cordotomy.[20] Most cordotomies can be performed percutaneously under local anaesthesia and fluoroscopic guidance using a radiofrequency probe.[9] This avoids the risks of an open operation and anaesthesia in patients in a poor medical condition. An open surgical approach may benefit patients in whom a percutaneous procedure has failed, those who cannot cooperate because of severe pain and confusion, those at risk of respiratory compromise and those with bilateral pain in whom a bilateral, high cervical cordotomy carries an additional risk of neurological impairment.[9] Potential complications include the unmasking of dysaesthetic pain, bladder, bowel, and sexual dysfunction, ataxia, paresis and sleep apnoea.[9]

Percutaneous cervical cordotomy

This technique is certainly chosen if the patient's physical status is poor. However, the simplicity and repeatability of this technique and the associated reduction in risks have made it the procedure of

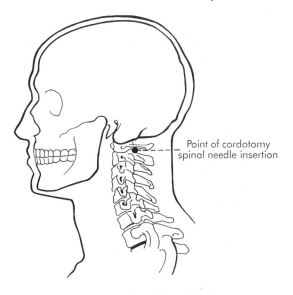

Point of cordotomy spinal needle insertion

Figure 13.3 Needle insertion site for C1–C2 cordotomy.

choice.[16] The patient is placed supine with the head immobilized by the forehead cushions of a head-holder.[21] C-arm fluoroscopy is arranged for lateral viewing. Under local anaesthesia and using X-ray image intensification, a short-bevelled spinal needle (20 gauge, 3.5 inch) is introduced into the intrathecal space anterior to the spinal cord between the C1 and C2 vertebrae (see Figure 13.3). Air or contrast medium (lipiodil) is injected to visualize the anterior border of the spinal cord, the dentate ligament and the posterior dura.[22] A second needle, the needle having been presized by passing it through and adjusting the sizing clamp to allow for complete exposure of the non-insulated tip, is now introduced.[21] The needle is placed in the ventral quadrant of the spinal cord just anterior to the dentate ligament. The needle is checked in an anteroposterior (open mouth view) projection under fluoroscopy. The thermocouple electrode is then passed though the spinal needle.[21] Under impedance monitoring and electrical stimulation, correct localization of the electrode tip is ensured.[16] Impedance is 300–500 ohms in the CSF and at 800–1200 ohms when it enters the spinal cord.[21] The final electrode position is determined by electrical stimulation at 75 Hz and 0.1–0.2 V.[21] This produces paraesthesia in the opposite side of the body including the affected dermatomes. Other sensations that can be experienced include warmth or coldness on the opposite side of the body, indicating that the tip is in the anterolateral spinothalamic tract.[21] The final electrode position is confirmed at 2 Hz and 1.0 V if no fasciculations in the opposite side of the body are obtained.[21] Using a radiofrequency generator, thermal lesioning is then made at 90°C for 10 seconds.[21] The temperature and pinprick sensation of the affected parts are rechecked, and, if the result is inadequate, repeat thermal lesioning is performed at 90°C for 10 seconds.[21] The patient should be awake and alert during the procedure, the extremities of the opposite side being elevated during thermal lesioning. If any weakness is experienced (e.g. sagging of the limbs), the procedure should be discontinued immediately.[21] Following each increment of current, the patient is tested for the analgesic level and for any signs of complications. A cooled roller to test for cold sensation has been found to be a better test of efficacy than pinprick, although there is still a definite association between a decrease in pinprick sensation and pain relief.[23]

In addition to relieving the pathological pain, the cordotomy abolishes the A delta fibre modalities of pinprick, cold sensation and skinfold pinch sensation.[23] The C fibre modality of warmth and heat pain is decreased to a lesser extent.[23] The greatest deficits produced are in the sensations of skinfold pinch and skin cooling. About 85 per cent of patients obtain good pain relief, which lasts realistically for 5–6 months, although relief may last for 1–2 years.[1,24,25] The complication rate is low, with an overall mortality rate of approximately 1.5 per cent.[24] Transitory ipsilateral limb weakness, ataxia, dysaesthesia and even mirror-image pain can, however, occur.[16,17] Urinary catheters occasionally have to be inserted. With cordotomies at the C2 level, pulmonary dysfunction with transient airway problems can occur. This procedure is recommended as the first line of treatment for progressive and advanced cancer affecting multiple dermatomes, including those of the lungs.[21] Stereotactic radiofrequency, current-selective thermocoagulation producing interruption of the nociceptive pathways can maintain a satisfactory quality of life for a relatively limited lifespan of afflicted cancer patients.[21]

Open surgical cordotomy

This is reserved for patients who are unable to lie still or have distorted anatomy and is usually performed under general anaesthesia.[17] A more precise lesion can be obtained as it is more accurate than other techniques. The secondary afferent fibres in the cord related to pain may be so diffusely distributed that lasting relief is more likely to be achieved by section of essentially the entire anterior quadrant on one or both sides.[14] This is more certainly accomplished by an open operation. Cancer pain referred to one or both sides of the torso and/or lower limbs remains the principal indication for this procedure.[14] A thoracic cordotomy incision is centred over T2–4 levels, while a midline incision from the inion to the C4 level is made for a cervical cordotomy.[16] The high cervical level is preferred for all unilateral incisions because complete crossover is more likely to have occurred and the pain tract is more accessible (more dorsal and compact) at this level.[14] To expose the dura, a laminectomy is performed and extended to the facet on the incision side.[16] An incision is made in the anterolateral quadrant (to a depth of 6 mm in the cervical area and 4–5 mm in the thoracic area), using the plane of the dentate ligament as the posterior extent of the incision.[2] This technique is less effective and has a higher incidence of complications than the percutaneous route. The main reason for inadequate pain relief is an inadequate incision in the anterior quadrant of the cord.[14] The mortality and lasting morbidity of unilateral cordotomy is low.[14] Bilateral surgery carries a much higher morbidity rate for the two major problems of ipsilateral weakness or paralysis of limbs and urinary tract, bowel and sexual dysfunction.[14] Postoperative radicular pain at the incision level usually disappears in a few weeks.[14] New dysaesthesias may appear, as may temporary hypotension.[14] The production of extensive analgesia up to the C4–5 level bilaterally is dangerous to voluntary respiratory pathways, which lie just lateral to the ventral horns of grey matter.[14] Late recurrences of pain may be caused by the redevelopment of some form of nociception via the anterior quadrant.[14] To relieve brachial plexus pain adequately, rhizotomies at the C2–4 levels on the painful side may additionally need to be performed.[2]

RARE NEUROSURGICAL INTERVENTIONS

Commissural myelotomy

Commissural myelotomy disrupts pain-conducting fibres as well as a polysynaptic pain pathway that runs through the centre of the spinal cord.[9] This is a controversial technique for the relief of bilateral and midline pelvic, perineal and rectal pain, especially of malignant aetiology and in the saddle area.[7,14] The procedure has a significant morbidity and risk of sphincter and motor dysfunction (visceroplegia and paraplegia).[7,9] The spinal cord is sectioned sagitally, dividing the spinothalamic fibres as they cross the anterior commissures from the dorsal horn to the spinothalamic tract.[2] Through a single cord incision, bilateral effects are thereby produced, providing the site of the pain is limited.[7] Open myelotomy requires a multilevel laminectomy and exposure of the appropriate lumbar and sacral segments of the spinal cord. By use of an operating microscope, a midline incision is made, and the spinal cord is divided vertically.[9] No reliable criteria exist on the length and depth of the incision to cut all fibres serving a given painful area.[19] It seems to produce mostly a temporary loss of pain and temperature in a corresponding girdle area.[14,19] Transient posterior column dysfunction can occur.[1] However, there is a real danger of spinal cord damage with an operative mortality rate of approximately 3 per cent.[3]

Percutaneous radiofrequency myelotomy techniques have been described.[19] A cervicomedullary junction (extralemniscal) myelotomy that is performed stereotactically with CT/MRI guidance, local anaesthesia and intraoperative physiological assessment can achieve pain relief over wide areas of the body, including midline structures.[9] The lesion is usually made 5 mm from the dorsal surface of the cord at sites at which threshold stimulation (usually 0.5–1.0 V at 50–75 Hz) evokes a tingling feeling in one or both distal lower limbs.[14] Potential complications include temporary dysaesthesia, pinprick and limb apraxia.[9,14]

Medullary spinothalamic tractotomy

Open medullary spinothalamic tractotomy is rarely used for the treatment of unilateral pain from malignant disease involving large areas as a high cervical cordotomy is preferable.[1] A unilateral suboccipital craniectomy is performed, and an incision is made 2–10 mm below the obex to interrupt the ascending pain paths.[19] A radiofrequency lesion technique for pontine spinothalamic tractotomy has been described.[19]

Mesencephalotomy

This technique interrupts the spinothalamic tract at the level of the mesencephalon. It is used for unilateral pain from malignant disease, which may include the shoulder, head and neck.[19] Stereotactic mesencephalotomy is indicated for cephalobrachial pain due to carcinoma that may involve the skull base or the proximal upper extremity.[7] A radiofrequency mesencephalotomy can be performed stereotactically under local anaesthesia after placement of the electrodes in the rostral midbrain.[7,19] This procedure relieves not only the pain itself, but also the suffering associated with it.

Cingulotomy

Cingulotomy is used mainly in the management of pain from malignant disease with a strong affective component (e.g. depression and suffering). The cingula is part of the limbic system and has cortical connections.[1] Currently, bilateral radiofrequency cingulotomy is performed stereotactically under local or general anaesthesia with few unwanted physical side-effects.[2] It provides significant short-term pain relief in half to three quarters of all patients.[26] The long-term benefits, particularly in cancer pain patients, are equivocal. The reported mortality is 0.1 per cent, the physical morbidity 0.3 per cent and the psychological morbidity 10–30 per cent.[2,26]

SYMPATHECTOMY

Except for the early intervention in CRPS type 2 and the temporary relief of pain achieved by sympathetic block in some patients, surgical sympathectomy is not an effective treatment for the pain of patients with CRPSs (see Chapter 10).[27] For lower extremity CRPS type 2, sympathectomy can be performed through a standard retroperitoneal flank approach.[2] The regeneration of sympathetic nerves is less likely if the L2–4 ganglia are removed.[8] For upper limb CRPS type 2, sympathectomy of the sympathetic cervical chain can be selectively performed (to avoid Horner's syndrome) via a posterior paraspinal approach.[2]

CANCER SURGERY

Operations for the curative excision or palliative debulking of a tumour have the potential to reduce pain, improve prognosis and even achieve a long-term, symptom-free survival.[9] On the other hand, a tumour may be recognized as an unresectable primary or a recurrence at the time of surgery.[28] Pain control is usually a secondary goal when curative tumour resection is performed.[9] In palliative surgery, pain control is frequently the operative indication.[9] Cancer pain may arise through a variety of mechanisms that are amenable to relief by surgery. During curative or palliative procedures, surgeons should use techniques to limit the development of chronic neuropathic pain such as nerve-sparing incisions, the avoidance of ischaemia and careful dissection around nerves.[9] The oncological surgeon should be familiar with the interactions of chemotherapy, radiotherapy and surgical interventions so that iatrogenic complications (e.g. multiple fistulas resulting from bowel resection performed after radiation) may be avoided.[9] The surgeon should recognize and treat characteristic pain syndromes that follow specific surgical procedures (e.g. mastectomy and nephrectomy).[9] Postoperatively, the patient is often left with major changes in anatomy and physiology (e.g. after laryngectomy or colostomy) that require further rehabilitation and continued attention to pain control.[9] Short- and long-term pain control may be enhanced by postoperative radiotherapy. Local tumour recurrence (e.g. soft tissue sarcoma or colorectal carcinoma) is not always the harbinger of disseminated disease and can be resected.[9] Prospective palliation, if undertaken before the onset of symptoms, may maximize surgical pain control (e.g. as seen in stabilizing a long bone with lytic metastases, in which fracture is likely, or decompressing a spinal canal to prevent impending paralysis or to relieve tumour nerve root entrapment).[9]

The palliative resection of the oesophagus, stomach, pancreas, small intestine and other organs can often be the most effective therapy in relieving chronic pain.[28] Patients who undergo total pelvic exenteration will avoid the occurrence of intestinal obstruction and also receive palliation for their pain. Many alimentary tract tumours become resectable after a course of radiotherapy and chemotherapy.[28] Many patients with mechanical obstruction secondary to malignant disease are able to undergo bypass surgery or a localized tumour resection, thus alleviating the mechanical obstruction. A significant proportion of patients with previous resection for abdominal malignancy present with mechanical obstruction not caused by malignancy.[28] The laparoscopic uterine nerve ablation procedure is effective in treating chronic pelvic pain.[28] Approximately 2–3 cm of the superior hypogastric plexus and the initial segments of the inferior hypogastric plexuses are resected.[28] The average operating time is 90 minutes. Unfortunately, fewer than half the patients experience adequate pain relief 12 months after surgery.[28] Surgeons now implant long-term central venous catheters (e.g. Hickman catheters) for the administration of medication, parenteral nutrition and chemotherapy, as well as for access for chronic blood withdrawal.[28] Other types of vascular access include Port-a-Caths, which are accessed via a needle inserted into the port through the overlying skin.[28] This reduces infection rate, increases patient acceptance and requires less care.[28] If the gastrointestinal tract can be used for feeding, it is generally more physiological, cheaper and less likely to develop infections or thrombotic complications.[28] In patients with head and neck, oesophageal or other tumours that make it difficult to swallow, the percutaneous placement of endoscopic gastrostomy tubes can be carried out under local anaesthesia and intravenous sedation to supplement the oral intake of protein and calories.[28]

OTHER TECHNIQUES

The ablation of the pituitary gland, as well as other stereotactic radiofrequency techniques, is described in Chapter 11. The implantation of peripheral nerve and spinal cord stimulatory devices is described in Chapter 12.

REFERENCES

1. **Kettler, R.E.** 1990: Neurosurgical management of cancer pain. In Abram, S.E. (ed.) *The pain clinic manual.* Philadelphia: J.B. Lippincott, 311–16.

2. **Freidberg, S.R.** 1992: The neurosurgeon's approach to pain. In Aronoff, G.M. (ed.) *Evaluation and treatment of chronic pain.* Baltimore: Williams & Wilkins, 229–37.

3. **Gybels, J.** 1990: Indications for the use of neurosurgical techniques. *Pain* (suppl. 5), S264.

4. **Loeser, J.D.** 1990: Introduction. In Bonica, J.J. (ed.) *The management of pain.* Philadelphia: Lea & Febiger, 2040–3.

5. **Campbell, J.N.** 1996: Pain treatment centers: a surgeon's perspective. In Cohen, M.J.M. and Campbell J.N. (eds) *Pain treatment centers at a crossroads: a practical and conceptual reappraisal, progress in pain research and management,* vol. 7. Seattle: IASP Press, 29–37.

6. **Burchiel, K.J.** 1996: Pain in neurology and neurosurgery: posttraumatic and postoperative neuralgia. In Campbell, J.N. (ed.) *Pain 1996 – an updated review.* Seattle: IASP Press, 31–9.

7. **Blumenkopf, B.** 1997: Neurosurgical approaches. In Parris, W.C.V. (ed.) *Cancer pain management: principles and practice.* Boston: Butterworth-Heinemann, 471–6.

8. **Loeser, J.D., Sweet, W.H., Tew, J.M., Van Loveren, H. and Bonica, J.J.** 1990: Neurosurgical operations involving peripheral nerves. In Bonica, J.J. (ed.) *The management of pain.* Philadelphia: Lea & Febiger, 2044–66.

9. **Jacox, A., Carr, D.B., Payne, R.** *et al.* 1994: *Management of cancer pain,* vol. 9. Publication No. 94–0592. Rockville: Agency for Health Care Policy and Research, 1–257.

10. **Koning, H.M., Koster, H.G. and Neimeijer, R.P.E.** 1991: Ischaemic spinal cord lesion following percutaneous radiofrequency spinal rhizotomy. *Pain* **45**, 161–6.

11. **Burchiel, K.J.** 1996: Pain in neurology and neurosurgery: tic douloureux (trigeminal neuralgia). In Campbell, J.N. (ed.) *Pain 1996 – an updated review.* Seattle: IASP Press, 41–60.

12. **Nashold, B.S.** 1990: The dorsal root entry zone operation: an update 1975–1990. *Pain* (suppl. 5), S415.

13. **Rawlings, C.E., El-Naggar, A.O. and Nashold, B.S.** 1989: The dorsal root entry zone procedure: an update on technique. *British Journal of Neurosurgery* **3**(6), 633–42.

14. **Sweet, W.H., Poletti, C.E. and Gybels, J.M.** 1994: Operations in the brainstem and spinal canal, with an appendix on the relationship of open to percutaneous cordotomy. In Wall, P.D. and Melzack, R. (eds) *Textbook of pain.* Edinburgh: Churchill Livingstone, 1113–35.

15. **Boivie, J.** 1996: Central pain syndromes. In Campbell, J.N. (ed.) *Pain 1996 – an updated review.* Seattle: IASP Press, 23–9.

16. **Rosomoff, H.L., Papo, I., Loeser, J.D. and Bonica, J.J.** 1990: Neurosurgical operations on the spinal cord. In Bonica, J.J. (ed.) *The management of pain.* Philadelphia: Lea & Febiger, 2067–81.

17. **Wells, J.C.D. and Miles, J.B.** 1991: Pain clinics and pain clinic treatments. *British Medical Bulletin* **47**(3), 762–85.

18. **Baumann, T.K. and Burchiel, K.J.** 1997: Intraoperative microneurographic recordings in patients with trigeminal neuralgia. In Jensen, T.S., Turner, J.A. and Wiesenfeld-Hallin, Z. (eds) *Proceedings of the 8th World Congress on Pain, progress in pain research and management,* vol. 8. Seattle: IASP Press, 459–67.

19. **Janetta, P.J., Gildenberg, P.L., Loeser, J.D., Sweet, W.H., Ojemann, G.A. and Bonica, J.J.** 1990: Operations on the brain and brain stem for chronic pain. In Bonica, J.J. (ed.) *The management of pain.* Philadelphia: Lea & Febiger, 2082–103.

20. **Di Piero, V., Jones, A.K.P., Iannotti, E.** *et al.* 1991: Chronic pain: a PET study of the central effects of percutaneous high cervical cordotomy. *Pain* **46**, 9–12.

21. **Kantha, S.** 1997: Stereotactic techniques. In Parris, W.C.V. (ed.) *Cancer pain management: principles and practice.* Boston: Butterworth-Heinemann, 181–95.

22. **Wiles, J.R., Wells, J.C.D., Buckley, P. and Hardy, P.A.J.** 1990: The use of lipiodol in the percutaneous anterolateral cervical cordotomy. *Pain* (suppl. 5), S411.

23. **Lahuerta, J., Bowsher, D., Campbell, J. and Lipton, S.** 1990: Clinical and instrumental evaluation of sensory function before and after percutaneous anterolateral cordotomy at cervical level in man. *Pain* **41**, 23–30.

24. **Stuart, G., Cramond, T. and Jamieson, K.G.** 1990: Percutaneous cordotomy for malignant pain. *Pain* (suppl. 5), S414.

25. **Bond, M.R.** 1984: Local analgesia, nerve blocks and surgical methods of pain relief. In Bond, M.R. (ed.) *Pain – its nature, analysis and treatment.* Edinburgh: Churchill Livingstone, 179–91.

26. **Bouckoms, A.J.** 1994: Limbic surgery for pain. In Wall, P.D. and Melzack, R. (eds) *Textbook of pain.* Edinburgh: Churchill Livingstone, 1171–87.

27. **Tasker, R.R.** 1990: Reflex sympathetic dystrophy: neurosurgical approaches. In Stanton-Hicks, M. Janig, W. and Boas, R.A. (eds) *Reflex sympathetic dystrophy.* Boston: Kluwer, 125–34.

28. **Richards, W.O. and Key, S.P.** 1997: Surgical approaches. In Parris, W.C.V. (ed.) *Cancer pain management: principles and practice.* Boston: Butterworth-Heinemann, 463–9.

14 PSYCHOLOGICAL INTERVENTION

Pain is a complex, personal, subjective and unpleasant sensory and perceptual experience that may or may not have any correlation with bodily injury or tissue damage.[1] As defined by the International Association for the Study of Pain, 'pain is unquestionably a sensation in part or parts of the body, but it is also always unpleasant and therefore an emotional experience'.[2] Pain is the outcome of a complex interplay of influences, including psychological factors, which may operate both as risk factors in and consequences of pain.[3] During the past half century, psychological thought has moved away from linear to multicausal models of pain.[4] When a psychological causation of pain is postulated, multiple determinants of pain are usually also discussed.[4] Research has failed to identify a typical personality profile in patients with chronic pain.[4] Chronic pain syndromes often serve no biological usefulness, and psychological factors can sustain or exacerbate these pain syndromes.[5]

Evidence has accumulated that psychological factors play a major role in the development and maintenance of many features of chronic pain in patients presenting for treatment, largely independent of the original cause of their pain. The level of disability is associated more with distress and maladaptive conditions than with pathophysiology.[6] Many problems are the result of inappropriate learning behaviours in dealing with pain and its consequences, for example pain complaints, resting, limping and taking medication. These behaviours are reinforced by their consequences or by the contingencies existing in the patient's current environment.[6] Emotional and cognitive factors are also involved, fear, anxiety, attributions, beliefs, self-efficacy and coping interacting in complex ways in the development of the problem.[7] Time is an essential ingredient, during which cognitive-behavioural factors may operate to establish the sick role.[7] These behaviours may include low levels of physical and social function, complaints, the overuse of medications, the use of passive coping strategies and beliefs that activity causes pain or injury.[7]

Pain is usually anxiety-provoking, and this creates fear avoidance, whereby anxiety about activities exacerbating the pain stimulates the avoidance of those activities. Activity patterns and daily routines become disrupted, while depression and catastrophizing thoughts may be obstacles to recovery.[7] Pain behaviours may be reinforced by the social response they bring (attention, sympathy, legitimization of the behaviour and a temporary reduction of pain or anxiety).[7] Passive behaviours such as resting, reading or watching television, which may be pleasant and associated with less pain, may become predominant. Pain behaviours may also buy time out of undesirable duties or activities. The process is typically gradual, and the patient may not realize that a drastic change in lifestyle is taking place. Thus, the basic tenet (secondary prevention) is to intervene early to prevent disruption of the patient's normal lifestyle, including work.[7] A person seeking help for chronic pain could therefore not only be experiencing persistent pain, but also be distressed, inactive with secondary physical deconditioning, and upholding unhelpful beliefs. He or she is overly passive or reliant on others for resolution of personal problems, and is most likely to be experiencing side-effects of various treatments besides the additional stress caused by the effects of the pain on the family and financial circumstances.[6]

PATIENT EDUCATION

Before treating patients in a pain clinic, it is important to provide them with information to clear up misperceptions about their pain.[8] The gate control model is often used as it explains pain as a perceptual event rather than just simple sensory stimulation (Figure 14.1).[5] Despite the fact that neurophysiology has moved on from the gate control theory, it remains a useful tool to explain to patients the nature of pain. It also explains why the surgical, electrical or neurolytic ablation of pain pathways does not always stop the pain. According to the gate control theory, pain perception is influenced by the net effect of large primary afferents, small primary afferents and higher brain function (top-down processing) for their pattern of action (or gating) on substantia gelatinosa neurones.[9]

Other educational topics include the difference between acute and chronic pain, the relationship of pain to anxiety and depression, the effect of stress on pain and the nature of the patient's illness. After overt injury, pain may only appear when reaction to the injury is biologically appropriate,[10] suggesting that expectation conditioning may be a factor determining the behaviour expressed.[10]

In the perioperative situation, education from the provision of information to patients and from various approaches to patient preparation results in a reduction of postoperative opioid requirements.[11–13] Four principal categories of preparatory procedure have been identified:[12]

1. the provision of information (e.g. regarding the procedure);
2. behavioural instructions (e.g. training the patient to relax or cough);
3. cognitive methods (e.g. positive thinking);
4. psychotherapeutic approaches (e.g. exploring emotional responses).

Patients are also less likely to refuse analgesia once this information has been provided.[11]

ASSESSMENT

A record of past treatments, interventions and investigations should be obtained and explained to the patient.[14] Inquiry should be made about the emotional state of the patient at the time of injury or onset of disease. Exceptional mental or physical stress before the painful event may be associated with acute stress reaction, post-traumatic stress disorder and adjustment disorders.[14] Questions to be asked include:

- When did your pain first start?
- Where do you feel your pain?
- When does your pain occur?
- How intense is your pain?
- Does it alter throughout the day?
- What is the effect of movement and posture change on your pain?
- What other factors increase or decrease your pain?
- What do you do less frequently and what do you do more since you developed the pain?
- Does your pain affect your mood, and does your mood affect your pain?
- What effect do drugs have on your pain?

The assessment requires an accurate evaluation of the degree and extent of organic pathology. It is not possible to assess whether the pain behaviour is appropriate unless the history of the painful complaint is known and a physical examination has been performed. Pain intensity can be measured using visual analogue, numerical or verbal category scales.[15] Pain location is typically assessed using a body chart or body map.[15]

A great deal of knowledge of the patient's past history, previous personality, recent life events and conflicts, and other cultural and social factors is needed to determine how far these affect the production of the pain complaint.[14] For example, severely injured veterans (patients with previous

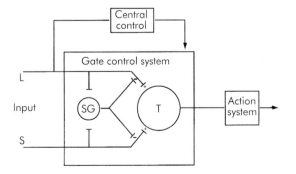

Figure 14.1 Gate control diagram. See text for details. T = transmission cell; SG = substantia gelatinosa; L = large nerve fibres; S = small nerve fibres.

long-term pain experiences) have a much higher pain threshold and tolerance than lightly injured veterans.[16] Questions to pose to determine the direction of further inquiry following examination include:[14]

- Is there any evidence of existing disease or past tissue damage?
- Is there any possibility of continuing physical pathology?
- Is there any evidence of psychiatric illness primary or secondary to the disabilities that have resulted from the events that caused the pain?
- Are there any emotional conflicts or psychosocial problems that were associated with pain onset or maintenance?
- Is there any suggestion of the intentional production, exaggeration or feigning of symptoms associated with the pain?

At the initial interview, much useful information can be gained by interviewing the partner or a close relative in order to gain a window on the psychosocial situation and stresses, the patterns of communication and conflict, the family beliefs and motivations.[17] Performing a physical examination allows the examiner to determine the current 'illness behaviour' and the influence of psychological factors on the presentation of medical symptoms. The mental status of the patient is assessed. Further enquiry is devoted to specific psychiatric symptoms (anxiety/panic and depression). A user-friendly interview schedule that can be completed in less than 10 minutes by a primary health care worker has recently been developed.[17] It is an excellent assessment training tool relevant to chronic pain clinic staff and is highly accurate in identifying affective disorders and somatoform conditions.[17]

If an assessment instrument is to be of value as an outcome measure, it must identify whether a patient has made progress towards an agreed goal.[18] For adequate assessments, outcome measures (e.g. pain, physical function, work and lifestyle goals, health care use, mood, beliefs, sleep and social relationships), as well as a description of the treatment population, must be identified. Patient and therapist expectations, adherence to treatment and treatment validity are also important.[18] Outcomes should be examined against criteria of health.

For pain measurements, the difficulties of separating the multidimensional experience of pain into measurable parts is enormous. Pain measures cannot be validated in any way that has meaning for clinical populations, and there is widespread neglect of the effect of context.[18] Verbal scales have a low error rate but a low sensitivity to change. VASs present some patients with problems of comprehension and are tiresome to score.

It is rare in treatment programmes for pain behaviours that are of significance in treatment to be identified, and for them to be measured systematically and with sensitivity to the context. Core pain behaviours for observers include the verbal report, facial, postural and movement cues, relative inactivity, taking analgesics and seeking help to relieve the pain.[18] The daily activity diary method (if the patient keeps accurate records) notes patient medication intake and the amount of time the patient spends sitting, walking or standing, and reclining.[15] A key measure of pain behaviour is 'daily down-time', the time spent in the reclining position. Assessment protocols include Keefe and Bock, the UAB scale, CHIP, the Cinciripini and Floreen scale, and facial expression analysis by videotaping.[18] The interaction of patient and partner behaviour may also be videotaped and measured. There is no evidence that expensive machinery provides better quality measurement than reliable and well-validated tests of physical performance such as walking tests and grip strength performed under standardized conditions.[18] Even the use of a 5–10 minute walk test in addition to the more usual self-report measures will greatly improve the quality of outcome measurements.[19] However, a new portable accelerometer, the Actigraph, can periodically sample movements over a period of 11 days and correlates well with physiological and self-report measures of activity.[20] Physiological measures such as dynamic EMGs at multiple sites are relevant and informative but challenging to process and interpret.[18] Indices of health care use, hospital admissions, investigations or their cost add significantly to data reliability.[18] Self-report measures of physical function include the Sickness Impact Profile, the Arthritis Impact Measurement Scales, and the SF-36.[18] Patients tend to underestimate activity by self-report in comparison with automated recordings.

The local level of employment of that age and skill group, the employer's willingness to accept a worker with a history of chronic pain, the length of time off work and disability options can have a major bearing on the patient's return to work and demand applied problem-solving.[18] External information sources (work absence records, disability payments and income) are helpful assessors of work and compensation. To assess sleep quality and quantity, self-ratings (difficulty in falling asleep and feeling rested on wakening), backed up by a sleeping partner report and the home use of automated instruments, are helpful.[18] Polysonographic recordings can also be used. To assess cognitive content and process, the areas of belief and behaviour are better sampled separately than mixed within a scale. Questionnaires with proven value in predicting behaviour include the Coping Strategies Questionnaire, the Pain Beliefs and Perceptions Inventory and the Fear Avoidance Beliefs Questionnaire.[18] Assessment of patients' expectations of pain relief or benefit from specific treatment components can be undertaken using a simple Linkert scale.[18]

Patients' social environments (family, friends and workmates) can be expected to have a major influence on how they fare during and after treatment, and useful information on this can be obtained from the Significant Others Scale.[18] A partner's supportive efforts may undermine the patient's own efforts to manage; the partner can be a potent source of both positive and problematic support. Patients overestimate treatment adherence, but adherence to drug regimens is generally low.[18]

In treatment studies, measures of treatment validity and patient and staff expectations have been neglected. Evidence-based medicine requires careful and systematic treatment evaluation. If the treatment aim is to return the patient to a reasonably independent lifestyle, measurement requires a combination of measures of function, health care use, pain and beliefs and moods.[18]

BEHAVIOURAL INTERVENTIONS

Overt behaviours are modified in behavioural therapy, covert behaviours in cognitive-behavioural therapy. Overt behaviours include:[21]

- physiological pain reactions, such as muscle tension, as a response to painful stimulation;
- respondent pain behaviours, such as bracing, limping, guarding, grimacing and sighing;
- operant pain behaviours, such as verbal complaints, temper tantrums and inactivity.

Covert behaviours include cognitions, which are subjective mental phenomena, such as perceptions, thoughts, images, beliefs, interpretations and expectations. The goal of behavioural and cognitive-behavioural therapy is to increase adaptive behaviours and cognitions, such as coping and problem-solving skills, and to decrease maladaptive

behaviours and cognitions, for example muscle tension, grimacing and catastrophizing.[21] The term 'maladaptive' refers to behaviours and cognitions that increase, rather than decrease, the suffering associated with pain.

Operant conditioning

Pain is not an isolated behaviour. It is to be understood in an interactional framework, which includes learning history, biological and genetic factors, and present environmental influences.[22] The aim of behavioural intervention is to increase the frequency of wellness (as opposed to sick) behaviours and decrease the frequency of pain behaviours. After the medical and psychological evaluations but before a behavioural programme can begin, the patient should grant informed consent. Behavioural interventional methods include self-monitoring and contingency management.[21] Self-monitoring is the ability to monitor one's behaviour; it allows patients to notice their dysfunctional reactions and to learn to control them. Continency management is the method of reinforcing 'wellness behaviours' only, thereby modifying dysfunctional operant pain behaviours associated with secondary gain.[21] Pain contingent reinforcers (medications, sympathetic attention, bed rest and the avoidance of aversive situations) are eliminated, while reinforcement contingent on 'wellness behaviours' (assumed to be incompatible with pain) is introduced.[4]

TECHNIQUE

Operant conditioning principles address behaviour in terms of the environmental consequences of a given response to a given stimulus environment.[22] A patient will respond to pain with a given behaviour when that behaviour has previously led to reinforcing consequences in a similar stimulus environment. If a behaviour is followed by a positive or desired response (i.e. it is reinforced), it will probably be used again in the same stimulus situation. If no reinforcement occurs, the frequency of this behaviour will decrease.[22] Pain behaviour includes verbal complaints, non-language sounds (e.g. groaning), body posture and gestures, and functional limitations (e.g. spending too much time in bed).[5] It may continue even in the absence of nociceptive stimulation.[3]

Two points are important here. First, for operant conditioning, pain behaviours that occur with adequate frequency are observed and identified by staff, by family or sometimes even by the patients themselves.[22] By monitoring the environment, the precipitating stimuli, reinforcement contingencies and behavioural consequences are identified and monitored.[22] For example, a 10-minute standardized sequence of movements can be videotaped and rated according to a set of pain behavioural categories (e.g. grimacing and guarding) by trained observers.[23] Another example is an inappropriate response to examination in low back pain, which can be identified and integrated into a systematic assessment.[23]

Second, activities and sensations that are pleasurable to the patient are identified and, if appropriate, substituted to provide positive reinforcement.[22] A patient's family, friends or health care providers may unwittingly reinforce pain behaviour by providing attention or by colluding in the avoidance of desirable activities.[5] Insurance companies may also reward pain behaviour financially (so-called 'compensation neurosis').

It is important to set specific goals for behavioural change. Examples include an increase in exercise or a decrease in opioid consumption. These can be reinforced with praise and attention initially each time the behaviour is shown in an appropriate situation.[22] Later, the number of positive responses required for reinforcement is increased in order to obtain the desired response even when there are long periods without reinforcement.[22] Conversely, pain behaviours do not receive undue attention. This will cause the behaviour to decrease until it ultimately stops. It is essential to feed back any progress noted to the patient as this allows the patient to experience success.[22]

A number of clinical studies provide evidence for the effectiveness of operant programmes in decreasing pain behaviour while increasing the level of function.[4] It has, however, been argued that patient needs are often neglected and that outcome is based on measures that may be unrelated to suffering.[4] Recent experimental evidence demonstrates that not only pain behaviours, but also the subjective experience of pain, as well as the physiological correlates of pain, are subject to operant learning mechanisms.[24] The N150/P260 component of the evoked cortical potential (a good correlate of subjectively experienced pain) is modifiable by operant learning. Subjects who learned to decrease the N150/P260 amplitude experienced less pain and vice versa.[24] Operant learning thus influences all levels of the pain experience and may establish powerful memories for pain-related responses.

Cognitive-behavioural interventions

A systems model views pain behaviour as controlled by multiple and interactive factors – environmental, psychological and biological.[20] The cognitive-behavioural approach focuses on the patient's pain and pain behaviour, and on how those patterns may vary in different situations. Attempts are made to analyse specific cognitive, affective and behavioural variables that may be controlling the patient's pain experience.[15] Assessment designs and guides are an integral part of the treatment process. Problems are targeted for intervention, treatments are matched to the patient's needs, and the effectiveness of the ongoing treatment is evaluated.[15] Through this, patients will suffer less and, although not cured, will find that their pain troubles them less, so they can resume a more active and fulfilling lifestyle.[6]

Pain beliefs have been defined as 'patients' own conceptualizations of what pain is and what pain means to them'.[25] Cognitive-behavioural interventions literally change the way in which patients think about their pain.[5] They emphasize cognitive factors as they affect perception and behavioural responses to pain. This helps patients to identify and correct distorted conceptualizations and unrealistic, irrational belief systems.[22] By changing behaviours, feelings, attitudes and beliefs, maladaptive behavioural and psychological ineffective belief systems are replaced with realistic and effective ones, and functional activity is increased.[26]

Anxiety and anger set up cyclical stress–pain and tension–pain patterns (see 'Biofeedback' below).[22] Depression undermines attempts to diminish pain behaviour and enhance functioning. The negative expectations and attitudes of patients can influence physiological processes and sustain or even increase pain.[5] Physically avoiding situations that cause pain can diminish overall activity and decrease muscle strength and flexibility.[5] Clinical experience suggests that the cognitive-behavioural approach is particularly helpful in patients who have become inactive because of their pain.[27] Patients' attitudes towards and beliefs about their pain may influence their compliance to treatment, their ability to cope with pain and the resultant treatment outcome.[25]

Cognitive-behavioural therapy is thus a therapeutic process to help individuals to modify their behaviours and feelings by altering their patterns of thought. Thus, the focus of such therapies is on monitoring and changing negative erroneous thinking or negative self-statements that lead to undesirable responses.[21] Eight styles of negative thinking are blaming, 'shoulds', polarized thinking, catastophizing, control fallacies, emotional reasoning, filtering and entitlement fallacy.[21] Blaming allows the patient to evade responsibility. Self-blame is self-defeating and is an excuse for inactivity. 'Shoulds' are irrational and are usually a putdown by admonishing oneself for creating expectations for others to meet. Polarized thinking is extreme thinking leading to damaging overgeneralizations. Catastrophizing is imagining the worst possible outcome, thus adding to anxiety. Control fallacies assign others (the doctor or clinic) total power over one's fate, thereby rendering one helpless. Emotional reasoning assumes feelings to be true, resulting in unrealistic reasoning. Filtering (tunnel vision pain) makes things appear worse. Entitlement fallacy is the feeling that no-one is 'entitled' to a totally pain-free existence. Each of these thinking styles can be modified through cognitive-behavioural therapy.[21]

Consistent programme application is obtained by using a programme based on a set of principles. Adequate programme information plus a visit to the programme site prepares patients for programme admission.[6] Establishing the patient's goals and associated motivations is useful at this stage. The different modalities of the pain experience (intensity, location and affect) are first assessed.[15] The affective subscale of the McGill Pain Questionnaire, cross-modality matching to psychophysically scaled descriptors and VASs have all been used to assess pain affect.[15] Pain behaviour can be assessed using a daily activity diary, videotaping or standardized observation methods.[15] Patients may use a wide range of cognitive and behavioural strategies to cope with, deal with and minimize their pain. The Coping Strategies Questionnaire is clinically useful in assessing the use and perceived effectiveness of coping strategies.[15] A five-factor structure (distraction, ignoring pain sensations, reinterpreting pain sensations, catastrophizing, and praying and hoping) is the most interpretable.[28] The prospective daily diary method has recently been used to assess pain coping in order to eliminate bias and assess rapidly changing coping processes closer to their real-time occupance.[15] The newly developed Daily Coping Inventory is proving to be a promising daily instrument in assessing coping changes.[5] The Meaning of the Illness Questionnaire showed that 56 per cent of pain patients had poor psychosocial adjustment to their pain.[29,30] A recent

factor analytic investigation of the Minnesota Multiphasic Personality Inventory –2 in the chronic pain population showed four interpretable factors: psychological and physical dysfunction, interpersonal isolation and psychomotor retardation.[31] Chronic pain patients recently completing both the Sickness Impact Profile and the Survey of Pain Attitudes showed that beliefs that emotions affect pain and disablement were associated positively with psychosocial dysfunction.[32] Beliefs of disablement and activity avoidance were associated positively with physical disability.[32]

Before embarking on any intervention, the therapist must show a readiness to understand and then negotiate with patients. This must be done in a manner that respects patients' capacity to understand, as well as their personal theories concerning their state of health. Most patients have expectations and questions that need to be dealt with.[22] Patients should be informed that all pain is the result of both physical and psychological factors and that their pain is believed to be 'real' pain.[22] It should be emphasized that the patient is undergoing what may be demanding therapy on a voluntary basis and that the responsibility for recovery remains with the patient.[22] Patient belief systems, as well as cognitive coping strategies, are then identified.

Activity levels (including physical exercises) must be increased and linked to restoration of function. Staff and patients themselves should verbally reinforce treatment progress.[6] Unhelpful thoughts and beliefs should be changed by explaining to patients that the programme is going to focus on those things which can be changed (activity level, mood, side-effects of medication and coping strategies) instead of focusing on pain (which has not yet been changed), resulting in a reduction of suffering.[6] Patients find the programme more acceptable if it initially concentrates on achieving behavioural changes along with learning specific exercise strategies, for example pacing and techniques such as relaxation, before progressing to cognitive aspects.[6] Usually by the end of the first week of a 4-week programme (as an in- or day-patient), most patients feel comfortable to move on to cognitive tasks.[6] Self-monitoring of conditions, mood and pain helps patients to see the links between them and then to progress to trying ways of identifying unhelpful cognitions when they occur, challenging them and changing them.[6] With a reduction in medication, patients must perceive that they are playing an active role in both the decision-making and implementation processes. In fact, with all behavioural changes made by patients, it is essential for them to take responsibility (or credit) rather than to attribute them to the programme staff.[6] This is in order to promote patients' confidence to deal with future difficulties and setbacks alone. Whenever possible, attempts should be made to contact significant others (spouse, partner or family), either directly or through the patient, and to seek their cooperation and participation in the programme as they might well have influential opposing views on the programme.[6] To prevent relapse in patients' normal environments, the following are undertaken:

- rehearsals of plans for dealing with flare-ups;
- setting specific goals (achievable in the eyes of the patient);
- identifying environmental difficulties with practice strategies to deal with them;
- giving patients written programme guidelines (which includes training in coping strategies and problem-solving skills) to equip them to deal with future problems.

In addition, the cooperation or partnership of other key reinforcement sources (employer, family and general practitioner) should be obtained. The general practitioner could review the patient's progress once a month, and constrain the patient from 'doctor shopping'.

TECHNIQUES

Cognitive-behavioural techniques also include relaxation training, biofeedback and hypnosis (see below).

Problem exploration and solving

Here, present attitudes and problem areas are identified and patients' methods of approaching and resolving problems assessed.[23] Basic problem-solving skills may be deficient in the chronic pain patient. The patient is instructed in planning and in goal-setting,[22] goals being broken down into manageable steps.

Cognitive restructuring

Cognitive restructuring requires patients to take responsibility for their feelings, thoughts and actions rather than externalizing them. Irrational beliefs are identified and reframed so that patients can evaluate their environment and themselves more rationally.[22] The therapist should also be direct in order not to allow patients to delude themselves that their problems are all physical.[1] The technique of thought-stopping and switching is also taught.

Self-efficacy

Self-efficacy is the personal conviction of the patient that he or she can successfully perform certain behaviours in a given situation.[5] It is not concerned with skills but with capability judgements.[33] It is an important predictor of a patient's ability to tolerate pain and is associated with decreased pain and disability.[5,33] Its validity has been shown in a variety of pain conditions, including temporomandibular joint syndrome, headaches, back pain and arthritis.[5] Associations have been found between efficacy and the perceived size of the pain problem, efficacy and exercise, and efficacy and relapse.[5] It is important that, during therapy, patients develop a sense of control over their pain.[5] Increased perceived control may be a underlying factor common to all psychological interventions in the management of pain.[13] In one study, activity-related self-efficacy beliefs were shown to be the best predictor of isokinetic trunk muscle strength.[33] An Arthritis Self-Efficacy Scale and a Pain Self-Efficacy Questionnaire have been used and validated.[33] A Chronic Self-Efficacy Scale has recently been developed and validated to measure self-efficacy beliefs in patients with chronic pain.[34]

Environmental factors

Pain has been found to be strongly influenced by environmental cues and can even be produced in the absence of peripheral stimulation.[35] If appropriate, a patient's environmental situation needs to be adjusted. For example, if the patient is unhappy in his or her job, there may need to be a change of jobs or some other adjustment.[8]

Stress management

Stress has been implicated in the development, exacerbation and maintenance of chronic pain syndromes by creating stress–pain–stress cycles.[36] Life stressors can lead to dysfunctional habits (e.g. clenching and guarding) that create chronic muscle tension and pain.[37] The role of stress should, however, not be conceptualized in terms of the occurrence of stressful life events but instead in terms of patients' cognitive or emotional appraisal of their negative impact on their life patterns.[17] Patients are instructed in stress management and are taught to identify stressors. Communication skills, conversation skills or assertiveness training can be given when necessary.[8] Such responses can be modelled by the therapist through role play.

Sleep disturbance

Behavioural techniques used to improve the quality of sleep include relaxation techniques, appropriate dietary adjustment and rising at the same time each morning.[8]

Distraction techniques

Humans have the ability to block and filter sensory messages. By using distraction techniques, patients are taught to focus their attention away from their pain.

It is important that patients correctly understand the factors affecting chronic pain.[22] Responses learned from therapy need to be applied in the home, work and social environments, and effective patient follow-up will discourage relapse.

Respondent (Pavlovian) conditioning

The assumption is that pain as an unconditioned stimulus may lead to numerous physiological reactions that will then be conditioned to all stimuli present along with the painful stimulation.[24] If these learned associations occur often and with great intensity, pain may develop that is maintained by the respondent learning process. This learned pain response is no longer related to the initial cause of the acute pain, although it may be localized at the same site and have comparable qualities.[24] Thus, many stimuli that were once associated with pain (certain body positions, movements, emotions, or external situations) may gain a pain-inducing function through respondent conditioning. Both operant and respondent conditioning, which are instrumental in creating psychophysiological dysfunction, can be used therapeutically.[24] For example, enhanced peripheral and physiological reactivity can be modified by biofeedback to reduce muscular reactivity or the operant conditioning of evoked cortical responses.[24] Further research should concentrate on demonstrating how these behavioural and psychophysiological methods change the biological substrate of response to pain.[24]

Psychophysiological interventions

Episodes of muscle tension, whether created through injury or stress, can cause pain. This can progress to a muscle–tension–pain cycle. Significant differences may be found in patients' EMG levels in the paravertebral muscles only when under stress, and in the latency of return to baseline after periods of prolonged tension.[5,22] Chronic pain patients are vulnerable to stressors and may respond to them with increased emotional distress and consequent arousal of the autonomic nervous system. This increases muscle tension and may even result in muscle spasms, which may progress to a stress–pain–stress cycle.[22]

ASSESSMENT

All patients must be orientated to the goals of autonomic nervous system regulatory techniques, namely how to recognize and control arousal stimuli.[22] Psychophysiological baseline response patterns to rest and stress can be obtained, which are useful in directing treatment and predicting outcome.[22] They include the use of heart rate, EMG, galvanic skin responses and changes in peripheral temperature.[22]

TREATMENT TECHNIQUES

Relaxation training

Relaxation training includes progressive muscle relaxation, autogenic training, mental imagery and systematic densitization.[21] Relaxation training teaches patients to become physically and mentally relaxed. It has a number of physiological effects.[8] It may slow heart and respiratory rate, and increase extremity temperature. It can improve sleep, diminish muscle tension and decrease pain. It also enhances coping ability by decreasing anxiety and increasing self-control. Tapes on relaxation training are often loaned to patients in order for them to practise at home.

Progressive muscle relaxation training

This is an 'active' exercise that involves systematically tensing and then relaxing all of the body's major muscle groups in turn.[8,21] This teaches awareness of the difference between tension and relaxation and how to learn to monitor and relieve muscle tension, as well as stretching the muscles. It requires regular practice, and sessions often begin with a standard 'cue' such as taking a deep breath or saying the word 'relax'.[21] The cue acts as a discriminative stimulus signalling that deep muscle relaxation is to follow, and it eventually elicits the entire relaxation response.

Cognitive relaxation training

This includes the use of imagery (mental images) and autogenic relaxation training. Relaxation with mental imagery involves using the imagination, such as in pleasant imagery, or transforming the context of pain while in a relaxed state.[21] The goal is to control the focus of attention away from the pain and to enhance patients' ability to control their pain. Having patients imagine a relaxing place or experience may relax them.[8] This technique can be used to desensitize patients to stressors.[22] In acute pain, the use of positive emotion induction, by re-creating a pleasant memory, results in lower ratings of pain, fear and anxiety.[38]

Autogenic relaxation training involves generating feelings of heaviness and warmth in the extremities.[21] It uses positive self-statements about body status (e.g. 'My legs feel warm and heavy') to induce relaxation.[8,22] The goal is to decrease heart and respiratory rates and muscle tension, as well as to increase blood flow.

Breathing

Chronic pain patients may breathe ineffectively (e.g. in a shallow and rapid manner).[22] To rectify this, patients are taught diaphragmatic exercises. They lie down, with their hands placed on their abdomen over their diaphragm in order to monitor respiratory movement.

Distraction techniques

In these, patients are taught to focus their attention away from their pain. The intermittent use of external stimulation (radio or television) is helpful.

Systematic desensitization

This involves constructing a hierarchy of anxiety-producing experiences and then pairing each with relaxation until the patient no longer associates anxiety with the previously anxiety-producing experience.[21] The goal is to extinguish anticipatory anxiety such as anxiety regarding medical problems.

Some patients exhibit considerable difficulty in relaxing.[21] Some people may have engaged in maladaptive thought processes throughout their lives until maladaptive thinking has become their perception of reality. For many, the concept of letting go and really relaxing can evoke fear. Some patients feel that 'something terrible will happen' if they really let go. They experience a sense of cognitive dissonance when asked to relax because they have been tense for so long.[21] Relaxation-induced anxiety can then occur. For them, anxiety has served as the energy to diffuse and keep out of awareness those things perceived as too frightening to process; thus, when they relax, they become flooded with primary thoughts (repressed thoughts and memories).[21] Using biofeedback-assisted hypnosis, the process can be graduated so that the patient is not too uncomfortable with the feelings of relaxation.[21]

Biofeedback

Biofeedback involves using electronic physiological monitoring equipment (usually computerized) to allow patients to see and hear changes in their body function, for the purpose of helping them to learn to increase, decrease or stabilize a targeted response.[21,22] This awareness enables patients to bring their body functions (e.g. muscle tension, heart rate and galvanic skin response) under voluntary control, thereby lowering their arousal.

EMG biofeedback uses the measure of the electrical charge in muscle fibres, which indicates contraction or relaxation of the muscles.[21] It is helpful in conditions with a muscular tension component, for example low back pain, temporomandibular joint syndromes and headaches (tension and migraine).[8] Thermal biofeedback is used to teach patients to increase their skin temperature in their extremities, thereby increasing vasodilatation and reducing sympathetic nervous system activity.[21] The premise is that sympathetic nervous system activity may result in vasoconstriction of the peripheral arterioles and that reduced sympathetic nervous system activity is associated with vasodilatation; however, the exact physiological mechanism of this is still unclear.[21] Thus, thermal biofeedback uses the vascular system to feed back extremity temperature changes. Generalized relaxation or imaging can induce changes in hand and foot temperature.[8] This technique has been used in the treatment of migraine and CRPS type 1.[8] It has also been successfully used in decreasing anal pain and in decreasing pain in labour.[39,40]

A major goal of using biofeedback with chronic pain patients is to help patients to refine their relaxation skills and increase their understanding of the link between thought processes and physiological responses.[21] During the process of biofeedback training, patients are taught to break up phenomena into small steps, each small segment being reinforced by visual or auditory feedback.[21] Patients are then trained to sustain a positive image or attach a relaxation response to an anxiety-producing stimulus, as in systematic desensitization. Through practice, patients build up a relaxation response equal in strength to the anxiety response.[21] Biofeedback is a way for the therapist, and patient, to monitor whether the patient is mastering the ability to control his or her physiological responses.

Biofeedback techniques are more effective when combined with relaxation training, cognitive-behavioural therapy or other autonomic nervous system regulatory techniques.[5] For example, EMG biofeedback augments long-term clinical improvements in headache patients who undergo autogenic relaxation training.[41] Older patients have been found to respond just as well as younger patients to biofeedback/relaxation training.[42]

Hypnosis

Hypnosis is a heightened state of concentration characterized by a markedly increased receptivity to suggestion and the capacity for the alteration of perception and the direct control of a variety of usually involuntary physiological functions, such as vasomotor activity.[21] This can be useful in pain control. Through hypnosis, patients can learn how to relax the affected areas that are physically causing pain, with an increase in circulation and a sense of overall lightness, warmth and well-being.[21] The conscious mind is relaxed and rested without being asleep. When a relaxed state is achieved by the patient, therapeutic suggestions are given in a manner expectant of a desired outcome, enabling the use of the imagination to produce the desired results.

Hypnotherapy techniques include progressive relaxation, imagery, glove anaesthesia, safe-place imagery and self-hypnosis. Progressive relaxation can be modified under hypnosis to produce a much greater depth of relaxation.[21] This technique will help patients to increase their concentration and redirect their attention to health and wellness. Imagery enables patients to dissolve and dismiss pain. Through imagery and hypnosis, patients can give the source of the pain and the size, shape and colour of the 'object', thereby managing their externalized pain problem.[21] Glove anaesthesia allows patients to anaesthetize a portion of their body by touching that portion with their hand. The hand is already made to feel numb through imagery and visualization, and that numbness is transferred from the hand to the area of discomfort.[21] With safe-place imagery, the hypnotist helps the patient to facilitate hypnotic analgesia. Hypnotic suggestions are given that patients are in another place and time.[21] That 'safe place' experienced is free of any discomfort or unpleasant sensation. Self-hypnosis is a technique that patients can easily learn and use to relieve chronic pain. Many different methods are used to teach the techniques involved.[21] Through self-hypnosis, patients can reinforce therapeutic suggestions at home or at work.

Hypnosis has been shown to be efficacious in the treatment of chronic pain. However, one third of patients are not hypnotizable, and other techniques therefore need to be used.[21] Hypnosis has been found to alleviate experimentally induced pain (induced by a cold pressor test).[43] It has recently been shown that hypnosis significantly attenuates a physiological measure – the nociceptive reflex elicited by electrical stimulation of the sural nerve.[44] Hypnosis was found to activate and attenuate a triple hierarchial pain control system: the nociceptive reflex (spinal and descending control mechanisms), the perceived intensity of evoked pain sensations (spinal and supraspinal inhibitory mechanisms) and the unpleasantness of the pain sensation (sensory and affective inhibitory systems).[44]

Psychotherapy

In addition to behavioural and cognitive-behavioural therapeutic techniques, supportive psychotherapy and family systems therapy are helpful with pain management.

SUPPORTIVE PSYCHOTHERAPY

This emphasizes empathetic understanding and unconditional positive regard, the primary goal being to help patients to achieve congruence between self and experience (e.g. between the ideal self and the experience of pain).[21] Empathetic understanding refers to the therapist's ability to understand the patient and to convey this. Methods used include nodding, eye contact and reflection of feeling. Unconditional positive regard indicates a genuine concern and care for the patient and involves affirming the patient's worth as a person and accepting that patient without evaluation.[21] Positive regard means the avoidance of any overt or covert judgement of the patient's behaviour. Because a judgement of any kind represents a 'condition of worth', positive judgements are considered to be as non-therapeutic as negative judgements. Genuineness means that the therapist must honestly communicate his or her feelings whenever it is appropriate to do so.[21] The desired outcome of supportive therapy is to help patients to incorporate their experience into the concept of self in order to become more fully functioning, self-actualized people.

SYSTEMS THERAPY

Behavioural, cognitive-behavioural and supportive therapy are most effective if applied within a systems framework.[21] A systems approach takes into account patients' role(s) in their concentric social circles (particularly the family). Once patients' behaviour has changed during the psychotherapeutic process, their modified behaviours will affect the homeostasis of the family system,[21] homeostasis referring to the reaction towards restoration of the *status quo* in the event of any change. Systematic attempts are made by the family to restore equilibrium, or homeostasis, when it is threatened in any way. The family is a system; all families have an implicit structure that determines how members relate to one another. Boundaries are the 'barriers' or rules that determine the amount of contact allowed between members. Overly rigid boundaries isolate members from one another. When boundaries are too diffuse, members are overly dependent.[21] The dysfunction is the result of an inflexible family structure that prohibits the family from adapting to situational changes, for example chronic pain.

Members of a dysfunctional family may be unwilling or unable to accept lifestyle changes in a member who is experiencing chronic pain.[21] They may expect the patient to continue functioning within the context of their role(s) (e.g. cleaning or cooking), with little or no help from other members. Conversely, the family system may be unable or unwilling to accept changes in a member who improves from chronic pain treatment. This is especially true if the pain member was regarded as the 'identified problem', thereby enabling the family to avoid dealing with other unprocessed conflicts and deeper unresolved issues while the family's energies were focused on the identified patient's care and treatment.[21] If the family is not involved in the treatment process, a patient whose pain improves may return to a dysfunctional family system and inadvertently be forced back into a patient role for no longer serving as a diversion for the family's unresolved problems.

The therapist must then first 'join' the family in a position of leadership in order to develop a therapeutic system.[21] Joining involves 'blending' with the family by adopting its affect, style and language. Second, the therapist must evaluate the family's structure, including its transactional patterns, power hierarchy, subsystems, boundaries and flexibility. The therapist must also evaluate possible unresolved problems that the family may be avoiding by focusing on the member in chronic pain. Based on this evaluation, specific goals are then formulated. Third, the therapist must use a number of techniques to restructure the family system. This may include 'reframing', which involves relabelling behaviours so that they can be viewed in more positive ways.[21]

PSYCHODYNAMIC PSYCHOTHERAPY

Psychodynamic psychotherapy refers to treatments derived from the psychodynamic theories of personality, whereby a therapist supports and helps patients to make sense of their problems.[8] Based on anecdotal evidence, psychodynamic psychotherapy seems helpful only to a limited degree in patients with chronic pain.[45] Outcome studies still need to be carried out. With abnormal pain behaviour, the conventional approach of instituting this psychotherapy is difficult.[27] Treatment may be more effective in combination with more action-orientated behavioural approaches.[46] Long-term psychotherapy is normally not undertaken in a pain clinic.[8]

Conclusion

Although it is a most useful adjunctive treatment modality, psychological intervention should never be considered a substitute for appropriate medical management.[21] A major component of psychological intervention is behavioural or cognitive-behavioural therapy, along with supportive psychotherapy, all applied within a systems framework. The goal of the behavioural and cognitive-behavioural therapies, relaxation training, biofeedback and hypnosis is to modify the patient's thoughts and feelings, and guide patients towards a sense of control over their pain.[21] The fundamental philosophy that motivates the application of cognitive-behavioural therapy is that pain and suffering are not the same. Suffering refers to a conscious state of mind determined by many different influences. Although pain is one of these influences, its presence does not necessary produce suffering. Patients can limit their suffering and enjoy aspects of their personal experience, even though they have pain, by acquiring substantial control over their conscious experience and behaviour.[21] The major goal of psychological intervention is not to eliminate pain, although pain levels may decrease. Instead, it is to help patients to regain a sense of control over managing their symptoms and improve their quality of life.

SECONDARY PREVENTION TACTICS

First, for secondary prevention, in the acute pain stage, adequate pain relief is essential for self-care, and to prevent fear avoidance.[7] A related goal is the reduction of anxiety and the fear of injury/movement to provide alternatives to maladaptive pain perceptions. A third goal is to help the patient to maintain everyday activities to reduce disruption and improve quality of life.[7] Fourth is to teach self-skills (increase self-efficacy) to reinforce coping skills. Finally, related health behaviours (smoking, exercise, obesity, coping style, type A behaviour and abuse) need improvements.[7]

MODES OF DELIVERY

Patients can be treated individually, as a group or as a combination of both according to their needs.

INDIVIDUAL BASIS

In this, the patient attends 12 weekly, 45-minute sessions run by a psychologist (or a psychiatrist) on an outpatient basis.[27] Following treatment, patients generally feel better and are less disabled, even though their pain level may remain the same.[27] No outcome studies have been published on this form of management.[46] A disadvantage is that patients are unable to share their experiences with other patients.

GROUP BASIS

Here, groups of up to 10 patients are seen twice weekly for 5 weeks (or once weekly for 10 weeks).[46] In order to qualify for group therapy, patients must be free of psychoses, be moderately motivated and compliant, and possess basic interactional skills.[8] An advantage of the group approach is that it facilitates the exchange of information and promotes therapeutic modelling.[27] The therapist is, however, less able to deal with specific issues raised by individual patients.[46] Disruptive patients are occasionally encountered.

Health care workers involved in running group sessions usually include a physiotherapist, a psychologist and, on occasion, an occupational therapist. The physiotherapist helps to develop patients' general fitness as well as prescribing specific exercises for improving individual muscle stretch and strength.[46] A Sickness Impact Profile Roland Scale can be used by the physiotherapist as a measure of physical dysfunction in chronic pain patients.[46,47] The psychologist plays a part in educating patients and in discussing their pain management. The psychologist can also teach distraction and relaxation techniques, and apply cognitive restructuring.[46] An occupational therapist can be used to set activity goals (e.g. walking for 30 minutes) and for relaxation training. All exercises and strategies taught should be practised at home. The cooperation of the family may therefore be needed.[46]

OUTPATIENT VERSUS INPATIENT TREATMENT

It is still unclear whether outpatient or inpatient treatment is more effective.[28] Inpatient treatment is obviously more costly but should be used in patients with a high level of medication usage.

EFFICACY OF PSYCHOLOGICAL TECHNIQUES

Various parameters can be used to assess the efficacy of psychological techniques.[46] A positive sign is an improvement in physical performance with less time spent resting. Mood elevation may also be apparent. Pain behaviour may diminish, with less groaning, limping, rubbing, bracing and talking about pain. The intake of all or some of the patient's drugs may decrease. Pain levels may decrease, but this may not be clinically significant.[46] The benefit of psychological approaches to pain management may lie in reducing the fear and depression associated with pain rather than in relieving the pain itself.[48] Other positive signs are the return to work and the decreased use of health facilities (with resulting substantial long-term savings).[49]

PAIN-ASSOCIATED PSYCHOLOGICAL/ PSYCHIATRIC ILLNESS

Factors predisposing to psychiatric illness in chronic pain

Social, economic, cultural, past history and personality features affect the predisposition of sufferers to develop a chronic painful state. People in boring, dissatisfying jobs, and those who are less educated and less intelligent, are prone to developing chronic pain.[14] There is an increased frequency of pain problems in the families of chronic pain sufferers.[17] Between 40 and 60 per cent of pain individuals also reported a parent in pain.[17] Information about pain and its effects is absorbed more accurately by the partner than by the person in pain.[14] Interviewing the partner of any pain patient is therefore essential. Also, oversolicitous spouses can increase the exhibition of pain behaviour markedly in comparison to partners who are less influenced by this behaviour.[14] Considering the serious impact of the pain patient's disability on the whole family and the impact of the psychological disturbance shared by the family members, family assessment and intervention should be available in the pain relief clinic as a standard service.

Anxiety fear

The fear of pain can be conceptualized as a multidimensional response that may contribute significantly to the chronic pain experience.[50] If patients are extremely anxious, either because of their previous experience or because they are constitutionally prone to anxiety, particular attention should be paid to reducing anxiety (relaxation treatment and antidepressants) before embarking on other therapeutic strategies.[14] Anxiety can disrupt the use of self-control strategies in coping with pain. A Pain Anxiety Symptoms Scale has recently been developed to measure the fear of pain and to clarify to pain patients their level of pain-related anxiety.[50] Two psychological processes mediating the influence of anxiety on pain have been proposed: an attributional process, in which the pain-relevance of anxiety is the essential factor, and an attentional process in which the focus of attention is the essential factor. Strong evidence has been found for

support for the role of attentional focus in the influence of anxiety on the pain experience.[51]

The preoperative visit is where the anaesthetist can reduce anxiety and provide pain relief.[52] The Amsterdam Preoperative Anxiety and Information Scale can provide anaesthetists with a valid, reliable and easily applicable instrument for assessing the level of patients' preoperative anxiety and their need for information.[53]

Depression

Depression is the most common emotional disorder in patients with chronic pain.[1] In persistent pain samples, various studies reported the frequency of major depression as ranging from 0 to 50 per cent (median 25 per cent), the frequency of psychotic depression as varying from 2 to 14 per cent (median 6 per cent), and the frequency of dysthymia as ranging from 4 to 51 per cent (median 27 per cent).[17] The relationship between chronic pain and depression is complicated and unclear.[33] Depression aggravates pain, and pain aggravates depression. Most surveys carried out show that patients who have chronic pain and depression exhibit their depression because of the demoralizing and debilitating effects of the pain itself.[14] In chronic pain patients, the presence of depressive symptoms seems to be much more common than the major syndrome of clinical depression.[33] First episodes of depression are more likely to follow closely the onset of chronic pain. Chronic pain leads to a loss of pleasure in previously enjoyable pursuits, affects domestic, social and leisure activities, and often terminates the person's occupation. There is a clear relationship between stress-provoking circumstances and the diagnosis of depression.[14] Clinicians must distinguish functional from organic causes of depression. There is a high frequency of depression (and alcoholism) in the families of chronic pain sufferers.[17] Abuse experiences may also promote the development of depression.[17] Depressive symptoms predict chronic pain with an odds ratio of 2.14 compared with non-depressed subjects.[17] There is growing evidence that depression decreases pain tolerance and results in more pain behaviours.[54] An inverse relationship between age and depression among chronic pain patients has been found, younger patients experiencing more depression.[55] This has recently been challenged by a greater association between pain and depression in the elderly, reflecting age-related changes in functional status along with a reduced availability of social support.[56] The effective treatment of depression significantly improves outcomes of pain management.[17] In a recent study in chronic pain patients, poor work, educational and marital status accounted for a significant amount of variance in depression scores.[57]

There are different types of depression classified in the standard psychiatric schedules. If the patient has a bipolar affective disorder, recurrent depressive disorder or persistent mood disorder (such as dysthymia or cyclothymia), different approaches are tried. Drug treatments are largely indicated in the former, while cognitive and behavioural strategies are more appropriate in the latter. In the International Association for the Study of Pain classification, pain of psychological origin associated with depression is recognized as a separate category, and the response to psychological treatments or antidepressants is more effective than that due to analgesic relief alone.[14] Pain patients often suffer from the vegetative signs of depression, including insomnia, appetite fluctuations, decreased libido and the increased use of drugs (alcohol, opioids and sedatives).[1]

Depression affects not only the patient, but also the patient's immediate family, who have to deal with the patient's pain, anger, limitations and altered role(s). Twenty per cent of the spouses of chronic pain patients are depressed, and 35 per cent report marital maladjustment.[17,58]

Self-rating scales are used as screening instruments. Those patients who score highly on these are interviewed in depth. If cognitive treatment is a considered option, the Beck Depression Inventory is useful as cognitive symptoms in depression are well represented among the items being presented.[59] Patients scoring 16 or more should benefit from referral to a psychologist/psychiatrist.[14] However, the total Beck Depression Inventory score may exaggerate cognitive and affective disturbances in patients with significant physical or medical problems.[60] Using the General Health Questionnaire, a higher cut-off point (above 11 on the 28-item questionnaire) is necessary for referral. To avoid contamination by physical factors in the assessment of depression, the Hospital Anxiety and Depression Scale is used specifically to measure anhedonia, the core symptom of depression.[14] The correct classification of psychiatric and non-psychiatric illness was recently achieved in 82 per cent of patients completing this questionnaire, using a cut-off score of 14 out of 15, for both the depressive and anxiety subscales of this instrument.[14] Other tools used include the Hamilton Rating Scale for Depression, the SCL-90 and the modified Zung Depression Scale.[18] The McGill Pain Questionnaire, the West Haven–Yale Multidimensional Pain Inventory and the Beck Depression Inventory have been found to be representative of the multidimensional nature of the pain experience, with minimal overlap between measures.[61] A strong association has been found between depression and McGill Pain Questionnaire sensory scores, loss of ability for activities and global evening pain ratings.[62] However, no consensus seems to exist concerning the validity and reliability of self-report questionnaires, nor concerning how the problems of pain-related symptoms should be solved.[33] More research is needed to clarify how various symptoms are to be interpreted and attributed.

Anger

The emotion of anger is quite frequently seen in patients with chronic pain.[14] It is a very salient feature of the chronic pain experience.[2] The more pain is felt to interfere with a person's life, the greater the degree of such anger. The precipitating factor in chronic pain is often an injury arising from a mishap or accident in which someone (an employer, a stranger or the patient) may be held answerable. Anger may thus be directed to the self or another. If the damage is seen as the result of something intentional and preventable, the anger will be intensified.[2] Anger has deleterious consequences on the physical and social well-being of the patient. This can arise out of inappropriately regulated overt anger or inhibited anger turned inward.[2] The adverse effects on depression and interpersonal relationships are especially noteworthy.[2] Anger undermines the therapeutic alliance that is critical to treatment success. Anger is closely associated with irritability and may indicate that the patient has a panic disorder or depressive illness.[14] New psychological approaches need to be developed to regulate anger. Further research is warranted to evaluate the effects of anger management on treatment outcome.

Pain-prone disorder

Pain-prone patients form a major subgroup within those suffering from chronic pain syndromes. These patients have often had stressful childhoods, have worked in several jobs and have a personal or family history of illness.[1] Pain proneness may be induced by early neglect, abuse (28 per cent reporting childhood sexual abuse), incest, parental loss, dependent families and the 'modelling' of ill relatives.[14,17] People with dependent, passive-aggressive and masochistic personalities have been shown to be prone to develop chronic pain.[14] Patients unemployed or receiving compensation at the start of treatment and those who have waited many years after the onset of their pain all have a poor prognosis in terms of their pain disability.

New discoveries concerning CNS plasticity call into question conceptualizations such as 'abnormal illness behaviour', 'pain-prone disorder' and 'masked depression', which are based on the assumption that if no (peripheral) injury is present, no sensory pain experience is possible.[33]

Somatoform disorders

There are several varieties, among which the important ones are chronic pain disorders, hypochondriasis, somatization disorders and conversion disorders.[17] In chronic pain disorders, the following occurs:[17]

- There is significant pain in one or more places causing major distress or impairment of functioning.
- Psychological factors seem to have an important role in the onset, severity, exacerbation and maintenance of the pain.
- The pain is not accounted for by dyspareunia, feigning or some other psychiatric disorder.
- There is pain of 6 months' or more duration.
- Significant contributing factors (medical, psychological or both) should be identified.

Psychiatric illness can affect the presentation of pain by hysterical or hypochondriacal mechanisms in the context of a depressive illness or occasionally a psychotic illness.

Hysteria means symptoms (or a reduction of physical functioning) that suggest a physical disorder but cannot be explained entirely on a physical basis. Persistent pain in the absence of normal laboratory and radiological investigations reinforces the patient's opinion that something must be wrong, and further symptom exaggeration and nonorganic signs may develop.[14] Hypochondriasis is a persistent preoccupation on the part of the patient based on a misinterpretation of bodily symptoms, that he or she has a serious disease.[17] The full triad of hypochondriacal neurosis, namely a persistent belief and fear of illness and a preoccupation with bodily symptoms, is rarely found in pain clinic patients. In the dissociative disorder multiple personality disorder, pain will fluctuate (in location and severity) according to the personal experiences with which it is associated.[63]

Conversion disorders present with sensory or motor symptoms suggesting but not supported by medical conditions or drug effects. They apparently arise from psychological conflicts or stressors, are not feigned, cause significant impairment and are not accounted for by other psychiatric or pain disorders.[17]

Somatization disorders are rare in chronic pain clinic work (perhaps accounting for 1–2 per cent of patients).[17] A continuous and long history of many physical complaints is found, beginning before the age of 30 and resulting in a significant medical history and in functional impairment. There must be at least 4 pain symptoms, 2 gastrointestinal complaints, 1 sexual problem and 1 pseudoneurological problem.[17] The complaints are not explained by medical illness or drugs, or are in excess of objective findings. Somatization is thus a tendency to experience and communicate somatic distress and symptoms unaccounted for by pathological findings, to attribute them to physical illness and to seek medical help for them.[14] Some patients express their emotional distress as physical symptoms as they are unable to comprehend and recognize psychological distress. However, the majority who somatise have the capacity to exhibit both psychiatric and physical symptoms.[14] The process of somatization involves experiential, cognitive and behavioural components. Somatizers experience emotional upsets as physical events and show excessive illness behaviour incongruent with the evidence for physical illness.[14] In the *International Classification of Diseases* (10th edition) and the *Diagnostic and Statistical Manual for Mental Disorders* (DSM IV), an attempt has been made to classify somatizers according to symptoms, signs and course of disease.[14] In the International Association for the Study of Pain classification of chronic pain, these patients are classified under 'Pain of psychological origin – hysteria, conversion or hypochondriacal'.[14] These patients constitute a clinical and economic challenge. It must, however, be established that there is no other mental disorder contributing to their disturbance.[1] For therapy, a multimodal combination of tricyclic antidepressants (amitriptyline) and psychotherapy has been used, which effectively increases patients' activity levels, decreases their pain and improves their productivity.[64]

Other psychiatric illness

Malingering is a voluntary fabrication of a physical or psychological symptom for personal gain.[1] These patients are occasionally encountered in a pain clinic, where they use pain to satisfy their drug-seeking behaviours. Rarely, patients with schizophrenia are sent to a pain clinic with pain as their primary complaint.[1]

Psychoactive substance abuse is found in patients presenting with chronic pain (see Chapter 3). These patients often use their pain to manipulate several clinicians into writing out prescriptions for sedatives, hypnotics, anxiolytics or opioids,[1] each clinician usually being unaware of the patient's other drug sources.

A factitious disorder with physical symptoms is defined by the American Psychiatric Association (DSM-IV) as the intentional production or feigning of physical symptoms (including pain). These patients have a psychological need to assume a sick role. In the chronic form of this disorder (Munchausen syndrome), the factitious physical symptoms are associated with multiple hospitalization.

OTHER PSYCHOLOGICAL INTERACTIONS AND PAIN

Social relationships

Anyone living with or offering social support to an individual with chronic pain must be affected by that pain but must also have some influence on the pain sufferer's self-concept and coping ability.[65] Spouse support has been shown to be important in reducing depression in the patient with chronic pain, adding to the quality of life and increasing the benefits from treatment.[65] However, the contribution of social relationships to pain intensity depends on the nature of the chronic disorder and on the type of interpersonal relationships (e.g. support or conflict).[66] Using an illness self-construct repertory grid (to investigate personal responses to chronic pain), it was found that the person closest to the patient placed the illness more centrally in the life of the individual with pain than did the pain patient him- or herself.[65] Learning to live with chronic pain is a family affair, and it is important in managing these patients that the role of the spouse (or person closest to the patient) and the family is not overlooked.[27]

Coping

Coping is the cognitive and behavioural effort an individual uses to manage a stressful situation such as a painful illness or disorder.[67] Active coping strategies occur when patients attempt to control their pain or to function in spite of their pain.[68] Passive coping involves relinquishing pain control to others or allowing other life areas to be adversely affected by the pain. Active coping is associated with activity level but is inversely related to the amount of distress.[68] Passive coping is strongly related to both distress and depression.[68] The way of coping is influenced by personal factors such as cognitive ability and pre-existing cognitive experiences or 'set'.[67] The context of a stressor and whether this is a threat, a change or a challenge has a major influence on the coping strategy used. Mood also influences coping ability. Although chronic pain can lead to dysfunction among some patients, others appears to adjust relatively well to the ongoing experience of pain.[69] In chronic benign pain, varying levels of disability are seen in patients with the same level of objective damage.[23] The role of distress and coping ability in chronic pain should be given an importance equal to that of the physical parameters.[23] A complex relationship exists between pain appraisals, coping strategies and adjustment to chronic pain.[69] The relationship between coping strategies and adjustment is studied using the Vanderbilt Pain Management Inventory, the Coping Strategies Questionnaire and the Ways of Coping Checklist (see Chapter 2). The Coping Strategies Questionnaire has been found to be a more psychometrically sound measure of active and passive coping than the Vanderbilt Pain Management Inventory.[68] A Chronic Pain Coping Inventory, with four scales (guarding, asking for assistance, resting and task persistence), has recently been developed and validated for use in patients coping with pain.[70] Patients' beliefs about internal and external factors controlling their pain have led to the concept of 'locus of control' to describe the dimension of generalized expectations; according to this, reinforcement is primarily dependent on one's own activity (internal control) or on the activity of others (external control).[33] Patient Locus of Control Scales have also been developed.[23] Patients who endorse an internal locus of control, and patients who believe that they have control over their pain, appear to function better than those who do not.[69] Adaptive coping and better psychological adjustment is thus associated with an increased sense of internal control; however, the trend is towards externality of control in domain-specific areas of health.[67] A belief in an external locus of control resulting from chance predicts greater disability.[67] In the elderly, emotion-focused, passive, mature styles of coping seem to be adaptive when the stressor is uncontrollable.[67] Fibromyalgia patients report a more frequent use of negative coping strategies (and lower levels of self-efficacy) relative to non-patients.[71] An overreliance on passive-avoidance coping activities is characteristic of depressed chronic lower back pain patients.[72] It has recently been found, in whiplash injury, that patients' psychological profiles were a consequence rather than a cause of somatic symptoms.[73] In back pain, well-designed, controlled studies provide clear evidence that cognitive-behavioural programmes help patients to cope more successfully with their pain.[74]

Although attention-based cognitive coping strategies are effective in altering pain perception and have potentially useful analgesic qualities, there is contradiction and equivocation over the role of various factors in analgesic production.[75] This is because of the variance in experimental pain procedures.[75] The endorsement of cognitive errors (especially catastrophizing) appears to be related to both psychological and physical dysfunction.[76] Self-efficacy expectancies appear to be related to coping and adjustment as patients generally engage in activities and coping strategies that they believe they are capable of performing.[69] Outcome expectations appear to be associated only weakly with activity level and coping behaviour.[65]

Compensation and litigation

Patients in receipt of compensation benefits or involved in litigation form a significant proportion of those attending pain clinics.[76] The effects of compensation on chronic pain patients are mediated by a complex interaction of biological, psychological, social and economic factors, as well as the legal characteristics of the particular compensation system. More marked anxiety and depression, however, occur among these patients, resulting in greater difficulties in coping with their pain.[76,77] The anxiety and depression can continue even after settlement.[75] Of interest is the fact that these patients experience pain of a severity similar to that of a comparable group of patients not in receipt of pain-related benefits, and that this pain is not necessarily cured following the settlement of claims.[76] There is now good evidence that the settlement of a claim does not usually result in a resolution of the disability or pain.[17] In most cases, the cost of being ill greatly outweighs the vague future of a legal settlement. However, many studies have found that compensation or litigation is not associated with a worse prognosis.[17]

Many compensation systems are a major source of stress for the patient. A pending financial windfall may discourage patients from resuming employment, and this increases the risk of the pain becoming chronic.[77] Compensation systems should thus be modified to direct their emphasis away from financial settlements towards finding suitable employment for injured workers.[77]

Relapse/non-compliance

The incidence of relapse following initial success in the treatment of chronic pain appears to be high, ranging from 30 to 60 per cent.[78] Why is this so? The adoption of new behaviours and skills is much easier than maintaining them. The translocation of treatment gains and skills to a patient's home environment may be partly hindered by the environment itself, especially if continuous reinforcement does not occur.[45] It is thus essential to plan realistically for a patient's re-entry into social and occupational life.

Patients often become discouraged with extended medical treatments that produce limited therapeutic results. Consequently, some become less compliant over time simply because they lose faith in the treatment.[78] These patients need extra encouragement and support. Long-standing personal habits (e.g. diet and exercise) are also notoriously resistant to change. Major contributors to non-compliance include the nature of the disease or injury, the complexity and duration of treatment, the extent of lifestyle changes required by the treatment, and the health care provider–patient relationship.[78] Strategies for assessing compliance include self-reporting, behaviour, and biochemical and clinical outcomes. A long-term therapeutic success may depend on regular adherence to self-care regimens.[5] The necessary self-care behaviours sufficient to maintain therapeutic benefits still need to be identified.[78]

'Shopping around'

Patients suffering chronic pain often 'shop around' the medical profession in an attempt to obtain relief. Failing to obtain relief from orthodox sources, they may seek help from outside the traditional medical profession. In this way osteopaths, homeopaths, chiropractors, aromatherapists, reflexologists and faith and traditional healers may be consulted. Unfortunately, such patients may also become victims of charlatans and quacks. However, it is worthwhile remembering that patients should nevertheless be given the final say and be granted the freedom to follow the treatment of their choice. The patient who is encouraged and supported is less likely to 'shop around'.

Complementary therapeutic approaches not in line with current scientific knowledge are becoming more popular. In parallel with an increasing body of evidence to suggest that these complementary approaches may be of value to patients, the readiness of the medical profession to consider such options seriously is growing.[79] However, the medical profession should insist on prospective clinical trials of effectiveness, reliable data on safety, and evidence for the professional competence of complementary practitioners.[79]

operationalized.[81] Because several treatments operate more or less simultaneously in pain clinic programmes, it is difficult to sort out the effectiveness of specific interventions. To promote further advances, research tools need to be sharpened in several areas.[82] Control groups should be comparable on all baseline measures except for the one under study. Because of selection bias, conclusions on the populations represented should be limited. Correlational data should not be overinterpreted. Psychological tests should be interpreted with caution, and results should convey clinical meaning. The lack of consistent findings across psychological studies continues to be a recurrent lament.[82] The increased use of standardized definitions, common tests and consistent methodology is needed.

CONCLUSION

Outcome research data support the efficacy of behavioural approaches in the management of chronic pain.[22] There is obviously a need to clarify the precise nature and role of psychophysiological variables in the development, maintenance and response to treatment of chronic pain.[23] In order to apply psychological assessment information to decision-making and treatment planning, there is a need to better integrate diverse psychological and behavioural information and to relate this to the physical findings.[5]

There is a need for an adequate multidimensional assessment of pain patients prior to therapy and also of the evaluation of outcome.[58] Grading chronic pain as a function of pain intensity and pain-related disability may be useful when a brief ordinal measure of global severity is required.[80] Recently, a multiaxial assessment of pain model has been described for the biomedical, psychosocial and behavioural assessment of patients with persistent pain.[5] To standardize communication in describing psychological and psychiatric syndromes, the nosology of the American Psychiatric Association (DSM-IV) should be used.[5] Further research needs to be carried out to explore the relationship of cognitive and behavioural factors to relapse and non-compliance.[5] Because of the multidimensional nature of pain, the importance of interdisciplinary cooperation cannot be overemphasized.

Treatment outcome research is complex, and consensus needs to be reached about what criteria should be used to measure treatments for chronic pain and how these constructs should be

REFERENCES

1. **Aronoff, G.M.** 1992: Psychological aspects of non-malignant chronic pain: a new nosology. In Aronoff, G.M. (ed.) *Evaluation and treatment of chronic pain.* Baltimore: Williams & Wilkins, 399–408.
2. **Fernandez, E. and Turk, D.C.** 1995: The scope and significance of anger in the experience of chronic pain. *Pain* **61**, 165–75.
3. **Gamsa, A. and Vikis-Freibergs, V.** 1991: Psychological events are both risk factors in, and consequences of, chronic pain. *Pain* **44**, 271–77.
4. **Gamsa, A.** 1994: The role of psychological factors in chronic pain. I: A half century of study. *Pain* **57**, 5–15.
5. **Rudy, T.E. and Turk, D.C.** 1992: Psychological aspects of pain. *Book Review*, 9–21.
6. **Nicholas, M.K.** 1996: Theory and practice of cognitive-behavioral programs. In Campbell, J.N. (ed.) *Pain 1996 – an updated review.* Seattle: IASP Press, 297–303.
7. **Linton, S.J.** 1996: Early interventions for the secondary prevention of chronic musculoskeletal pain. In Campbell, J.N. (ed.) *Pain 1996 – an updated review.* Seattle: IASP Press, 305–11.
8. **Taylor, M.L.** 1990: Psychological treatment of chronic pain. In Abram, S.E. (ed.) *The pain clinic manual.* Philadelphia: J.B. Lippincott, 225–33.
9. **Hoffert, M.J.** 1992: The neurophysiology of pain. In: Aronoff, G.M. (ed.) *Evaluation and treatment of chronic pain.* Baltimore: Williams & Wilkins, 10–25.
10. **Wall, P.D.** 1992: The placebo effect: an unpopular topic. *Pain* **51**, 1–3.
11. **Wilder-Smith, C.H. and Schuler, L.** 1992: Postoperative analgesia: pain by choice? The influence of patient attitudes and patient education. *Pain* **50**, 257–62.
12. **Shipton, E.A. and Van der Merwe, C.** 1993: The perioperative pain care of patients – an update. *South*

African Journal of Continuing Medical Education **11**(3): 459–66.

13. **Van Dalfsen, P.J. and Syrjala, K.L.** 1990: Psychological strategies in acute pain management. *Critical Care Clinics* **6**(2), 421–31.

14. **Tyrer, S.** 1996: Psychological and psychiatric assessment of patients in pain. In Campbell, J.N. (ed.) *Pain 1996 – an updated review.* Seattle: IASP Press, 495–504.

15. **Keefe, F.J.** 1996: Cognitive-behavioral approaches to assessing pain and pain behavior. In Campbell, J.N. (ed.) *Pain 1996 – an updated review.* Seattle: IASP Press, 517–23.

16. **Dar, R., Ariely, D. and Frenk, H.** 1995: The effect of past-injury on pain threshold and tolerance. *Pain* **60**, 189–193.

17. **Tunks, E.** 1996: Comorbidity of psychiatric disorder and chronic pain. In Campbell, J.N. (ed.) *Pain 1996 – an updated review.* Seattle: IASP Press, 287–96.

18. **De C. Williams, A.C.** 1996: Assessment of pain, psychological impact and disability. In Campbell, J.N. (ed.) *Pain 1996 – an updated review.* Seattle: IASP Press, 269–77.

19. **Harding, V.R., De C. Williams, A.C., Richardson, P.H.** *et al.* 1994: The development of a battery of measures for assessing physical functioning of chronic pain patients. *Pain* **58**, 367–75.

20. **Keefe, F.J. and Lefebvre, J.** 1994: Pain behavior concepts: controversies, current status, and future directions. In Gebhart, G.E., Hammond, D.L. and Jensen, T.S. (eds) *Proceedings of the 7th World Congress on Pain, Progress in pain research and management.* vol. 2. Seattle: IASP Press, 127–47.

21. **Livengood, J.M.** 1996: Psychological techniques for chronic pain management. *Pain Digest* **6**, 77–82.

22. **Ott, B.D.** 1992: Behavioral interventions in the management of chronic pain. In Aronoff, G.M. (ed.) *Evaluation and treatment of chronic pain.* Baltimore: Williams & Wilkins, 440–54.

23. **Main, C.J.** 1991: Pain: psychological and psychiatric factors. *British Medical Bulletin* **47**(3), 732–42.

24. **Flor, H. and Borbaumer, N.** 1994: Basic issues in the psychobiology of pain. In Gebhart, G.E., Hammond, D.L. and Jensen, T.S. (eds) *Proceedings of the 7th World Congress on Pain, progress in pain research and management*, vol. 2. Seattle: IASP Press, 113–24.

25. **Strong, J., Ashton, R. and Chant, D.** 1992: The measurement of attitudes towards and beliefs about pain. *Pain* **48**, 227–36.

26. **Tauschke, E., Merskey, H. and Helmes, E.S.** 1990: Psychological defence mechanisms in patients with pain. *Pain* **40**, 161–70.

27. **Pilowsky, I.** 1992: Abnormal illness behaviour (dysosognosia) and the management of chronic non-malignant pain. In Aronoff, G.M. (ed.) *Evaluation and treatment of chronic pain.* Baltimore: Williams & Wilkins, 409–15.

28. **Swartzman, L.C., Gwadry, F.G., Shapiro, A.P. and Teasell, R.W.** 1994: The factor structure of the Coping Strategies Questionnaire. *Pain* **57**, 311–16.

29. **Weir, R., Browne, G., Roberts, J., Tunks, E. and Gafni, A.** 1994: The meaning of the Illness Questionnaire: further evidence for its reliability and validity. *Pain* **58**, 377–86.

30. **Pilowsky, I. and Katsikitis, M.** 1994: A classification of illness behaviour in pain clinic patients. *Pain* **57**, 91–4.

31. **Deardorff, W.W., Chino, A.F., and Scott, D.W.** 1993: Characteristics of chronic pain patients: factor analysis of the MMPI-2. *Pain* **54**, 153–8.

32. **Jensen, M.P., Turner, J.A., Romano, J.M. and Lawler, B.K.** 1994: Relationship of pain-specific beliefs to chronic pain adjustment. *Pain* **57**, 301–9.

33. **Estlander, A.M.** 1996: Assessment of cognitive variables and depression in patients with chronic pain. In Campbell, J.N. (ed.) *Pain 1996 – an updated review.* Seattle: IASP Press, 505–15.

34. **Anderson, K.O., Dowds, B.N., Pelletz, R.E., Edwards, W.T. and Peeters-Asdourian, C.** 1995: Development and initial validation of a scale to measure self-efficacy beliefs in patients with chronic pain. *Pain* **63**, 77–84.

35. **Bayer, T.L., Baer, P.E. and Early, C.** 1991: Situational and psychophysiological factors in psychologically induced pain. *Pain* **44**, 45–50.

36. **De Benedittis, G., Lorenzetti, A. and Pieri, A.** 1990: The role of stressful life events in the onset of chronic primary headache. *Pain* **40**, 65–75.

37. **McCreary, C.P., Clark, G.T., Meril, R.L., Flack, V. and Oakley, M.E.** 1991: Psychological distress and diagnostic subgroups of temporomandibular disorder patients. *Pain* **44**, 29–34.

38. **Bruehl, S.B., Carlson, C.R. and McCubbin, J.A.** 1993: Two brief interventions for acute pain. *Pain* **54**, 29–36.

39. **Grimaud, J.C., Bouvier, M., Naudy, B., Guien, C. and Salducci, J.** 1991: Manometric and radiologic investigations and biofeedback treatment of chronic idiopathic anal pain. *Diseases of the Colon and Rectum* **34**(8), 690–95.

40. **Duchene, P.** 1989: Effects of biofeedback on childbirth pain. *Journal of Pain and Symptom Management* **4**(3), 117–23.

41. **Cott, A., Parkinson, W., Fabich, M., Bedard, M. and Marlin, R.** 1992: Long-term efficacy of combined relaxation: biofeedback treatments for chronic headache. *Pain* **51**, 49–56.

42. **Middaugh, S.J., Woods, S.E., Kee, W.G., Harden, R.N. and Peters, J.R.** 1991: Biofeedback-assisted relaxation training for the ageing chronic pain patient. *Biofeedback and Self Regulation* **16**(4), 361–77.

43. **Moret, V., Forster, A., Laverriere, M.C.** *et al.* 1991: Mechanism of analgesia induced by hypnosis and acupuncture: is there a difference? *Pain* **45**, 135–40.

44. **Gracely, R.H.** 1995: Hypnosis and hierarchical pain control systems. *Pain* **60**, 1–2.

45. **Merskey, H.** 1986: Traditional individual psychotherapy and psychopharmacology. In Holzman, A.D. and Turk, D.C. (eds) *Pain management: a handbook of psychological treatment approaches.* New York: Pergamon.

46. **Pither, C.E. and Nicholas, M.K.** 1991: Psychological approaches in chronic pain management. *British Medical Bulletin* **47**(3), 743–61.

47. **Jensen, M.P., Strom, S.E., Turner, J.A. and Romano, J.M.** 1992: Validity of the Sickness Impact Profile Roland scale as a measure of dysfunction in chronic pain patients. *Pain* **50**, 157–62.

48. **Malone, M.D., Strube, M.J. and Scogin, F.R.** 1988: Meta-analysis of non-medical treatments for chronic pain. *Pain* **34**(3), 231–44.

49. **Caudill, M., Schnable, R., Zuttermeister, P., Benson, H. and Friedman, R.** 1991: Decreased clinic use by chronic pain patients: response to behavioral medicine intervention. *Clinical Journal of Pain* **7**(4), 305–10.

50. **McCracken, L.M., Zayfert, C. and Gross, R.T.** 1992: The Pain Anxiety Symptoms Scale: development and validation of a scale to measure fear of pain. *Pain* **50**, 67–73.

51. **Arntz, A., Dreessen, L. and De Jong, P.** 1994: The influence of anxiety on pain: attentional and attributional mediators. *Pain* **56**, 307–14.

52. **Roizen, M.F.** 1996: How much do they really want to know? Preoperative patient interviews and the anesthesiologist. *Anesthesia and Analgesia* **82**, 443–4.

53. **Moerman, N., Van Dam, F.S.A.M., Muller, M.J. and Oosting, H.** 1996: The Amsterdam Preoperative Anxiety and Information Scale. *Anesthesia and Analgesia* **82**, 445–51.

54. **Sullivan, M.J.L., Reesor, K., Mikail, S. and Fisher, R.** 1992: The treatment of depression in chronic low back pain: review and recommendations. *Pain* **50**, 5–13.

55. **Haythornthwaite, J.A., Sieber, W.J. and Kerns, R.D.** 1991: Depression and the chronic pain experience. *Pain* **46**, 177–84.

56. **Turk, D.C., Okifuji, A. and Scharff, L.** 1995: Chronic pain and depression: role of perceived impact and perceived control in different age cohorts. *Pain* **61**, 93–101.

57. **Averill, P.M., Novy, D.M., Nelson, D.V. and Berry, L.A.** 1996: Correlates of depression in chronic pain patients: a comprehensive examination. *Pain* **65**, 93–100.

58. **Schwartz, L., Slater, M.A., Birchler, G.R. and Atkinson, J.H.** 1991: Depression in spouses of chronic pain patients: the role of patient pain and anger and marital satisfaction. *Pain* **44**, 61–7.

59. **Novy, D.M., Nelson, D.V., Berry, L.A. and Averill, P.M.** 1995: What does the Beck Depression Inventory measure in chronic pain?: a reappraisal. *Pain* **61**, 261–70.

60. **De C. Williams, A.C. and Richardson, P.H.** 1993: What does the BDI measure in chronic pain? *Pain* **55**, 259–66.

61. **De Gagne, T.A., Mikail, S.F. and D'Eon, J.L.** 1995: Confirmatory factor analysis of a 4-factor model of chronic pain evaluation. *Pain* **60**, 195–202.

62. **Doan, B.D. and Wadden, N.P.** 1989: Relationships between depressive symptoms and descriptions of chronic pain. *Pain* **36**, 75–84.

63. **Merskey, H.** 1993: Pain and dissociation. *Pain* **55**, 281–2.

64. **Pilowsky, I. and Barrow, C.G.** 1990: A controlled study of psychotherapy and amitriptyline used individually and in combination in the treatment of chronic intractable, psychogenic pain. *Pain* **40**, 3–19.

65. **James, F.R. and Large, R.G.** 1992: Chronic pain, relationships and illness self-construct. *Pain* **50**, 263–71.

66. **Faucett, J.A. and Levine, J.D.** 1991: The contributions of interpersonal conflict to chronic pain in the presence or absence of organic pathology. *Pain* **34**, 35–43.

67. **Melding, P.S.** 1995: How do older people respond to chronic pain? A review of coping with pain and illness in elders. *Pain Reviews* **2**, 65–75.

68. **Snow-Turek, A.L., Norris, M.P. and Tan, G.** 1996: Active and passive coping strategies in chronic pain patients. *Pain* **64**, 455–62.

69. **Jensen, M.P., Turner, J.A., Romano, J.M. and Karoly, P.** 1991: Coping with chronic pain: a critical review of the literature. *Pain* **47**, 249–53.

70. **Jensen, M.P., Turner, J.A., Romano, J.M. and Strom, S.E.** 1995: The Chronic Pain Coping Inventory: development and preliminary validation. *Pain* **60**, 203–16.

71. **Bradley, L.A., Alarcon, G.S., Alexander, R.W., Triana, M., Aaron, L.A. and Stewart, K.E.** 1994: Pain thresholds, symptom severity, coping strategies, and pain beliefs as predictors of health care seeking in fibromyalgia patients. In Gebhart, G.E., Hammond, D.L. and Jensen, T.S. (eds) *Proceedings of the 7th World Congress on Pain, progress in pain research and management*, vol. 2. Seattle: IASP Press, 167–76.

72. **Weickgenant, A.L. Slater, M.A., Patterson, T.L., Atkinson, J.H., Grant, I. and Garfin, S.R.** 1993: Coping activities in chronic low back pain: relationship with depression. *Pain* **53**, 95–103.

73. **Radanov, B.P., Begre, S., Sturzenegger, M. and Augustiny, K.F.** 1996: Course of psychological variables in whiplash injury – a 2-year follow-up with age, gender and education pair-matched patients. *Pain* **64**, 429–34.

74. **Linton, S.J.** 1994: The role of psychological factors in back pain and its remediation. *Pain Reviews* **1**, 231–43.

75. **Eccleston, C.** 1995: The attentional control of pain: methodological and theoretical concerns. *Pain* **63**, 3–10.

76. **Mendelson, G.** 1992: Compensation and chronic pain. *Pain* **48**, 121–3.

77. **Guest, G.H. and Drummond, P.D.** 1992: Effect of compensation on emotional state and disability in chronic back pain. *Pain* **48**, 125–30.

78. **Turk, D.C. and Rudy, T.E.** 1991: Neglected topics in the treatment of chronic pain patients – relapse, noncompliance, and adherence enhancement. *Pain* **44**, 5–28.

79. **Ernst, E.** 1995: Bitter pills of nature: safety issues in complementary medicine. *Pain* **60**, 237–8.

80. **Von Korff, M., Ormel, J., Keefe, F.J. and Dworkin, S.F.** 1992: Grading the severity of chronic pain. *Pain* **50**, 133–49.

81. **Turk, D.C., Rudy, T.E. and Sorkin, B.A.** 1993: Neglected topics in chronic pain treatment outcome studies: determination of success. *Pain* **53**, 3–16.

82. **Gamsa, A.** 1994: The role of psychological factors in chronic pain. II: A critical appraisal. *Pain* **57**, 17–29.

15 REHABILITATION

For all pain patients, a return to normal function, reflecting effective pain management, is the most important therapeutic objective during first and subsequent encounters.[1] The restoration of normal mobility and metabolism after injury is associated with a decrease in pain and inflammation.[1] Local anaesthetic axonal blockade, when used in combination with behavioural modification and the restoration of full range of motion, can have a positive impact on the recovery and rehabilitation of patients suffering acute and chronic pain.[1] Local anaesthetic blockade can allow mobility without pain. All patients with chronic pain should be referred for comprehensive physical therapeutic evaluation to identify any dysfunction.[2] Many pain patients can learn to function normally despite low to moderate levels of daily pain. Yet, evidence from back pain suggests that, on rigorous outcome measures, physiotherapy and other forms of manipulation have but limited success.[3,4] Such analyses, however, did not include any measure of quality of life.[3] Also, when used in short courses, these techniques may allow for earlier involvement in exercise and other restorative programmes.[4]

The primary therapeutic objectives are the reduction of pain and associated disability, the promotion of optimal function in everyday living and enabling meaningful family and social relationships.[5] The promotion of health and well-being through the prevention of pain, and disability or handicap resulting from pain, are fundamental concerns. It is essential that an holistic and collaborative view be taken of the needs of patients in pain. The goal of all rehabilitative interventions is, however, an expedient return to work, or to a productive life, by relieving pain, by minimizing impairment, by improving function and by restoring the patients' confidence in their ability to move.[1,6] The rehabilitative team may consist of a physiatrist, a physiotherapist, an occupational therapist and a social worker.[7] These therapists play a major role in decreasing the patient's fear and building confidence by gradually increasing activities.[8] The physiatrist is a physician specializing in physical medicine and rehabilitation. Both the physiatrist and the physiotherapist (also known as physical therapist) are trained to administer a wide range of physical and behavioural modalities to reduce pain and prevent dysfunction.[9] Their roles include:[9]

■ Assessment of the primary and secondary chemical (infection/inflammation), biochemical (stress/strain) and behavioural factors that contribute to pain, the pain–activity cycle and overall function.
■ The development of a physical therapy programme directed at modifying the effect of primary and secondary contributors to pain, the promotion of tissue healing and the reduction of factors that may lead to the recurrence of pain and dysfunction. Intervention may include education, exercise, manual therapy, movement facilitation techniques and the application of electro/physical agents based on thermal, mechanical, electrical or phototherapeutic modalities. Education is focused on understanding pain and on improved posture, body mechanics and gait. Exercise is directed towards

strengthening specific muscle groups as well as counteracting the effects of generalized deconditioning. Movement is used as a mechanism to control and decrease pain, and to increase mobility.

■ Liaison and referral within an interdisciplinary team approach. A flare-up plan is also provided.[8] Proper body mechanics in daily activities are encouraged.

Occupational therapists mobilize patients in an effort to occupy their minds and bodies in purposeful activities.[10] They focus on increasing patients' ability to perform specific tasks necessary at home or at work.[8] Occupational therapists are primarily concerned with the psychosocial and environmental factors that contribute to pain and the impact of pain on an individual's everyday life.[9] Their roles include:[9]

■ Assessment of the impact of pain on occupational performance in the areas of self-care, paid and unpaid work, interests and leisure pursuits, customary habits and routines, and family relationships. Assessment will include evaluation of the psychosocial and environmental factors aggravating pain in the home and workplace.

■ The development of an occupational therapy programme to increase self-esteem, restore self-efficacy and promote optimal occupational function despite pain. Intervention strategies may include assistive devices and adaptive equipment, purposeful and productive occupations/activities and vocational rehabilitation or work hardening in order to improve endurance and work skills, and re-establish the roles, habits and routines of everyday life. Education about pain and supportive individual, family or group counselling are used as needed.

■ Liaison and referral within an interdisciplinary team approach. Exercises taught are thus related to the activities of daily living.[11] Mental activities practised include music therapy, and visualization and relaxation techniques. Appropriate problem-solving and work skills are taught by the occupational therapist, thus facilitating a safe and successful return to work.[12]

The social worker will assess the patient's home environment and support system, and assist in work placement and functioning.[7] The social worker can also address issues such as the patient's cognitive and emotional functioning, the interpersonal dynamics of communication, marital dysfunction, family disruption and the facilitation, education and advocacy necessary to empower the pain patient. Future research needs to be under-

taken to establish how social work services can benefit the rehabilitation of the chronic pain patient.

While selection criteria for successful rehabilitation have not been established, physical rehabilitation programmes have certainly been found to play an important part in the rehabilitation of chronic back pain patients.[13] Rehabilitation programmes can be run on an inpatient or outpatient basis.[14] Outpatient rehabilitation programmes help to control costs. In injured hospital employees, it has been found that aggressive early intervention by a physiatrist decreases working time lost as a result of injury.[15]

The question of how ethnicity is related to pain experience, and the patients' reaction to their disability *per se*, will influence the rehabilitation process. Cultural dysruption of physiotherapy, occupational therapy and counselling, and the use of assistive devices, is important to the planning of rehabilitative strategies.

The specific goals in the treatment of patients with chronic persistent pain are as follows:[8]

1. to return to their usual role in daily life;
2. to eliminate or decrease pain-induced behaviours;
3. to teach skills to cope with pain;
4. to increase physical activity, flexibility and endurance;
5. to increase independence;
6. to eliminate or decrease the use of dependence-producing (and non-essential) medications;
7. to improve sleep patterns and control depression;
8. to improve socialization and the enjoyment of recreational activities;
9. to support the patient with a good follow-up and support programme.

Functional rehabilitation may involve postural correction, activities of daily living rehabilitation, sport-specific rehabilitation, work-specific rehabilitation, work hardening, ergonomic correction, balance and coordination rehabilitation, proprioceptive rehabilitation, and endurance and fitness rehabilitation.

MULTIMODAL APPROACH TO POSTOPERATIVE REHABILITATION

The key pathogenic factor in postoperative morbidity is the surgical stress response, with increased demands on organ function.[16] The development of pain-alleviating regimens that allow early ambulation, techniques to reduce nausea, vomiting and ileus, the realization that early enteral nutrition is important for recovery and the reduction of infective complications, and the use of well-established antithrombotic and antimicrobial regimens represent a global approach to perioperative care.[16] Adequate pain scores at rest are not good enough to improve outcome; instead, patients must be comfortable and alert enough to get up and walk.[17] Analgesic regimens need to provide analgesia adequate for movement while minimizing the side-effects that prevent early mobilization, including confusion and somnolence. Before surgery, detailed information about the accelerated stay programme must be provided. Stress response must be reduced by available techniques (high-dose opioid anaesthesia, pain alleviation, neural blockade, pharmacological reduction of the inflammatory response and heat loss prevention).[16] Sufficient pain relief should be given by currently available multimodal regimens (e.g. epidural opioid–local anaesthetic combinations plus systemic NSAIDs).[17] Pain relief must be used for early aggressive ambulation and enforced enteral nutrition to avoid conventional postoperative impairment.[16] In some high-risk patients, the use of growth factors or other anabolic supportive agents may be indicated.[16] Slow-wave sleep is significantly depressed on the first 2 nights after surgery.[17] Episodic night-time hypoxaemia is common after surgery and may contribute to postoperative confusion and major cardio-respiratory events.[17] There is room for great improvement in analgesia techniques that minimize the effects on ventilatory effort, particularly during sleep. Postoperative fatigue may be prevented by improved analgesic regimens that more than adequately suppress the stress response and by a more aggressive rehabilitative approach to postoperative care.[15]

MANUAL THERAPY

Movement and exercise are essential for the development, maintenance and continuing strength of the musculoskeletal system throughout life and form a vital part of treatment directed toward improving the function of or reducing the pain from the musculoskeletal system after inactivity, trauma or disease.[18] The techniques of manual therapy all use movement and the alteration of stress and loading to the body.[18] Treatment strategies in manual therapy include soft tissue massage (including friction massage), mobilization, manipulation, therapeutic exercises and muscle training, muscle stretching and traction techniques.[19] When exercising, exercises carried out can be passive, active or active–assistive. Passive exercises are carried out by the therapist for the patient.[7] The patient actively exercises when moving a body part against gravity. If this is assisted by the therapist, it is known as an active–assistive exercise.[7]

The four major approaches in manual therapy have been espoused by Maitland, Cyriax, Kaltenborn and Mennell.[19] Individual researchers and practitioners, however, define mobilization, manipulation and stretching in different ways.[20] A common denominator is the degree of force in the hands of the therapist when applying passive exercises to the musculoskeletal structures with the intent of restoring body structure and/or function.[20] Only very few controlled studies have been conducted to clarify the efficacy of these techniques.[20] The manual therapies (massage and manipulation) remain the most universally applied techniques for relieving pain.[21] It is possible to group these techniques according to the position within the range of motion of the joint where the treatment is being applied, the depth, direction and nature of the tissue being massaged and mobilized, and whether stretching or thrusting motions are applied to a joint.[21]

Massage

Massage is the systematic manipulation (effluerage) of soft tissues (usually muscles, tendons or ligaments) without changing the joint position, for therapeutic purposes (Figure 15.1).[22,23] Classic massage consists of stroking and gliding, kneading and percussion. Stroking involves the light movement of the hands over the skin in a slow, rhythmic fashion.[23] Kneading massage involves the deep handling of tissues in preparation for the stretching of muscles. Tapotement is the use of percussion, clapping, shaking and vibration. Friction massage is applied parallel or perpendicularly to muscle, tendon or ligament fibres.[22]

Massage includes connective tissue massage, myofascial release and trigger point therapy. It is frequently used to relieve pain, reduce oedema and minimize adhesion formation after soft tissue injury.[22] It is also used in the treatment of muscle spasm, myofascial pain, back pain and arthritis.[7,22,23]

Massage increases superficial blood flow in the

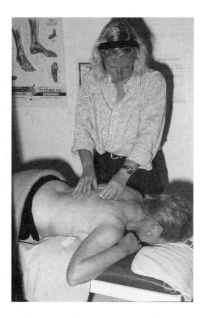

Figure 15.1 Massage of the upper back of a patient to relieve muscle spasm.

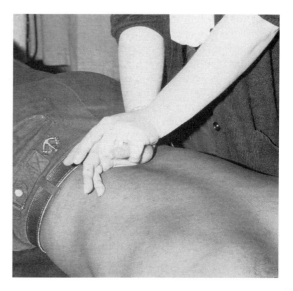

Figure 15.2 Mobilization of the lower spine to relieve joint pain.

treated area and improves venous and lymph return.[7,22] Friction techniques prevent or break up adhesions as well as softening scar tissue.[22] The stimulation of peripheral receptors by massage enhances muscle relaxation and well-being, and causes sedation.[22] It is contraindicated in thrombophlebitis, over malignancies, open wounds and over inflamed and infected tissues.[22] Despite patient satisfaction and acceptance of the technique, there are no controlled studies to show its effectiveness.[23]

Mobilization

Here, the therapist uses hands and fingers to handle tissues.[23] The mobilization increases the range of motion beyond the resistance that limits passive range of motion or exercises (Figure 15.2). There is no forceful or jerking motion. It is used to correct joint dysfunction by taking a joint passively through its range, aided by stretching and strengthening exercises (e.g. for headaches).[2]

Manipulation

This controversial technique has generally been defined as an accurately localized, single, quick, decisive but forceful passive movement of small amplitude, following careful positioning of the patient.[19] This is known as high-velocity, low-amplitude manipulation (or thrusting). It is, however, difficult to confirm the efficacy of its various forms as its effect seems to be largely a result of the skills of the therapist.[20] The goal of manipulation is to restore normal motion, eliminate pain caused by altered biomechanics (e.g. malposition of the intervertebral discs and facet joints) and increase the range of spinal motion.[22] It should be preceded by a heat modality to relax soft tissues around the area, followed by passive exercises to the joint.[7] Generally speaking, pain of recent onset is more responsive to manipulation.[6]

In non-thrust (isometric) manipulation, the therapist first removes slack motion.[22] The patient then exerts moderate forces against the therapist in a direction opposite to the limitation for 5–10 seconds, which is followed by relaxation.[22]

The most commonly accepted theory on manipulation is based on the concept of restricted barriers in joint range of motion.[21] It is assumed to improve range of motion, with subsequent positive effects on the intervertebral disc, joints, muscles and ligaments. Manipulation and massage are also felt to increase pain thresholds and circulation, relax muscles, reduce oedema and in this way provide pain relief.[21] There is growing objective evidence that patients have high satisfaction with and confidence in manipulation.[21]

Manipulation has been used in conditions such as chronic back pain, acute low back pain (with a bulging intervertebral disc), piriformis syndrome and posterior facet syndrome.[6] Contraindications include infection, malignancy, inflammation, fracture, osteoporosis and joint instability.[25] It should be avoided in systemic anticoagulation, vertebrobasilar arterial disease or any condition that may lead to spinal cord compression.[6,22] Clinical research can now substantiate a role for manipulation in the treatment of acute, uncomplicated back pain.[21,23] Lesser evidence is available to justify its use in the management of chronic back pain, sciatica, neck pain and headaches.[21] Patients with chronic back and neck pain treated with manipulation or physiotherapy (exercise, massage and physical therapy) were recently followed up after 1 year.[24] It was found that, in the particular manipulative therapy used, patients were only slightly better off than the physiotherapy patients.[24]

Therapeutic exercises

Immobilization can reduce the strength and function of muscles, ligaments and tendons. Prescribed exercises that increase the forces being transmitted to muscles, ligaments, tendons and bones will maintain and gradually increase the strength and functional capacity of these structures.[23] Exercise is necessary for the preservation of the optimal function and structure of muscle, bone, joints and the cardiovascular system at all stages of life, including old age (Figure 15.3).[18] The goals of therapeutic exercise include increased strength, endurance, range of motion, coordination and balance to reduce pain, spasm, oedema and postural deviations.[23] Therapeutic exercises are thus used in the rehabilitation of acute and chronic pain patients by maintaining muscle strength, range of motion and general conditioning with various pain problems. During acute pain, immobilization may be indi-

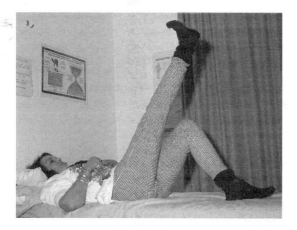

Figure 15.3 Therapeutic exercises.

cated, except for the passive range of movements of all extremities and the trunk.[7] Therapeutic exercises help to enhance joint range of motion, promote flexibility, increase muscle strength to achieve good body alignment, and correct muscle imbalance.[6] Pain, if caused by the malfunction of any of these entities, can thus be relieved. After patient evaluation, the exercise plan and its goals need to be individualized.

There are three types of exercises isotonic, isometric and isokinetic. Isotonic exercises are performed against a steady load with joint movement and are used to build up muscle power after an injury.[7] One form of isotonic exercise – progressive resistance exercise – is widely performed.[7]

Isometric exercises are performed against resistance without joint movement, maintaining the same muscle length throughout the exercises.[7] They are used to increase muscle volume and strength in acute pain, especially involving joints or immobilized fractures.[7] For example, an isometric progressive resistance quadriceps exercise programme with iliotibial band and hamstring stretching exercises has been successfully used in treating the patellofemoral pain syndrome.[25]

Isokinetic exercises are performed against a variable resistance with joint movement occurring and muscles exerting a maximal force throughout the range of movement.[7] It allows a pain-free and safe range of movement exercises after injury. The advent of isokinetic testing equipment allows the measurement of strength in a particular joint throughout the range of movement.[26] This allows for improvements in physical functioning to be documented.[26] Relaxation and general aerobic conditioning exercises increase cardiovascular endurance.

Engineering skills are increasingly being used in rehabilitative medicine. The principles of mechanics include such concepts as statics (where bodies are in static or dynamic equilibrium with no great acceleration) and dynamics (where bodies are in motion but not in equilibrium).[27] Dynamics are further divided into kinematics (the study of the characteristics of motion) and kinetics (the study of the relationship existing between forces acting on the mass of the body). Biomechanical investigations play a role in the analysis of walking patterns, the development of orthotics and prosthetics, the analysis of the role that muscles play in functional activities, tendon transfers and sport injuries.[27]

Many of the therapeutic exercise programmes are still based on empirical evidence.[27] In back pain, it is still not clear whether therapeutic exercises are better than other conservative measures and whether a specific type of exercise is better.[28] For years, lumbar spine flexion exercises were used for lumbar disc disease, although a substantial number of patients found that these increased their sciatica.[29] Lumbar extension exercises (e.g. the McKenzie approach) push the nucleus pulposus anteriorly and may decrease the neuropathic pain component.[29] However, there is evidence that patients with a herniated nucleus pulposus with low back pain and leg pain can benefit from an aggressive physical exercise programme.[23] After acute neck sprains, a programme of early exercises has been found to decrease the number of symptomatic patients at 2 years and to be superior to manipulative physiotherapy.[30]

Group exercise programmes (e.g. back schools) benefit chronic pain patients with widespread muscle weakness and stiffness secondary to prolonged inactivity.[2] Increased aerobic fitness is necessary when patients need to perform movements or tasks repetitively.[26] For this, ergometer bicycling, treadmill running and group training with aerobics, swimming, paddling, hiking and riding can be used.[31] Progress in muscle power (of the arms and legs) can be measured using isokinetic techniques, and aerobic capacity can be estimated (e.g. with an Aastrand's bicycle test).[31] Aerobic exercises that increase cardiopulmonary capacity, fitness and endurance include rhythmic, repetitive, dynamic exercises such as running, cycling and swimming.[23] Further studies on how therapeutic exercise affects the cell, tissue, organs and systems will enhance the development of movement therapy and its effects on the reduction of pain.[27]

STRETCHING

The most common muscle-stretching techniques used are as follows:[32]

- ballistic stretch, in which momentum is used to place a muscle on stretch (although the use of this technique is controversial);
- static stretch, which is a slow-speed, passive movement to place a muscle on stretch;
- contract relax, in which passive movement takes place to the onset of muscle stretch and then a maximal voluntary contraction is performed against resistance, before being passively moved further into the range;
- reciprocal relaxation, where the agonist produces the stretching force on the opposite muscle (antagonist) (Figure 15.4).

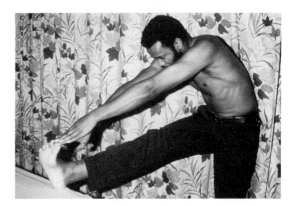

Figure 15.4 Stretching the hamstrings.

The contract relax and reciprocal relaxation techniques are collectively referred to as proprioceptive neuromuscular facilitation relaxation techniques.[32] These techniques increase EMG activity yet paradoxically result in greater gains in range than those obtained from passive stretching techniques.[32] The most effective protocol for normal muscle is a reciprocal relaxation stretch (for 15 seconds, repeated 2–4 times) with or without a preceding contract relax phase.[32]

Stretching exercises are important for muscles that cross joints (hamstrings, gastrocnemius, hip flexors and the pectoral and paraspinal muscles).[23] Stretching exercises should be performed slowly and steadily without bouncing and jerking movements. In the rehabilitation of low back pain patients, stretching manoeuvres can increase the static strength of back extensors and increase functional ability without necessarily an immediate corresponding decrease in pain.[20] Aerobic exercises should be preceded and followed by stretching exercises. There is evidence that stretching exercises and aerobic conditioning exercises can help some patients with chronic pain of musculoskeletal origin.[23]

For myofascial pain with trigger point isolation, spray and stretch techniques are used to inactivate the trigger points.[6] This technique involves sustained progressive stretching of tight muscles with active trigger points while a vapocoolant (fluoromethane or ethyl chloride) is applied to the overlying skin.

Traction

Traction is the act of pulling or is a pulling force (by manual, mechanical, motorized or gravity techniques)[22] (Figure 15.5). It results in the distraction of

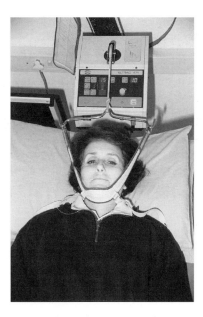

Figure 15.5 The use of traction. A patient undergoing cervical traction for nerve entrapment.

the tissues and is an adjunct in the treatment of soft tissue problems. Traction can be intermittent variable, intermittent static or just static. Traction in a swimming pool (pool traction) can also be used.[31] Traction is generally limited to the cervical and lumbar spine, where it distracts vertebral bodies, enlarges neural foramina, stretches muscles and ligaments, and separates facet joints.[7] It is usually applied to relieve pain and overcome muscle spasm in painful disorders of the neck and back (e.g. acute disc herniation).[22] Overhead cervical traction is one of the most effective methods for the treatment of cervical radiculopathy.[23] Important medical contraindications include cervical ligamentous instability, underlying malignancy, severe osteopaenia and vertebrobasilar arterial disease.[22]

THERMOTHERAPY

Temperature modalities should rarely be used alone but instead in conjunction with appropriate exercises, such as stretching for range of motion and for strengthening after pain reduction.[23] Heat and cold have special physiological effects. They can raise the pain threshold significantly.[23] Both heat and cold are useful in reducing the pain and spasm of neurological and musculoskeletal pathologies and in nerve root irritations.[23] Heat is used to reduce pain, relax muscles and enhance sedation.[2] Superficial skin heating produces muscle relaxation from decreased gamma fibre activity and results in decreased spindle excitability, thus decreasing pain and spasm.[23] The physiological effects of heat include decreasing the vasomotor tone, increasing tissue metabolism, increasing blood flow (which eliminates muscle waste products), increasing capillary permeability, increasing the extensibility of connective tissue, increasing enzymatic activity and increasing the threshold of sensory nerve endings.[7,23] Heat decreases joint stiffness and helps to resolve inflammatory infiltrates (once the initial process has subsided).[6] Superficial tissue heating causes marked skeletal muscle relaxation.[6] When vigorous responses are desired, local heat is preferred.[33] Factors determining the intensity of the physiological reaction locally are temperature elevation level (40–50°C) and duration of temperature elevation (5–30 minutes).[33] The safe dosage is dependent on the patient's cardiorespiratory reserves (for hypermetabolism and heat dissipation). Heat may accelerate the destructive joint process in rheumatoid arthritis and promote neurological deterioration in patients with multiple sclerosis.[7] It is also contraindicated in acute trauma as it may increase the bleeding tendency and oedema.[23] It is relatively contraindicated in patients with sensory impairment and where circulation is decreased over active malignancies, gonads or a developing foetus.[7,23] With heat, the approximate therapeutic tissue temperature ranges from 40 to 45.5°C.[6] The duration of therapy ranges from 3 to 30 minutes.[5]

Heat therapy

CONDUCTION HEAT

The superficial heating agents such as hot packs (e.g. hydrocollator packs with silica gel), electrical heating pads, hot water bottles, hot compresses, chemical packs, paraffin wax and electric heating pads can increase skin temperature above 44°C, the highest temperature being in the most superficial tissues[6,33] (Figure 15.6). Care must therefore be taken to avoid burns. These modalities are effective in reducing the pain of muscle spasm, tendonitis and bursitis.[7] For arthritis of the small joints of the hands and feet, the affected extremity can be repeatedly dipped into wax mixed with mineral oil (at 47.5–52.0°C).[6]

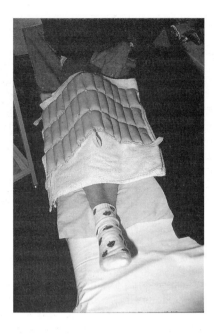

Figure 15.6 Hot packs for the relief of knee pain.

CONVECTION HEAT

For patients with multiple joint pains, convection heat can be provided by water at temperatures of 36.6–43.0°C.[7] Hydrothermal environments (32–38°C) are provided by a whirlpool bath, Hubbard tank or hydrotherapy pool (see Figure 15.7).[6] Agitation of the water creates a massage-like effect, and the elimination of gravity stress pain in the joints enhances

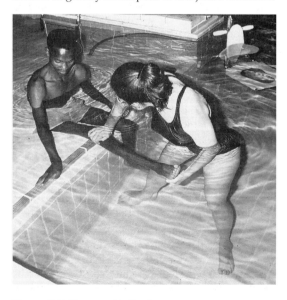

Figure 15.7 The use of hydrotherapy.

mobility. Caution is, however, advised in the first trimester of pregnancy.[7]

With fluidotherapy, warm dry air is blown through a container of glass beads to produce a warm semifluid mixture in which the treated part is immersed.[7] Sauna heat has rarely been found to lead to heat allodynia and hyperalgesia in patients with peripheral neuropathic pain or pain of central or rheumatoid origin.[34] Superficial heat (e.g. radiant heat lamps) produces heating of only the superficial tissues up to 0.5 cm from the surface of the skin, while deep heating modalities heat to a depth of 3–5 cm.[23]

CONVERSION HEAT

When infrared radiation, shortwaves, microwaves or ultrasound interact with tissues, some energy is converted into heat, which is used for its therapeutic effects.[7]

Infrared radiation

Infrared radiation (7000–12 000 Angstroms wavelength) is generated by luminous and non-luminous lamps (of various wattage) and penetrates the skin surface superficially (less than 10 mm) before being converted to heat.[5] Treatment lasts for 20–30 minutes, and abrasions, scars and the eyes may need protection by wet compress pads.[7]

Shortwave diathermy

In this technique, the patient is placed in an electromagnetic field created by a high-frequency alternating current.[7] The conversion of electromagnetic energy to thermal energy results from tissue resistance to the current. The frequency most commonly used is 27.12 MHz.[35] Shortwave energy can be delivered in either a continuous or pulsed mode. Pulsed shortwave diathermy is delivered in the form of a train of pulses with pulse lengths of 25–400 microseconds.[35] The number of pulses lies between 15 and 800 per second.[35]

The level of heat developed depends on tissue properties. The greatest heating occurs in the subcutaneous tissues and superficial musculature. This method helps to relieve pain associated with muscle spasm (e.g. low back pain).[6] It is also used to treat joint conditions (osteoarthritis).[35] Pulsed shortwave diathermy is thought to facilitate tissue healing.[35] The pelvic organs are selectively heated using internal vaginal or rectal electrodes.[33]

Contraindications to the use of shortwave diathermy include pregnancy (as it can induce abortions), metallic implants and internal stimulators and pacemakers. When used over the lower back, it may increase menstrual blood flow.[35] Contact lenses cause hot spots and should be removed.[7] Burns and scalds can arise from overdosage.[35] Few clinical trials have examined the efficacy of this form of treatment.[35]

Microwave diathermy

Microwave is a form of electromagnetic radiation with certain frequencies (2456 and 915 MHz) approved for medical use. However, these frequencies may not be optimal.[7] Microwaves are selectively absorbed in tissues of high water content, allowing selective tissue heating (e.g. of the muscles).[6] Similar contraindications apply as for shortwave diathermy.

Ultrasound

Ultrasound consists of high-frequency sound waves (i.e. 0.8–1.0 MHz) that lie above those heard by the human ear.[6,7] They are converted to provide deep, localized heat. Ultrasound selectively heats muscles, tendons, tendon–bone junctions and deep-seated fibrous scars within soft tissues.[23,33] Ultrasound is a most effective heating agent, with little temperature elevation in the superficial tissues.[6] A coupling agent (gel or mineral oil) is applied to the skin to ensure the efficient transmission of energy.[7] The applicator overlaps the treatment area for 5–10 minutes. For a thermal effect, a machine with continuous output should be used and a slow circulatory movement applied. There are also machines that have a pulsed, intermittent output control.[7] If the patient complains of pain, the pulsed mode can be used or the intensity turned down.

Experimental studies have found that ultrasound accelerates the restoration of tissue regeneration, increases pain thresholds, stimulates bone growth and increases tendon extensibility.[36] Ultrasound is used for myofascial pain, pain from muscle spasms, pain from neuromata and post-herpetic pain (Figure 15.8).[7] Joints and periarthritic areas can be selectively heated.[6] This technique been widely used in treating soft tissue injuries (tennis elbow, pressure sores, leg ulcers and post-oral surgery).[37] It seems to improve pain and range of motion in acute periarticular disorders and osteoarthritis but not in chronic periarticular inflammatory disorders.[36] Any possible beneficial effect of ultrasound as a supplement to exercise therapy still remains unanswered.[36] Ultrasound should not be applied over areas containing fluid (the eye, heart, amniotic fluid or joints with active effusions), the spinal cord after

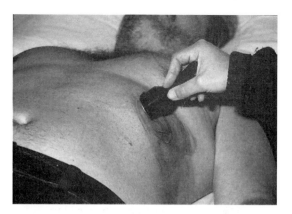

Figure 15.8 The use of ultrasound.

laminectomy or materials used for total joint replacement.[6,7,23] The use of ultrasound in the treatment of musculoskeletal disorders is based on empirical experience but lacks substantial support from controlled studies.[36] Future studies should resolve the question of whether ultrasound can supplement exercise therapy in well-designed, placebo-controlled studies.

Cold therapy

The application of cold therapy relieves the pain of muscle spasm by an effect on the muscle spindle itself.[6] In acute trauma or an inflammatory reaction, a reduction of pain and oedema occurs because of vasoconstriction and diminished nerve conduction velocity from the cold therapy.[7] A decrease in tissue metabolism, histamine release, lymph production and capillary permeability further help to decrease the formation of oedema.[2] Cold can also act as a direct counterirritant to relieve pain. However, cold may increase muscle and joint stiffness, which can be minimized by exercises immediately after treatment.[2]

Cold therapy can be administered in various ways. Cold reduces pain, bleeding and swelling because of its vasoconstrictive properties.[23] After 1–2 days, heat application causes vasodilatation, helping in healing and haematoma resolution. The prolonged application of cold therapy can be used to treat spasticity but has the potential of freezing the skin and may cause frostbite (especially over bony prominences).[2] Most commonly, a rubber bag containing ice cubes in water is applied as a compress.[33] With ice massage, a block of ice is moved over the surface to be cooled.[7] The initial phases of cooling is followed in 2–3 minutes by a period of burning, and then by analgesia.[23] Ice massage has been used to treat myofascial pain.[23] The use of vapocoolant sprays has already been discussed. The involved part can also be repeatedly dipped for 20–30 seconds in ice water over a period of 5–6 minutes.[5] Use is also made of cold wet packs (consisting of gel enclosed in a plastic pouch), which are placed in the refrigerator.[7] Towelling protects the skin from the cold pack. Contraindications to cold therapy include hypersensitivity to cold, vascular insufficiency, an anaesthetic area, cryoglobulinaemia, paroxysmal cold haemoglobinuria and patients with a marked cold pressor response.[2,7,33] For the relief of chronic low back pain, ice massage has been found to be more effective than cold packs.[38]

Laser therapy

Low-level laser therapy has been used to treat a variety of conditions by reducing pain and joint swelling, and improving function.[39] Conditions include ulcers, burns, headaches, sinus pain, wound management and different arthritic and musculoskeletal conditions (e.g. rheumatoid and osteoarthritis, tennis elbow, nerve inflammation and muscle spasm) (Figure 15.9).[39–42] Lasers may have some therapeutic effect on underlying musculoskeletal conditions and may aid resolution of the pathological condition.[39] This may be because of red light being absorbed by cytochromes in the cell mitochondria, affecting cell membrane permeability and the transport of calcium across the cell membrane.[39] A sequence of events is set in motion to restore the cell to its normal function.[43] The relief of neuropathic pain with lasers in some patients is thought to be due to the laser affecting serotonin metabolism.[44]

Two of the low-level lasers used are the infrared gallium aluminium arsenide laser and the visible helium–neon laser.[7] The low energy levels used do not increase the temperature in the tissues treated. Direct eye exposure should be avoided. Pain can also be relieved by using the laser on acupuncture points as well as on hyperaesthetic areas, which are less irritated by subliminal treatment.[39]

The number of well-controlled studies using laser therapy is, however, limited.[40] There is no scientific evidence to show that laser light at the applied intensity and wavelength can penetrate deeper structures.[45] A placebo effect amounting to approximately 20 per cent has been reported with low-level laser treatment.[40] An increase in collagen formation and vasodilatation in the soft tissue are shown to occur after laser irradiation.[40] However, no universally accepted theory has so far explained the mechanism of either laser analgesia or laser biostimulation.[40] Optimal doses still need to be established. A recent meta-analysis concluded that low-level laser therapy has no effect on pain in musculoskeletal syndromes.[45] Contraindications include pregnancy, photosensitivity, malignancy and the fontanelles of growing children.[7] More controlled studies that give the specific parameters of laser application will be necessary to assess the technique's efficacy.

ELECTROTHERAPY

The stress of pain, besides affecting the segmental and suprasegmental reflexes, also affects sympathetic tone and the endocrine and metabolic response in humans.[39] The modulation of pain can be assisted by the use of low-frequency electromagnetic fields.[39] Electrical currents are known to have physical effects on the body, for example chemical, magnetic, mechanical, thermal and electrostatic effects, and the stimulation of other electrical fields, because the cells and tissues respond to a wide range of externally applied electrical and magnetic energies, and are themselves weak emitters of electromagnetic energy.[39]

TENS

This has been discussed more fully in Chapter 12. The most probable mechanism underlying TENS is

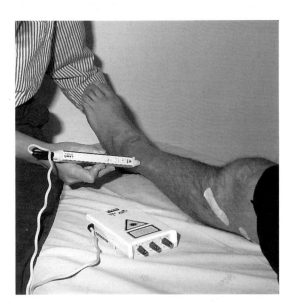

Figure 15.9 The use of laser in wound healing.

the activation of segmental inhibitory circuits in the spinal cord, supplemented by descending inhibitory pathways.[39] From the TENS device (e.g. the Biostim Sportmed, Pulsmed 240[R]), electrodes are placed on the skin, either in the painful area on the spinal region, which may affect the somatic/autonomic supply to the painful region, or as a combination of both.[39] New cordless TENS machines with stay-on patches and no wires are now available. In chronic pain states, using TENS for about 8 hours a day for 3 days with large pads, approximately 10 per cent of patients respond (P. Berger, 1998, personal communication). These usually are the 'rubbers', namely patients who rub, brush or hold their painful part, inadvertently stimulating their mechanoreceptive sensory fibres.[39] This direct mechanical inhibition of an excited, abnormally firing nerve creates presynaptic inhibition; enkephalin- and dynorphin-containing neurones in the substantia gelatinosa contribute to segmental analgesia.[39] TENS may release pituitary and hypothalamic opioid peptides into the CSF.[46] TENS may also lessen the sensitizing action of noradrenaline on injured axons and their terminals in inflamed tissue, interrupting the reflex sympathetic circuit.[39] It could also increase blood flow, thus aiding wound healing.[39] TENS has been found to be effective in treating detrusor overactivity when electrodes were applied alternatively to the quadriceps and hamstring muscles of one or both legs for 20 minutes.[47]

A trial of TENS therapy is initially applied for 8 hours per day over a 3-day period.[39] If this aggravates the pain, treatment in the chosen region is changed to another region until success or pain exacerbation and discontinuation is achieved.[39] If some pain relief occurs, TENS is continued for a while, especially for a few hours a day, during the most painful periods.[39] Over many months, this may further improve the condition.[39] Nevertheless, TENS introduces another measure of self-help for patients to control their pain, improve their quality of life and reduce their medication level.[39]

The long-term use of TENS is associated with a significant reduction in the utilization of pain medication (reducing medication costs by 55 per cent) and physical/occupational therapy (reducing these costs by up to 69 per cent).[48] Nevertheless, using evidence-based resources, TENS has been found to be ineffective for postoperative pain of limited value in labour pain but possibly useful in chronic pain, although a large multicentre randomized trial of TENS with sufficient dose and duration is needed.[49–51]

Acupuncture and electroacupuncture

This has been discussed in greater detail in Chapter 12. Written records of traditional Chinese medicine provide ample evidence for a science based on centuries of inductive logic, observation and painstaking classification.[52] Recent biomedical research on the neural modulation of pain has rekindled an interest in acupuncture as a mode of peripheral sensory stimulation. Analgesia from acupuncture may occur as a result of activation at the level of the spinal cord, the periaqueductal grey matter and the hypothalamic pituitary system, inhibiting incoming nociception.[39] Counter-irritation produced peripherally even by needling trigger points or pecking the periosteum can raise central and CSF beta-endorphin levels.[39,53] In addition, peripheral stimulation of the A delta mechanoreceptors affects the spinal enkephalinergic interneurones, inhibiting pain transmission.[39] It has recently been proposed that stretch-activated ion channels and mechano-electrical transduction cause opening or closing of the membrane channel in response to mechanical displacement of the needle.[54] It is notable that, when abnormal reverberating circuits within the CNS are disrupted with needling, pain relief occurs that often results in an improvement in motor patterns.[39] This has important connotations in CRPS.[39] Sympatholytic effects may occur after needle (or electromagnetic) stimulation over skin areas containing total body information (e.g. the scalp, hands, feet and ear).[39] Electroacupuncture has recently been found to provide more effective analgesia than manual acupuncture.[53] Furthermore, electrical stimulation via patch electrodes is as effective as electroacupuncture.[53] Electroacupuncture with surface electrodes has potential application in modulating pain, augmenting muscle strength and enhancing blood flow in the management of patients with peripheral vascular disease.[55] After lower abdominal surgery, high transcutaneous acupoint electrical stimulation significantly decreases postoperative PCA opioid requirements and opioid-related side-effects.[56] Following electroacupuncture, endorphins are released into the CSF.[53] In addition, low-frequency (2 Hz) and high-frequency (100 Hz) electroacupuncture selectively induce the release of enkephalins and dynorphins in both animals and humans.[53] Electroacupuncture (at 2 Hz and 100 Hz) accelerates preproenkephalin gene transcription.[57]

Clinical research on acupuncture analgesia often

lacks adequate controls, randomization, double-blinding and descriptive detail for replicability.[52] Peripheral sensory stimulation techniques are recognized as being useful for the treatment of pain. Acupuncture analgesia has a traditional basis but is also a technique of peripheral sensory stimulation because it targets the neural network for endogenous pain modulation. It is effective against some forms of chronic pain, where it may occasionally offer significant long-term benefits, but it is not a blunderbuss for treating all pain.[52] Three systematic reviews on acupuncture analgesia in chronic non-malignant pain showed an effect that was often short-lived (93 days).[3] Pain pathophysiology and selection of the optimal parameters of acupuncture determine its effectiveness. Episodic nociceptive pain, as in dysmenorrhoea, may be pre-empted by acupuncture, but acupuncture exacerbates rather than pre-empts acute pain following dental extraction.[52] Long-term pain reduction can be obtained in chronic nociceptive musculoskeletal pain, while chronic idiopathic pain is comparatively unresponsive to acupuncture.[52]

Functional electrical stimulation

Functional electrical stimulation is a system whereby functional movements of muscles are produced by electrically elicited motor responses. The technique acts as an electronic splint, allowing for neuromuscular re-education, so that the patient can increase specific movements necessary for functional activity.[58,59] By increasing muscle strength and decreasing spasticity, it is an effective and safe way for patients with spinal cord injury to regain musculoskeletal and cardiovascular fitness.[58,59]

High-voltage galvanic stimulation

This is used to decrease swelling, muscle tension and spasm. It is thought to act by creating an osmotic effect by ionizing the salts in the tissue fluid.[2] Altered nerve ending polarization may also lead to pain relief.

Interferential therapy

Interferential therapy (with alternating current) is used for the relief of acute and chronic pain, and for muscle stimulation (Figure 15.10).[7] Two pairs of

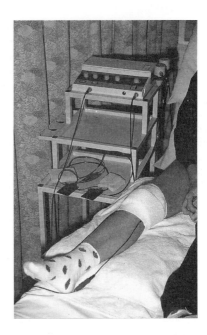

Figure 15.10 The use of interferential therapy for swelling of the ankle.

electrodes are placed perpendicularly to each other and adjusted so that the cross-point of the currents is located at the point of pain.[7] This is the quadripolar technique and is most often used for well-defined, deeper pain. A bipolar technique (with two electrodes placed opposite each other) can be used for the treatment of less-defined superficial pain.

Action potential simulation therapy

The action potential simulator is a device that was invented and manufactured in South Africa in 1992 theoretically to simulate the body's natural nerve impulse. The current produced has a continuous, monophasic square pulse with a waveform of a simulated action potential (P. Berger, 1998, personal communication). The low pulse frequency is 151 Hz and has a width of between 800 microseconds and 6.6 milliseconds. When the current of the action potential simulation device flows into the patient at the point of the electrodes, it produces cycle-synchronous depolarization of the nerve fibre; that is, it moves with the natural action potential through the fibre. With pathology (from the 'inflammatory soup' or damage to the Schwann sheath), a blockage occurs along the impulse path, producing a weakened or absent current and inhibiting the muscular response. The simulated action potential of the device is much stronger (in voltage) than the natural nerve impulse (P. Berger, 1998, personal communication). The negative current from the negative electrode reduces the voltage immediately outside the membrane, drawing this voltage nearer to the voltage across the membrane, and allows activation of the sodium channels, (theoretically) resulting in an action potential. The current produced by the TENS machine increases the difference between the resting and threshold membrane potentials, while the action potential simulator (theoretically) narrows the gap and makes the membrane more excitable. Another difference is that action potential simulation therapy penetrates deeper into the tissues than does TENS. It is claimed (but not proven) that the action potential simulation device stimulates the electrolysis of biochemical 'waste' build-up, resulting in the removal of waste products by the blood and their subsequent excretion. When swelling, inflammation, poor circulation and pain occur as a result of mechanical, chemical or electrical disturbances, these conditions are encouraged to resolve, by stimulating the body's natural regenerative processes (as in depolarization).[39]

Action potential stimulation therapy is claimed to cause vasodilatation, improve sleep patterns and prevent jet lag (P. Berger, 1998, personal communication). Various neuroendocrine changes associated with its use have been studied, including those of melatonin, leu-enkephalin and beta-endorphin.[57] It has been used to treat a variety of painful conditions, ranging from inflammatory joint disease (osteoarthritis, ankylosing spondylitis and gout), tendonitis and osteoporosis with stress fractures, to fracture non-union, phantom pain, migraine, diabetic peripheral neuropathy and myofascial pain. The device offers a 4-, 8- or 16-minute treatment. In inflammatory arthritis (ankylosing spondylitis), sinusitis and post-fracture trauma, there have been rapid improvements within the first 1–3 treatments.[39] With local application, the negative electrodes are placed on the most painful area (e.g. the knee) for 8 minutes.[39] In chronic conditions, a daily spinal treatment for 16 minutes daily for at least 6 days is recommended.[39]

Double-blind, randomized controlled studies comparing the efficacy of this technique against that of TENS are now being carried out. One involving 99 patients with osteoarthritis of the knee, examining the effects of action potential stimulation, TENS and a placebo, has recently been completed (P. Berger and L. Matzner, 1999, unpub-

lished data).[39] Another recently completed double-blind, randomized controlled study of the neuro-hormonal consequences of action potential stimulation therapy showed clinically relevant levels of melatonin after the second treatment and leu-enkephalin after the fourth treatment, with a reduction in beta-endorphins after five treatments and the normalization of serotonin and cortisol after six treatments (E.H. De Wet and J.M.C. Oosthuizen, 1997, unpublished data).[39] Leu-enkephalin may produce analgesia because of its interaction with delta opioid receptors and the inhibition of substance P; it may also relieve inflammation at the sites of tissue damage/hypoxia.[39] Because of its effects on prostaglandins and free oxygen radicals, melatonin may produce analgesia, anxiolysis, sedation, vasodilatation and anticoagulation, with limitation of inflammation at the sites of tissue damage.[39]

Neuro Stim 2000r®

The Neuro Stim 2000,[R] which was manufactured in South Africa late in 1997, generates a variable amplitude, triangular form of waveform, which is offset by a variable direct current (DC) level.[60] The triangular waveform is responsible for the TENS effect and is also used to determine the correct DC level at the application site. The DC offset is responsible for the microcurrent electrical treatment effect and also causes a DC current to flow through the application site, producing electrolysis.[60] It is theorized that the electrolysis (similar to that from the action potential simulator) stimulates the breakdown of 'unwanted body chemicals', which are then excreted by the body (including the lymphatic system).[60] The DC current causes vasodilatation, which aids the excretion of these 'unwanted body chemicals', thereby lessening pain and swelling.[60] Double-blind randomized controlled studies comparing its efficacy against that of TENS and the action potential simulator need to still be carried out to verify these claims. An open prospective trial using the Neuro Stim 2000® to treat cetain types of acute and chronic pain has recently been completed (M. Zipfel and E.A. Shipton, 1999, unpublished).

Transdermal microcurrent patches

Microcurrent therapy is normally 1000 times weaker than TENS and is mostly subliminal.[39] It is closer to the naturally occurring low frequency that normally exists in the body (10 μA) and may align with naturally occurring action potentials in the neurones, as it passes through the injured area.[39] It has beneficial effects in patients normally irritated by other low- or medium-frequency currents and could possibly assist those with hyperaesthesia or allodynia.[39] Microcurrent therapy is claimed to work along the same lines as TENS and to offer drug-free pain relief in a wide range of acute and chronic soft tissue injuries, arthritis, back and neck problems, as well as in postoperative pain. The principle stated is:[61]

> the application of extremely minute electrical charges to cells, increasing amino acids and ATP production within the cells, as well as accelerating the transport of nutrients and wastes through the cell walls. There is more electrical resistance in injured cells, so that the normal energy flow through these cells is lower, impeding the healing process, and maintaining the pain. Microcurrent energy can be stored, and used by the injured cells to lower their electrical resistance, and provide additional energy to aid the body's natural healing process, and the relief of pain.

One such electromembrane provides a microcurrent stimulation of between 10 and 30 μA. The polymer membrane is designed to retain an electrical charge, which is released when brought into contact with the skin for a period of 48 hours.[61]

Another applicator of microcurrent consists of two self-adhesive skin contact electrodes, one of aluminium/copper and the other of copper/aluminium.[62] When in contact with the electrolyte salt found in normal perspiration, the electrodes will generate a weak potential difference. The two electrodes are connected by a flexible connecting wire. Prior to use, the electrolyte gel within the electrodes is isolated, and the cells are held inactive. A thin breakable membrane covering the electrolyte gel is broken when the electrode is applied to the skin by pressing on the electrode cap.[62] The rupturing of the thin breakable membrane allows the gel to contact the gel contact layers of the electrode, completing the circuit and beginning the action of the natural galvanic battery. Self-adhesive plastic foam rings serve as insulators around the rims of the electrodes, creating a sealed chamber for the electrolyte gel of the natural galvanic battery.[62] The electrode produces a stable 10 μA current for continuous treatment extending over several days. Well-designed placebo-controlled studies need to be carried out to verify the efficacy of transdermal microcurrent patches.

Transcranial electrostimulation

Transcranial electrostimulation is described in Chapter 7. This current, when applied via a headset anteriorly over the frontalis muscle, and bilaterally over the mastoid regions, produces quasi-resonance with the antinociceptive system in the brain.[39] This low-frequency current (maximum 4 A but usually 2 A is used) increases beta-endorphin secretion in the brain, CSF and blood up to three times normal levels.[39] As well as its analgesic effects, it is claimed to normalize blood pressure and accelerate tissue repair processes.[39] It is used in the treatment of spondylosis, whiplash, migraine headaches, post-traumatic and cancer-associated neuropathic pain.[39] Ten treatments on consecutive or alternate days are given for 30 minutes per treatment.[39] The patient's pain may only resolve a couple of weeks after treatment has been completed. Contraindications include glaucoma, acute cerebral trauma, epilepsy, CNS disease and the presence of a pacemaker.[39]

Magnetic fields

The same microcurrent frequency is produced by the earth's magnetic field.[39] If magnetic fields are introduced to an injured region of the body (e.g. by the Medicur®), action potentials may be encouraged owing to the fact that magnetic forces are an inevitable consequence of the movement of charges.[39] This may be because living tissues contain many moving charges, as a result of blood or lymph flow, cell movement and nerve impulses.[63] Normal homeostatic mechanisms within the tissues may be induced by evoking many neurological effects.[39]

Multimodal approach

A multimodal approach means that if one type of treatment is only partially successful in achieving pain relief and increased mobility, other therapies can be added in a systematic manner for maximum patient benefit.[39] The ability for the patient to be advised by health care professionals who understand the pain process and its negative effects on the psyche does much to engender patient confidence and cooperation in this planned approach.[39] The use of devices such as TENS, electroacupuncture and microcurrent apparatus, the action potential simulator the Neuro Stim 2000[R] and the Pulsatilla[R] represents a multimodal approach to the patient with acute pain and swelling in which massage and mobilization would only aggravate the pain. All patients are different, and these currents may assist or even irritate some patients; they make it necessary to explore the patient's tolerance and response to different electrical and magnetic impulses.[39] An algorithmic approach could first be TENS, followed in non-responders by electroacupuncture, microcurrent stimulation, action potential simulation, Neuro Stim 2000® laser application, or ultrasonography to determine which one works for the patient concerned (P. Berger, 1998, personal communication). Once mobilization can occur, it may be accompanied by TENS, faradic currents or biofeedback, followed by assisted active movements and finally by daily aerobic activities. It may be possible to have many symptoms relating to a particular condition, as in CRPS, each symptom (e.g. circulatory problems, pain and dysfunction) possibly requiring its own treatment.[39] Patient encouragement in the form of hand and eye contact, and continual praise also plays a role in the rehabilitation process.

To summarize, electrotherapy that arrests pain, decreases inflammation and improves mobility and strength empowers patients and improves their quality of life. Once the patient's pain reaches a level that no longer impinges on function, the physiotherapist can resume normal attention to mobilization, re-education of posture and strengthening exercises.[39]

Self-help

Many of these devices can be used by patients in their homes or worn during normal daily activities, allowing them complete control of the pain situation.[39] The benefits of all the above treatments are that they are non-invasive, have almost no side-effects and may improve the quality of life of the patient to permit a return to normal working and social activities.

MOBILIZATION OF THE NERVOUS SYSTEM

If the nervous system is examined in terms of the features required to maintain normal impulse conduction and axonal transport systems, it becomes clear that many of these relate to body movements. Yet things can very easily go wrong with these

movement mechanics.[64] Just as the sensibility of a muscle and its ability to stretch can be tested, so also can the mechanical abilities of the nervous system. The nervous system structures to be tested include nerves in non-neural tissues (such as nerve fibres in ligaments) up to and including the cortex. Thus the nervous system, just like joints, muscle and fascia, can be physically mobilized.[65] The concept of mobilization of the nervous system facilitates the treatment of non-neural tissues, including target and interfacing tissues. Neurodynamics (the preferred term to neural tension) is the mechanics and physiology of the nervous system as they relate to each other. Neural pathodynamics refers to adverse neural or mechanical tension.[64] The techniques of neural mobilization are unproven at this stage and rely on the clinical reasoning framework; there are, as yet, no randomized controlled studies.

To test the mechanosensitivity and pathomechanics of the nervous system, a series of base tests covering major areas of neural tissue are performed.[64] These include the straight leg raise (testing the tibial, peroneal and sciatic nerves, lumbar sympathetic trunk, lower lumbar roots and meninges and spinal cord); passive neck flexion (which tests the pons, spinal cord and meninges); prone knee bend (testing the femoral tracts, mid and upper lumbar roots, meninges and spinal cord); slump (testing the pons, spinal cord, meninges and sciatic tract); and upper limb tension test (with subdivisions based on individual nerves and sensitizing manoeuvres). An analysis of the test responses should consider the hypothesized mechanisms behind the symptoms evoked. These include peripherally evoked (e.g. nerve entrapment and neuritis), centrally evoked (e.g. heightened dorsal horn sensitivity from persistent peripheral input), motor/autonomic and affective mechanisms.[64] After examination of the patient, if the physiotherapist decides that there is a relevant tension component related to the patient's disorder that needs changing, there are three related approaches:[64]

1. direct mobilization of the nervous system;
2. treatment via interfacing tissues (joints, muscles, fascia and skin);
3. the incorporation of postural advice and ergonomic design.

The latter can be incorporated into a programme of self-treatment as a progression and continuation of hands-on treatment.[64] Precautions against neural mobilization include worsening neurological signs, marked injury or abnormality in the interfacing tissues, inflammatory and infective states, and patients in severe pain.[65]

Pathodynamics of the sympathetic nervous system, especially of the trunk, rami and ganglia, may be a potent source of pain maintenance.[65] Injury that occurs in the presence of sympathetic neurone pathodynamics takes longer to heal, with a greater chance of re-injury. Neural mobilizing techniques can be directed at the sympathetic nervous system (including the trunk, rami and ganglia).[65]

SUPPORTIVE DEVICES

A variety of types of apparatus (splints, plaster of Paris, lightweight casts and orthoses) are used to immobilize parts of the body or joints in the management of acute pain caused by musculoskeletal conditions (muscle sprain, muscle spasm and fracture).[7]

In more chronic pain, supportive devices are often used to reduce pain and to assist weak muscles.[6] They may enable a patient to remain active even with a painful condition. By partially immobilizing the area treated, supportive devices can protect against further injury and prevent or help correct a deformity.[6] Examples of such devices are braces, collars, crutches, canes and even wheelchairs. A spinal orthosis (e.g. lumbosacral corset or cervical collar) provides the biomechanical effects of trunk and neck support, motion control and spinal realignment.[4] Lumbar braces and supports decrease stress on the spine (by increasing intra-abdominal pressure).[7,8] In the past, corsets and braces were used extensively in the treatment of low back pain, but the current recommendation is to avoid these support devices.[8] At times, a simple lumbosacral corset may be provided for the patient more as a reminder than as a specific treatment. Other supportive devices used include patellar tendon weight-bearing devices (for painful heels, arthritis of the ankle joints and numbness of the sole of the foot), ankle–foot orthoses and proper shoeing with total contact orthotics and soft inserts (for sensory neuropathies).[8,66]

It is, however, important frequently to re-evaluate the necessity of using a supportive device as restrictions in body movement will result in muscle shortening and weakening, joint limitation and postural adaption.[2] These may create further disability and pain. Patients can become psychologically dependent on supportive devices and may use them to sustain their invalid role. To prevent this, a rehabilitation treatment plan (e.g. an isometric exercise programme) should be started at the same time as a supportive device is prescribed. The aim of treatment should always be the restoration of functional muscle strength and movement patterns, and the reinforcement of correct posture and body mechanics.[2]

CLINICAL CONDITIONS

To illustrate the practicality of rehabilitation therapies, their application in a few clinical conditions is mentioned briefly.[67]

Arthritis

In the acute inflammatory stage of arthritis, correct joint immobilization plus isometric exercises are important.[7] In the chronic stage, thermotherapy and therapeutic exercises are prescribed.[7] In rheumatoid arthritis, the use of heat, electrical stimulation, splints, bracing, exercises, activities of daily living training and psychological counselling can reduce suffering and disability.[68]

Back pain

In the acute stage of back pain, bed rest, traction, hot and cold therapy (for muscle spasm), the use of a supportive device and gentle exercises have all been used.[7] Surgery for low back pain is currently undergoing significant re-evaluation. It is only necessary in clear nerve compression from disc herniation, posterior disc herniation causing a cauda equina syndrome, and gross instability of the spine.[8] Reassurance, rest for 3–4 days, gradual exercises including flexibility and aerobic strengthening exercises, along with the judicious use of some medications, are sufficient to relieve back pain in most patients.[8] A physical approach plays an important role in the rehabilitation of patients disabled by chronic low back pain.[13] In a recent study, a rehabilitation programme (consisting of mobilizing physiotherapy, isokinetic testing, physical reconditioning, work hardening and psychological testing) was carried out 7 hours a day, 5 days a week, for 4 weeks.[13] Fifty-five per cent of the patients were successfully returned to work.[13] The Oxford Rehabilitation Programme for low back pain includes functional activities and general aerobic, mobilizing and stretching exercises, and is based on the principles of circuit training.[28]

A physical therapy model for the treatment of low back pain has recently been described.[69] Its objective is to modify the pain, to introduce non-destructive forces into the injured area in order to increase activity, to enhance neuromuscular performance and to counsel the patient on biomechanics.[69] To improve rehabilitation, it has been felt that such a programme should be introduced earlier on (i.e. in the subacute stage following injury).[31] A graded activity programme in the subacute stage has been shown to improve mobility, strength and fitness in these patients.[70] A recent task force examining low back pain in the workplace suggested that patients should start with low-stress aerobic activities (swimming, walking and cycling) to improve their general stamina.[71] Exercises to condition specific trunk muscles can be added a few weeks later. Finally, specific training to perform activities required at home or at work can begin. Worksite-based interventions are, however, necessary to minimize and limit disability.[71] The task force found that disability programmes were a major contributor to the explosion in disability as a result of non-specific low back pain and called for a new paradigm for the assessment and management of disability ascribed to non-specific low back pain.[71] The most important things for patients with low back pain to learn are to practise appropriate lifting techniques and to gain an understanding of the effects of back posture on their symptoms.[8]

Headaches

With primary headaches (migraine, cluster and tension), there is no known specific cause for the pain. Secondary headaches result from an underlying problem (tumours, infections, injuries, sinus, jaw and teeth conditions, and visual problems).[8] Despite advances in technology and medicine, no specific diagnosis can be identified in over 90 per cent of chronic headache patients.[8]

A stepped care approach in managing acute headaches is helpful, starting with simple analgesics and moving to combination products and finally to prescription products.[72] Rehabilitation goals include the elimination of non-essential medications (hypnotics and tranquillizers), the normalization of sleep patterns and the treatment of depression.[8] Physical and occupational therapy increases flexibility, strength and endurance as well as general conditioning through a graded therapy programme.[8] Non-pharmacological approaches for

pain relief include the use of heat and cold, massage, TENS and stretching exercises of the neck and shoulder muscles.[8] Coping skills (stress management), relaxation training of the muscles of the scalp, shoulders and neck, and biofeedback (EMG and thermal) enable patients to gain control over their pain.[8] In migraine, a thorough exploration of possible trigger factors and advice on their avoidance may help to reduce the frequency of attacks.[73] Patients need reassurance that their headache does not have a sinister cause, and should have a correct understanding of the way in which a drug works, its potential side-effects, drug interactions and its appropriate use regarding dosing and frequency.[72,73]

Tension myalgia/myofascial pain syndromes

The recommended therapeutic approach to tension myalgia includes reassurance, the elimination of contributory factors, physical therapy, conditioning and medication.[74] In addition to the spray and stretch technique, trigger points can be treated by local anaesthetic injection, acupuncture, low-level laser treatment, ultrasound, interferential therapy or with microwave diathermy (Figure 15.11).[7] Between six and eight treatments of deep heat (e.g. ultrasound) can be given to the tender and tight muscles, followed by vigorous massage and stretching

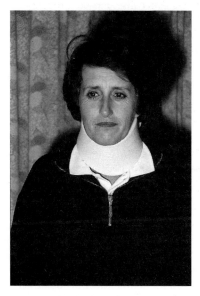

Figure 15.11 Supportive devices. A patient wearing a cervical collar for support.

(facilitated by a fluoromethane or ethyl chloride spray), and finally by vigorous aerobic conditioning exercises.[8]

Joint sprains/muscle strains

The injured part should be immobilized (e.g. with a splint) and cold therapy applied (to reduce muscle spasm).[7] After 48–72 hours, heat therapy (ultrasound or hot packs) can be introduced, followed by active exercises.[7]

Fibromyalgia

Fibromyalgia is a distinct and one of the three top rheumatic disorders, affecting about 2 per cent of the population (3.4 per cent females, 0.5 per cent males; usually in the middle aged, but recently seen in children) with widespread pain/stiffness and tender points on examination.[75] There is a familial aggregation (e.g. fibromyalgia being found in about 25 per cent of children with fibromyalgic mothers) and significant linkage to a disease susceptibility gene to human leucocyte antigen.[75] The American College of Rheumatology Diagnostic Criteria include widespread pain (right and left, above and below the waist and in axial areas), plus 11 out of 18 tender points (no control points and a generalized decreased pain threshold) and with or without other rheumatic disorders (e.g Sjögren's syndrome, lupus erythomatosus and rheumatoid or osteoarthritis).[75] Clinical features include pain (at rest, cold and humid weather, with emotional stress or with poor sleep), fatigue (non-restorative sleep, awakening and problems falling asleep), and miscellaneous features (decreased concentration, headaches, irritable bowel syndrome, postural dizziness, endometriosis, pre-menstrual syndrome, restless leg syndrome and mitral valve prolapse).[75] Fibromyalgia has a poor prognosis, with a disability equal to that of rheumatoid arthritis and depression coupled to disease duration.[75] This is hopefully because of past undertreatment of nociceptive pain, an iatrogenic psychiatric diagnosis and an underuse of non-drug therapy. Trigger stressors on a hypoactive stress system include the physical (trauma, illness and surgery) and the psychological (stress, anxiety, depression and sexual abuse).[75] The main pathophysiology in fibromyalgia consists of changes in sleep patterns, sensory processing disturbances and neuroendocrine dysfunction. Four main endocrine deficiencies (with low basal levels and a decreased exercise response) are thought to exist: decreased cortisol, serotonin and growth hor-

mone levels and a decreased autonomic response.[76] Related to these, other alterations occur, including decreased CSF substance P and melatonin levels, decreased androgen/oestrogen levels, decreased calcium metabolism and thyroid function, and increased prolactin levels.[75,76]

Drug therapy for sleep disturbances includes the use of tricyclic/tetracyclic antidepressants (also for pain) and hypnotics (zopiclone).[75] Adequate control of nociceptive pain (e.g. from injury, arthritis or lupus erythomatosus) is mandatory.[75] Non-nociceptive pain is treated with secondary analgesics (e.g. antiepileptics including the new sodium channel blockers, and NMDA receptor antagonists).[77] Drug therapy for neuroendocrine deficiencies, includes:[75]

- for serotonin – tricyclic antidepressants and selective serotonin uptake inhibitors (SSRIs);
- for growth hormone – pyridostigmine pre-exercise;
- for autonomic disturbances – clonidine, levodopa and pemoline;
- for substance P – clonidine;
- for sex steroids – oestrogen; dehydroepiandrosterone sulphate supplements often lead to a marked improvement in general physical and psychological well-being (P.H. Dessein and E.A. Shipton, 1999, unpublished data);
- for prolactin – levo-dopa or bromocriptine.

Rehabilitation therapy consists of:[8,75]

- sleep hygiene;
- 30 minutes' daily gentle aerobic exercises (walking or swimming), affecting growth hormone, serotonin and androgen levels and autonomic dysfunction;
- weight control (a special high-protein, low-fat, low-carbohydrate diet has been developed and tested; P.H. Dessein and E.A. Shipton, 1998, unpublished data);
- cognitive-behavioural therapy to increase self-efficiency and reduce negative cognitions;
- relaxation techniques (affecting serotonin, androgens and delta wave sleep activity);
- learning pacing skills.

Peripheral neuropathies

The painful dysaesthesias of sensory neuropathies (e.g. from AIDS) may be managed with the use of physical modalities, TENS and orthotics.[66] Motor weakness may require gait aids, bracing, splinting and adaptive equipment.[66] A resistive exercise programme may be instituted if lesions are incomplete and stable.[66]

Burns

In the acute stage in patients with burns, splinting is used to prevent contractures (e.g. of the hands or feet).[78] Later on, pressure garments are used to flatten hypertrophic scarring.[78] An exercise programme is instituted as soon as possible to maintain a full range of movement, either actively or passively.[78,79] Effective pain management is essential for patient compliance to enable successful rehabilitation to be carried out.

CRPS and the physiotherapist

There should be no increase of pain during the physiotherapy treatment (e.g. by examination and handling of the limb). There should be no attempt to massage or subject to ultrasound a region of hyperaesthesia, and no attempt should also be made to force a limb passively into the painful range of movement.[80] Taping a hyperaesthetic joint increases pain. Interferential therapy also appears to increase pain in this condition.[80] Electrophysiotherapy (especially with microcurrent devices) and/or acupuncture has often relieved the pain of CRPS conditions.[80] This allows rehabilitation to proceed. Faradic current does not require movement through the range of motion to develop strength and is well suited to strengthening and gently mobilizing such painful limbs.[80] Once the pain and hyperaesthesia have disappeared, and the limb can be handled normally, all the usual physiotherapeutic aids can be employed to reduce inflammation, swelling and induration, and mobility can be encouraged. The environment and enthusiasm of the care-giver are important in order to motivate the patient to develop the correct attitude to the treatment. Patients are exhorted, 'If you don't use it, you lose it.'[80] Setbacks are regarded as learning curves. Patients are encouraged to take responsibility for their pain and improvement. The use of a TENS machine at home gives patients a sense of achievement and the satisfaction of controlling their own pain. CRPS has a powerful effect on a patient's mental attitude, and, once alleviated, the personality is restored to its normal state. As medical science progresses and the understanding of the body's natural electromagnetic system increases, there may be other modalities that will improve pain relief and dysfunction for the CRPS patient.

Miscellaneous conditions

Physical therapy is being increasingly used to decrease pain and improve function in the treatment of temporomandibular joint disorders, chronic headaches and other orofacial pains.[81] Postoperatively, following temporomandibular joint arthroscopy, physical therapy (moist heat, ultrasound, ice, electrical stimulation, mobilization and therapeutic exercises) has been found to reduce pain and inflammation, and to increase the range of movement.[82] In sympathetically maintained pain (see Chapter 10), intensive physical rehabilitation is essential for pain relief, as surgical attempts almost always fail to relieve pain, by producing further neuronal changes, both peripherally and centrally.[83] In polio patients, stretching exercises can maintain the extensibility of muscle and connective tissue, as well as the joint range.[84] A low-intensity exercise programme (e.g. swimming) can increase muscle strength and movement, and improve aerobic fitness.[84] Supportive devices can maintain postural alignment, and mobility devices (e.g. wheelchairs and scooters) may enable patients to fulfil their social obligations.[84]

PATIENT EDUCATION

In rehabilitation, patient education is critical in affecting long-term improvements in function.[2] In order to assume responsibility for their rehabilitation, patients must understand the nature and mechanics of their disability. The emphasis should be on the prevention of disability through self-participation.[85] Education in ergonomy, pain physiology, the importance of correct posture, self-care and the prevention of further injury (e.g. by lifting techniques) should be given.[31] Ergonomics is the science of the workplace. Adjustable workbenches, adaptable chairs and other alterations can reduce pain. Where a job activity or an environmental condition cannot be modified, the patient can be taught to do the same job in a more efficient manner through proper body mechanic training.[8] With the evolution of formalized educational programmes for back pain sufferers, back schools have proved to be one of the most effective methods of treatment – even better than manipulative therapy.[86–88] In one back school, the best predictor of outcome was found to be job satisfaction![89]

Steps taught to patients in order to enable them to learn to live with their pain and to find pleasure in life again include:[8]

1. acceptance of the fact that they have chronic pain;
2. the setting of specific goals in their work and recreational and social activities;
3. the direction of their anger at their pain;
4. focusing on achieving good physical health;
5. increasing but balancing their physical activities, and pacing themselves;
6. seeking support (not sympathy) from their family, friends and co-workers, and including them in the recovery process;
7. not expecting the medical profession and the healthcare system to provide all the pain relief that they seek;
8. eliminating non-essential medications;
9. changing negative lifestyle habits (excessive coffee intake, smoking and poor nutrition);
10. seeking experienced, supportive, professional help when needed.

Gaining control over their pain is a large part of their pain management. Knowledge, the right attitude and commitment are the three key ingredients enabling patients to gain and maintain control over their pain.[8] Excessive stress can contribute to the pain intensity. Stress management may involve deep breathing exercises, autogenic training (concentrating on positive behaviours) and movements such as stretching.

Prioritizing, planning, pacing, positioning and problem-solving are skills that patients should be taught in order to handle flare-ups in their pain.[8] It is important for patients to set priorities for activities that may produce the pain. Planning involves reviewing carefully the steps needed to perform the activity. Patients may have to pace themselves and only carry on an activity for a certain period of time before resting. It is important for patients to use proper body mechanics, placing their bodies and joints in the best position to use the body most efficiently. If a symptom recurs, patients need to problem-solve and ask themselves what this means and what the options are. Physical activity should be halved but should be built up to the previous level once the pain is under control again.[8] Chronic pain can either be an obstacle or an opportunity. Regaining a positive outlook on life may be the single most important factor for patients in learning to manage their pain.[8]

HOME CARE

It is important that patients continue their rehabilitation programme when at home.[2,6] Patient empowerment, pain control, functional restoration and return to work and leisure activities remain some of the guiding principles of rehabilitation.[90] Physical modalities such as hot packs, electrical heating pads, cold packs and electrical nerve stimulation (TENS, microcurrent therapy, action potential stimulation and the Neuro Stim 2000®) can easily be applied at home.[91] If necessary, home traction can be provided. The McKenzie approach to manual therapy actively involves patients in their own management at home.[15,19] Other self-help therapies include cognitive-behavioural techniques (such as diaphragmatic breathing, positive visualization rehearsal and autogenic training), self-hypnosis and biofeedback.[91] Patients should be weaned early from one-on-one physical therapy to group classes, and thereafter on to an individual independent home programme.[90] The group setting provides friendship between patients and encourages mutual support.[90] The home exercise programme may consist of aqua-aerobics (allowing aerobic exercise, range of motion and weight-bearing that would not be possible out of the water) or aerobic exercises in a gym facility.[90] Specific simulated work activities (work hardening) can be practised at home 2–6 weeks before returning to work.[90] Progression to self-help home programmes is always the goal, with the understanding that exercise should become a daily routine, often for the rest of the patient's life.[4]

In treating repetitive strain injuries with tissue microtrauma, a vital step is the elimination of aggravating factors (e.g. improper posture), inadequate attention to ergonomic factors at work and contributory habits (e.g. jaw or hand clenching).[92] The use of simple joint-protection measures can alleviate much of the discomfort. Appropriate self-help strategies used at home may restore flexibility and strength with a minimum of medical intervention (ice packs, massage, topical NSAIDs or local anaesthetic injections).[92]

At discharge, by providing written instructions or an audiotape (after adequate demonstration), patients can be helped to continue their exercise (and relaxation) programmes at home. In rheumatoid arthritis patients, 85 per cent were found to be continuing their exercise programme 6–18 months after discharge.[93] Home compliance is enhanced by repeated information and instruction, and by the stimulation of the patient and nearest relative.[93] Various support groups (e.g. arthritis and cancer support groups) are available in many countries, and the patient should be placed in contact with, and encouraged to join, such a group. Variables that affect patient adherence, both positively and negatively, include patient motivation, the nature and chronicity of the disorder, treatment variables and the quality of the doctor–patient relationship.[91] Physician behaviours may encourage or discourage patient adherence.[91]

REFERENCES

1. **Korevaar, W.C.** 1992: Talk, nerve blocks and exercise: modern concepts in pain management. *American Society of Anesthesiologists' Annual Refresher Course Lectures* **11**, 123–31.
2. **Yeh, C., Shiell, M., Lamke, J. and Volpe, M.** 1992: Physical therapy: evaluation and treatment of chronic pain. In Aronoff, G.M. (ed.) *Evaluation and treatment of chronic pain*. Baltimore: Williams & Wilkins, 285–90.
3. **McQuay, H.J. and Moore, R.A.** 1998: *An evidence-based resource for pain relief*. Oxford: Oxford University Press 23, 195–200.
4. **Rauck, R.L.** 1998: Chronic low back pain. In Rawal, N. (ed.) *Management of acute and chronic pain*. London: BMJ Books, 139–71.
5. **Unruh, A., Baxter, G.D., Casale, R.** *et al.* 1995: *Outline curriculum on pain for schools of occupational therapy and physical therapy*. Seattle: IASP Press, 1–14.
6. **Wilensky, J.** 1992: Physiatric approach to chronic pain. In Aronoff, G.M. (ed.) *Evaluation and treatment of chronic pain*. Baltimore: Williams & Wilkins, 176–201.
7. **Lee, M.H.M., Itoh, M., Yang, G.F.W. and Eason, A.L.** 1990: Physical therapy and rehabilitation medicine. In Bonica, J.J. (ed.) *The management of pain*. Philadelphia: Lea & Febiger, 1769–88.
8. **Vasudevan, S.V.** 1993: *Pain: a four-letter word you can live with*, 2nd edn. Milwaukee: Montgomery Media, 1–225.
9. **Berde, C.B.** 1994: Pain curriculum for students in occupational therapy or physical therapy. *IASP Newsletter* (Nov/Dec), 3–8.
10. **McCormack, G.L.** 1988: Pain management by occupational therapists. *American Journal of Occupational Therapy* **42**(9), 582–90.
11. **American Occupational Therapy Association** 1992: Statement: Use of adjunctive modalities in occupational therapy. *American Journal of Occupational Therapy* **46**(12), 1075–81.
12. **American Occupational Therapy Association** 1992: Statement: Occupational therapy services in work

practice. *American Journal of Occupational Therapy* **46**(12), 1086–91.
13. **Edwards, B.C., Zusman, M., Hardcastle, P., Twomey, L., O'Sullivan, P. and McLean, N.** 1992: A physical approach to the rehabilitation of patients disabled by chronic low back pain. *Medical Journal of Australia* **156**, 167–72.
14. **Rosomoff, R.S.** 1990: Inpatient and outpatient chronic pain programs can be successful in returning patients to gainful employment. *Clinical Journal of Pain* **6**(1), 80–3.
15. **Haig, A.J., Linton, P., McIntosh, M., Moneta, L. and Mead, P.B.** 1990: Aggressive early medical management by a specialist in physical medicine and rehabilitation: effect on lost time due to injuries in hospital employees. *Journal of Occupational Medicine* **32**(10), 966.
16. **Kehlet, H.** 1997: Multimodal approach to control postoperative pathophysiology and rehabilitation. *British Journal of Anaesthesia* **78**, 606–17.
17. **Berde, C.B.** 1998: Staying in bed: harmful to your health? *IASP Newsletter* (Mar/Apr), 3–4.
18. **Towmey, L.T.** 1992: A rationale for the treatment of back pain and joint pain by manual therapy. *Physical Therapy* **72**(12), 885–92.
19. **Farrell, J.P. and Jensen, G.M.** 1992: Manual therapy: a critical assessment of role in the profession of physical therapy. *Physical Therapy* **72**(1), 843–52.
20. **Khalil, T.M., Asfour, S.S., Martinez, L.M., Waly, S.F., Rosomoff, R.S. and Rosomoff, H.L.** 1992: Stretching in the rehabilitation of low back pain patients. *Spine* **17**(3), 311–17.
21. **Haldeman, S.** 1994: Manipulation and massage for the relief of back pain. In Wall, P.D. and Melzack, R. (eds) *Textbook of pain*, 3rd edn. Edinburgh: Churchill Livingstone, 1251–62.
22. **Giringer, S.D. and Lateur, B.J.** 1990: Physiatric therapeutics. 3: Traction, manipulation, and massage. *Archives of Physical and Medical Rehabilitation* **71**, S264–S266.
23. **Fields, H.L.** (ed). Physical medicine and rehabilitation. In *Task Force on Professional Education. Core curriculum for professional education in pain*. Seattle: IASP Press. 45–8.
24. **Koes, B.W., Bouter, L.M., Van Mameren, H.** *et al.* 1992: Randomised clinical trial of manipulative therapy and physiotherapy for persistent back and neck complaints: results of one year of follow-up. *British Medical Journal* **304**, 601–5.
25. **O'Neill, D.B. Micheli, L.J and Warner, J.P.** 1992: Patellofemoral stress: a prospective analysis of exercise treatment in adolescents and adults. *American Journal of Sports Medicine* **20**(2), 151–6.
26. **Davis, V.P., Fillingim, R.B., Doleys, D.M., and Davis, M.P.** 1992: Assessment of aerobic power in chronic pain patients before and after a multi-disciplinary treatment program. *Archives of Physical Medicine and Rehabilitation* **73**, 726–9.
27. **Wells, P. and Lessard, E.** 1994: Movement education and limitation of movement. In Wall, P.D. and

Melzack, R. (eds) *Textbook of pain*, 3rd edn. Edinburgh: Churchill Livingstone, 1263–76.

28. **Frost, H. and Moffett, J.K.** 1992: Physiotherapy management of chronic low back pain. *Physiotherapy* **78**(10), 751–4.

29. **Abram, S.E. and Hebar, R.L.** 1990: Radiculopathy. In Abram, S.E. (ed.) *The pain clinic manual*. Philadelphia: J.B. Lippincott, 105–17.

30. **McKinney, L.A.** 1989: Early mobilisation and outcome in acute sprains of the neck. *British Medical Journal* **299**, 1006–8.

31. **Oland, G. and Tveiten, G.** 1991: A trial of modern rehabilitation for chronic low back pain and disability: vocational outcome and effect of pain modulation. *Spine* **16**(4), 457–9.

32. **Wilkinson, A.** 1992: Stretching the truth: a review of the literature on muscle stretching. *Australian Physiotherapy* **38**(4), 283–7.

33. **Lehmann, J.F. and De Lateur, B.J.** 1994: Ultrasound, shortwave, microwave, laser, superficial heat and cold in the treatment of pain. In Wall, P.D. and Melzack, R. (eds) *Textbook of pain*, 3rd edn. Edinburgh: Churchill Livingstone, 1237–49.

34. **Nurmikko, T. and Hietaharju, A.** 1992: Effect of exposure to sauna heat on neuropathic and rheumatoid pain. *Pain* **49**, 43–51.

35. **Kitchen, S. and Partridge, C.** 1992: Review of shortwave diathermy continuous and pulsed patterns. *Physiotherapy* **78**(4), 243–52.

36. **Gam, A.N. and Johannsen, F.** 1995: Ultrasound therapy in musculoskeletal disorders: a meta-analysis. *Pain* **63**, 85–91.

37. **Everett, T., McIntosh, J. and Grant, A.** 1992: Ultrasound therapy for persistent post-natal perineal pain and dyspareunia: a randomised placebo-controlled trial. *Physiotherapy* **78**(4), 263–7.

38. **Roberts, D.J., Walls, C.M., Carlile, J.A., Wheaton, C.G. and Aronoff, G.M.** 1992: Relief of chronic low-back pain: heat versus cold. In Aronoff, G.M. (ed.) *Evaluation and treatment of chronic pain*. Baltimore: Williams & Wilkins, 299–301.

39. **Berger, P.** 1999: Electrical pain modulation for the chronic pain patient. *South African Journal of Anaesthesiology and Analgesia* **5**(1), 14–19.

40. **Vasseljen, O.** 1992: Low-level laser versus traditional physiotherapy in the treatment of tennis elbow. *Physiotherapy* **78**(5), 329–34.

41. **De Lateur, B.J. and Hinderer, S.R.** 1990: Physiatric therapeutics. 2: Therapeutic heat and cold, electrotherapy, and therapeutic exercise. *Archives of Physical Medicine and Rehabilitation* **71**, S260–S263.

42. **Klein, R.G. and Eek, B.C.** 1990: Low-energy laser treatment and exercise for chronic low back pain: a double-blind controlled trial. *Archives of Physical Medicine and Rehabilitation* **71**, 34–7.

43. **Seitz, L. and Kleinkort, J.A.** 1986: Low-power laser: its application in physical therapy. In Michlovitz, S.L. (ed.) *Thermal agents in rehabilitation*. Philadelphia: F.A. Davies, 217–37.

44. **Mester, E., Mester, A.E. and Mester, A.** 1995: The biochemical effect of laser application. *Lasers in Surgery and Medicine* **5**, 31–9.

45. **Gam, A.N., Thorsen, H. and Lonnberg.** 1993: The effect of low-level laser therapy on musculoskeletal pain; a meta-analysis. *Pain* **52**, 63–6.

46. **Facchinetti, F., Sandrini, G., Petralgia, F.** *et al.* 1984: Concomitant increase in nociceptive flexion reflex threshold and plasma opioids following transcutaneous nerve stimulation. *Pain* **19**, 295–307.

47. **Okada, N., Igawa, Y., Ogawa, A. and Nishizawa, O.** 1998: Transcutaneous electrical stimulation of thigh muscles in the treatment of detrusor overactivity. *British Journal of Urology* **81**(4), 560–4.

48. **Chabal, C., Fishbain, D.A., Weaver, M. and Heine, L.W.** 1998: Long-term transcutaneous electrical stimulation (TENS) use: impact on medication utilization and physical therapy costs. *Clinical Journal of Pain* **14**(1), 66–73.

49. **McQuay, H.J. and Moore, R.A.** 1998: *An evidence-based resource for pain relief*. Oxford: Oxford University Press 22, 187–92.

50. **McQuay, H.J. and Moore, R.A.** 1998: *An evidence-based resource for pain relief*. Oxford: Oxford University Press 25, 207–11.

51. **Kaplan, B., Rabinerson, D., Krieser, R.U. and Neri, A.** 1997: Transcutaneous electrical nerve stimulation (TENS) as a pain-relief device in obstetrics and gynaecology. *Clinical and Experimental Obstetrics and Gynecology* **24**(3), 123–6.

52. **Thomas, M. and Lundeberg, T.** 1996: Does acupuncture work? *Pain – Clinical Updates* **4**(3), 1–4.

53. **Ulett, G.A., Han, S. and Han, J.S.** 1998: Electro-acupuncture: mechanisms and clinical application. *Biological Psychiatry* **44**(2), 129–38.

54. **Kho, H.-G. and Robertson, E.N.** 1997: The mechanisms of acupuncture analgesia: review and update. *American Journal of Acupuncture* **25**(4), 261–81.

55. **Balogun, J.A., Biasci, S. and Han, L.** 1998: The effects of acupuncture, electroneedling and transcutaneous electrical stimulation therapies on peripheral haemodynamic functioning. *Disability Rehabilitation* **20**(2), 41–8.

56. **Wang, B., Tang, J., White, P.F.** *et al.* 1997: Effect of the intensity of transcutaneous acupoint electrical stimulation on the postoperative analgesic requirement. *Anesthesia and Analgesia* **85**(2), 406–13.

57. **Guo, H.F.** 1996: Comparative study of the expression and interaction of oncogene c-fos/c-jun and three opioid genes induced by low and high frequency electroacupuncture. *Sheng Li Ko Hsueh Chin Chan* **27**(2), 135–8.

58. **Ferguson, A.C.B. and Granat, M.H.** 1992: Evaluation of functional electrical stimulation for an incomplete spinal cord injured patient. *Physiotherapy* **78**(4), 253–6.

59. **Arnold, P.B., McVey, P.P., Farrell, W.J., Deurloo, T.M. and Grasso, A.R.** 1992: Functional electric stimulation: its efficacy and safety in improving pulmonary

function and musculoskeletal fitness. *Archives of Physical Medicine and Rehabilitation* **73**, 665–8.

60. **Neuro Stim 2000 (PTY) LTD.** 1998: Neuro Stim 2000 Mk1. *User manual.* Johannesburg: Benoni Neuro Stim 2000 (PTY) LTD, 1–3.

61. **Kreft, J.** 1996: Acustat – transdermal micro-current patch for pain relief. *Pharmaceutical enterprises manual,* Cape Town, 1–6.

62. **Bergner, M.** 1995: Painmaster: therapeutic results of a new method of stable galvanization with current of 10 μA. *Universal medical products manual,* 1–4.

63. **Low, J. and Reed, A.** 1994: *Electrotherapy explained: principles and practice,* 2nd edn, vol. 10. Oxford: Butterworth Heineman, 272.

64. **Butler, D.S. and Jones, M.A.** 1994: *Mobilisation of the nervous system.* Edinburgh: Churchill Livingstone, 1–265.

65. *Mobilisation of the nervous system: part of a neuro orthopaedic approach.* 1994: Falmouth: Neuro Orthopaedic Institute International/Longmans, 1–97.

66. **Levinson, S.F. and O'Connell, P.G.** 1991: Rehabilitation dimensions of AIDS: a review. *Archives of Physical Medicine and Rehabilitation* **72**, 690–6.

67. **Cohen, M.L.** 1996: Arthralgia and myalgia. *Pain 1996 – an updated review.* Seattle: IASP Press, 327–37.

68. **Swezey, R.L.** 1990: Rheumatoid arthritis: the role of the kinder and gentler therapies. *Journal of Rheumatology* **25**(suppl.), 8–13.

69. **DeRosa, C.P. and Porterfield, J.A.** 1992: A physical therapy model for the treatment of low back pain. *Physical Therapy* **72**(4), 261–9.

70. **Lindstrom, I., Ohlund, C., Eek, C., Wallin, L., Petersen, L.E. and Nachemson, A.** 1991: Mobility, strength, and fitness after a graded activity program for patients with subacute low back pain. *Spine* **17**(6), 641–9.

71. **Fordyce, W.E.** (ed.) *Back pain in the workplace: management of disability in nonspecific conditions.* Task Force on Pain in the Workplace. Seattle: IASP Press, 1–75.

72. **Sheftell, F.D.** 1997: Role and impact of over-the-counter medications in the management of headache. *Neurology Clinics* **15**(1), 187–98.

73. **Macgregor, E.A.** 1997: The doctor and the migraine patient: improving compliance. *Neurology* **48**(suppl. 3), S16–S20.

74. **Thompson, J.M.** 1990: Tension myalgia as a diagnosis at the Mayo Clinic and its relationship to fibrositis, fibromyalgia, and myofascial pain syndrome. *Mayo Clinic Proceedings* **65**(9), 1237–48.

75. **Dessein, P.H.** 1998: Fibromyalgia. *South African Journal of Anaesthesiology and Analgesia* **4**(4), 29–32.

76. **Dessein, P.H. Shipton, E.A. and Cloete, A.** 1997: Fibromyalgia as a syndrome of neuroendocrine deficiency: a hypothetical model with therapeutic implications. *Pain Reviews* **4**(2), 79–88.

77. **Dessein, P.H. Shipton, E.A.** 1998: Pain in rheumatological disorders – new developments in the understanding of mechanisms and treatment implications.

South African Journal of Anaesthesiology and Analgesia **4**(3), 2–8.

78. **Raeside, F.** 1992: Physiotherapy management of burned children: a pilot study. *Physiotherapy* **78**(12), 891–5.

79. **Blassingame, W.M., Bennett, G.B., Helm, P.A., Purdue, G.F. and Hunt, J.L.** 1989: Range of motion of the shoulder performed while patient is anesthetised. *Journal of Burns Care and Rehabilitation* **10**(6), 539–42.

80. **Berger, P.** 1997: The contribution to pain management in complex regional pain syndromes by the physiotherapist: a physiotherapy algorithm and treatment. *South African Journal of Anaesthesiology and Analgesia* **3**(4), 14–18.

81. **McDonald, J.S., Pensak, M.L. and Phero, J.C.** 1990: Thoughts on the management of chronic facial, head, and neck pain. *American Journal of Otology* **11**, 378–82.

82. **Waide, F.L., Bade, D.M., Lovasko, J. and Montana, J.** 1992: Clinical management of a patient following temporomandibular joint arthroscopy. *Physical Therapy* **72**(5), 355–64.

83. **Girgis, F.L. and Parry, C.B.** 1989: Management of causalgia after peripheral nerve injury. *International Disability Studies* **11**(1), 15–20.

84. **Dean, E.** Clinical decision making in the management of the late sequelae of poliomyelitis. *Physical Therapy* **71**(10), 752–61.

85. **American Occupational Therapy Association, Inc.** 1992: Position paper: physical agent modalities. *American Journal of Occupational Therapy* **46**(12), 1090–1.

86. **Martin, L.** 1992: Back basics: general information for back school participants. *Occupational Medicine* **7**(1), 9–16.

87. **White, L.A.** 1992: The evolution of back school. *Occupational Medicine* **7**(1), 1–8.

88. **Koes, B.W., Bouter, L.M., Beckerman, H., Van der Heijden, G.J. and Knipschild, P.G.** 1991: Physiotherapy exercises and back pain: a blinded review. *British Medical Journal* **302**, 1572–6.

89. **Hurri, H.** 1989: The Swedish back school in chronic low back pain: Part II. Factors predicting the outcome. *Scandinavian Journal of Rehabilitation Medicine* **21**(1), 41–4.

90. **Trumble, E.A. and Krengel, M.P.** 1996: Physical therapy. In Raj, P.P. (ed.) *Pain medicine – a comprehensive review,* vol. 33. St Louis: C.V. Mosby **33**: 335–8.

91. **Moskowitz, L.** 1996: Psychological management of postsurgical pain and patient adherence. *Hand Clinics* **12**(1), 129–37.

92. **Sheon, R.P.** 1997: Repetitive strain injury: 2. Diagnostic and treatment tips on six common problems. The Goff Group. *Postgraduate Medicine* **102**(4), 72–8.

93. **Terpstra, S.J., De Witte, L.P. and Diederiks, J.P.M.** 1992: Compliance of patients with an exercise program for rheumatoid arthritis. *Physiotherapy Canada* **44**(2), 37–41.

16

THE FUTURE

Pain is indeed a complex phenomenon, psycho-social and behavioural parameters interacting with the physical pathology to produce an integrated perceptional experience and behavioural response.[1] The transmission of pain is an interplay between a number of transmitter systems, both excitatory and inhibitory, at many levels of the CNS but which converge especially on the spinal cord.[2] The main processes contributing to chronic pain are peripheral mechanisms leading to an abnormal excitation of peripheral nociceptive afferent fibres, and central mechanisms resulting in facilitated transmission in the dorsal horn or higher up the nociceptive pathway.[3] Inflammation and nerve damage give rise to changes in sensory processing at both a peripheral and central level, with resulting sensitization.[4]

The concept that injury can induce both peripheral and central hypersensitivity has important consequences for pain control strategies. It is clear that, even within the definition of acute pain as pain that lasts up to 3 months, there are many time-related alterations, both increases and decreases, in

the levels of both excitation and inhibition.[2] For several decades, basic research into the mechanisms underlying pain and pain inhibition has been conducted using a combination of biochemical, pharmacological, electrophysiological and behavioural techniques.[5] The spinal cord processes nociceptive input in very specific ways that are not static but change with time.[6] These changes manifest themselves as an increased sensitivity of the spinal cord to afferent input and an expansion of the peripheral fields termed spinal hyperexcitability.[6] Spinal cord neurone excitability depends on the balance of inputs from primary afferent nociceptors, intrinsic spinal cord neurones and descending systems projecting from supraspinal sites.[6] The neurotransmitter role comes from experiments measuring neurotransmitter release and the effect of neurotransmitter antagonists, and from gene expression in neurotransmitter systems.[6] Advances in molecular biological technology, notably the development of the polymerase chain reaction and large-capacity DNA vectors, have recently led to the study of biological systems at the level of the gene.[5] Many of these genes are up- or downregulated in models of inflammatory and neuropathic pain, suggesting that they are important in initiating or maintaining spinal components of pain.[6] The potential of this type of research lies in identifying possible new targets for analgesic therapy and in understanding the timing of events contributing to spinal cord hyperexcitability.[6] Timing drug administration targeted at individual neurotransmitter systems (receptors or enzymes involved in neurotransmitter synthesis) to pre-empt or coincide with known changes in neurotransmitter gene expression may provide a useful approach to the management of pain.[6]

The previous chapters have hopefully provided an insight into the present management of acute and chronic pain, but what of the future? There should be potential progress in a number of areas. The current, and final, chapter affirms some of the possibilities already discussed but goes on to explore these further.

NEUROPHYSIOLOGY OF PAIN

The components of the pain system may be traced from sensory receptors to sensory areas in the cerebral cortex by mapping the density of nociceptive nerve endings, by labelling of GAP-43 produced by axonal growth cones in peripheral nerves and the spinal cord, by monitoring the activity of primary afferents and by the biochemical measurement of neurotransmitters in the dorsal horn (e.g. substance P, somatostatin, leukotrienes and met-enkephalin).[7] Microneurography can accurately document the activity of a single nociceptor in the peripheral nervous system.

PERIPHERALLY ACTING AGENTS AND PERIPHERAL SENSITIZATION

At peripheral levels, most of the nociceptive signalling of thermal and mechanical pain arises from the activation of polymodal nociceptors that are innervated by C fibres. In the presence of inflammation, local tissue damage (oedema and synovial effusion), these fibres become sensitized to chemical, thermal and mechanical stimuli. They are readily excited by non-noxious stimuli (allodynia) or show an enhanced response to noxious stimuli (primary hyperalgesia).[6] During inflammation, blood vessels become leaky as a result of the actions of some of these chemical mediators so that other mediators gain access to the damaged tissue site from the vasculature.[2] Tissue damage generates the synthesis of arachidonic acid metabolites from adjacent membranes, the cleavage of the precursor of bradykinin to release active peptide from the circulation, and the release of peptides such as substance P and from the C fibres via the axon reflex. This inflammatory soup also contains 5-HT, potassium ions and hydrogen ions, activates and sensitizes the peripheral endings and causes vasodilatation and plasma extravasation, thus eliciting pain, swelling and tenderness.[2] These chemicals then act to sensitize high-threshold nociceptors such that continuous low-frequency firing (at about 1 Hz) can be detected in the afferent axons of these nociceptors.[6] The sensitivity of nerve endings to mechanical and thermal stimuli is altered.[6] Following sensitization, low-intensity stimuli that would not normally cause pain are perceived as painful. This series of events that follows tissue injury is termed peripheral sensitization.[4] It is characterized by an increased responsiveness to thermal stimuli at the site of injury.

There is a class of unmyelinated primary afferent fibres, the so-called 'silent nociceptors', that become responsive in the presence of inflammation and chemical sensitization. They then become responsive and discharge vigorously even during ordinary movement.[4] A blockage or reduction of nociceptive messages at the first stage in the periphery prevents some of the central alterations that occur.

CENTRAL SENSITIZATION AND WIND-UP

Nociceptor stimuli that produce tissue damage and a subsequent inflammatory response result in alterations in the processing of sensory information at the spinal cord level. This 'plasticity' is expressed as changes in the physiology and neurochemistry of spinal neurones.[8] This has been shown most exclusively in neurones located in the deep dorsal and ventral horns, which receive input from both nociceptors and low-threshold mechanoreceptors, that is, WDR neurones.[6] The transmission and modulation of nociception at the level of the spinal cord involves interactions between a variety of neurones and neurotransmitters that may have both excitatory and inhibitory effects.[9] This leads to the potential for convergence and modulation on a large scale.

There is evidence that the transmission of nociception at the dorsal horn level involves a variety of amino acid and peptide molecules. These are present in the primary afferent nerve terminals and are released on noxious stimulation. The principal neurotransmitters are the excitatory amino acids aspartate and glutamate, and the neurokinins (NK A) and substance P.[9] However, other peptides, including CGRP, somatostatin, galanin, vasoactive intestinal peptide, bombesin and neurotensin, have also been implicated.[9] The excitatory amino acids glutamate and aspartate act at a variety of receptors and are of the utmost importance in the transmission of acute and chronic pain. Glutamate is used by most neurones in the CNS as their excitatory transmitter. It acts on a number of receptors, including the NMDA receptor, the alpha-amino-3-hydroxy-5-methyl-4-isoxazole-propionic acid (AMPA) receptor, the metabotropic receptor and the kainate receptor.[2] A proportion of primary afferent nerve fibres also express and synthesize neuropeptides such as substance P, CRGP and NK A that are co-released with glutamate.[6] Recent preclinical animal studies have attempted to functionally define the role of NMDA receptors in nociceptive processing from neurophysiological, pharmacological and behavioural perspectives using both acute and chronic pain models.[10] In particular, NMDA receptor activation after nociceptive challenge has been associated with the phenomenon of wind-up. Wind-up after sustained C fibre afferent stimulation is predominantly driven by activated NMDA receptors, localized on the dorsal horn WDR neurones. The evoked release of the excitatory amino acids glutamate and aspartate, and neuromodulatory peptides such as substance P, from primary afferent nerve terminals effectively removes the magnesium voltage-dependent sensory block of the NMDA receptor, resulting in a form of central sensitization to peripheral nerve stimuli.

Transmission from C fibres after brief acute mechanical or thermal stimuli involves only glutamate, which acts on the AMPA receptor to produce short-lasting excitation. If the stimulus is maintained and/or its frequency or intensity increased, the release of peptides then contributes to transmission and allows the NMDA receptor to become activated, the resulting amplification of the response underlying many forms of hyperalgesia.[2] The increased release of both excitatory amino acids and peptides in inflammatory pains will facilitate these processes. The NMDA receptor not only sets up enhanced pain transmission, but also maintains this state.

The signal transduction pathways that are involved in central sensitization appear to include those activated by NMDA receptors and several G protein-mediated pathways through the metabotropic glutamate receptors and tachykinin receptors. One of the second messenger systems involved is that mediated by phopholipase C, the action of which increases inositol triphosphate and diacylglycerol levels. These substances cause intracellular calcium release and the activation of protein kinase C respectively. Protein kinase C can enhance cation current flow, including calcium ion current through the NMDA receptor.

NO is another mediator. Calcium ions entering the cell bind to the cytosolic calmodulin, which in turn participates in the activation of NO synthetase. The consequence of this is the intracellular production of NO from its L-arginine precursor.[5] NO is a small reactive molecule that can pass easily through membranes and has a very short half-life. This makes NO an ideal gaseous transmitter, which can be produced in increased amounts in inflammation. The known effects of NO include: antinociception in the periphery; the modification of cell membranes; the inhibition of eicosanoid production; free radical scavenging; and the stimulation of guanidine cyclase to increase cyclic guanidine monophosphate (cGMP) and activate protein kinase levels.[5] NO is required for wind-up and inflammation-produced spinal neuronal responses. It has been suggested that NO feeds back in a positive way to increase the release of C fibre transmitters, thus further enhancing pain transmission.[2] These also result in the increased expression of immediate-early genes such as *C-Fos*.

Centrally generated prostanoids can also contribute to central sensitization. Arachidonic acid metabolites, generated by the action of phopholipase, break down to prostanoids, which is the basis for potential central actions of the NSAIDs.[2]

Afferents that induce central sensitization produce slow synaptic potentials in spinal neurones. Following low-frequency repetitive afferent activation, the slow potentials, summate to produce a cumulatively increasing postsynaptic depolarization. With peripheral inflammation, there is persistent firing in the afferent nociceptors, which continuously release neurotransmitters into the synapse.[6] The amount of glutamate released increases, which elicits AMPA receptor- and NMDA receptor-dependent excitatory postsynaptic potentials, which, together with other neurotransmitters (such as substance P, NK A and CGRP), leads to prolonged depolarization of the postsynaptic neurone and a progressive increase in the action potential discharge on repeated stimulation.[6] An enhanced response of spinal cord neurones to successive stimuli occurs because of the summation of excitatory postsynaptic potentials, which results in a progressive depolarization and enhanced cell firing following each stimulus.[6] This hyperexcitable state and neuronal plasticity in the dorsal horn neurones has already been defined as 'wind-up'.[8] This is clearly a frequency-dependent effect and can be observed at stimulus frequencies as low as 0.5 Hz, a frequency that is not dissimilar to the background firing rate of sensitized nociceptive afferents.[6] Using PET, changes in the cortical and subcortical areas have been shown to occur.[11] Therefore, with nociceptive input, there is not a simple stimulus–response relationship but a 'wind-up' of spinal cord neurone activity, this wind-up making these neurones more sensitive to other inputs.[4] Sustained C fibre barrage in primary afferent fibres leads to other morphological and biochemical changes in the dorsal horn, with central sensitization.[4] First, there is an expansion in receptive field size so that the spinal neurone will respond to stimuli that would normally be outside the region reacting to nociceptive stimuli. Second, there is an increase in the magnitude and duration of response to stimuli that are above the threshold in strength. Last, there is a reduction in threshold so that stimuli that are not normally noxious activate neurones that usually transmit nociceptive information. These changes are important in acute pain states and in the development of chronic pain. Central sensitization is thus manifested by the enlargement of primary receptive fields, automaticity and alterations in stimulus–response relationships, resulting in a greater amplitude of depolarization. Central sensitization is clinically perceived as allodynia and hyperpathia. Wind-up and central sensitization are not, however, identical processes, although they share many features.[6] In humans, electrical stimulation at an intensity sufficient to elicit pain produces temporal summation, which can be blocked by NMDA antagonists.[6]

Following peripheral nerve injury, the terminals of myelinated afferents sprout into neighbouring regions of the dorsal horn.[4] In the dorsal horn, both nociceptive-specific and WDR neurones have enlarged receptive fields.[12] Similar hypersensitivity of the trigeminal brain stem nociceptive neurones occurs.[12] Central sensitization allows the recruitment of low-threshold mechanoreceptor afferent input, which begins to produce pain (something it never normally does).[13] The expanded receptive fields lead to a greater number of nociceptive neurones being activated by a stimulus and may ultimately be perceived as more intense pain.[14] A persistent pain state will then develop.

GENETIC INFLUENCES

The CGRP gene and the NMDA receptor NR1 subunit gene are the two genes involved in nociceptive transmission.[15] CGRP is found in many small primary afferent neurones in the dorsal ganglion and is a co-transmitter there with the pretachykinin-derived peptides, substance P and NK A, and glutamate. It thus plays a role in nociceptive primary afferent neurotransmission. The NMDA NR1 gene codes for the subunit of the NMDA receptor obligatory for generating a functional receptor. The multisubunit receptor is involved in glutamate excitatory neurotransmission and is the binding site for ketamine and dizocilpine (MK-801).[15] NMDA-mediated activation of protein kinase activity in the dorsal horn can produce changes outlasting the initial stimulus by phosphorylating target proteins, ion channels, receptors and enzymes.[13] Brief pain inputs may also produce long-lasting changes by altering gene expression.[8,13]

This has been shown for immediate-early genes and for dynorphin.[13] The consequences of such changes for the nociceptive pathways could be far reaching.

Noxious stimulation is followed by a rapid change in gene expression within the postsynaptic neurones of the dorsal horn.[16] These postsynaptic events are detectable for several hours after stimulation.[16] The immediate-early gene *C-Fos* appears rapidly within the spinal cord after noxious stimulation. This gene codes for a protein (Fos). This Fos expression is a useful marker of the effect of peripheral noxious stimulation on postsysnaptic spinal cord neurones. Fos activation may result directly in the activation of analgesic compounds in the spinal cord.[16] As such, it may be a useful tool after nociceptive stimulation to examine the effectiveness of different analgesic regimens. An increased understanding of *C-Fos* as well as other upregulated genes (e.g. *Fos B, FRA-1, FRA-2, Jun B, Jun D* and *NGF1-A*) is likely to lead to many novel targets to restore spinal cord function in pain states and after nerve injury.[16]

Dynorphin is one of the genes that is induced by persistent nociceptive states. Persistent nociceptive states such as those encountered in tissue injury or inflammation are characterized by the induction of a network of genes in neurones in the dorsal spinal cord that commences within minutes of the onset of a persistent noxious stimulus.[15] During peripheral inflammation, the dynorphin gene is markedly upregulated in the dorsal spinal cord neurones.

C-Fos is rapidly transcribed and translated to yield the protein product. The *C-Fos* gene codes for a cellular bZIP transcription factor protein Fos. Fos is induced in a matter of minutes following a persistent noxious input, but the induction is transient: the mRNA has a half-life of approximately 4 hours, although the Fos protein may have a much more prolonged lifetime depending on the duration of the persistent input.[15] There are four genes coding for four Fos-like proteins: *C-Fos, Fos-B*, Fos-related antigen (*Fra-1*) and *Fra-2*.[15] The Jun family contains three members C-Jun, Jun-B and Jun-D.

The stimulation of nociceptive primary afferent neurones transynaptically turns on the expression of immediate-early genes, including the *C-Fos* proto-oncogene.[17] In response to nociceptive signalling by the A delta and C fibres, Fos-like proteins form homo- or heterodimeric transcription complexes, which then bind to specific DNA sequences to regulate the transcription of target genes.[17] Thus, changes in the transcriptional regulation of *C-Fos* may identify neuronal regions important in nociceptive processing.[17] The influx of calcium into neurones through the NMDA channel may be one means by which genes can be activated in dorsal horn neurones 15 minutes after noxious stimulation, either mechanical, thermal or inflammatory.[2] Thus, even with the most acute pains, there is the potential for marked alterations in the mechanisms of processing and even in the ultrastructure of neurones via gene expression. Since gene induction cannot be counteracted once set in motion, this has been used as a good reason for the use of pre-emptive analgesia: giving the analgesics before the pain is established.[2] However, not only are the physiological consequences of gene induction still unclear, but also animals are still completely

sensitive to analgesics in the presence of new genes.[2]

Dextromethorphan is available as an oral antitussive preparation with demonstrated clinical safety. Its ability to block a multiplicity of postsynaptic calcium channels, and thereby suppress neuronal excitability, may underlie its ability to suppress nociceptive behaviour and the induction of *C-Fos* mRNA.[17] Studies of dextromethorphan in the clinical management of chronic pain disorders are still needed.

Transgenic pain studies

A revolution in molecular biology has allowed, for the first time, the study of pain at the level of the gene, using transgenic mice that overexpress, or do not express, pain-related proteins.[5] Gene therapy overcomes specificity limitations of existing pharmacological ligands.[5] Gene therapy is the treatment of a disease or genetic defect by the insertion of DNA into the cells of a patient. Future possibilities in the case of pain control include conferring a new level of physiological modulation through the expression of a gene. Nociceptors are functional early in postnatal life, and the topographical pattern of their termination on second-order neurones is similar to that of adults.[18] Fos-like immunoreactive neurones are found in the superficial and deeper layers of the dorsal horn and in the ventral horn neurones.[18] Twenty-five different kinds of mutant mice – lacking neurotrophins and their receptors, peripheral mediators of nociception and hyperalgesia, opioids and their receptors, nonopioid transmitter receptors and intracellular molecules participating in signal conduction – have been produced and tested in behavioural assays of nociception.[5] New advances in molecular biological technology include:

- the cloning, sequencing and mapping of genes mediating biological phenomena;
- the study of gene expression in a tissue-specific, temporally specific and experience-dependent manner;
- the alteration of gene expression by antisense mRNA injection, or the creation of transgenic animals.[5]

Genetically altered mice have been subject to *in vivo* algesiometric testing.[5]

To create genetically altered transgenic animals, exogenous genes can be added to a genome, or endogenous genes can be inactivated (a null mutation) or otherwise functionally compromised.[5] A popular strategy is the creation of 'knock-out' mice by targeted gene disruption. DNA strands targeting vectors are usually designed with portions showing sequence identity to the targetted DNA, and portions of foreign sequence.[5] The targeting vector can be designed to integrate within the targeted sequence or to replace the targeted sequence so that it will no longer encode a functional protein.[5] Transgenic embryonic stem cells are microinjected into the blastocoele cavity of a pre-implantation mouse embryo, and the blastocyst is surgically implanted into the uterus of a pseudopregnant foster mother.[5] There is complete selectivity obtained in a knock-out mouse. Five classes of pain-relevant molecules have been studied using these techniques: neurotrophins and their receptors, peripheral mediators of nociception and hyperalgesia, opioids and their receptors, non-opioid neurotransmitter receptors and intracellular signal transduction molecules.[5]

Neurotrophins are necessary for the development and survival of peripheral neurones, and nociceptive neurones are the major targets of nerve growth factor (NGF) and other neurotrophins.[5] *In vivo* evidence for the involvement of NGF in the development of inflammatory and neuropathic hyperalgesia abounds.[5] After sciatic nerve section in the neonatal rat, the death of primary sensory neurones can be prevented by brain-derived neurotrophic factor (BDNF) and neurotrophin-3 (NT-3), which exert analgesic actions.[5] They bind to three tyrosine kinase receptors called trk (NGF only), trB (BDNF and NT-4) and tkC (NT-3), and to the p75 receptor.[5] Nociceptive testing has been performed on null mutants for NGF, trkA and p75 receptors, and on NGF transgenic mice.[5] 'Sense' mice with an increased NGF levels exhibit decreased thresholds to mechanical force, whereas NGF 'antisense' mice display analgesia.[5] NGF-overexpressing mice showed thermal hyperalgesia and allodynia, producing novel sympathetic projections to primary sensory neurones (similar to those seen in peripheral nerve injury), suggesting the involvement of NGF in neuropathic hyperalgesia.[5] TrkA-deficient mice display reduced sensitivity to thermal, mechanical and chemical stimulation, similar to the type IV hereditary sensory neuropathy seen in humans.[5] Mice lacking p75 receptors exhibit a tonic analgesia to both mechanical and heat stimuli.[5]

Substance P and its precursor, preprotachykinin-A (PPT-A) are upregulated by inflammation, and normally silent A beta fibres begin to express PPT-A and substance P, as well as increasing central excitability.[5] Knock-out mice lacking substance P

were found to exhibit relative analgesia, suggesting substance P to be involved in supraspinal pain modulation.[5] Data from PPT-A and NK_1 knock-out mice considered together are consistent with a proposed role for NK_2 receptors in mediating acute nociception.[5] Adenosine-2a receptors knock-out mice were found to display a relative tonic analgesia.[5]

The cloning of the mu opioid receptor, which followed the cloning of the kappa receptor, does not lend support to the existence of separate mu_1 and mu_2 subtypes.[19] Do these receptors result from the post-translational modification of a common protein?[19] This remains to be determined.[19] Endomorphins 1 and 2, displaying extremely high affinity and selectivity for mu receptors and producing spinal and supraspinal analgesia in mice, have recently been identified in the human brain.[19] When given intrathecally in rats, endomorphin 1 reduced C fibre and A beta fibre responses, while endomorphin 2 reduced C fibre responses only.[19] Endomorphins inhibit calcium ion entry through voltage-sensitive calcium channels and inhibit cAMP formation in cells expressing recombinant mu opioid receptors, also resulting in a decreased cardiac output and total peripheral resistance.[19] The clinical significance of these peptides in anaesthesiology and pain management will be carefully evaluated in the future.

Stress-induced analgesia has been found to be mediated by the endogenous opioids (endorphins, enkephalins and dynorphins), although considerable cross-reactivity has been documented across the opioid receptor gene family.[5] Enkephalin knock-out mice as well as neutral endopeptidase knock-out mice exhibit behaviours suggestive of tonic analgesia.[5] Mu opioid receptor knock-out mice display a complete absence of morphine analgesia as well as hypolocomotion, reward/reinforcement, physical dependence and immunosuppression.[5] No alterations in mu or kappa receptor binding properties, opioid peptide levels or morphine analgesia have been noted in delta receptor knock-out mice, and delta-preferring peptides exert their analgesic effects through mu receptors in delta knock-out mice.[5] Analgesia from the prototypical kappa-receptor agonist U50,488H is abolished in kappa receptor knock-out mice.[5]

A fascinating new orphanin FQ/nociceptin (OFQ/N) and its receptor (ORL1) have recently been identified.[19] OFQ/N and its receptor are related structurally, in terms of evolution and functionally to the classical opioids and opioid receptors respectively.[5] Rat localization studies reveal the receptor's mRNA and protein to be widely distributed throughout the CNS (especially in the hypothalamus and locus coeruleus in the brain).[20] The receptor is found in the pain pathways but does not bind to conventional opioids.[19] The endogenous peptide nociceptin, or orphanin FQ, produces a range of effects in animals, including analgesia, hyperalgesia and anti-opioid actions, but this is controversial.[19] The microsequence of this heptadecapeptide (similar to dynorphin) is: phe-gly-gly-phe-thr-gly-ala-arg-lys-ser-ala-arg-lys-leu-ala-asn-gln.[20] The peptide was named FQ-orphanin because its receptor had been known as the orphan receptor.[20] FQ represents the N-terminal (phenylalanine; abbreviated F) and C-terminal (glutamine; abbreviated Q) residues of the peptide.[20] Although OFQ/N receptor knock-out mice showed an unaltered morphine analgesic magnitude after acute injection, they displayed an impaired development of morphine analgesic tolerance after daily injections, which supports the involvement of OFQ/N as an anti-opioid peptide.[19] An antagonist for the orphan receptor with affinity at the peripheral type receptor has recently been described.[19] Nocistatin from the precursor protein of orphanin, prepronociceptin or prepro-orphanin FQ, which appears to reverse nociceptin action, has been described.[19] In OFQ/N receptor mutants, the absence of analgesia from the kappa$_3$ receptor ligand naloxone benzoylhydrazone strongly implicates this compound as an antagonist of the OFQ/N receptor.[5] There are reports of novel mutants lacking the OFQ/N precursor propeptide and corticotrophin releasing hormone with pain-relevant phenotypical alterations.[5] The sheer abundance of OFQ peptide in the brain and spinal cord implies that it is a major neurotransmitter.[20] The expression pattern of prepro-orphanin FQ and its receptor, as well as the anti-opioid effects that OFQ produced in rodents exposed to morphine, strongly suggest that the pharmacological manipulation of this system may have important clinical applications, ranging from pain management to the treatment of tolerance and dependence.[20]

Transgenic mice overexpressing or not expressing adrenergic receptor (AR) subtypes (AR$_{alpha\ 1a,1b,2a,2b,2c}$ and AR$_{beta\ 1,2}$) have been extensively tested for a variety of phenotypes.[5] The pharmacological tools for dissociating the three AR$_{alpha\ 2}$ subtypes are not presently available. The involvement of the AR$_{alpha\ 2}$ subtypes in the modulation of morphine analgesia remains unclear.[5] AR$_{alpha\ 2b,\ 2c}$ knock-out mice are, however, sensitive to the analgesic and antihyperalgesic effects of dexmedetomidine.[5]

Pharmacological evidence implicates 5-HT or serotonin subtypes 5-HT$_{1a}$ and 5-HT$_{1b}$ in nociceptive processing in the spinal cord.[5] Knock-out mice were found to be 10-fold more sensitive to morphine than wild-type alleles, a finding consistent with the 5-HT$_{1b}$ receptor's known status as an autoreceptor and the positive relationship between spinal cord serotonin levels and analgesic magnitude.[5] Increased serotonin release in the midbrain raphe nuclei of 5-HT$_{1b}$ knock-out mice has been shown; this area is known to be especially relevant to opioid analgesic magnitude.[5]

Transgenic technology has been used to study intracellular transduction systems in the changes that accompany inflammatory or chronic pain.[5] Two particular second messenger transduction cascades have been implicated – the cyclic adenosine 3'-5'-monophosphate (c-AMP)-dependent protein kinase A system, and the calcium ion-dependent protein kinase C system – in the postsynaptic mediation of peripheral and central sensitization.[5] Protein kinase A is a tetrameric molecule made up of two regulatory (containing the cAMP binding site) and two catalytic subunits. Regulatory subunit isoenzymes (R I alpha, R I beta, R II alpha, R II beta) with distinct expression have been characterized.[5] R I beta knock-out mice display significant reductions in the tonic phases of the formalin test, in capsaicin-evoked neurogenic inflammation and in prostaglandin E$_2$-evoked cAMP-dependent thermal hyperalgesia.[5] R I beta-containing protein kinase A thus plays a critical role in the expression of neurogenic inflammation, oedema and persistent pain following tissue injury, but does not contribute to pain from peripheral nerve injury.[5] Both protein kinase A (using null mutations) and protein kinase C have been found to be involved in tissue injury nociceptive pain.[5] Neuropathic pain (invoked by nerve injury), however, involves protein kinase C gamma (rather than protein kinase A R I beta), suggesting that these intracellular transduction systems are an attractive target for drug development in chronic pain.[5] The absence of thermal hyperalgesia occurs from the spinal administration of prostaglandin E$_2$ in mice lacking the epsilon 1 and epsilon 4 subunits of the NMDA receptor.[5] Unaltered thermal and mechanical hyperalgesia was observed in intraplantar complete Freund's adjuvant injection in mice lacking the cytokine/leukaemia inhibitory factor despite large increases in Freunds' adjuvant inflammation in the mutants.[5]

In contrast to work using NO synthetase inhibitors, mice lacking the neuronal form (nNOS) of the enzyme synthethizing NO displayed a normal sensitization of nociceptive neurones as assessed by an unaltered formalin test behaviour.[5] It was concluded that, although NO is clearly involved in nociception, it is not necessarily required for the development of noxious stimulation-induced sensitization.[5]

The involvement of the G_i/G_o proteins in opioid analgesia has been repeatedly shown using pertussin toxin.[5] Antisense studies have demonstrated a complicated pattern of specific opioid receptor types to G protein subtypes.[5] G_o knock-out mice show hyperalgesia on the hot-plate test.[5]

Knock-out mice lack the targeted gene throughout development, leading to a plethora of compensatory reactions explaining the mild phenotypes seen.[5] Phenotypical differences in knock-out mice have also been attributed to the inheritance of 129-derived alleles of hitchhiking genes, which may confound some existing knock-out studies of pain.[5] Yet recent advanced techniques have been developed (called 'conditional'/'inducible' knock-outs), in which a spatial and/or temporal control over gene disruption is afforded.[5] Genetic rescue or the elimination of knock-out mice on pure genetic backgrounds should completely eliminate this problem.[5] To eliminate gene disruption by the genetic background on which it is placed, the moderately scoring DBA/2 strain of mice has been proposed as a more appropriate genetic background for transgenic pain studies.[5] Alternate approaches in the future study of the mechanisms of pain, include:[5]

- pharmacological studies using newly developed, more selective ligands;
- antisense strategies;
- gene mapping efforts using inbred mouse strains;
- human association and sib-pair linkage studies of gene variants.

With this in mind, transgenic technology should contribute greatly to pain research.

AUTONOMICALLY MEDIATED PAIN

The autonomic nervous system modulates inflammation, pain transmission, pain perception and the response to analgesics, and may be involved in the perpetuation of pain.[21] Cytokines are important triggers of the stress response, and the autonomic nervous system is one of the axes of stress response.[21] After certain injuries, cutaneous nociceptors develop an enhanced α_1-adrenergic response to sympathetic efferent activity. Thus a peripheral α-adrenergic mechanism has been found to operate in sympathetically maintained pain (see Chapter 10).

NEUROCHEMISTRY OF CENTRAL PAIN

The pathophysiology of central pain, that is, pain resulting from CNS damage along the spinothalamo-cortical pathway, has so far eluded the efforts of many investigators.[22] It may be caused by a deranged neurotransmission between the sensory thalamus and sensory cortical areas.[22] It is speculated that a relative hypofunction of GABAergic inhibition at both thalamic and cortical levels leads to a sectorial excitatory hypertonus in those same areas.[22] A blend of the two should mark each patient. A proposed protocol of evaluation and therapeutic intervention is as follows:[22]

1. Central pain should initially be assessed with a GABAergic agent (e.g. propofol);
2. a trial of intrathecal midazolam or baclofen is the next step, and being followed, if successful, by chronic programmable pump infusion of the drug;
3. a ketamine test (intravenously or intramuscularly) as a second assessment, followed by a continuous subcutaneous infusion if successful, watching for psychomimetic side-effects;
4. oral lamotrigine and other antiglutaminergic drugs (felbamate, high-dose dextromorphan, GABApentin and memantine);
5. other drugs (clonidine for spinal cord pain, amitriptyline, opioids and mexilitene).

Potent new brain imaging techniques (PET, SPECT, fMRI, SQUID/MEG) will help to delineate which brain stations are involved in central pain and optimize the ability to modulate such deranged biochemistry.[22]

PRE-EMPTIVE ANALGESIA

Pre-emptive analgesia implies that analgesia given before the painful stimulus prevents or reduces subsequent pain. Its purpose is to prevent or reduce any 'memory' of the pain stimulus in the nervous system, thereby lowering any subsequent analgesic requirement.[23] There is clear basic scientific evidence for pre-emptive analgesia in terms of reduced CNS excitation.[23] Physiology and behaviourial animal studies show that noxious stimulus-induced neuroplasticity can be prevented, or 'pre-empted', by the administration of analgesics prior to injury.[24] The pre-emptive use of local anaesthetics delays the development of autotomy after peripheral nerve section by several weeks.[23] Bathing the peripheral nerves with local anaesthetic prior to transection decreases the incidence of behaviours indicative of pain in the weeks after neurectomy. Pre-treatment with mu-opioid agonists or local anaesthetics prevents the development of injury-induced spinal hyperexcitability and pain-related behaviour.[24,25] When given after prolonged central excitability, they are, however, much less effective.[24]

Pre-emptive analgesia may protect patients from the deleterious effects of surgical incision and other noxious perioperative events, long after the operation has been performed, by attenuating or preventing central sensitization. In a small number of patients, a reduction in the incidence of phantom limb pain occurred after elective amputation for ischaemic vascular disease when, for 3 days before operation, the pain was reduced by epidural local anaesthetic and opioid.[26] Numerous studies have confirmed the short-term benefit of pre-emptive interventions aimed at blocking nociceptive input from the periphery to the CNS.[27] Additional benefits have been seen in selected patient populations, including decreased long-term postoperative pain at iliac crest bone donor sites in patients undergoing spinal fusion surgery, and a reduction in the severity of phantom limb pain in post-amputation patients. Other studies point to a lack of benefit or a less than anticipated benefit. These negative results are most probably caused by continuous afferent input from the surgical area, leading to pain and the re-establishment of neuroplasticity after the initial pre-emptive analgesia has disappeared, or by an inadequate level of block in the beginning.[27] This underscores some of the current controversies surrounding pre-emptive analgesia: how intense and how long must the pre-emptive intervention be sustained in the postoperative period to guarantee a prolonged benefit? The initial enthusiasm for the idea of pre-emptive analgesia has diminished somewhat as clinical studies have so far failed to support the concept,[28] most probably because of a number

of confounding factors and the use of study designs that have made it difficult to find any reliable answers. The evidence from randomized controlled trials has now been reviewed.[29] Four studies with paracetamol or NSAIDs did not show any pre-emptive effect. Of the 7 studies using local anaesthetic, 6 did not show a pre-emptive effect. In the 4 opioid studies, there was weak evidence of a pre-emptive effect in 3. It may be that any pre-emptive effect of opioids is counteracted by the induction of acute tolerance. Meta-analysis is very difficult in this field because of the outcome measures investigators are using.[29]

Complete local anaesthesia that prevents afferent impulses from the injured tissue reaching the spinal cord will, of course, prevent central sensitization, but only for as long as the blockade is effective.[28] Local anaesthetic blockade of peripheral nerves will not decrease or eliminate the central sensitization once it has been established. Systemic opioids act both presynaptically, to reduce transmitter release, and postsynaptically, to hyperpolarize the cell membrane of the dorsal horn neurones. Low doses of morphine have been shown to prevent the establishment of central sensitization, but, once established, about 10 times the dose is required to suppress it.[28] Appropriate pre-injury treatment can probably reduce postoperative pain and hyperalgesia. However, there is an ongoing nociceptive input into, and sensitization of, the CNS from the injured tissue during and after surgery. This requires that a pre-emptive analgesia regimen should continue from before the onset of the surgical insult until wound healing is well established. A clinically more relevant study design than giving a single-shot bolus before or after surgery is the use of a pharmacokinetically guided infusion to ensure that all patients have similar organ concentrations at the time of outcome measurement.[28]

The prevention of chronic postoperative neuropathic pain is a very important aspect of pre-emptive analgesia. The NMDA receptors are probably involved in the development of persistent postoperative neuropathic pain. Combining an NMDA receptor antagonist with an opioid or a local anaesthetic may be a strategy to give adequate acute pain relief and inhibit the process of central sensitization and hyperalgesia. Prospective, correctly designed and well-controlled studies are needed to clarify whether a continuous pre-emptive analgesia regimen for postoperative pain will reduce the incidence of chronic pain after surgery. The prevention of postoperative pain is based on two phenomena:[30]

1. The effective blockade of noxious stimuli generated during surgery and during the initial postoperative period (inflammatory phases) reduces subsequent postoperative pain (the phenomenon of pre-emptive analgesia in the broad sense).

2. An antinociceptive treatment started before surgery is more effective in the reduction of postoperative pain than is treatment given on recovery from general anaesthesia (the phenomenon of pre-emptive analgesia in the narrow sense).

It was found that both phenomena can be induced by neural blockade with local anaesthetics, and by systemic or epidural opioids. Clinically impressive results are observed when the blockade of noxious stimuli is complete and extended into the initial postoperative period (a combination of both phenomena).[30]

NSAIDs may be better able to break down central sensitization once it is established than may opioids used in postoperative doses.[31] It makes sense to ensure that adequate opioids are active before severe surgical stimulation in the patient during inhalational general anaesthesia, since inhalational anaesthesia does not protect against central sensitization.[31] A correct definition of pre-emptive analgesia should emphasize the importance of treatment that prevents the development of central hyperexcitability even if it occurs after surgery.[30] Allodynia and hyperalgesia observed in postsurgical patients may be related to the postoperative sensitization of central neurones. A recent study showed increased sensitivity to noxious sural nerve stimulation in postoperative patients using subjective parameters and nociceptive flexion reflexes compared with a control group of volunteers.[25] Another study showed that thoracotomy patients receiving epidural fentanyl before incision have less pain and need fewer analgesics postoperatively compared with patients receiving the same dose of epidural fentanyl after incision.[24]

Opioid peptides are effective in reducing windup, but only when applied pre-emptively, by activating receptors on the spinal cord neurones (mu, delta and kappa) or on the primary afferent nerve fibres (mu and delta).[6] Opioid peptides probably exert their effects by blocking voltage-gated calcium channels that will prevent neurotransmitter release from the primary afferent nerve fibres, or by opening potassium channels, which will result in neuronal hyperpolarization, or both.[6] Opioid premedication has been found to reduce the sustained

hyperexcitability of the CNS to intraoperative stimuli, prolonging the pain-free period immediately postoperatively and decreasing the frequency of analgesic demands.[32] The NSAIDs (naproxen and indomethacin) given as premedicants have also been found to decrease postoperative pain and to lessen postoperative analgesic requirements.[33,34] An interesting question posed is whether the NMDA antagonists (ketamine and pentazocine) will also confer protection from needless pain if given to patients before surgical incision?[24] In future, the provision of pre-emptive analgesia should engender multiple benefits not only in the acute perioperative pain situation, but also in preventing the development of neuropathic painful states.

MULTIMODAL ANALGESIA

The provision of pre-emptive analgesia is advantageous, but, to be completely successful, the following components are necessary: an opioid, an NSAID, afferent sensory blockade, sympathetic blockade and anxiolysis.[35] The plasticity in opioid controls illustrates the advantage of combining opioids with local anaesthetics, α_2-adrenergic agonists and NMDA antagonists where reducing excitability or enhancing inhibition improves opioid efficacy.[8,36] The rationale is that each drug exerts its analgesic effect via a different mechanism. Thus, a low-dose combination might offer the best therapeutic effect while minimizing the risk of the unwanted side-effects seen with high doses of each of these drugs. This is known as multimodal analgesia.

There is clinical evidence that the neuraxial combination of local anaesthetics and opioids produces improved analgesia in a variety of acute pain states compared with systemic opioids.[37] Preliminary evidence suggests that increases in perioperative coagulability can be reduced and the recovery of gastrointestinal functions hastened after epidural analgesia.[37] Preliminary data also suggest that epidural analgesia is beneficial for patients at high risk of cardiac, pulmonary and infectious morbidity, especially after major surgery.[37] Combination therapy is useful in neuropathic (and other chronic pain states) where there is a reduction or loss of opioid sensitivity. Here, combination therapy may restore pain relief without the need to augment the dose and risk side-effects. Multimodal analgesia will have a powerful influence on the injury response and may even prevent the development of chronic pain syndromes in surgical patients.

NERVE GROWTH FACTOR

Recent evidence shows that NGF regulates nociception in health and disease.[38,39] NGF is a protein normally produced by cells in target organs (e.g. skin, blood vessels and bladder). It is secreted and taken up by sympathetic and small sensory fibres. NGF acts on trk-A receptors. The high-affinity form of trk-A receptors is associated with a tyrosine kinase. The NGF–receptor complex is internalized and transported to the soma of the neurone, where it alters gene transcription in the nucleus.[40] The result in primary afferent nociceptive neurones includes an increased synthesis of substance P and CGRP. An excess of NGF (as found in animal models of inflammation) may produce hyperalgesia by sensitizing nociceptors, by increasing levels of substance P and CGRP, and by the release of histamine.[38,39] In such conditions, anti-NGF treatment (e.g. with trkAIgG) may reduce hyperalgesia. Paradoxically, however, NGF may play a different role in the development of chronic pain (e.g. neuropathic pain) that results from cell death or atrophy and failure of adaption in the spinal cord.[38,39] In such cases, NGF may, at the appropriate time, dose, site and mode of administration, provide prophylaxis and treatment in conditions that lead to chronic pain.[38,39]

PERIPHERAL ACTION OF OPIOIDS AND THE CENTRAL ACTION OF NSAIDs

Human peripheral nerves have been found to contain endogenous opioid ligands (beta-endorphin and met-enkephalin) as well as opioid receptors.[41] Opioid receptors have been demonstrated on the peripheral terminals of thinly myelinated and unmyelinated sensory nerves in animals and humans. The opioid receptor messenger RNA has been detected in dorsal root ganglia.[42] These findings are in line with functional studies indicating that C fibre neurones mediate the peripheral antinociceptive effects of morphine.[42] Recent animal and human studies reveal that immune cells produce endogenous opioids during inflammation.[42] This production of opioids is matched by an increased expression of different opioid receptors on primary afferent nociceptors, where they can exert analgesic activity. Endogenous ligands of peripheral opioid receptors, opioid peptides (endorphin, enkephalin and dynorphin) and their respective mRNAs have been discovered in inflamed tissue.[42] These peptides can be produced by immune cells, including T- and B-lymphocytes, monocytes and macro-phages. The injection of mu-, delta- and kappa-selective agonists produces selective peripheral antinociceptive effects that can be blocked by the respective selective antagonists.[42] Opioids also act peripherally on sympathetic fibres.[42] These data suggest that both primary afferent nociceptors and sympathetic fibres could be targets for peripherally acting opioids, which would avoid the sedative and psychotropic effects of existing opioids, as well as the problem of dependence. Opioids (fentanyl) injected as very low doses into the rat brachial plexus sheath give rise to a localized, potent and prolonged antinociceptive effect, which is naloxone reversible.[43] Opioids (fentanyl and pethidine) can block peripheral conduction.[36,44] A growing number of controlled clinical studies examining the local analgesic effects of opioids is emerging. A wide variety of regional analgesic techniques could be enhanced by using exogenous opioids to bind to endogenous peripheral nerve opioid receptors.[42] In humans, studies show prolonged regional analgesia after giving opioids (morphine, fentanyl and buprenorphine) combined with local anaesthetics.[45] Several laboratories have recently developed a number of opioid compounds that do not cross the blood–brain barrier, some of which have already shown promising results in preclinical testing.[42]

Recent experiments have indicated that, in addition to their peripheral actions, NSAIDs may exert an important central action in hyperalgesic states,[46] and a central mode of action (in addition to the peripheral effects) of the NSAIDs now seems certain.[47,48] A greater understanding of enantiomer pharmacology may lead to the development of safer drugs. The discovery of an inducible cyclo-oxygenase offers additional insight into NSAID activity.[47] Great interest is currently being placed in the potential for COX-2 inhibitors, which might avoid the adverse effects of damage to the gastric mucosa and kidney, while retaining their analgesic properties.[9] Prototypes such as SC-58125 and

L-745,337 seem, in the rat, to fulfil these hopes. R-Ketoprofen reduces gastrointestinal side-effects compared with racemic ketoprofen. The intrathecal administration of NSAIDs has been shown to cause inhibition of the late phase behavioural and electrophysiological responses to formalin.[47] Low intrathecal doses of NSAIDs also reverse the thermal hyperalgesia elicited by intrathecal NMDA or substance P.[47] The spinal effects of selective COX-2 inhibitors have not yet been reported.[47] The discovery of a second form of cyclo-oxygenase offers potential for the development of a novel, safe and effective antihyperalgesic agent, even though a COX-2 inhibitor will produce only the same analgesic relief as the current NSAIDs, which clearly show a ceiling effect in their analgesic action in humans.[49] Celecoxib inhibits COX-2 with a 375-fold selectivity over COX-1 (B.D. Schwartz, 1998, unpublished data). There is still a major requirement for the development of more efficacious analgesics to treat arthritic pain. The successful management of cancer-related pain often requires the use of NSAIDs, either alone or in combination with other analgesic drugs.[50] They have some efficacy in malignant neuropathic pain. Inhibitors of the lipo-oxygenase pathway products (leukotrienes), for example CP-105,696, have been lacking in analgesic activity (although they do reduce the symptoms and signs of inflammation).[9] CP-105,696 (the novel leukotriene B$_4$ antagonist) attenuates the progression of collagen-induced arthritis.[3] Unanswered questions include the use of long-term continuous NSAID infusions, the use of neuraxial NSAIDs and the development of NSAIDs with a better profile than that of existing agents.

Cytokine-suppressive anti-inflammatory drugs such as SKF 86002 inhibit the production of interleukin-1 and tumour necrosis factor-alpha, and show analgesic activity in acute and chronic pain models.[3] SKF 86002 blocks the activity of the serine/threonine protein kinases.[3] Cytokine suppressive anti-inflammatory drugs, by blocking the activity of these kinases, may provide new analgesic or anti-inflammatory drugs for clinical use.

ADRENAL MEDULLARY IMPLANTS

Adrenal medullary tissue transplanted into the intrathecal space of experimental animals not only survives, but also continues to produce adrenergic agonists and opioid peptides, and, more importantly, produces analgesia.[51] In the rat model, this method was found to decrease the onset and frequency of autotomy.[52] CSF levels of noradrenaline and met-enkephalin are markedly increased. In humans, preliminary data indicate that this technique decreases terminal cancer pain.[51,53] In the future, there is the potential for transplants into the CNS to provide a local source of neuroactive substances for reducing pain sensitivity. This will provide a new therapeutic approach to the treatment of chronic pain.[52,54]

NEUROTRANSMITTERS, AGONISTS AND ANTAGONISTS/BLOCKERS

In addition to opioids, for which the mu, delta and kappa receptors represent useful analgesic targets, a wide range of agents have been shown to modulate nociceptive processing, with some selectivity. Agonists at the α-adrenergic, serotoninergic, adenosine (A$_1$ and A$_2$), GABA$_B$, muscarinic, neuropeptide Y, neurokinin, somatostatin, neurotensin and calcitonin receptors exert antinociceptive effects in behavioural tests.[46]

Agonists

ADENOSINE AGONISTS

The endogenous neuromodulator adenosine exerts its effects by activating specific extracelluar receptors (A$_1$, A$_{2A}$, A$_{2B}$ and A$_3$). In the dorsal horn, the adenosine receptors are involved in mediating an antinociceptive effect from A$_1$ and A$_2$ agonists.[42,45,55] Studies suggest that the antinociceptive action results from activation of A$_1$ receptors, which are known to exert pre- and postsynaptic inhibitory effects on the dorsal horn. Adenosine or adenosine agonists interact (like NMDA antagonists) with the release of glutamate in dorsal horn interneurones, blocking the allodynia to low-threshold tactile stimuli. Adenosine agonists (like NMDA antagonists) have been shown to be powerful anticonvulsants. Of interest is that the tricyclic antidepressants are also potent inhibitors of adenosine uptake. In rats, intrathecal injections of R-phenyl isopropyladenosine, a selective A$_1$ receptor agonist induces significant antinociception without inducing motor impairment.[56] A$_1$ receptor agonists might prove to be useful analgesic agents, either as systemic agents, provided that the problems of cardiovascular side-effects and effective penetration into the CNS can be overcome, or for use neuraxially, possibly in combination with opioids.[42,55] Agents that inhibit adenosine metabolism may have a similar analgesic and anti-inflammatory profile, with the advantage of a reduced side-effect profile compared with direct agonists.

α_2-ADRENERGIC AGONISTS

α_2-Adrenergic agonists are likely to be used more and more in anaesthesia and analgesia. With α_2-adrenergic isoreceptors (α_{2A}, α_{2B} and α_{2C}), it may be possible to differentiate spinal analgesia from side-effects using receptor subtype-selective agents. The future of the α_2-adrenergic agonists will be enhanced by the clinical availability of an α-adrenergic receptor antagonist and isoreceptor-selective agonists (without sedation or hypotension).[45,55] There is evidence that two pharmacologically discernible components contribute to α_2-adrenergic agonist-elicited analgesia.[46] These may be found to correspond to the subtypes of the α_2 receptor as defined by molecular cloning techniques.

CAPSAICIN

Capsaicin, the active ingredient in hot chili peppers, is a polymodal nociceptor agonist but has selected actions on unmyelinated C fibres and thinly myelinated A delta primary sensory neurones.[57,58] It is a cell-specific peripheral analgesic. Agonism, that is, the ability to open capsaicin-operative channels, is required for its efficacy. Although the initial topical application of capsaicin (0.025–1 per cent) is algesic, repeated application leads to desensitization. It is calcium dependent and probably involves the activation of a phosphatase that inactivates the capsaicin channel. Functional desensitization is a loss of sensitivity to a range of noxious stimuli and underlies the analgesic effects of capsaicin (because of the depletion of neurotransmitters such as substance P and CGRP).[9] This is reversible and may also depend on the calcium-dependent dephosphorylation of other intracellular proteins such as enzymes or ion channels.[58] High concentrations can block C fibre conduction and result in long-lasting sensory deficits.[58] Neurotoxicity is induced by high doses of capsaicin.[58] Topical application causes an initial burning pain and hyperalgesia, followed by a

late selective local anaesthesia. Topical applications are effective in treating post-herpetic neuralgia, diabetic neuropathy, cluster headaches, CRPSs and arthritis (rheumatoid and osteoarthritis), and are without side-effects.[57] Topical capsaicin is used in the treatment of pruritus, which is believed to be mediated by a subset of capsaicin-sensitive nociceptive neurones.[58] There is potential therapeutic usefulness in an analogue of capsaicin, which retains its selective action on primary afferent neurones and analgesic activity but is devoid of unwanted side-effects'. A better window between analgesic doses and doses that produce side-effects is required for an orally active therapeutic drug. Three such examples are olvanil, nuvanil and resiniferatoxin.[58] The effects of topical capsaicin in doses of 1–2 orders of magnitude higher than are commercially available are currently being investigated, with encouraging results (J.N. Campbell, 1998, unpublished data).

Neurotransmitter antagonists/blockers

NMDA ANTAGONISTS

The NMDA complex is thus involved in sustaining or even magnifying pain transmission in the cord.[55,59] NMDA antagonists have been shown to reduce the heightened excitability of the flexion reflex produced by inflammatory agents.[11] Non-competitive and competitive antagonists have been tested. Both non-competitive antagonists (dizocilpine and 5-amino phosphovalerate,[60,61] HU211[62] and ketamine) and the highly specific competitive antagonist 3(R-2-carboxypiperazin-4 yl)-propyl-1-phosphonic acid (or D-CPP, which binds to the NMDA receptor-gated ion channel) prevent wind-up and central sensitization (in the rat spinal cord).[59,63,64] This suggests that autotomy in rats is mediated by long-lasting NMDA receptor-related spinal disinhibition. NMDA antagonists may also be involved in hippocampal long-term potentiation or 'pain memory'.[59] Selective NMDA receptor antagonists are anticonvulsant in many seizure models.[65] The clinical use of NMDA antagonists could present problems such as amnesia, psychotomimesis and sedation.[66] Ketamine and 5-amino phosphovalerate can cause motor toxicity. Nevertheless, for optimal pain relief, any change occurring at the NMDA receptor complex should be prevented (for acute pain) or reversed (for chronic pain).[59]

NMDA antagonists such as ketamine,

dextromorphan, MK-801 (acting at the PCP site and blocking the channel), 2-amino-5-phosphonopentoic acid (AP-5), CPP (acting at the NMDA site), 7-chlorokynurenate (acting at the glycine site) and CNQX (acting on AMPA sites needed for activation) have been shown to attenuate the neuronal and behavioural response to noxious stimuli.[9] Expansion of the dorsal horn neurone receptive fields is a manifestation of plasticity and is reduced by NMDA receptor antagonists. In patients with neuropathic pain, hyperalgesia and spreading pain have been reduced and the afterdischarges in the dorsal horn neurones abolished. Pretreatment in animal models has been shown to reduce the increased expression of Fos in response to noxious stimuli. Although NMDA receptor antagonists have found a place in the treatment in chronic pain, their usefulness is likely to be limited by the distribution of the receptor within the CNS.[9]

Data from preclinical and clinical studies support the intimate association between wind-up, spinal NMDA receptors and the centralization of nociceptive stimuli in neuropathic pain states.[67] Clinical trials indicate that the practical uses of non-competitive NMDA receptor blockers, such as ketamine, dextromethorphan and memantine, will become part of accepted therapeutic regimens in the management of neuropathic pain.[67] These prevent or block central hypersensitive states. They have no effect on the inputs onto the cells but abolish wind-up, thus converting the potentiated response to a steady response. As a result of the different but complementary effects of opioids and NMDA antagonists on wind-up events, profound inhibitions of nociceptive responses can predictably be seen with threshold doses of morphine combined with NMDA antagonists in both short-term inflammatory and neuropathic models.[2] The marked heterogenicity in the molecular structures and anatomical distribution of glutamate receptor subtypes throughout the CNS indicates the potential use of non-NMDA receptor antagonists for the treatment of pain.[67]

SUBSTANCE P AND NEUROKININ ANTAGONISTS

Substance P and NK A mediate their pharmacological actions at distinct receptor subtypes and play a critical role in a number of physiological and pathophysiological processes, including nociception and the processing of sensory information.[49] Blockers of specific mediators may provide novel classes of analgesic agent. The tachykinins (substance P, NK A

and NK B) act on tachykinin receptors (NK_1, NK_2 and NK_3). Positive data have been obtained from electrophysiological studies in which antagonists reduce certain nociceptive inputs.[49] Highly selective substance P (or NK_1) antagonists, such as CP-96345, CP-99,994, RP-67580, RP-100893, L-733,060 and SR-140333, show good analgesic activity (in animal models).[3,49,68] A number of pharmaceutical companies have NK_1 antagonists in clinical development, with pain and inflammation as major targets.

Of more relevance to chronic pain is the evaluation of the non-peptide NK_2 receptor antagonists (SR-48968 and SR-159897) in models of persistent hyperalgesia.[49] SR-48968 is effective in both electrophysiological and behavioural models of brief nociceptive responses and has led to the new, and now directly testable, hypothesis of NK_2 blockade for clinical pain relief.[46] It has been proposed that combining NK_1 and NK_2 antagonists (and blocking substance P and NK A simultaneously), might yield a more efficacious analgesic agent.[49] Also, optimal physiological blockade may result from the combined administration of NMDA and NK_1 receptor antagonists.

BRADYKININ RECEPTOR ANTAGONISTS

Evidence that bradykinin is physiologically a mediator of pain and inflammation comes from the fact that competitive antagonists at bradykinin receptors ($beta_1$ and $beta_2$) show antinociceptive and anti-inflammatory activity in the animal model.[69] Bradykinin receptor antagonists provide potential for analgesia because of the prominence of bradykinin in the production of pain and inflammation. Bradykinin $beta_1$ receptor antagonists could potentially have a role in the treatment of chronic pain, in which they have been shown to modulate the hyperalgesia associated with chronic inflammation.[55] Some of the newly developed bradykinin $beta_2$-receptor antagonists, NPC 16731, NPC 567, HOE 140, CP 0127, and the non-peptide antagonist WIN 64338, may prove clinically useful in the inhibition of pain and inflammation in the acute setting.[3,9]

CCK ANTAGONISTS[45]

CCK is an endogenous inhibitor of opioid-mediated analgesia. It mobilizes calcium from intracellular stores on the spinal terminals of C fibres, thus counteracting the opioid inhibition of transmitter release.[70] The postsynaptic CCK receptors are mainly of the CCK_B type in the rat but of the

CCK$_A$ type in the primate.[70] CCK$_A$ antagonists (devazepide and lorglumide) may enhance the analgesic potency of opioids.[3] However, the presynaptic receptors are of the CCK$_B$ type in all species, and it is probable that these receptors interfere with opioid actions.[70] CCK$_B$ antagonists have been shown to potentiate the actions of opioids in rodent nociceptive tests.[49] CCK antagonists may well enhance morphine analgesia in non-pathological pain states, as well as restoring morphine analgesia in humans with neuropathic pain.[2,70]

CGRP ANTAGONISTS

CGRP is released in the dorsal horn in response to noxious stimuli. Antagonists to this peptide still need to be developed and tested, so its exact role in pain processing is unknown.[70] CGRP shares the same degrading peptidases as substance P, its presence allowing substance P to escape degradation and diffuse over greater distances in the cord.[70] An antinociceptive effect of anti-CGRP antiserum has been reported.[46]

NEUROPEPTIDE Y ANTAGONISTS

The level of neuropeptide Y is markedly elevated in the dorsal horn following peripheral nerve injury.[49] There is a strong correlation between the magnitude of hyperalgesia and the elevation of neuropeptide Y expression in laminae III/IV of the dorsal horn, suggesting a linkage. NMDA antagonists (MK-801) and α_2-adrenegic agonists (clonidine) delay the onset of hyperalgesia as well as neuropeptide Y expression.[49] The development of a selective neuropeptide Y antagonist is necessary for further understanding of this peptide.

SEROTONIN (5-HT) ANTAGONISTS

Subtypes of the serotonin receptor appear to exert quite different effects on nociceptive processing: 5-HT$_{1B}$ sites exert an antinociceptive influence, whereas 5-HT$_2$, 5-HT$_3$ and probably also 5-HT$_{1A}$ sites facilitate nociceptive responses.[48] Serotonin may sensitize or directly activate some nociceptors. This can be inhibited by the 5-HT$_3$ antagonist ICS 2051930.[69] The possibility exists that other subtypes of 5-HT receptor, such as the 5-HT$_4$ receptor (which is also blocked by ICS 2051930), are also involved in hyperalgesia.[69]

The 5-HT$_2$ antagonist ketanserin has been used in the treatment of algodystrophy and in certain collagen diseases (Raynaud's disease).[71] The activity of ketanserin is essentially peripheral, and the availability of centrally acting congeners such as ritanserin will not only be of value clinically, but also shed some light on the part that serotonin plays in nociception and its possible sites of activity.[40,66] A full characterization of 5-HT receptor subtypes in nociceptive processing, together with the development of highly selective agents, clearly has the potential to lead to useful new analgesics.[48]

Inhibitory neuropeptides

GALANIN

Galanin is a putative inhibitory peptide that is localized with substance P and CGRP in a large proportion of primary afferents. Galanin exerts a tonic inhibitory effect on nociceptive transmission in the dorsal horn in studies of thermal nociception,[42,55,70] but there is also evidence that it has pronociceptive effects. Galanin-like agonists may be used for developing new analgesic drugs, but the development of selective antagonists is necessary for the further understanding of this peptide.

SOMATOSTATIN

Somatostatin is released into the dorsal horn by noxious stimuli, apparently originating from a subpopulation of fine afferent fibres.[48] The iontophorectic application of somatostatin results in the hyperpolarization of dorsal horn neurones and a reduction in spontaneous firing.[70] This peptide is a potential primary afferent inhibitory transmitter. Intrathecal somatostatin may be analgesic in animals and humans[43] but can show neurotoxicity at high doses. Octreotide produces analgesia in humans when given systemically.[3] Molecular cloning techniques have revealed the existence of at least five types of somatostatin receptor,[48] for which discriminately pharmacological agents are unknown. The development of such agents (especially in non-peptide forms) may in future provide an important addition to analgesic therapy.

Others

Although vasoactive intestinal polypeptide is present in the primary sensory neurones, its role during the spinal nociceptive processing of noxious cutaneous or visceral stimuli is unknown.[70] Selective vasoactive intestinal polypeptide antagonists need to be developed.

Another substance, bombesin, present in small

afferents, also modifies dorsal horn neurone excitability and nociceptive behaviour.[46] Its role in processing sensory input still needs further exploration.

MODULATION OF ION CHANNELS

Sodium channel blockers

It has been found that systemic lignocaine silences ectopic neuroma and dorsal root ganglion discharge without blocking nerve conduction, which is a useful property for treating neuropathic pain.[72] Like lignocaine, anticonvulsants (phenytoin and carbamazepine) and other class I antiarrhythmics also block voltage-sensitive sodium ion channels, suppressing the ectopic discharge in injured peripheral nerves.[72] In future, an important advance would be the synthesis of active derivatives of these drugs that do not cross the blood–brain barrier.

The effectiveness of anticonvulsants, antiarrhythmics and local anaesthetics in the treatment of neuropathic pain reflects the fact that they are sodium channel blockers and that neuronal activity is ultimately dependent on the depolarization of cells by the ingress of sodium ions.[9] The finding that specific types of sodium channel are present at the site of nerve injury (type III) and in small polymodal nociceptors (tetrodotoxin resistant) brings the hope that more specific drugs could become available in the future.[52] Thus, the tetrodotoxin-resistant sodium channel (of small diameter slow-conducting cells) offers an attractive target for novel analgesic drugs. Selectivity for sensory versus motor, and for nociceptive versus non-nociceptive sensory afferent fibres, is a highly desirable and long-sought-after property for local anaesthetics. The steroidal alkaloid veratridine holds sodium channels open rather than blocking them (in the rabbit).[36,73] It appears preferentially to block unmyelinated C fibres, although it does inhibit motor function (in the rat).[73,74] In the future, it might serve as an adjuvant to the more traditional local anaesthetics.

Potassium channel openers

Opening potassium channels results in membrane hyperpolarization and an inhibition of membrane excitability, effects that might be exploited in analgesia. The analgesic effects of maxi-potassium openers (dehydrosaponins and the substituted benzimidazolones – NS 004 and NS 1619) or the ATP-sensitive potassium channel openers (cromakalim, pinacidil and aprikalim) still need to be adequately assessed.[3]

Cholinergic channel modulators

Emerging knowledge related to the diversity of neuronal nicotinic acetylcholine receptors suggests that the modulation of distinct cellular and tissue functions is mediated by neuronal nicotinic acetylcholine receptor subtypes. Epibatidine (isolated from frog skin) is a potent nicotinic agonist, about 100 times more potent than and equally efficacious to morphine in producing antinociceptive effects.[42,55] However, it is extremely toxic, causing hypertension, respiratory paralysis and seizures, with death at doses not much higher than those required for antinociception.[75] Epibatidine can exist as two enantiomers, R(+) or S(–), with little difference in pharmacological activity and with similar affinity and potency as antinociceptive agents.[75] In all rodent experimental paradigms, epibatidine is equiactive and more effective than morphine.[75] It does not bind to opioid receptors but has a high affinity for nicotinic acetylcholine receptor binding sites, labelled by [³H] nicotine or its derivatives.[75] The antinociceptive action of epibatidine (prevented by mecamylamine but not hexamethonium) is mediated by activation through central (neuronal nicotinic acetylcholine receptors, and such receptors may mediate many other actions of nicotinic agonists, such as the release of catecholamines (by a calcium-dependent mechanism), excitatory amino acids and 5-HT (which may contribute to the antinociceptive actions).[75] The noradrenergic system is implicated in the antinociceptive actions of epibatidine, but its actual role remains unclear.[75] In peptidergic cells expressing ganglionic-type receptors, epibatidine enhances the release of substance P and may conceivably be responsible for antinociception by depleting stores of nociceptive transmitters.[75] Agents raising the intracellular calcium ion concentration significantly potentiate nociception.[75]

Unlike nicotine, there is no substantial tolerance developed to epibatidine (in mice), and it is considerably more potent.[75] In rodent antinociceptive tests, epibatidine is an effective antinociceptive at about 5 μg/kg; nicotine is about 200–300 times less potent given by various routes, and morphine is about 1000 times less potent.[75] Its analgesic action is rapid in onset (3–5 minutes) and lasts up to 1 hour.[75]

There is considerable interest in nicotinic agonists as analgesic agents, and the wide diversity of neuronal nicotinic acetylcholine receptors suggests that many nicotinic actions are mediated by different receptors.[75] Although toxicities related to interactions with ganglionic and neuromuscular neuronal nicotinic acetylcholine receptors preclude the clinical development of epibatidine, safer, neuronal nicotinic acetylcholine receptors subtype-selective cholinergic channel modulators could represent a major breakthrough in treating severe acute and neuropathic pain. Two compounds, A-85380 and ABT-594, have the same affinity as epibatidine for the alpha$_4$, beta$_2$ subtype but have, respectively, over 3000 or over 100 000 times lower affinity for the alpha$_7$ and neuromuscular subtypes.[75] ABT-594 inhibits capsaicin-induced substance P release from spinal slices, selectively inhibits thermal and mechanical noxious stimuli in the dorsal horn neurones, and may activate descending pain pathways after brain stem injection.[75] It will soon be undergoing safety and then efficacy studies in humans.

Calcium channel blockers

A novel neurone-specific N-type calcium channel blocker, the omega conopeptide SNX-111, has been used in the treatment of malignant, non-malignant and AIDS neuropathic pain states refractory to opioids (R.R. Luther, 1998, unpublished data).

ENZYME INHIBITORS

Acetyl cholinesterase inhibitors

The analgesic effects of acetyl cholinesterase inhibitors have been demonstrated by well-organized animal studies followed by meticulous phase I human studies using intrathecal neostigmine.[76]

NO synthetase inhibitors

Inhibitors of NO synthetase are effective against the hyperalgesia produced by NMDA and substance P, and also more natural stimuli, such as inflammatory and neuropathic nociception in animals at spinal sites of action.[70] NO may feed back from post-synaptic neurones to increase the release of C fibre transmitters such as glutamate.[70] An induction of NO synthetase in sensory afferents has been reported to occur after nerve damage, and ectopic activity in damaged nerves appears to be mediated by NO.[70] Various NO synthetase antagonists (L-NAME and L-NMMA) have been shown to reverse hyperalgesia in rat models, but clinically useful drugs are some way off.[9] It has been possible to separate the neuronal from the vascular effects of NO by the synthesis of agents such as 7-nitroindazole, which is a selective inhibitor of neuronal NO synthetase with antinociceptive actions.[70] Drugs specific to NO synthetase involved in stage 3 or 4 sensory levels could be developed, providing more selective analgesics.

OPIOIDS

Opioid receptor combinations

All three subtypes of opioid receptor [i.e. mu(OP3), delta (OP1) and kappa (OP2)] have been cloned and can interact to produce antinociceptive synergy.[77,78] This has allowed many questions to be answered by expressing receptor cDNAs in cell lines that lack endogenous receptors.[79] Multiple isoforms of each subtype have been proposed.[78] However, the molecular nature of desensitization remains largely unresolved.[79] Studies of chimeric receptors have shown that the third loop of the delta opioid receptor, the first and third extracellular loops of the mu receptor, and the second extracellular loop and top half of the fourth transmembrane domain in the kappa opioid receptor are important in their agonist selective binding, but they were unable to reveal key residues in the receptor binding sites.[79] All cloned opioid receptors have been expressed in cell lines and have been found to inhibit adenylyl cyclase (involving G$_i$ and G$_o$ proteins with G$_q$ being implicated in kappa-mediated analgesia) and to couple to various calcium channels.[79] Mu and delta receptors inhibit L-type calcium ion channels, and kappa agonists modulate calcium ion currents in isolated neuroendocrine nerve terminals.[79] Opioid receptors are shown to regulate inwardly rectifying potassium channels.[79] Different agonists could have different effects on G-protein coupling, leading to different biological responses.[79]

To summarize, opioid receptors belong to the family of guanine-nucleotide binding protein (G protein)-coupled receptors, consisting of seven transmembrane-spanning domains, an extracellular N-terminus and an intracellular C-terminus.[78] G proteins consist of alpha (16 types), beta (7 or more types) and gamma (5 types) subunits, which activate G protein second-messenger systems such as adenyl cyclase-cAMP and phopholipase$_3$-inositol 1,4,5 triphosphate [Ins(1,4,5)P$_3$]-Ca^{++}.[78] cAMP activates cAMP-dependent protein kinase for phosphorylating intracellular calcium release channels.[78] The hydrolysis of phosphadidylinositol 4,5 biphosphate (PIP$_2$) by the membrane-bound enzyme phospholipase C (PLC) yields the second messengers Ins(1,4,5,)P$_3$ and diacylglycerol.[78] Ins(1,4,5,)P$_3$ can release calcium from specialized intracellular stores.[78] The released calcium may bind to calmodulin or cause further calcium release.[78] Diacylglycerol may than be cleaved to produce arachidonic acid or cause the activation of protein kinase C, which also phosphorylates cellular proteins such as ion channels in neurones.[78] Opioid analgesia occurs via an inhibitory effect of excitatory neurotransmission (substance P and glutamate) by the closure of voltage-sensitive calcium channels and the activation of potassium currents, thus slowing the action potential, reducing the cAMP level, inhibiting the inwardly rectifying cation current and resulting in a reduction in neuronal firing.[78] Opioid stimulation of a variety of second-messenger systems (adenylyl cyclase activity, phosphoinositide hydrolysis and intracellular calcium elevation) may underlie the opioid stimulation of neuronal activity.[78] The C-terminus of the delta receptor appears to be important in acute phospholipase C coupling.[78] Opioid-induced increases in protein kinase C activity have been shown to modulate potassium ion channels.[78] As well as the opioid mobilization of intracellular calcium ions from inositol (1,4,5) P$_3$-sensitive stores, the delta receptor may regulate the activity of ryanodine receptors on intracellular calcium stores.[78] All the physiological consequences of the opioid-induced mobilization of intracellular calcium remain unclear, and further work is needed to clarify this. Both inhibitory and excitatory effects of opioids have been observed as a result of high versus low concentrations of opioid agonist, acute versus chronic agonist administration, and a change in experimental conditions.[78] These bimodal opioid actions may be involved in tolerance to and dependence on opioids.[78]

Opioids thus exert a variation of stimulatory effects on signal transduction. These include cAMP stimulation, phophoinositide hydrolysis and elevation of intracellular calcium by mobilization from intracellular stores and by stimulating influx.[78] At a cellular level, these changes may underlie an opioid stimulation of neuronal activity and play a part in the development of opioid drug tolerance.[78] Studies aimed at unravelling these signalling events will contribute to the understanding of opioid action.

Desensitization is defined as a loss of function under prolonged exposure to an agonist.[79] Opioid receptor regulation is fundamental for signalling control and involves internalization, downregulation and possible receptor modifications.[79] Opioid receptors (expressed in heterologous cells) undergo rapid internalization upon agonist treatment; approximately 50 per cent are internalized within 6 minutes.[79] Receptor monomerization precedes internalization (in delta opioid receptors), suggesting this to be a prerequisite for receptor internalization.[79] The C-tail is also important in opioid receptor internalization.[79] Downregulation is characterized by a generalized loss of both cell surface and intracellular receptors.[79] High affinity G complex formation may be necessary for downregulation and internalization, and phosphorylation by G protein-coupled receptor kinases or cAMP-responsive kinases, or both, could play a significant part in receptor downregulation.[79] The presence of spare receptors with the ability to inhibit adenylyl cyclase may yield clues to the specific desensitization of the opioid receptor.[79] Exploration of receptor regulation is still at an early stage;[79] future work should unravel unanswered questions and lead to an explanation of the molecular mechanisms of opioid tolerance.[79] In clinical practice, opioid tolerance is rarely a limiting factor.[80] Patients and their families should be reassured that morphine will continue to relieve their pain for many months or years.[80] Worsening pain in a patient previously stable on a dose of opioid should never be attributed to tolerance unless a comprehensive evaluation fails to reveal an alternative explanation.[80] The prevention of tolerance by NMDA antagonists, and the recognition that there is incomplete cross-tolerance to both the analgesic and non-analgesic effects of opioids, have important potential clinical implications.[80] The pre-eminent question – whether the very presence of pain has some modulatory effect on the development of tolerance – has yet to be answered.[80]

The intrathecal combination of [D-Ala,[2] MePhe,[4] Gly-ol] enkephalin (or DAGO, a selective mu agonist) and [D-Pen,[5] D-Pen[5]] enkephalin (or DPDPE, a selective delta agonist) produces significant synergistic suppressive effects on the evoked activity of the WDR neurones.[81] Weaker analgesia after kappa opioids, together with psychotomimetic effects, is reflected in the initial preclinical human studies.[70] Delta-mediated analgesia is less associated with respiratory depression, dependence and tolerance. The delta receptor appears to have considerable potential as a target for drugs that produce good analgesia but with a reduced probability of side-effects.[2] The recent availability of non-peptide delta agonists has provided encouraging results in the animal model, and subtypes of the delta receptor have been described pharmacologically.[49] A newer, highly selective delta opioid, SNC 80, effective via central and systemic (including oral) routes, has been produced. SNC 80 leads to analgesic effects, reversed by a number of delta, but not mu, opioid receptor antagonists.[70] The potential for delta opioids to act as analgesics in nociceptive and even neuropathic pain is high.[70] Delta opioids may eventually become clinical alternatives to morphine.

An alternative lead into the discovery of safer opioids may come from the identification of additional subtypes of opioid receptors using molecular technologies.[49] A receptor with significant (approximately 50 per cent) homology to the mu, kappa and delta receptors has been cloned, although the endogenous ligand for this opioid-like receptor has not been identified as yet.[49] The future of neuraxially administered opioids for pain management may be enhanced by the use of highly selective opioid subtype agonists in a multidrug combination to reduce the occurrence of complications.[36]

Endogenous opioid peptides

The modification of endogenous peptides may be possible in the future, resulting in compounds with long-lasting analgesic properties. Prolonged analgesia has been obtained with intrathecal beta-endorphin.[36] Aside from beta-endorphin, intrathecal D-ala-D-leu enkephalin is another peptide that has been used for chronic spinal administration in terminal cancer patients who have displayed an apparent tolerance to morphine.[82]

Many of the experimental drugs for probing opioid function are modified endogenous opioid peptides, as enkephalins themselves have brief actions since they are rapidly downgraded by membrane-bound peptidases.[70] This has led to the synthesis of peptidase inhibitors with no physical or psychological dependence. Kelatorphan, a mixed peptidase inhibitor, provides almost complete protection to the enkephalins.[70] Its neuraxial application reduces nociceptive cell response, reversible by a selective delta antagonist.[70] The systemic use of a new active mixed peptidase inhibitor, RB 101, is a novel approach to analgesia, whereby delta opioid receptor activation is produced by a natural transmitter.[70] The efficacy of these agents for severe pain remains to be determined.

Exogenous opioids

MORPHINE-6-GLUCURONIDE

Renal failure *per se* has little effect on morphine parent drug clearance but does result in the accumulation of the analgesically active metabolite morphine-6-glucuronide, accounting for profound analgesia and sedation in uraemic patients receiving large morphine doses because of the long half-life of morphine-6-glucuronide (89–136 hours).[83] Recently, intrathecal morphine-6 glucuronide has been found to have greater analgesic activity than intrathecal morphine in man,[84] persisting in the CSF. This may make it useful as an intrathecal analgesic when prolonged pain relief is required. However, in the postoperative situation, respiratory depression is a problem; hence the efficacy of morphine-6-glucuronide is clear, but its safety is questionable.[83]

TRAMADOL

Among the atypical 'opioids' is tramadol hydrochloride (see also Chapter 3).[85] Tramadol [tramadol hydrochloride: (1RS, 2RS)-2-[(dimethylamine) methyl)-1-(3 methoxyphenyl)-cyclohexanol HCL] is a synthetic 4-phenyl-piperidine analogue of codeine.[86] It is the most recently introduced analgesic in many countries, although it has been available in Germany since the late 1970s.[87] Throughout the world, some 50 million patients have received tramadol, and hence a large pool of knowledge has been gathered concerning its behaviour in terms of both efficacy and safety.

The drug is available in formulations suitable for oral, rectal and parenteral administration.[87] The marketed formulations of tramadol contain a racemic (50:50) mixture of two enantiomers, each one displaying differing affinities for various receptors.[86] The complementary and synergistic mode of action of these two enantiomers is both opioid and monoaminergic, so that its analgesic effect extends to both opioid-sensitive and opioid-insensitive pain.[86] The opioid and 5-HT reuptake inhibitory effect (increasing the central neuronal synaptic 5-HT levels and displacing stored 5-HT from nerve endings), is located in the (+) enantiomer, while the noradrenaline reuptake inhibitory effect lies in the (–) enantiomer.[83,88,89] The activity of tramadol is only partially (about 30 per cent)[90] reversed with naloxone, and 5-HT and α_2-adrenergic receptor antagonists will remove the remainder.[91,92] Tramadol achieves spinal modulation of pain through indirect activation of the postsynaptic α_2-adrenoceptors, preventing impulses reaching the brain.[93] The synergy of monoaminergic and opioid activity achieves analgesic effects.[93]

Tramadol possesses a weak affinity for the mu opioid receptor and even less for the kappa and delta receptors. This affinity is some 6000 times less than that of morphine, 100-fold less than that of dextropropoxyphene, 10-fold less than that of codeine and equivalent to that of dextromethorphan.[88,94] Tramadol is metabolized to an active metabolite, O-Desmethyl tramadol by a polymorphic isoenzyme of the debrisoquine type, cytochrome P450 2D6 (CYP2D6).[86,95] O-Desmethyl tramadol has a greater (200-fold) affinity for the mu opioid receptor than does tramadol itself[86,96] but clinically plays little role in the production of analgesia. Tramadol has a potency about one fifth to one tenth that of morphine.[83]

In terms of human pharmacokinetics, tramadol is rapidly absorbed after oral administration and demonstrates a bioavailability of 68 per cent, peak serum concentrations being reached within 2 hours.[86,93] Regular dosing will achieve a steady state within 2 days.[93] It has a high tissue affinity with a volume of distribution of 306 and 203 L after oral and intravenous administration, respectively.[93] There is 1 per cent placental transfer,[93] and approximately 20 per cent is protein bound.[97] The elimination kinetics of tramadol are appropriately described by a two-compartment model, with a reported elimination half-life of 5.1 (SD ± 0.8) hours for tramadol and 9 hours for the O-desmethyl derivative after a single oral dose of 100 mg.[86,98] This explains the approximately two-fold accumulation of the parent drug and its O-desmethyl derivative that is observed during multiple dose treatment with tramadol.[86] The recommended oral daily dose is between 50 and 100 mg every 4–6 hours.[86] The duration of analgesia is about 6 hours after a single oral dose of 100 mg.[86] Postoperatively, an initial dose of 100 mg intravenously and then 50 mg every 10–20 minutes up to a maximum of 250 mg in the first hour and 600 mg in 24 hours may be given.[93]

Eighty-six per cent of the absorbed tramadol is metabolized in the liver, and 90 per cent is excreted in the kidneys.[93] Consequently, malfunction of either organ may affect plasma levels of tramadol (e.g. necessitating a change of dose to 200 mg per day in 12-hourly divided doses in chronic renal failure, and to 50 mg every 12 hours with hepatic cirrhosis).[93] With drug-induced hepatic enzyme induction, the dose of drug can be doubled.[98] Tramadol has a minor delaying effect on colonic transit but no effect on upper gastrointestinal transit or gut smooth muscle tone.[99] There has been no correlation shown between plasma tramadol and analgesic effect.[93]

Clinically, in the acute situation, tramadol compares favourably with a range of analgesic agents, from paracetamol to morphine, in terms of both efficacy and the occurrence of adverse events. Comparative studies have generally shown tramadol to be more effective than oral agents such as NSAIDs, pentazocine, dextropropoxyphene and combination formulations containing paracetamol.[87,100–103] Parenteral administration is mainly concerned with postoperative pain. The lack of analgesic efficacy limits tramadol as a sole agent to treat severe pain after surgery.[93] Here, it may well have a place in combination with another drug (e.g. paracetamol) or after control of the worst pain by a regional local anaesthetic technique.[93]

Although tramadol is substantially haemodynamically stable, transient haemodynamic effects have been seen after intravenous injection.[93] Tramadol has shown significant efficacy in continuous intravenous infusion,[104,105] in PCA (with wide individual variations)[86,106,107] and in subcutaneous PCA.[108,109] Tramadol would appear to lend itself particularly to use in the day case surgical environment. Its efficacy and safety are most appropriate for a combined preoperative, perioperative and postoperative sequence.[106,110–113] Oral tramadol is effective for the relief of acute dento-alveolar surgical pain.[114,115]

Postoperatively, intravenous and intramuscular tramadol has been used with good efficacy in moderate surgical pain.[116] Orally, in postsurgical pain, tramadol in doses of 50, 100 and 150 mg gave rise to NNTs for over 50 per cent maximal total pain relief of 7.1 (95 per cent confidence intervals 4.6–18), 4.8 (3.4–8.2) and 2.4 (2.0–3.1), comparable to aspirin 650 mg plus codeine 60 mg (NNT 3.6 [2.5–6.3]), and paracetamol 650 mg plus propoxyphene 100 mg (NNT 4.0 [3.0–5.7]).[117] Tramadol has been well evaluated in all the surgical fields including the cardiothoracic,[118,119] orthopaedic,[102,109] general[104,106,120] and paediatric.[121–124] In this last area, tramadol has real potential as a safe and effective agent to treat moderate pain. Intramuscular tramadol has been used with good results being as effective as intramuscular pethidine for the management of labour pain without respiratory depression of the neonate.[114,116] Neuraxially, in epidural administration for pain after abdominal surgery, it is more effective than bupivacaine but less effective than morphine.[114] It is also effective in the treatment of pain from myocardial ischaemia, ureteric colic and acute trauma.[116] However, used intraoperatively as part of a balanced anaesthetic technique, it has been associated with a high incidence of intraoperative recall and dreaming.[116] It has been successfully used in the treatment of postoperative shivering.[125]

In the treatment of chronic pain, tramadol has been shown to be effective across a wide range of conditions (even neuropathic pain),[126] as could be predicted on account of its modes of analgesic action. In both cancer and non-cancer pain, it has been shown to have a comparable analgesic effect to morphine and other commonly used analgesia agents, with significantly fewer adverse events.[127–134] For the treatment of cancer pain, it occupies step 2 of the WHO ladder.[86]

In all areas of practice, the adverse event profile of tramadol is a mixture of the opioid (nausea, vomiting, tiredness and drowsiness) and the monoaminergic (headache, dizziness, sweating and dry mouth), with an overall incidence of between 1 and 6 per cent.[135] It is also associated with a low incidence of cardiac depression, and significantly less dizziness and drowsiness than morphine.[87] In comparison to other strong analgesics, the incidence of adverse events is lower, and many of these events can either be prevented or readily treated.[102,136,137] In children, the incidence of adverse events with tramadol is much less than that seen in adults.[138]

Particularly in the therapy of chronic pain, the commencement of dosing at a low level with a gradual increase frequently prevents the onset of adverse events, especially in the elderly. One of the more outstanding aspects of tramadol is its extremely low liability to produce clinically relevant respiratory depression, which is negligible in comparison with other opioids used for postoperative pain management.[116,139,140] However, when used in combination with other CNS depressants, respiratory changes can be seen.

Tramadol, similarly to the other opioids, may induce seizures, especially when used in the presence of proconvulsive drugs (such as MAOIs and tricyclic antidepressants), and this should be avoided.[86,141] Much of the toxicity in tramadol overdose appears to be attributable to the monoamine uptake inhibition rather than to its opioid effects.[142]

Agitation, tachycardia, confusion and hypertension suggest a possible mild 5-HT syndrome.[142] A 5-HT syndrome may occur with the concomitant administration of tramadol with sertraline.[95]

The frequency of euphoria and dysphoria with tramadol is negligible.[97] It thus has the pharmacodynamic and pharmacokinetic properties that are highly unlikely to lead to dependence.[86] Both controlled and postmarketing surveillance studies have confirmed the liability of the development of tolerance and dependence with tramadol to be extremely low.[86,130,143]

Tramadol is a centrally acting analgesic that has been shown to be effective and well tolerated.[86] It appears to be a valuable addition to the analgesic armamentarium as a safe and effective agent across a wide spectrum of acute and chronic painful conditions. When compared to the NSAIDs, it does not aggravate hypertension or provoke asthma, gastrointestinal mucosal damage, renal impairment or congestive heart failure.[93,144] When compared with other opioids, it does not induce significant respiratory depression, constipation, histamine release or cross-tolerance, or have significant abuse potential, and it is a prescription-only medicine rather than a drug controlled by the Misuse of Drugs Act.[93,144] The most important side-effects of tramadol are nausea and vomiting, which can often be prevented by slow dose titration and the administration of a prophylactic antiemetic.[87]

The unique composition of this agent will promote further research in this area. A series of compounds related to tramadol has been prepared by linking one of the N-methyl to the 3-position of the cyclohexane ring (J.R. Carson, 1997, unpublished data). These 4-aryloctahydroisoindoles showed antinociceptive effects in rats and mice. They did not bind to the mu opioid receptor, nor did their activity parallel their effects on monoamine reuptake.

NEW SHORT-ACTING OPIOIDS

Remifentanil

Remifentanil[145] is a new opioid with a difference. It is a fentanyl derivative (within the 4-anilopiperidine series) with an ester linkage and is the hydrochloride salt of 3[4-methoxycarbonyl-4-(1-oxpropyl) phenylamino]-1-piperidine propanoic acid methyl ester.[146] It is a mu opioid agonist that incorporates the methyl ester group at position 1 of the piperidine ring.[147] This makes it readily susceptible to rapid hydrolysis by non-specific esterases (not entirely known) in the plasma and tissues. Its analgesic potency is similar to that of fentanyl and 20–30 times that of alfentanil.[146,148] Its analgesic effect is mediated through coupling to a G protein, which concomitantly results presynaptically in an inhibition of excitatory neurotransmitter release and postsynaptically in an inhibition of cyclic adenosine monophosphatase, a suppression of voltage-sensitive calcium channels and hyperpolarization of the postsysnaptic membrane through increased potassium conductance.[148] The effects of remifentanil are antagonized by naloxone.[146]

Although differing in potency (being 16 times more potent), remifentanil exhibits alfentanil-like pharmacodynamics with a shorter-acting pharmacokinetic profile.[83,149] The preparation is a white crystalline powder, readily soluble in water, with a pKa of 7.07.[93] Remifentanil (molecular weight = 413) is lipophilic, with an octanol/water partition coefficient of 17.9 at a pH of 7.4.[148] It has a very rapid onset of action, comparable with that of alfentanil.[147] The $t_{1/2}k_{eo}$ (a parameter that characterizes the speed of equilibration between the blood and a theoretical compartment) in human volunteers studies (using the EEG spectral edge) was 1.4 minutes, and 1.3 minutes using an experimental pain model.[150,151] The $t_{1/2}k_{eo}$ was 1.3 minutes for the effect on minute ventilation.[93] It is 70 per cent bound to alpha-1-acid glycoprotein.[93] It has a volume of distribution at steady state of 25–40 L, a rapid metabolic clearance of 3–5 L per minute and a systemic half-life of 9–11 minutes.[146–148] It is not a substrate for butyrylcholinesterases (pseudocholinesterase), and thus its clearance should not be affected by cholinesterase deficiency, anticholinergics or the administration of anticholinesterases.[146,148]

Remifentanil is predominantly metabolized via non-specific red blood cell and tissue esterases to an acid metabolite, Gl-90291 (a mu agonist with 1/2000–1/4000 less potency, with a half-life of 19 minutes in dogs), and to a lesser extent by N-dealkylation to Gl-94219 (a minor metabolite).[93,148] Extensive metabolism occurs in blood cells and muscle that is unaffected by isolated organ failure.[93] Available evidence suggests that neither the pharmacokinetics nor the pharmacodynamics (e.g. respiratory effects) of remifentanil are significantly altered in patients with severe hepatic or renal disease.[93,152] However, as the renal elimination of the metabolite Gl-90291 may be as high as 90 per cent, preliminary data suggest its clearance to be greatly reduced in patients with renal failure.[153] The clinical relevance of this remains to be determined because

of its lack of potency relative to remifentanil. Interestingly, the same rate of clearance of remifentanil during the anhepatic stage of liver transplantation has been observed.[154] Preliminary findings in children suggest that remifentanil has a pharmacokinetic profile similar to that in adults.[155] *In vitro*, haemodilution can affect the metabolism of remifentanil (crystalloids less than colloids).[156] It is speculated that albumen binds to remifentanil and protects it from red cell esterases.[156]

The value of the context-sensitive half-time, rather than the terminal elimination half-life, in describing drug offset is shown with remifentanil.[157] Computer simulations have predicted its context-sensitive half-time to be independent of the duration of infusion.[147] The measured context-sensitive half-time after a 3-h infusion was 3.2 ± 0.9 minutes.[157] The pharmacodynamic offsets, defined as time to 50 per cent recovery of the baseline minute ventilation when breathing 7.5 per cent carbon dioxide, was 5.4 ± 1.8 minutes.[147,157] When a rapid decrease in blood concentration is the goal, it is beneficial to have a small central volume and a larger central clearance. The high clearance of the drug, combined with its small steady-state distribution volume, results in a rapid decline in blood concentration after the termination of an infusion.[149]

Studies that have compared remifentanil with alfentanil have reported greater haemodynamic stability with remifentanil irrespective of the dose rate.[158] Nevertheless, the cardiovascular effects of remifentanil are similar to those observed with the other fentanyl analogues, that is, mild bradycardia and a decrease of 15–20 per cent in blood pressure.[148] Escalating doses of 2–30 μg/kg injected as a bolus over 1 minute during general anaesthesia decreased blood pressure by 25–40 per cent but were not associated with changes in plasma histamine concentration.[159] Remifentanil blocks the stress hormone response in a dose-dependent manner.[148]

In non-intubated patients, respiratory depression produced by remifentanil is dose dependent but is not expected to last for more than 10–15 minutes after discontinuation of the infusion.[148] The EEG effects of remifentanil are similar to those of other opioids, but there is a more rapid recovery in cerebral blood flow and EEG patterns after the termination of remifentanil infusions.[146,148] Human studies with remifentanil and nitrous oxide revealed an intact cerebral vascular reactivity to carbon dioxide and a cerebral blood flow similar to that with anaesthesia with isoflurane/nitrous oxide or fentanyl/nitrous oxide.[160] No changes in intracranial pressure have been found in patients with space-occupying lesions treated with remifentanil.[161]

As with all opioids, nausea, vomiting, pruritus, sedation, muscle rigidity and cardiopulmonary depression may be consequences of remifentanil administration.[148] The adverse effects are short lived and are antagonized by naloxone.[93] Because of its rapid clearance, however, the incidence of some of these side-effects may prove to be less compared with other opioids.[146] The incidence of muscle rigidity is similar to that of alfentanil, most cases being described as mild to moderate yet depending on the dose and rate of administration.[146,148] In patients breathing spontaneously, the onset of life-threatening muscle rigidity and apnoea can be alarmingly rapid and may be avoided by spreading the injection of single doses over 30 seconds and changing remifentanil infusion rates no more frequently than at 10 minute intervals.[93]

Remifentanil is formulated in glycine, an inhibitory neurotransmitter. This can produce reversible, naloxone-insensitive motor dysfunction after continuous intrathecal administration.[148] Hence neuraxial administration is not recommended.

One of the problems with the use of opioid infusions is that a rate that will be sufficient for the most intense stimulus will result in overdosage at times of lesser stimulation. This can result in prolonged recovery and postoperative respiratory depression. This problem should not arise with remifentanil. The fast decay in plasma concentration even after high doses and long infusions will ensure a rapid recovery. With infusion rates of $2\,\mu g/kg$ per minute for 3 hours, patients resumed spontaneous ventilation on average 4 minutes after stopping the remifentanil infusion, and no patient required more than 10 minutes to breathe spontaneously.[162] Over an 80-fold range of infusion rates, patients awoke, breathed and were extubated within minutes of discontinuing remifentanil.[147] The pharmacokinetics of remifentanil make blood concentrations predictable.[93]

Preliminary evidence from volunteer and patient studies suggests that remifentanil may constitute the first ultrashort acting opioid for use as a supplement to general anaesthesia.[149] It does not reliably produce loss of consciousness.[93] Remifentanil would generally not be considered suitable as a sole anaesthetic agent and should be given in association with an intravenous or inhalational anaesthetic agent, and similarly for sedation during surgical procedures under local anaesthesia.[93] The amount of anaesthetic supplement required to achieve anaesthesia is considerably reduced by remifentanil.[93] Remifentanil exerts synergy with hypnotic drugs. It is associated with an age-related reduction in the mean alveolar concentration of isoflurane.[163] Remifentanil also reduces auditory and somatosensory evoked responses during isoflurane anaesthesia in a dose-dependent manner.[158] Opioid potency, as determined by EEG, can be related to clinical measures of potency (the so-called EEG–clinical potency fingerprint).[164] Simulations based on the EEG model show that bolus doses should be halved and infusion rates decreased to one third in the elderly compared with the young.[165,166] Remifentanil's favourable titration characteristics are independent of age, although there is an increased variability in recovery in elderly individuals. Based on the EEG model, age and lean body mass are significant demographic factors that must be considered when determining a dose regimen.[165,166] This remains true even when interindividual pharmacodynamic and pharmacokinetic variability is incorporated into the analysis.[166] Gender, however, does not influence any pharmacokinetic or pharmacodynamic parameter.[165] In a dose-ranging study during propofol and nitrous oxide anaesthesia in unpremedicated American Society of Anesthesiologists class I or II adult patients undergoing surgery for at least an hour, the dose at which 50 per cent of patients did not respond to skin incision varied between 0.02 and $0.087\,\mu g/kg$ per minute.[162] The dose at which 50 per cent did not respond to all surgical stimuli was $0.52\,\mu g/kg$ per minute.[162]

Anaesthesia with remifentanil can be induced with a slowly delivered bolus dose of $1\,\mu g/kg$ over 60–90 seconds or with a gradual starting up of the initial infusion (0.5–$1.0\,\mu g/kg$ per minute 10 minutes prior to intubation) and a standard dose of an hypnotic agent (propofol, thiopentone or isoflurane).[148] Induction of anaesthesia can also take place as an infusion of 0.5–$1.0\,\mu g/kg$ per minute (with or without $1\,\mu g/kg$ injected intravenously over 30 seconds).[93] Pre-administration with glycopyrrolate will reduce the incidence of bradycardia (especially with abdominal surgery and strabismus surgery in children).[93] For the maintenance of analgesia after endotracheal intubation, the infusion rate can be titrated according to the patient's requirements and the anaesthetic technique, usually as an analgesic infusion of 0.05–$2.0\,\mu g/kg$ per minute with supplemental doses as required.[93,148]

The pharmacology of remifentanil suggests that the rapid onset and recovery of its effect will be a unique tool in certain clinical circumstances, for example day case surgery, short painful interventions (e.g. lithotripsy), monitored anaesthesia care (e.g. the wake-up test in spinal surgery), long inpatient surgery or surgery of unknown duration, and surgical procedures in which high levels of surgical stimulation persist until the end of surgery, all these being cases where rapid recovery is desirable.[148,167,168] Remifentanil has successfully been used for the maintenance of anaesthesia in a 1:4 ratio compared with alfentanil for total intravenous anaesthesia in ambulatory surgery.[167] This dose of remifentanil provided a more effective suppression of intraoperative responses and did not result in prolonged awakening.[167] Remifentanil at a dose of 0.1–0.123 μg/kg per minute, or remifentanil 0.05–0.065 μg/kg per minute combined with midazolam 2 mg provided effective analgesia and adequate comfort (without compromising respiratory function) during superficial surgery in patients under monitored anaesthetic care.[169] Open heart surgery using a total intravenous anaesthesia technique with remifentanil instead of fentanyl allows a faster extubation.[148] In patients undergoing coronary bypass surgery, total intravenous anaesthesia with remifentanil and propofol provided marked intraoperative reflex suppression.[170] Remifentanil attenuates increases in catecholamine levels during coronary bypass surgery.[83] The relative short-lasting analgesia after cessation of the remifentanil infusion might demand new techniques to prevent the immediate onset of postoperative pain; these include the administration of longer-acting opioids as the analgesic effects of remifentanil begin to fade, and the increased use of regional local anaesthetic techniques. Remifentanil (0.1 μg/kg per minute) has been used as an alternative to propofol for supplemental sedation in patients undergoing surgery under local anaesthesia.[171] Remifentanil easily crosses the placenta but continues to be rapidly metabolized in the fetus with an umbilical arterial-to-venous ratio of 0.29.[172] This rapidly metabolized opioid may find a unique place in obstetric anaesthesia.

Remifentanil is a highly effective opioid analgesic with a short half-life, predictable pharmacokinetics and a close concentration–effect relationship.[93] However, care must be taken to ensure that infusion rates are set appropriately to control pain and responses to surgical stimuli without inducing life-threatening respiratory depression and muscle rigidity, the onset of which can be rapid.[93] Remifentanil may be used widely because of its predictability and reversibility. Its independence of the concentrations infused, of their duration, and of liver and kidney function makes it a drug that

should potentially find a unique place in clinical practice. Future clinical use will determine whether the theoretical advantages associated with this short-acting opioid are realized.

Trefentanil

Trefentanil (A3665)[147] is a substituted anilidopiperidine opioid derivative currently undergoing phase 1 evaluation in human.[153] It is a full mu opioid agonist. Its pharmacokinetic profile is similar to that of alfentanil, with a similar potency but a higher metabolic clearance (0.44 L per minute compared with 0.18 L per minute) and a slightly larger volume of distribution.[83] At doses up to 32 μg/kg, it causes significant analgesia, with a peak effect 3 minutes after dosing.[83] At doses of up to 32 μg/kg and above, there is significant respiratory depression but cardiostability.[83] The $t_{1/2}k_{eo}$ is 1.2 ± 0.5 minutes. Recovery from trefentanil is faster than from alfentanil irrespective of the duration of the infusion.[83] Its context half-time varies between 10 and 20 minutes. Its blood–brain equilibration time is slightly longer than that of alfentanil (1.2 versus 0.6 minutes).[83] Its pharmacokinetic and pharmacodynamic characteristics are intermediate between those of alfentanil and remifentanil. Computer recovery simulations suggest that it may have advantages over alfentanil and fentanyl but not over remifentanil.[83]

NEW DRUGS

Butamen

A suspension of butamen, a highly non-water soluble local anaesthetic, has been used spinally and peripherally to successfully treat patients with metastatic cancer or chronic low back pain.[173] Further investigations with this promising drug preparation are underway.

Gabapentin

The antiepileptic gabapentin can exert powerful antihyperalgesic effects in models of surgical and inflammatory pain, although it possesses negligible intrinsic analgesic activity (see Chapter 4). Its antihyperalgesic effect appears to be located at the segmental level and may involve a selective modulation of a calcium channel and also possibly of glutamate-mediated neurotransmission. This may represent a new avenue for the treatment of neuropathic and chronic inflammatory pain.

Ropivacaine

There is a growing awareness of employing enantiomers in clinical anaesthesiology. Ropivacaine[174] is a new, long-acting local anaesthetic chemically homologous to bupivacaine and mepivacaine. It is the first enantiomerically pure local anaesthetic and exists as an S-enantiomer.[175] The relative lipid solubility of ropivacaine is intermediate between that of lignocaine and bupivacaine. The plasma protein binding of ropivacaine is marginally less than that of bupivacaine, but its pK_a is identical.[176]

In animal models, low concentrations of ropivacaine (25–50 μmol/L) produce a profound and rapid block of both A delta and C fibres (responsible for pain transmission), and have been shown to be more potent than similar low concentrations of bupivacaine in blocking these fibres.[176] *In vitro* studies showed that ropivacaine blocked A delta fibres more completely than those which control motor function (A beta fibres).[177] Using desheathed rabbit vagus nerves, it was found that ropivacaine blocked C fibres more quickly than A delta fibres and was a potent producer of frequency-dependent block.[176] Both these properties offer considerable clinical advantages in providing analgesia with minimal motor blockade.

In vitro studies confirm that ropivacaine has a vasoconstrictive effect in low doses, an effect that may be minimal with the doses used in clinical practice.[176] *In vitro* studies also indicate that ropivacaine is less cardiotoxic than equimolar concentrations of bupivacaine (but more cardiotoxic than equimolar concentrations of lignocaine) as it dissociates from the sodium channels more rapidly and produces less accumulation of sodium channel blockade.[177–181] In animal studies, overdoses of ropivacaine were better tolerated than overdoses of bupivacaine but not of lignocaine.[177] Substitution of bupivacaine by ropivacaine should decrease the potential for irreversible cardiovascular toxicity.

Animal studies have shown that ropivacaine (0.5–1.0 per cent) consistently produces effective sensory and motor anaesthesia in sciatic and brachial plexus nerve blocks albeit with a shorter onset and duration of action than equal concentrations of bupivacaine.[176] Human studies in brachial plexus block have shown that ropivacaine 0.5 per cent and bupivacaine 0.5 per cent provide equivalent motor and sensory blockade with a comparable onset time, long duration and analgesic efficacy.[182] Neuraxial animal studies have shown equipotent sensory blockade but shorter motor blockade for ropivacaine compared with bupivacaine.[176]

CNS toxicity is related directly to the anaesthetic potency of local anaesthetic drugs, and similar doses of ropivacaine and bupivacaine have been found to cause convulsions in conscious dogs.[183] Overall, however, in preclinical studies, ropivacaine shows a better therapeutic ratio, producing less CNS and cardiotoxicity (to depress myocardial contractility and conduction and to trigger ventricular arrhythmia) than bupivacaine.[182,184] The fatal cardiotoxic dose ratio in sheep is 1:2:9 for bupivacaine:ropivacaine:lignocaine.[182] A CNS toxicity study showed that humans can tolerate a slow infusion of 30 per cent more ropivacaine than bupivacaine before symptoms occur (mean 124 mg versus 99 mg).[182] Also, the incidence of neuropathic symptoms is lower with ropivacaine than bupivacaine. A few patients have received accidental intravenous injections of a range of doses of ropivacaine without any long-term sequelae.[182] The toxic blood concentration for ropivacaine has not yet been documented in humans.[182]

Ropivacaine administered by intravenous infusion was found to be less toxic than bupivacaine in human volunteers in terms of producing CNS and cardiovascular changes.[176,183] Compared with bupivacaine, its clearance is higher (reducing systemic toxicity), and its plasma protein binding (94 ± 1 per cent) and volume of distribution at a steady state (59 ± 7 L) are slightly lower.[176] The terminal elimination half-life (111 ± 62 minutes) is less than that of bupivacaine.[176]

A large number of open and double-blind studies have been performed in humans to determine the efficacy and degree of differential blockade with ropivacaine compared with bupivacaine in central and peripheral neural blockade. The addition of adrenaline has been found to have no more effect on systemic concentrations in both volunteer and clinical studies than on block profiles. It does not alter the block intensity or duration.[182] In peripheral neural blockade, ropivacaine was maximal in effect at concentrations between 0.5 and 0.75 per cent.[185] With intercostal blockade, ropivacaine 0.25 per cent showed a faster T_{max}, a similar C_{max} and a shorter elimination half-life compared with bupivacaine.[186] Ropivacaine has been shown to induce successful brachial plexus anaesthesia when given at a concentration of 5 mg/mL (but not 2.5 mg/mL) and was as effective as bupivacaine in comparative studies for this indication.[177] Ropivacaine also controls postoperative pain when infiltrated directly into surgical wound sites.[177]

The greater part of the clinical evaluation of ropivacaine for surgical anaesthesia has been carried out using epidural injections. About 10 000 patients in 25 separate studies have received the drug for a wide variety of lower limb and lower abdominal operations.[176,177] Employing equal doses of ropivacaine and bupivacaine has shown that there is no detectable difference in the onset or frequency of sensory blockade.[176,177] The duration of action of ropivacaine was slightly shorter. There was also a measurably slower onset of motor blockade with ropivacaine, and both the degree and duration of that motor blockade were less than with bupivacaine.[177] Higher concentrations (0.75–1.0 per cent) of ropivacaine were required to achieve the same degree and duration of motor blockade in epidural anaesthesia compared with bupivacaine.[182] Nevertheless, during various surgical procedures (with one exception), none of the clinical studies of epidural ropivacaine (with different doses) have revealed any consistent dose-related changes with respect to sensory blockade.[177] Motor block, however, did become more intense with dose increases.[177] The safety margin of ropivacaine narrows if the dose is increased substantially to augment motor block density.[182] Analgesic efficacy for postoperative pain management proved dose dependent, but even with 0.3 per cent at 10 mL per hour, systemic opioid supplementation was necessary to achieve satisfactory analgesia.[182]

Epidural ropivacaine has an adverse event profile similar to that of bupivacaine, including hypotension, nausea, bradycardia, transient paraesthesia, back pain, urinary retention and fever.[177] For postepidural analgesia, there are obvious advantages in avoiding excessive motor blockade that limits mobilization. The potential advantages of reducing motor block with low-dose ropivacaine infusions have been demonstrated in volunteers using fixed-rate infusions over 21 hours.[187] Ropivacaine 0.1 per cent produced limited analgesia and motor blockade, making ambulation possible.[187] With ropivacaine 0.2–0.3 per cent, analgesia was more extensive and motor blockade more moderate.[187] Ropivacaine epidural infusions have been given for up to 72 hours in clinical studies.[188] Although the total plasma ropivacaine level rose transiently, free levels plateaued and declined thereafter, being well below the toxic range.[188] However, motor block developed over time even with lower concentrations.[182] Following major abdominal or orthopaedic surgery, in patients with access to intravenous PCA (with morphine), the ropivacaine groups of patients consumed significantly less morphine over the infusion periods.[175,184,189] Ropivacaine also provided postoperative analgesia superior to

that with PCA morphine alone.[175,184,189] Therefore, after major abdominal or orthopaedic surgery, ropivacaine (2–3 mg/mL at 8–10 mL per hour) provides the best balance of analgesia, opioid-sparing and minimal motor blockade.[174,175,184,190] Higher infusion rates (10–14 mL per hour) cause an increase in motor blockade and urinary retention without providing significantly improved analgesia.[11] Alternatively, ropivacaine 0.1 per cent combined with an epidural opioid might produce adequate analgesia with a lower risk of motor blockade, but study results are still pending.[182] At present, the 0.2 per cent solution is commercially available as a Polybag® epidural infusion kit with 100 mL and 200 mL doses, or as 20 mL (10 mg/mL) or 0 mL (2.5 mg/mL).[182]

The intrathecal administration of 3 mL 0.5 per cent and 0.75 per cent plain ropivacaine has been studied.[176] The incidence of complete motor blockade and the duration of analgesia was higher with 0.75 per cent ropivacaine. A high proportion of patients did not achieve complete motor blockade with 0.5 per cent ropivacaine. This may have implications in terms of a 'test dose' as the absence of motor blockade may not exclude intrathecal catheter placement.[176]

Maternal deaths resulting from the use of epidural bupivacaine have highlighted the risks associated with this local anaesthetic. A meta-analysis of six obstetric studies of patents in labour has confirmed a lower incidence of motor blockade and consequently a reduced rate of instrumental deliveries with ropivacaine (0.2–0.25 per cent at 6–8 mL per hour).[191,192] Moreover, possibly because of the drug's shorter half-life in maternal plasma, neonates born to mothers who had received ropivacaine had better neurobehavioural scores 24 hours after birth compared with those whose mothers had been given bupivacaine.

Studies published so far show an equal efficacy of epidural ropivacaine and bupivacaine in caesarean section deliveries.[176,193–195] Sensory blockade and surgical conditions appear to be similar. One open study has shown the effectiveness of 150 mg ropivacaine (7.5 mg/mL).[196] Assessment of the uteroplacental circulation by Doppler ultrasound has shown evidence of some vasoconstriction with the use of bupivacaine but not with ropivacaine. No side-effects could be demonstrated in either mother or newborn. Apgar and post-delivery neurological adaptive capacity scores showed no signs of any local anaesthetic influence on the neonate.

Based on available clinical data, ropivacaine appears to be as effective and well tolerated as bupivacaine when equianalgesic doses are compared.[177] A greater separation between motor and sensory blockade is seen with ropivacaine relative to bupivacaine at lower concentrations. This profile of blockade with low doses of ropivacaine in terms of its greater sensory–motor separation and higher clearance than bupivacaine makes it suitable for use as a continuous epidural infusion.[176] Ropivacaine can also be considered to be a genuine advance in epidural analgesia/anaesthesia for labour and caesarean section deliveries. The maximum recommended dose is 2.5–3.0 mg/kg for peripheral nerve, brachial plexus and epidural blocks.[182] Ropivacaine thus offers distinct advantages over bupivacaine.

BENZODIAZEPINES

Despite their extensive use in anaesthesia and chronic pain management, the involvement of the benzodiazepines in pain mechanisms and their method of modulation is not well established. The intrathecal injection of midazolam provides analgesia that is clearly segmental and is therefore spinally mediated. The analgesic effects are specific for somatic pain.[197] Flumazenil blocks this antinociceptive effect. The selective GABA antagonist bucuculline, when given intrathecally, markedly attenuates the segmental analgesic effect of midazolam.[198] Benzodiazepines injected into the periaqueductal grey matter antagonize morphine analgesia, showing an interaction between the benzodiazepines and the opioid system in the modulation of nociceptive inputs.[199] The possible involvement of the benzodiazepines in the modulation of nociceptive transmission at the level of the dorsal horn has recently been presented.[200] Further research in this area needs to be undertaken.

INTRAVENOUS REGIONAL ANAESTHESIA

Since systemic toxicity is dose dependent, new approaches aim to reduce the dose of lignocaine and supplement with an opioid, non-depolarizing muscle relaxant or an NSAID.[182] Morphine 6 mg and pethidine 100 mg (with intrinsic local anaes-

thetic properties) have been used with local anaesthetics, with varying degrees of success.[182] Low-dose non-depolarizing muscle relaxants (pancuronium 0.5 mg; atracurium 2 mg and mivacurium 0.6 mg) have been successfully used to improve the onset time and intensity of motor blockade with intravenous regional anaesthesia.[182] Intravenous regional anaesthesia with a combination of lignocaine 1.5 mg/kg, fentanyl 1 μg/kg and pancuronium 0.5 mg gives rise to an anaesthetic effect similar to that of lignocaine 3 mg/kg at 20 minutes.[182] Ketorolac 60 mg, an injectable NSAID added to lignocaine 190 mg, can prolong analgesia to a mean of 10 hours by its anti-inflammatory response at peripheral nerve endings.[182] A similar response is seen after direct wound infiltration with ketorolac.[182]

NEW APPROACHES IN PERIPHERAL NERVE BLOCKADE

The continued refinement of new blocking techniques will enhance the potential for success of blockade and patient safety, benefitting both patient care and the health care economy.[182] Target nerves and local anaesthetic spread can be localized using ultrasound.[182] The mid-humeral approach to the brachial plexus uses a single needle puncture in the upper third of the arm by individually anaesthetizing the median, radial, ulnar and musculocutaneous nerves with 10 mL local anaesthetic, with 88 per cent success rates in 4–8 minutes.[182] For a 93 per cent success rate in shoulder and arm surgery, a novel supraclavicular intersternocleidomastoid technique can be used by passing the needle (and later a catheter) between the sternal and clavicular heads towards the mid-clavicular point to contact the superior brachial plexus trunk.[182] Eliciting proximal paraesthesia at the shoulder with interscalene blocks is as reliable as distal paraesthesia.[182] Axillary blockade provides surgical anaesthesia in 89 per cent of patients undergoing elbow surgery.[182]

Parasacral sciatic nerve block (at the greater sciatic foramen) blocks other plexus branches (e.g. the obturator nerve), facilitating catheter placement for postoperative analgesia.[182] In posterior sciatic nerve blockade, midline needle insertion with inversion and dorsiflexion via a nerve stimulator ensures success.[182] The classical approach 10 cm above the crease may, because of a surrounding epineural sheath, allow complete blockade when only one nerve branch is contacted.[182] A new compartment block below the popliteal fossa blocks both the tibial and common peroneal nerves individually in separate osteofascial compartments.[182] Selective blockade of the posterior popliteal nerve and the posterior cutaneous nerve of the thigh gives surgical anaesthesia and a faster recovery for short saphenous vein stripping.[182] Blockade of the femoral and genitofemoral nerves for stripping of the long saphenous vein results in fast-track recovery.[182]

NEURAXIAL ANAESTHESIA

Transient radicular irritation, a syndrome of back and leg pain after intrathecal local anaesthesia, common with lignocaine (16–37 per cent), may be a mild form of neurotoxicity increased by lithotomy and the addition of phenylephrine.[182] The current recommendation is to use dilute lignocaine (1.5 per cent or less) in a dose of not more than 100 mg (some recommending less than 60 mg).[182] The onset, quality and duration of intrathecal hyperbaric lignocaine are clinically indistinguishable from those seen with the 5 per cent solution (which should never be used).[182] The mean effective anaesthetic concentration of hyperbaric lignocaine to produce complete sensory and motor block in 50 per cent of human subjects has been found to be 0.54 per cent when a dose of 48 mg is given, and this value is dose dependent.[182] The addition of opioid to supplement low-dose intrathecal local anaesthetics (e.g. fentanyl to lignocaine/bupivacaine) is also new.

DRUG DELIVERY SYSTEMS

Great use is made by the hospice movement of small syringe drivers for continuous subcutaneous opioid infusions. PCA equipment ranges from simple disposable pumps (Baxter Health Care, United Kingdom; Go-Medical – Subiaco, Western Australia) to very sophisticated microprocessor systems.[201–204] Catheters have been implanted into perivascular sheaths where continuous infusions of local anaesthetic have been used. Catheters can also be implanted into the epidural and intrathecal spaces with or without permanent infusion devices. Intrathecal pumps range from a simple intrathecal pump, where a little reservoir is placed subcutaneously on top of a rib and the morphine is pumped into the intrathecal space via a catheter, to permanent intrathecal pumps (Deltic Pump – Pharmacia Deltic, United States; Cordis Secor – Cordis Corporation United States; Synchromed – Medtronic, United States; and Infusaid Continuous Infusion Pump).[205–207]

Novel routes of opioid administration for acute pain include aerosol inhalation (morphine), intranasal spraying (with butorphanol, fentanyl and sufentanil), the oral transmucosal route (fentanyl) and the transdermal route (slow-release fentanyl patches).[45] Fentanyl patches have also been used in the treatment of cancer pain.[45] The transdermal drug delivery of ionized drugs can be enhanced by iontophoresis, whereby transfer can be facilitated using a small current across two electrodes.[205] Recent work with EMLA cream has shown the efficacy of the method in preventing pain on the injection of propofol.[208] Morphine is a water-soluble opioid that is absorbed transdermally by iontophoresis by the application of 2 mA of pulsed direct current (2.5 kHz).[208] It was detectable after 5 minutes with a t_{max} of about 1 hour and a peak concentration ranging from 11.4 to 19.8 ng/mL.[208] The future development of iontophoretctic delivery techniques may provide an effective and non-invasive system for PCA. The delivery of fentanyl by iontophoresis enables the rapid achievement of steady state and the ability to vary the delivery rate.[208] This would potentially be beneficial not only in patients suffering chronic pain with breakthrough symptoms, but also for the treatment of acute pain.[208]

The inhalational route is non-invasive and is associated with a rapid but large variation in absorption.[208] Inhalational opioids given by wet nebulization have been investigated in a variety of opioids in a wide range of doses, concentrations and volumes (2–6 mL).[208] Morphine (with its bitter taste) was detected in the plasma after 1 minute, with a plasma t_{max} for morphine and diamorphine at about 10 and 6 minutes, respectively.[208] Fentanyl (causing cough and nasal pruritus) is also absorbed rapidly (t_{max} approximately 2 minutes).[208] Inhaled fentanyl for postoperative pain has been associated with plasma concentrations 95 per cent lower than those regarded as analgesic, but there is no evidence that this mode of delivery is more effective than other parenteral methods.[208]

For providing prolonged regional analgesia, the application of a timed-release local anaesthetic preparation adjacent to nerves could potentially be a useful alternative to catheter infusions or neurolytic blocks.[205] Some of the local anaesthetics and opioids (bupivacaine and fentanyl) are being prolonged by incorporating them in a variety of encapsulation matrices. These include liposomes, iophendylate, biodegradable polymers and transfersomes.[205] Perhaps inhaled liposome-encapsulated fentanyl may offer a future method of opioid administration.[147] Novel cell therapy systems are being designed to deliver therapeutic substances to the CNS for the treatment of chronic (including cancer) pain.

Continuous intrathecal anaesthesia, using microcatheters (28 and 32 gauge) in the intrathecal space, provides a route of administration of drugs with additive or synergistic effects (e.g. local anaesthetics, opioids and and α_2-adrenergic agonists).[205] The advantage is that these catheters keep the risk of postdural puncture headaches to a minimum. They could prove beneficial, especially in high-risk patients, by providing excellent analgesia while causing minimal changes in blood pressure and minimal motor blockade.[55] Problems with microcatheters include difficulty in placement and the maldistribution of local anaesthetics. Cauda equina syndromes as a result of the neurotoxic effect of high concentrations of local anaesthetic administration have been reported.[55,205]

PCEA (using fentanyl, hydromorphone or morphine) has been successfully used for postsurgical pain.[55] Continuous infusion lumbar epidural infusions as well as PCEA with bupivacaine (0.0625–0.125 per cent) or ropivacaine, plus fentanyl (1–2 μg/mL), has been successfully used for analgesia during labour and delivery.[205,209] In one institution, PCEA is first established as a basal infusion using bupivacaine 0.1 per cent and fentanyl 4 μg/mL (or hydromorphone 0.03 mg/mL) at 4–8 mL per hour (although at a lower rate for thoracic catheters).[182] The PCEA dose is about 30 per cent of the hourly basal infusion rate with a lockout time of 15–30 minutes.[182] PCEA is also used in chronic cancer pain.

Combined spinal–epidural or double-needle techniques provide the speed and reliability of neuraxial analgesia or anaesthesia with the advantages of a continuous catheter technique.[55,209,210] This gives

greater flexibility in providing high-quality analgesia and anaesthesia, before, during and after surgery (especially for labour, caesarean section and outpatient lower limb surgery).[182] To lower the risk of hypotension, a small intrathecal dose of local anaesthetic (e.g. lignocaine 30–40 mg) is given first.[182] Adrenaline 15 μg injected epidurally after the induction of intrathecal anaesthesia remains a reliable test dose.[182] The extension of intrathecal anaesthesia is rapid after epidural drug injection.[182] The rate of flux of an epidural opioid (and also catheter penetration) through the dural hole depends on the size of the hole rather than on the physicochemical properties of the drugs given.[182] Catheter penetration remains rare unless dural puncture by a 22 gauge or larger needle occurs.[182]

The introduction of small diameter 'pencil point' needles (Whitacre, Sprotte, Gertie Marx and Portex) is associated with a small incidence of headaches (less than 1 per cent in the obstetric patient).[209,210]

The balanced approach of using combined epidural and general anaesthesia for major vascular, thoracic and abdominal surgery needs diligent attention to epidural placement, test dose administration and the choice of top-up agents.[182] An epidural test dose (e.g. lignocaine 45 mg and adrenaline 15 μg producing an increase in heart rate of 20 beats per minute or a systolic blood pressure of 15 mmHg, respectively, if given intravenously) is blunted under general anaesthesia by volatile cardiovascular depression.[182] Haemodynamic stability under general anaesthesia is preserved by giving less epidural local anaesthetic and more epidural opioid (e.g. bupivacaine 0.1 per cent continuous solution with morphine 0.05 mg/mL or fentanyl 4 μg/mL).[182] Using postoperative epidural analgesia, several (but not all) studies report improved cardiorespiratory function after major vascular, thoracic and abdominal surgery.[182] Gastrointestinal recovery is accelerated using epidural local anaesthetics, early enteral feeding, patient ambulation and systemic ketorolac.[182]

CHONDROMODULATION IN JOINT DISEASE

Chondromodulation implies the capacity of therapeutic and/or biological agents to modify the progression of cartilage breakdown and joint destruction.[211] Hyaluronan and glycosaminoglycans are being used experimentally to inhibit cartilage degeneration, with materials containing sulphated proteoglycans having potential therapeutic, symptomatic and disease modification effects.[211] Clinical efficacy studies are in progress with artepon, rumalon, pentosan and chondroitin sulphate.[211] The metalloproteases collegenase and stromolysin, produced by articular chondrocytes, are critical enzymes involved in cartilage destruction.[211] Doxycycline binds zinc, an important co-enzyme in collagenase activation at a site distant from its antibiotic action, and is able to ameliorate cartilage destruction in the anterior cruciate-resected dog model of osteoarthritis.[211] Multicentre human trials in osteoarthritis of the knee are currently in progress. Diacerein acts via lymphokine inhibition (particularly interleukin-1 production) as an analgesic and anti-inflammatory agent.[211] It stimulates proteoglycan, glycosaminoglycan and hyaluronic acid synthesis while reducing metalloprotease activity on articular cartilage.[211] Clinical trials have found it to reduce pain, improve mobility and retard the progression of osteoarthritis.[5] The rational therapeutic use of chondromodulatory agents will relieve pain and suffering in joint disease in the future.

CANNABIS

The discovery of cannabinoid receptors was undoubtedly facilitated by the synthesis of novel cannabinoid ligands (delta⁹-tetrahydrocannabinol [THC], levonatradol, nabilone, CP55,940, WIN 55,212-2 and HU210).[212] Cannabinoid receptors (CB1 and CB2) are coupled to a pertussis toxin-sensitive G protein that, when activated, results in agonist inhibition of adenylyl cyclase in a pertussis toxin-sensitive manner and inhibits N-type calcium currents.[212] CB1 receptors can also activate potassium ion currents.[212] CB1 receptors are present in the brain (olfactory areas, cortex, hippocampus, cerebellum and basal ganglia) at very high concentrations, as well as in the spinal cord.[212] The few CB1 receptors in the brain stem may explain the lack of respiratory depression.[212] CB2 receptors are found mainly in the peripheral tissues (spleen, macrophages and peripheral nerve terminals).[212] CB1-selective receptor antagonists include SR141716A (with over 1000-fold selectivity) and LY320135 (with 100-fold selectivity).[212] The first CB2 antagonist is SR144528 (with a 700-fold selectivity

for the CB2 receptor).[212] The rank order binding affinity of cannabinoid ligands is as follows: SR141716A > CP55,940 > WIN55–212–2 = delta⁹-THC > anandamide.[212] Cloning of the cannabinoid receptor has led to anandamide being described as the endogenous agonist of the CB1 receptor and palmitoylethanolamide as the endogenous agonist at the CB2 receptor.[212] In future, it will be important to determine whether these two endogenous agonists are involved in acute and chronic pain syndromes. Case reports only have described the therapeutic uses of cannabinoids: as antimetics in cancer chemotherapy (nabilone, starting with 0.25 mg by opening the 1 mg capsule and dividing the resultant powder accordingly); as potential analgesics; in the treatment of glaucoma; epilepsy and movement disorders; and as appetite suppressants.[212]

Cannabinoids are likely to produce antinociception at both spinal and supraspinal sites.[212] Delta⁹-THC, WIN 55,212, and CP55,940 all possess analgesic activity at the CB1 receptor.[212] Intravenous, intraperitoneal and intrathecal anandamide produce antinociception in mice.[212] Intrathecal cannabinoid agonists may have the potential to produce antinociceptive effects without psychotropism.[212] WIN 55,212 suppresses formalin-induced C-Fos expression in the rat spinal cord, indicating that cannabinoids also inhibit the spinal processing of noxious stimuli.[212]. In a controlled trial in humans, THC 20 mg was found to be comparable to codeine 60 mg or 120 mg in cancer pain. Patients prefer cannabis to nabilone (which results in drowsiness and dysphoria) for analgesia (the success rate of pain relief in neurogenic pain is less than 30 per cent with nabilone), for pain distancing, compressing the pain, sleep, the relief of muscle and bladder spasms, the relief of constipation, relaxation, anxiolysis, the amelioration of depression and euphoria.[212]

For cannabinoids, both a central and a peripheral receptor have been cloned and endogenous agonists identified.[212] Animal work and limited clinical trials suggest a great analgesic therapeutic potential for cannabinoids.

NEUROSURGERY

Much progress has been made in the improvement of spinal cord stimulation devices. The percutaneous placement of spinal cord stimulation electrodes has reduced morbidity and facilitates proper patient selection following a trial period. The application of functional neuroaugmentation of pain is still in its infancy.[213] As new methods become established, they should contribute to the understanding of cerebral pain mechanisms.

EDUCATION IN CANCER MANAGEMENT AND PALLIATIVE CARE

The Network Project is a 2-week observership programme in cancer pain management, psychosocial oncology and cancer rehabilitation, which has proved to be an effective means of improving and disseminating knowledge regarding the multidisciplinary management of pain and psychological distress in cancer patients.[214] The Patient Care Travelling Record is a passport-like health care summary that has been found to be a feasible and acceptable tool to convey important clinical information about the palliative care patient, reducing patient uncertainty, specifically in adults under 65 years.[215]

ALTERNATIVE THERAPIES AND COMPLEMENTARY MEDICINE

Alternative and complementary medicine includes a vast array of both modalities in which the patient is a passive recipient, as well as self-care techniques.[216] As a result of individuals taking more charge of their health, as well as becoming disenchanted with the costs and outcomes of allopathic care, interest in this area is rapidly growing.[216] These therapies include meditation, music, guided imagery, massage, vitamin and mineral supplementation, and relaxation techniques.[217] A survey of the use of alternative therapies by rehabilitation outpatients showed that one or more alternative medical therapies had been used by 29.1 per cent of subjects in the past 12 months for their problem, 53 per cent of whom reported some degree of efficacy.[217] Musculoskeletal pain syndromes involving the spine and extremities were the most common problems for which patients sought care.[217] In another recent survey in a family practice population, more than 28 per cent used alternative medicine.[218] Common

methods were chiropractic (64 per cent), massage therapy (36 per cent), herbal therapy (32 per cent) and acupuncture (16 per cent).[218] The most common problems for which patients sought alternative care were back pain (56 per cent) and other musculoskeletal pain (22 per cent).[218] Most had not informed their family practitioner of their use of alternative health care.[218] Although most (82 per cent) derived some benefit, many (under 50 per cent) were not satisfied with the results, which demands further study in the future.[218] The majority of alternative medicine users, however, appear to be following such treatment as they find these health care alternatives to be more congruent with their own values, beliefs and philosophical orientations towards health and life.[219]

The techniques of mindfulness meditation (e.g. Christian meditation and prayer) may represent a powerful method of transforming the ways in which patients respond to and cope with painful life events, with the potential for preventing relapse.[216,220] The what of suffering is unclear.[221] It is pain, fear, despair, lack of strength, lack of freedom and non-motion.[221] It is a struggle between wanting and knowing, and between guilt and responsibility.[221] In a caring culture, to be physically touched by a care-giver can help alleviate the deepest suffering.[221] Compassion always helps to alleviate suffering.[221]

Music is a nursing intervention with the potential to decrease patient perception in the post-anaesthesia care unit.[222] Following surgery, repeated measures analysis of variance showed an interaction between the distress of pain on day 1 and the sensation of pain on day 2.[223] Cross-culturally, compared with the USA, fewer Taiwanese found the music calming, choosing more harp and less jazz music that their American counterparts.[223] It is thus important for culturally acceptable music to be used in future such trials.

Burn injury patients undergoing debridement were found to benefit from massage therapy.[224] Debridement sessions were less painful after the massage therapy as a result of a reduction in anxiety, and the clinical course was probably enhanced because of a reduction in pain, anger and depression.[224] For geriatric and hospice care, the use of aromatherapy with massage may be beneficial.[225] Articles extolling the use of essential oils reflect subjective, individual findings and do not account for the multitude of influencing environmental factors (e.g. the degree of pain).[225] Future research needs to be conducted so that scientific, qualitative measurements can be proved and documented.

Pain management programmes assist patients in using their behavioural and cognitive skills for the purpose of rendering their experience of pain in some way more tolerable.[226] Thus, hypnosis can best be conceived as a set of skills to be deployed by the individual rather than as a state.[226] Hypnotic analgesia is an active process that requires inhibitory effort, dissociated from conscious awareness, in which the anterior frontal cortex participates in a topographically inhibitory feedback circuit that cooperates in the allocation of thalamocortical activities.[227] There are different strategies of modulation operative during effective hypnotic analgesia, and these are subject dependent.[228] Although all patients may shift their attention away from the painful stimulus (leading to the decrease in late somatosensory evoked potentials), some inhibit their motor reaction to the stimulus at the spinal level, while in others this reaction is facilitated.[228] Self-efficacy can be developed through the successful transfer by participants of newly learned skills of experimental pain reduction to a reduction of their own chronic pain.[228]

THE PSYCHOLOGICAL FACTOR

In recent years, in patients suffering pain, psychological factors and their importance have increasingly been realized,[45] although not all of the available psychological tests have been adequately constructed or validated.[45] There is a need to do this, as well as to continue studying the psychological factors that influence the experience of pain. It is critical for patients to understand why they have pain, what the potential causes are, and the way to manage it.[229] The goal of pain management is to enhance function and improve quality of life. To facilitate this, it is necessary that the patient be educated to understand and accept pain, reduce stress, stay active, learn the difference between hurt and harm, and understand the myths about chronic pain.[229] This is most often provided by the patient attending pain classes on a contractual basis. The patient's immediate family (and employer) are often included in this process.[229]

CONCLUSION

Advances need to be made in the establishment of more appropriate clinical models of pain.[49] The more effective use of techniques such as microneurography, argon laser excitation and somatosensory evoked potential recording is warranted. A better understanding of the molecular pathology of human pain using molecular technologies to advance the understanding of human genetics and disease processes is essential.[49] Understanding the relationship between the change in chemical phenotype and the mechanisms underlying the development of persistent hyperalgesia represents one of the major challenges for current pain research.[49] New pain conditions, such as AIDS-related neuropathic pain, need to be promptly recognized and effectively treated. Novel new opioids (acting peripherally), new NMDA and NK receptor antagonists, CCK antagonists, leukotriene antagonists, NO synthetase inhibitors, new adenosine A_1 receptor agonists, novel α_2-adrenergic receptor agonists and new COX-2 selective NSAIDs are awaited in the short and medium terms. In the long term, new bradykinin B_2/B_1 receptor antagonists, cytokine suppressive anti-inflammatory drugs, novel sodium channel blockers and potassium channel openers, new CGRP-receptor antagonists, somatostatin receptor agonists, galanin receptor agonists and nicotinic receptor agonists are being sought. The clarification of the mechanisms involved in the establishment of chronic painful conditions (in which pain persists even though the precipitating cause has disappeared) should reveal new targets for drug discovery.[3] Many will be conventional targets (receptors, enzymes, transport systems and channels), yet the targeting of regulatory events at the level of gene transcription will advance therapeutic intervention at this level.[3]

For acute pain management, the public are increasingly demanding first-class post-traumatic and perioperative pain management, which should be a quality assurance item in every hospital.[230] There are very few standardized, tested algorithms for the diagnosis or treatment of any painful condition, and studies looking directly at treatment outcomes for common painful conditions are needed.[230] The biomedical model has largely given way, especially for chronic diseases, to the biopsychosocial model, which implies an interaction between personal, psychological and social factors to explain individual differences in illness and disability.[230] Physicians should recognize the important roles of affective and environmental factors in symptom generation and remission.[230] There has been a shift from inpatient to outpatient care, as well as a shift towards outcome-based medical practice and research of pain management.[230] If pain management specialists and pain relief units are to survive, their efficacy and relative value compared with other forms of health care will have to be demonstrated.[230] Epidemiological studies are starting to show the true incidence of painful illnesses, and health services research is beginning to study resource allocation for the management of different painful conditions to reduce costs and provide effective rehabilitation.[230] Health services research is identifying varieties, costs and outcomes of treatment.[230] Those who provide pain management services will have to learn about the illness they treat, how to determine treatment outcomes compared with other treatment methods and how to collect treatment data in a clinically meaningful and scientifically valid way.[230] Yet the most important role of the physician, to listen and educate, to provide guidance, prognostication, support and sympathy, must not be lost.[230]

To conclude, future progress in pain management will come from strengthening the alliance between basic science, which suggests therapeutic options, and clinical epidemiology, which evaluates them.[231] In recent years, psychological factors and their importance have increasingly been realized. Advances in receptor pharmacology, the synthesis of different classes of active drugs, the increasing sophistication of drug delivery systems and research seeking to clarify the psychological processes that affect the pain experience have all helped in understanding the neurophysiological and neuropsychological aspects of pain.[232,233] Relief for patients will come from ensuring that practice is based on the best available knowledge. What an exciting challenge this provides to all health care professionals to alleviate suffering and to improve the pain care of patients responsible for their control.

REFERENCES

1. **Rudy, T.E., Turk, D.C., Brena, S.F., Stieg, R.L. and Brody, M.C.** 1990: Quantification of biomedical findings of chronic pain patients: development of an index of pathology. *Pain* **42**, 167–82.
2. **Dickenson, A.H.** 1996: Pharmacology of pain transmission and control. In Campbell, J.N. (ed.) *Pain 1996 – an updated review*. Seattle: IASP Press, 113–21.
3. **Rang, H.P. and Urban, L.** 1995: New molecules in analgesia. *British Journal of Anaesthesia* **75**, 145–56.
4. **Cousins, M.J. and Siddal, P.J.** 1996: Postoperative pain: implication of peripheral and central sensitisa-

tion. In Keneally, J.P. and Jones, M.J. (eds) *150 years on – a selection of papers presented at the 11th World Congress of Anaesthesiologists*. Rosebery, NSW: Bridge Printery, 73–81.
5. **Mogil, J.S. and Grisel, J.E.** 1998: Transgenic studies of pain. *Pain* **77**, 107–28.
6. **Grubb, B.D.** 1998: Peripheral and central mechanisms of pain. *British Journal of Anaesthesia* **81**, 8–11.
7. **Jain, S.** 1995: Current concepts in chronic pain management. *American Society of Anesthesiologists' Annual Refresher Course Lectures* **272**, 1–7.
8. **Traub, R.J., Pechmann, P., Iadarola, M.J. and Gebhart, G.F.** 1992: Fos-like proteins in the lumbosacral spinal cord following noxious and non-noxious colorectal distension in the rat. *Pain* **49**, 393–403.
9. **Jagger, S.I. and Rice, A.S.C.** 1996: Novel vistas in analgesic pharmacology for the treatment of chronic pain. *Anaesthetic Pharmacology and Physiology Review* **4**, 66–73.
10. **Ren, K.** 1994: Wind-up and the NMDA receptor: from animal studies to humans. *Pain* **59**, 157–8.
11. **Shipton, E.A.** 1993: Sensitisation, pre-emptive and total analgesia. *South African Medical Journal* **83**, 555–6.
12. **Dubner, R.** 1992: Hyperalgesia and expanded receptive fields. *Pain* **48**, 3–4.
13. **Woolf, C.J.** 1991: Generation of acute pain: central mechanisms. *British Medical Bulletin* **47**(3), 523–33.
14. **Dubner, R.** 1990: Neuronal plasticity and pain. *Pain* (Suppl. 5), S263.
15. **Iadarola, M.J.** 1996: Functional analysis of cloned genes and regulation of gene-expression: examples from pain-related studies. In Campbell, J.N. (ed.) *Pain 1996 – an updated review*. Seattle: IASP Press, 533–48.
16. **Munglani, R. and Hunt, S.P.** 1995: Molecular biology of pain. *British Journal of Anaesthesia* **75**, 186–92.
17. **Elliot, K.J., Brodsky, M., Hynansky, A.D., Foley, K. and Inturrisi, C.E.** 1995: Dextromethorphan suppresses both formalin-induced nociceptive behavior and the formalin-induced increase in spinal cord c-fos mRNA. *Pain* **61**, 401–9.
18. **Yi, D.K. and Barr, G.A.** 1995: The induction of Fos-like immunoreactivity by noxious thermal, mechanical and chemical stimuli in the lumbar cord. *Pain* **60**, 257–65.
19. **Lambert, D.G.** 1998: Recent advances in opioid pharmacology. *British Journal of Anaesthesia* **81**(1), 1–2.
20. **Darland, T. and Grandy, D.K.** 1998: The orphanin FQ system: an emerging target for the management of pain? *British Journal of Anaesthesia* **81**, 29–37.
21. **Cepeda, M.S.** 1995: Autonomic nervous system and pain. *Current Opinion in Anaesthesiology* **8**(5), 450–4.
22. **Canavero, S. and Bonicalzi, V.** 1998: The neurochemistry of central pain: evidence from clinical studies, hypothesis and therapeutic implications. *Pain* **74**, 109–14.
23. **McQuay, H.J.** 1992: Pre-emptive analgesia. *British Journal of Anaesthesia* **69**(1), 1–3.
24. **Katz, J., Kavanagh, B.P., Sandler, A.N. *et al.*** 1992: Pre-emptive analgesia: clinical evidence of neuroplasticity contributing to postoperative pain. *Anesthesiology* **77**, 439–46.

25. **Dahl, J.B., Erichsen, C.J., Fuglsang-Frederiksen, A. and Kehlet, H.** 1992: Pain sensation and nociceptive reflex excitability in surgical patients and human volunteers. *British Journal of Anaesthesia* **69**, 117–21.

26. **Bach, S., Noreng, M.F. and Tjellden, N.U.** 1988: Phantom limb pain in amputees during the first 12 months following limb amputation, after preoperative lumbar epidural blockade. *Pain* **33**, 297–301.

27. **Atanassoff, P.G. and Jarret, J.M.** 1996: The physiological and pharmacological aspects of pre-emptive analgesia. *Anaesthetic Pharmacology and Physiology Review* **4**, 6–20.

28. **Breivik, H., Breivik, E.K. and Stubhaug, A.** 1996: Clinical aspects of pre-emptive analgesia: prevention of post-operative pain by pretreatment and continued optimal treatment. *Pain Reviews* **3**, 63–78.

29. **McQuay, H.J.** 1995: Pre-emptive analgesia: a systematic review of clinical studies. *Annals of Medicine* **27**, 249–56.

30. **Kissin, I.** 1996: Preemptive analgesia: why its effect is not always obvious. *Anesthesiology* **84**(5), 1015–19.

31. **Penning, J.P.** 1996: Pre-emptive analgesia: what does it mean to the clinical anaesthetist? *Canadian Journal of Anaesthesia* **43**(2), 97–101.

32. **Kiss, I.E. and Kilian, M.** 1992: Does opiate premedication influence postoperative analgesia? *Pain* **48**, 157–8.

33. **Comfort, V.K., Code, W.E., Rooyney, M.E. and Yip, R.W.** 1992: Naproxen premedication reduces post tubal ligation pain. *Canadian Journal of Anaesthesia* **39**(4), 349–52.

34. **Nissen, I., Jensen, K.A. and Ohrstram, J.K.** 1992: Indomethacin in the management of postoperative pain. *British Journal of Anaesthesia* **69**, 304–6.

35. **Budd, K.** 1992: A rational approach to acute pain. *South African Society of Anaesthetists Annual Refresher Course Lectures*, 1–13.

36. **Dickenson, A.H.** 1995: Spinal cord pharmacology of pain. *British Journal of Anaesthesia* **75**, 193–200.

37. **Carpenter, R.I.** 1995: Does outcome change with pain management? *American Society of Anesthesiologists Annual Refresher Course Lectures* **273**, 1–6.

38. **MacMahon, S.B., Dmitrieva, N. and Koltzenburg, M.** 1995: Visceral pain. *British Journal of Anaesthesia* **75**, 32–44.

39. **Anand, P.** 1995: Nerve growth factor regulates nociception in human health and disease. *British Journal of Anaesthesia* **75**, 201–8.

40. **Willis, W.D.** 1996: Signal transduction mechanisms. In Campbell, J.N. (ed.) *Pain 1996 – an updated review.* Seattle: IASP Press, 527–31.

41. **Brooks, J.H.J., Rattan, A.K., Gupta, B. and Tejwani, G.** 1991: Opioid peptides in human peripheral nerves. *Anesthesiology* **75**(3A), A591.

42. **Stein, C. and Yassouridis, A.** 1997: Peripheral morphine analgesia. *Pain* **71**, 119–21.

43. **Kayser, V., Gobeaux, D., Lombard, M.C., Guilbaud, G. and Besson, J.M.** 1990: Potent and long-lasting antinociceptive effects after injection of low doses of a mu-opioid agonist, fentanyl, into the brachial plexus sheath of the rat. *Pain* **42**, 215–25.

44. **Wildsmith, J.A.W.** 1989: Developments in local anaesthetic drugs and techniques for pain relief. *British Journal of Anaesthesia* **63**, 159–64.

45. **Shipton, E.A.** 1994: Pain care – new developments. *South African Medical Journal* **84**, 188–9.

46. **Fleetwood-Walker, S.M.** 1995: Nonopioid mediators and modulators of nociceptive processing in the spinal horn as targets for novel analgesics. *Pain Reviews* **2**, 153–73.

47. **Ballantyne, J.C. and Dershwitz, M.** 1995: The pharmacology on non-steroidal anti-inflammatory drugs for acute pain. *Current Opinion in Anaesthesiology* **8**(5), 461–8.

48. **Wall, P.D.** 1995: Inflammatory and neurogenic pain: new molecules, new mechanisms. *British Journal of Anaesthesia* **75**(2), 123–4.

49. **Birch, P.J.** 1995: Clinical relevance of receptor pharmacology in the nociceptive pathway. *Pain Reviews* **2**, 13–27.

50. **Eisenburg, E. and Birkhan, J.** 1995: Non-steroidal anti-inflammatory drugs for cancer-related pain. *Current Opinion in Anaesthesiology* **8**(5), 469–72.

51. **Winnie, A.P., Krolick, T.J., Sagen, J., Pappas, G.D. and Wang, H.** 1991: Subarachnoid adrenal medullary transplantation. *Anesthesiology* **75**(3A), A695.

52. **Ginzburg, R. and Seltzer, Z.** 1990: Allografting the adrenal medulla of adult rats into the lumbar subarachnoid space suppresses autotomy: a model of deafferentation-induced pain. *Pain* (suppl. 5), S462.

53. **Martinez, R., Vaquero, J. and Reig, E.** 1990: Transplantation of chromaffin tissue into medullary arachnoid for relieving malignant pain in humans. *Pain* (suppl. 5), S413.

54. **Sagen, J., Wang, H. and Pappas, G.D.** 1990: Adrenal medullary implants in the rat spinal cord reduce nociception in the chronic pain model. *Pain* **42**, 69–79.

55. **Shipton, E.A.** 1996: New concepts in pain management. *South African Journal of Anaesthesiology and Analgesia* **2**(1), 4–8.

56. **Karlsten, R., Gordh, T., Hartvig, P. and Post, C.** 1990: Effects of intrathecal injection of the adenosine receptor agonists R-phenyl isopropyl adenosine and N-ethyl carboxamide-adenosine on nociception and motor function in the rat. *Anesthesia and Analgesia* **71**, 60–4.

57. **Fusco, B.M. and Alessandri, M.** 1992: Analgesic effect of capsaicin in idiopathic trigeminal neuralgia. *Anesthesia and Analgesia* **74**, 375–7.

58. **Winter, J., Bevan, S. and Campbell, E.A.** 1995: Capsaicin and pain mechanisms. *British Journal of Anaesthesia* **75**, 157–68.

59. **McQuay, H.J. and Dickenson, A.H.** 1990: Implication of nervous system plasticity for pain management. *Anaesthesia* **45**, 101–2.

60. **Aanonsen, L., Lei, S. and Wilcox, G.L.** 1990: Excitatory amino acid receptors and nociceptive neurotransmission in the rat spinal cord. *Pain* **41**, 309–21.

61. **Murray, C.W., Cowan, A. and Larson, A.A.** 1991: Neurokinin and NMDA antagonists (but not a kainic acid antagonist) are antinociceptive in the mouse formalin model. *Pain* **44**, 179–85.

62. **Zelster, R., Seltzer, Z., Eisen, A., Feigenbaum, J.J. and Mechoulam, R.** 1991: Suppression of neuropathic pain behavior in rats by non-psychotropic synthetic cannabinoid with NMDA receptor-blocking properties. *Pain* **47**, 95–103.

63. **Yamamoto, T. and Yaksh, T.L.** 1992: Spinal pharmacology of thermal hyperesthesia induced by constrictive injury of sciatic nerve: excitatory amino acid antagonists. *Pain* **49**, 121–8.

64. **Woolf, C.J. and Thompson, W.N.** 1991: The induction and maintenance of central sensitisation is dependent on N-methyl-D-aspartic acid receptor activation: implications for the treatment of post-injury pain hypersensitivity states. *Pain* **44**, 293–9.

65. **Dubner, R.** 1991: Pain and hyperalgesia following tissue injury: new mechanisms and new treatments. *Pain* **44**, 213–14.

66. **Fraser, H.M., Chapman, V. and Dickenson, A.H.** 1992: Spinal local anaesthetic actions on afferent evoked responses and wind-up of nociceptive neurones in the rat spinal cord: combination with morphine produces marked potentiation of antinociception. *Pain* **49**, 33–41.

67. **Sukiennik, A.W. and Krean, R.M.** 1995: N-methyl-D-aspartate receptors and pain. *Current Opinion in Anaesthesiology* **8**(5), 445–9.

68. **Hill, R.G.** 1996: Discovery of new analgesic drugs: issues relating to centrally acting agents given systemically. In Campbell, J.N. (ed.) *Pain 1996 – an updated review*. Seattle: IASP Press, 377–80.

69. **Rang, H.P., Bevan, S. and Dray, A.** 1991: Chemical activation of nociceptive peripheral neurones. *British Medical Bulletin* **47**(3), 534–48.

70. **Dickenson, A.** 1995: Novel pharmacological targets in the treatment of pain. *Pain Reviews* **2**, 1–12.

71. **Budd, K.** 1989: Recent advances in the treatment of chronic pain. *British Journal of Anaesthesia* **63**, 207–12.

72. **Devor, M., Wall, P.D. and Catalan, N.** 1992: Systemic lidocaine silences ectopic neuroma and DRG discharge without blocking nerve conduction. *Pain* **48**, 261–8.

73. **Schneider, M., Datta, S. and Strichartz, G.R.** 1991: A preferential inhibition of impulses in C-fibres of the rabbit vagus nerve by veratridine, an activator of sodium channels. *Anesthesiology* **74**, 270–80.

74. **Strichartz, G.R., Drachmann, D.E., Latka, C. and Feldman, H.S.** 1991: Sensory and motor block of rat sciatic nerve in vivo produced by the sodium channel activator veratridine. *Anesthesiology* **75**(3A), A771.

75. **Traynor, J.R.** 1998: Epibatidine and pain. *British Journal of Anaesthesia* **81**, 69–76.

76. **Abram, S.E.** 1996: Analgesia in the clinic. In: Campbell, J.N. (ed.) *Pain 1996 – an updated review*. Seattle: IASP Press, 375–6.

77. **Miaskowski, C., Sutters, K.A., Taiwo, Y.O. and**

78. **Levine, J.D.** 1992: Antinociceptive and motor effects of delta/mu and kappa/mu combinations of intrathecal opioid agonists. *Pain* **49**, 137–44.

78. **Harrison, C., Smart, D. and Lambert, D.G.** 1998: Stimulatory effects of opioids. *British Journal Anaesthesia* **81**, 20–8.

79. **Jordan, B. and Devi, L.A.** 1998: Molecular mechanisms of opioid receptor signal transduction. *British Journal of Anaesthesia* **81**, 12–19.

80. **Collett, B.-J.** 1998: Opioid tolerance: the clinical perspective. *British Journal of Anaesthesia* **81**, 58–68.

81. **Omote, K., Kitahata, L.M., Collins, J.G., Nakatani, K. and Nakagawa, I.** 1990: The antinociceptive role of mu and delta-opiate receptors and their interaction in the spinal dorsal horn of cats. *Anesthesia and Analgesia* **71**, 23–8.

82. **Stevens, C.W. and Yaksh, T.L.** 1992: Studies of morphine and DADLE cross-tolerance after continuous intrathecal infusion in the rat. *Anesthesiology* **76**, 596–603.

83. **Sear, J.W.** 1998: Recent advances and developments in the clinical use of i.v. opioids during the perioperative period. *British Journal of Anaesthesia* **81**, 38–50.

84. **Hanna, M.H., Peat, S.J., Woodham, M., Knibb, A. and Fung, C.** 1990: Analgesic efficacy and CSF pharmacokinetics in intrathecal morphine-6-glucuronide: comparison with morphine. *British Journal of Anaesthetics* **64**, 547–50.

85. **Budd, K. and Shipton, E.A.** 1999: Tramadol – towards the ideal analgesic? *International Journal of Acute Pain* (in press).

86. **Dayer, P., Desmeules, J. and Collart, L.** 1997: Pharmacology of tramadol. *Drugs* **53**(suppl. 2), 18–24.

87. **Lehmann, K.A.** 1997: Tramadol in acute pain. *Drugs* **53**(suppl. 2), 25–33.

88. **Raffa, R.B.** 1996: A novel approach to the pharmacology of analgesics. *American Journal of Medicine* **101**(1A), 40S–46S.

89. **Raffa, R.B. and Friederichs, E.** 1996: The basic science aspect of tramadol hydrochloride. *Pain Reviews* **4**, 249–71.

90. **Collart, L., Luthy, C.** 1993: Partial inhibition of tramadol antinociceptive effect by naloxone in man. *British Journal of Clinical Pharmacology* **35**, 73P.

91. **Raffa, R.B., Nyak, R.K.** 1993: The mechanisms of action and pharmacokinetics of tramadol hydrochloride. *Reviews in Contemporary Pharmacotherapeutics* **6**, 485–97.

92. **Desmeules, J.A., Piguet, V., Collart, L. and Dayer, P.** 1996: Contribution of monoaminergic modulation to the analgesic effect of tramadol. *British Journal of Clinical Pharmacology* **41**(1), 7–12.

93. **Duthie, D.J.R.** 1998: Remifentanil and tramadol. *British Journal of Anaesthesia* **81**, 51–7.

94. **Raffa, R.B. and Friederichs, E.** 1992: Opioid and non-opioid components independently contribute to the mechanism of action of tramadol, an 'atypical' opioid analgesic. *Journal of Pharmacology and Experimental Therapeutics* **260**, 275–85.

95. **Mason, B.J. and Blackburn, K.H.** 1997: Possible serotonin syndrome associated with tramadol and sertraline coadministration. *Annals of Pharmacotherapeutics* **31**(2), 175–7.

96. **Seveik, J., Nieber, K., Driessen, B. and Illes, P.** 1993: Effects of the central analgesic tramadol and its main metabolite – desmethyltramadol on rat locus coeruleus neurons. *British Journal of Pharmacology* **110**, 169–76.

97. **Bono, A.V. and Cuffari, S.** 1997: Effectiveness and tolerance of tramadol in cancer pain: a comparative study with respect to buprenorphine. *Drugs* **53** (suppl. 2), 40–9.

98. **Lintz, W., Barth, H., Osterloh, G. and Schmidt-Bothelt, E.** 1986: The bioavailability of enteral tramadol formulations – first communication: capsules. *Arzneimittel Forschung/Drug Research* **36**, 1278–83.

99. **Wilder-Smith, C.H. and Bettiga, A.** 1997: The analgesic tramadol has minimal effect on gastrointestinal motor function. *British Journal of Clinical Pharmacology* **43**(1), 71–5.

100. **Sunshine, A., Olsen, N.Z., Zighelboim, I., De Castro, A. and Minn, F.L.** 1992: Analgesic oral efficacy of tramadol hydrochloride in postoperative pain. *Clinical Pharmacology and Therapeutics* **51**, 740–6.

101. **Jensen, E.M. and Ginsberg, F.** 1994: Tramadol versus dextropropoxyphene in the treatment of osteoarthritis. *Drug Investigation* **8**, 211–18.

102. **Kupers, R., Callebaut, V., Debois, V., Camu, F., Verbogh, C., Coppejars, H., Adriaensen, H.** 1995: Efficacy and safety of oral tramadol and pentazocine for post-operative pain following prolapsed intervertebral disc repair. *Acta Anaesthesiologica Belgica* **46**, 31–7.

103. **Lebedeva, R.N. and Nikoda, V.V.** 1994: Postoperative analgesia with tramadol, ketorolac, and their combination: comparison of efficacy and safety. *IX European Congress of Anaesthesiology*, 11.

104. **Rud, V. and Fischer, M.V.** 1994: Postoperative analgesia with tramadol: continuous infusion versus repetitive bolus administration. *Anaesthetist* **43**, 316–21.

105. **Rodriguez, M.J. and de la Torre, M.R.** 1993: Comparative study of tramadol versus NSAIDs as intravenous continuous infusion for post-operative pain. *Current Ther Res Clinical Exp* **54**, 375–83.

106. **Vickers, M.D., O'Flaherty, D., Szekely, S.M., Read, M. and Yoshizumi, J.** 1992: Tramadol: pain relief by an opioid without depression of respiration. *Anaesthesia* **47**, 291–6.

107. **Stamer, U.M., Maier, C., Grond, S., Veh-Schmidt, B., Klaschlik, E. and Lehmann, L.A.** 1997: Tramadol in the management of post-operative pain: a double-blind, placebo- and active-controlled study. *European Journal of Anaesthesiology* **14**(6), 646–54.

108. **Alfonso Megido, J. and Valasco, L.** 1994: Utilidad clinica dela administracion de tramadol por via subcutanea. *Cienc Pharm* **4**, 22–4.

109. **Hopkins, D., Shipton, E.A., Potgieter, D.** *et al.* 1998: The comparison of tramadol and morphine by subcutaneous PCA. *Canadian Journal of Anaesthesia* **45**, 435–42.

110. **Makanday, S. and Wilson, A.** 1997: *Integrated clinical and statistical report for a randomised, double-blind, multicentre study to compare intravenous Zydol (tramadol)/oral Zydol with intravenous fentanyl/Co-codamol in day case patients following groin/testicular surgery.* Clinical Research Report No. U90–97–06–029. High Wycombe: Searle.

111. **Melish, D.R. and Minn, F.** 1990: Tramadol hydrochloride; efficacy compared to codeine sulphate, acetaminophen with dextropropoxyphene and placebo in dental extraction pain. *Pain* **40**(suppl. 5), 41.

112. **Thomson, P.J. and Rood, J.P.** 1994: Investigation of pre-operative tramadol in the prevention of post-operative pain for day case surgery. *7th World Congress on pain.* Seattle: IASP Press, 54.

113. **Couthard, P. and Snowdon, A.T.** 1996: The efficacy and safety of postoperative pain management with tramadol for day case surgery. *Ambulatory Surgery* **4**, 25–9.

114. **Lewis, K.S. and Han, N.H.** 1997: Tramadol: a new acting central analgesic. *American Journal of Health and Systemic Pharmacology* **54**(6), 643–52.

115. **Collins, M., Young, I., Sweeney, P.** *et al.* 1997: The effect of tramadol on dento-alveolar surgical pain. *British Journal of Maxillofacial Surgery* **35**(1), 54–8.

116. **Radbruch, L., Grond, S. and Lehmann, K.A.** 1996: A risk-benefit assessment of tramadol in the management of pain. *Drug Safety* **15**(1), 8–29.

117. **Moore, R.A. and McQuay, H.J.** 1997: Single-patient data meta-analysis of 3453 postoperative patients: oral tramadol versus placebo, codeine, and combination analgesics. *Pain* **69**(3), 287–94.

118. **Lomona, J.** 1995: Is tramadol a suitable analgesic for high risk patients after heart surgery? *British Journal of Anaesthesia* **74**(suppl. 2), 7.

119. **James, M.F., Heike, S.A. and Gordon, P.C.** 1996: Intravenous tramadol versus epidural morphine for post thoracotomy pain. *Anesthesia and Analgesia* **83**, 87–91.

120. **Canepa, G., Di-Somma, C., Ghia, M., Vadala, A., Real, M., Cerruti, S., Stasi, M. and Trezzi, P.** 1993: Post-operative analgesia with tramadol. *International Journal of Clinical Pharmacology and Research* **13**, 43–51.

121. **Barsoum, M.W.** 1995: Comparison of the efficacy and tolerability of tramadol, pethidine, and nalbuphine in children with post-operative pain. *Clinical Drug Investigations* **9**, 183–90.

122. **Schaffer, J. and Pipenbrock, S.** 1986: Nalbuphine und tramadol zur postoperativen schmertzkampfung bei kindern. *Anaesthetist* **35**, 408–13.

123. **Schaffer, J. and Hagemann, H.** 1989: Investigation of paediatric postoperative analgesia with tramadol. *Fortschrift Anaesthesiologie* **3**, 42–5.

124. **Bosenberg, A. and Ratcliffe, S.** 1999: Respiratory effects of tramadol in children under halothane anaesthesia. *Anesthesia and Analgesia* (in press).

125. **de Witte, J., Deloof, T., de Veylder, J. and Housemans, P.R.** 1997: Tramadol in the treatment of

postanesthetic shivering. *Acta Anaesthesiologica Scandinavica* **41**(4), 506–10.

126. **Mackin, G.A.** 1997: Medical and pharmacologic management of upper extremity neuropathic pain syndromes. *Journal of Hand Therapy* **10**(2), 96–109.

127. **Osipova, N.A. and Novilov, G.A.** 1991: Analgesic effect of tramadol on cancer patients with chronic pain: a comparison with prolonged action morphine. *Current Therapeutic Research and Clinical Experience* **50**, 812–21.

128. **Wilder-Smith, C.H., Schimke, J., Osterwalde, B. and Senn H.J.** 1994: Oral tramadol, a non-opioid agonist and monoamine reuptake blocker and morphine in strong cancer related pain. *Annals of Oncology* **5**, 141–6.

129. **Grond, S., Zech, D. et al.** 1992: Tramadol – a weak opioid in the relief of cancer pain: a double-blind comparison against sustained release morphine. *Pain Clinics* **5**, 241–7.

130. **Budd, K.** 1994: Chronic pain – challenge and response. *Drugs* **47**(suppl. 1), 33–8.

131. **Pavelka, K., Peliskova, Z. et al.** 1999: Intraindividual differences in pain relief and functional improvement in osteoarthritic patients receiving diclofenac or tramadol. *Annals of Rheumatic Disease* (in press).

132. **Roth, S.** 1998: Efficacy and safety of tramadol hydrochloride in breakthrough osteoarthritic pain. *Journal of Rheumatology* **25**(7): 1358–63.

133. **Rauck, R.L. and Ruoff, G.E.** 1994: Comparison of tramadol and acetaminophen with codeine for long term management in elderly patients. *Current Therapeutic Research and Clinical Experience* **55**, 1417–31.

134. **Price, P.M. and Budd, K.** 1995: Tramadol in the treatment of spinal pain. *British Journal of Medical Economics* **9**, 17–20.

135. **Cossmann, M., Kohnen, C., Langford, R. and McCartney, C.** 1997: Tolerance and safety of tramadol use: results of international studies and data from drug surveillance. *Drugs* **53**(suppl 2), 50–62.

136. **Cossmann, M. and Kohnen, C.** 1995: General tolerability and adverse event profile of tramadol hydrochloride. *Reviews in Contemporary Pharmacotherapeutics* **6**, 513–31.

137. **Cossman, D. and Wilsmann, K.M.** 1987: Wirking und Begleitwerkungen von Tramadol. Offene Phase-IV-Prufung mit 7198 Patienten. *Therapiewoch* **37**, 3475–85.

138. **Ratcliffe, S. and Repas, C.** 1994: A comparison of adverse effects of tramadol in children and adults. *3rd International Symposium of Paediatric Pain*, 182.

139. **Lee, C.R., McTavish, D. and Sorkin, E.M.** 1993: Tramadol: a preliminary review of its pharmacodynamic and pharmacokinetic properties, and therapeutic potential in acute and chronic pain states. *Drugs* **46**, 313–40.

140. **Tarkkila, P., Tuominen, M. and Lindgren, L.** 1998: Comparison of respiratory effects of tramadol and pethidine. *European Journal of Anaesthesiology* **15**, 64–8.

141. **Committee on Safety of Medicines/Medicines Control Agency** 1996: *Current Problems in Pharmacovigilance* **22**, 11.

142. **Spiller, H.A., Gorman, S.E., Villalobos, D. et al.** 1997: Prospective multicenter evaluation of tramadol exposure. *Journal of Toxicology and Clinical Toxicology* **35**(4), 361–4.

143. **Gibson, T.P.** 1996: Pharmacokinetics, efficacy, and safety of analgesia with a focus on tramadol HCL. *American Journal of Medicine* **101**(1A), 47S–53S.

144. **Katz, W.A.** 1996: Pharmacology and clinical experience with tramadol in osteoarthritis. *Drugs* **52**(suppl. 3), 39–47.

145. **Shipton, E.A.** 1997: Remifentanil – a new opioid with a difference. *South African Journal of Anaesthesiology and Analgesia* **3**(2), 1–5.

146. **Thompson, J.P. and Rowbotham, D.J.** 1996: Remifentanil – an opioid for the 21st century. *British Journal of Anaesthesia* **76**(3), 341–3.

147. **Bovill, J.G.** 1996: New drugs. *Current Opinion in Anaesthesiology* **9**, 318–22.

148. **Burkle, H., Dunbar, S. and Van Aken, H.** 1996: Remifentanil: a novel, short-acting, u-opioid. *Anesthesia and Analgesia* **83**, 646–51.

149. **Egan, T.D., Minto, C.F., Hermann, D.J. et al.** 1996: Remifentanil versus alfentanil: comparative pharmacokinetics and pharmacodynamics in healthy adult male volunteers. *Anesthesiology* **84**, 821–33.

150. **Egan, T.D., Minto, C.F., Lemmens, H.J.M. et al.** 1994: Remifentanil versus alfentanil: comparative pharmacodynamics. *Anesthesiology* **81**, 374.

151. **Glass, P.S.A., Hardman, D., Kamiyama, Y. et al.** 1993. Preliminary pharmacokinetics and pharmacodynamics of an ultra-short-acting opioid: remifentanil (GI-87084B). *Anesthesia and Analgesia* **77**, 1030–40.

152. **Egan, T.D.** 1995: Remifentanil pharmacokinetics and pharmacodynamics: a preliminary appraisal. *Clinical Pharmacokinetics* **29**, 80–94.

153. **Rosow, C.E.** 1995: Newer opioid agonists. *Baillière's Clinical Anaesthesiology* **9**, 67–82.

154. **Navapurkar, V.U., Archer, S., Frazer, N.M. et al.** 1995: Pharmacokinetics of remifentanil during hepatic transplantation. *Anesthesiology* **83**, A382.

155. **Davis, P.J., Ross, A., Stiller, R.L. et al.** 1995: Pharmacokinetics of remifentanil in anesthetised children 2–12 years of age. *Anesthesia and Analgesia* **80**, S93.

156. **Davis, P.J., Scierka, M.S., Stiller, R.L. et al.** 1997: In vitro metabolism of remifentanil: the effects of hemodilution. *Anesthesia and Analgesia* **84**, S474.

157. **Kapila, A., Glass, P.S.A., Jacobs, J.R. et al.** 1995: Measured context-sensitive half-times of remifentanil and alfentanil. *Anesthesiology* **83**, 968–75.

158. **Crabb, I., Thornton, C., Konieczko, K.M. et al.** 1996: Remifentanil reduces auditory and somatosensory evoked responses during isoflurane anaesthesia in a dose-dependent manner. *British Journal of Anaesthesia* **76**, 795–801.

159. **Sebel, P.S., Hoke, J.F., Westmoreland, C. et al.** 1995: Histamine concentrations and hemodynamic responses after remifentanil. *Anesthesia and Analgesia* **80**, 990–3.

160. **Baker, K.Z., Ostapkovich, N., Jackson, T. et al.** 1995:

Cerebral blood flow activity is intact during remifentanil/N$_2$O anesthesia. *Anesthesia and Analgesia* **80**, S27.

161. **Hindman, B., Warner, D., Todd, M.** *et al.* 1994: ICP and CPP effects of remifentanil and alfentanil. *Journal of Neurosurgical Anesthesiology* **6**, 304.

162. **Dershwitz, M., Randel, G.I., Rosow, C.E.** *et al.* 1995: Initial clinical experience with remifentanil, a new opioid metabolised by esterases. *Anesthesia and Analgesia* **81**, 619–23.

163. **Kapila, A., Lang, E., Glass, P.** *et al.* 1994: MAC reduction of isoflurane by remifentanil. *Anesthesiology* **81**, A378.

164. **Egan, T.D., Muir, K.T., Stanski, D.R. and Shafer, S.L.** 1996: The EEG versus clinical measures of opioid potency: defining the EEG-clinical potency fingerprint with application to remifentanil. *Anesthesiology* **85**(3A), A349.

165. **Minto, C.F., Schnider, T.W., Egan, T.D.** *et al.* 1997: Influence of age and gender on the pharmacokinetics and pharmacodynamics of remifentanil: I. Model development. *Anesthesiology* **86**, 10–23.

166. **Minto, C.F., Schnider, T.W. and Shafer, S.L.** 1997: Pharmacokinetics and pharmacodynamics of remifentanil: II. Model application. *Anesthesiology* **86**, 24–33.

167. **Philip, B.K., Scuderi, P.E., Chung, F.** *et al.* 1997: Remifentanil compared with alfentanil for ambulatory surgery using total intravenous anesthesia. *Anesthesia and Analgesia* **84**, 515–21.

168. **Sa Rego, M.M., Inagaki, Y. and White, P.F.** 1997: Use of remifentanil during lithotripsy: intermittent boluses vs. continuous infusion. *Anesthesia and Analgesia* **84**, S540.

169. **Gold, M.I., Watkins, W.D. and Sung, Y.F.** 1996: Evaluation of remifentanil vs. remifentanil/midazolam during monitored anesthesia care (MAC). *Anesthesiology* **85**(3A), A4.

170. **Royston, D., Kirkham, A., Adt, M.** *et al.* 1996: Remifentanil based total intravenous anesthesia (TIVA) in primary CABG surgery patients: use as a sole induction agent and hemodynamic responses throughout surgery. *Anesthesiology* **85**(3A), A83.

171. **Smith, I., Avramov, M. and White, P.F.** 1995: Remifentanil versus propofol for monitored anesthesia care-effects on ventilation. *Anesthesiology* **83**, A4.

172. **Hughes, S.C., Kan, R.E., Rosen, M.A.** *et al.* 1996: Remifentanil: ultra-short acting opioid for obstetric anesthesia. *Anesthesiology* **85**(3A), A894.

173. **Shulman, M., Ivankovich, A.D., Braverman, B. and Lubenow, T.R.** 1991: Treatment of chronic intractable back pain with injection of a 10% butamen suspension. *Anesthesiology* **75**(3A), A739.

174. **Shipton, E.A.** 1997: Ropivacaine – an advance over bupivacaine? *South African Journal of Anaesthesiology and Analgesia* **3**(1), 1–2.

175. **Schug, S.A., Scott, D.A., Payne, J., Mooney, P.H. and Hagglof, B.** 1996: Postoperative analgesia by continuous extradural infusion of ropivacaine after upper abdominal surgery. *British Journal of Anaesthesia* **76**, 487–91.

176. **McClure, J.H.** 1996: Ropivacaine. *British Journal of Anaesthesia* **76**, 300–7.

177. **Markham, A. and Faulds, D.** 1996: Ropivacaine – a review of its pharmacology and therapeutic use in regional anaesthesia. *Drugs* **52**(3), 429–49.

178. **Pitkanen, M., Feldman, H.S., Arthur, G.R. and Covino, B.G.** 1992: Chronotropic and inotropic effects of ropivacaine, bupivacaine, and lidocaine in the spontaneously beating and electrically paced isolated, perfused rabbit heart. *Regional Anesthesia* **17**, 183–92.

179. **Reitz, S., Haggmark, S., Johansson, G. and Nath, S.** 1989: Cardiotoxicity of ropivacaine – a new amide local anaesthetic agent. *Acta Anaesthesiologica Scandinavica* **33**, 93.

180. **Moller, R. and Covino, B.G.** 1990: Cardiac electrophysiologic properties of bupivacaine and lidocaine compared with those of ropivacaine, a new amide local anaesthetic. *Anesthesiology* **72**, 322.

181. **Arlock, P.** 1988: Actions of three local anaesthetics, lidocaine, bupivacaine and ropivacaine, on guinea pig papillary muscle sodium channels (V$_{max}$). *Pharmacology and Toxicology* **63**, 96.

182. **Chan, V.** 1998: Advances in regional anaesthesia and pain management. *Canadian Journal of Anaesthesia* **45**(5), R49–R57.

183. **Feldman, H.S., Arthur, G.R. and Covino, B.G.** 1989: Comparative systemic toxicity of convulsant and supraconvulsant doses of intravenous ropivacaine, bupivacaine, and lidocaine in the conscious dog. *Anesthesia and Analgesia* **69**, 794–801.

184. **Turner, G., Blake, D., Buckland, M.** *et al.* Continuous extradural infusion of ropivacaine for prevention of postoperative pain after major orthopaedic surgery. *British Journal of Anaesthesia* **76**, 606–10.

185. **Nolte, H., Fruhstorfer, H. and Edstrom, H.H.** 1990: Local anaesthetic efficacy of ropivacaine (LEA 103) in ulnar nerve block. *Regional Anesthesia* **15**, 118–24.

186. **Kopacz, D.J., Emanuelsson, B.M., Thompson, G.E., Carpenter, R.L. and Stephenson, C.A.** 1994: Pharmacokinetics of ropivacaine and bupivacaine for bilateral intercostal blockade in healthy male volunteers. *Anesthesiology* **81**, 1139–48.

187. **Zaric, D., Nydahl, P.A., Philipson, L., Samuelsson, L., Heierson, A. and Axelsson, K.** 1996: The effect of continuous lumbar epidural infusion of ropivacaine (0.1%, 0.2%, and 0.3%) and 0.25% bupivacaine on sensory and motor block in volunteers. *Regional Anesthesia* **21**(1), 14–25.

188. **Scott, D.A., Emanuelsson, B., Mooney, P.H., Cook, R.J. and Junestrand, C.** 1997: Long term epidural ropivacaine infusion for postoperative analgesia. *Anesthesia and Analgesia* **85**(6), 1322–30.

189. **Scott, D.A., Chamley, D.M., Mooney, P.H., Deam, R.K., Mark, A.H. and Hagglof, B.** 1995: Epidural ropivacaine infusion for postoperative analgesia after

lower abdominal surgery – a dose finding study. *Anesthesia and Analgesia* **81**, 982–6.

190. **Muldoon, T., Milligan, K., Quinn, P. and Connolly, J.D.R.** 1996: Analgesia and motor block during postoperative epidural infusion of ropivacaine or bupivacaine at equal doses after total knee replacement. *Anesthesiology* **85**(3A), A747.

191. **McCrae, A.F., Jozwiak, H. and McClure, J.H.** 1995: Comparison of ropivacaine and bupivacaine in extradural analgesia for the relief of pain in labour. *British Journal of Anaesthesia* **74**, 261–5.

192. **Stienstra, R., Jonker, T.A., Bourdrez, P., Kuijpers, J.C., Van Kleef, K.W. and Lundberg, U.** 1995: Ropivacaine 0.25% versus bupivacaine 0.25% for continuous epidural analgesia in labor: a double-blind comparison. *Anesthesia and Analgesia* **80**, 285–9.

193. **Alahuhta, S., Rasanen, J., Jouppila, P. *et al.*** 1995: The effects of epidural ropivacaine and bupivacaine for cesarean section on uteroplacental and fetal circulation. *Anesthesiology* **83**, 23–32.

194. **Datta, S., Camann, W., Bader, A. and Van der Burgh, L.** 1995: Clinical effects and maternal and fetal plasma concentrations of epidural ropivacaine versus bupivacaine for cesarean section. *Anesthesiology* **82**, 1346–52.

195. **Griffin, R.P. and Reynolds, F.** 1995: Extradural anaesthesia for caesarean section: a double blind comparison of 0.5% ropivacaine with 0.5% bupivacaine. *British Journal of Anaesthesia* **74**, 512–16.

196. **Morton, C.P.J., Bloomfield, S., Magnusson, A., Jozwiak, H. and McClure, J.H.** 1995: Ropivacaine 0.75% for epidural anaesthesia in elective Caesarean section: an open clinical and pharmacokinetic study in mother and neonate. *International Monitor on Regional Anaesthesia*, A28.

197. **Serrao, J.M., Stubbs, S.C., Goodchild, C.S. and Gent, J.P.** 1989: Intrathecal midazolam and fentanyl in the rat: evidence for different spinal antinociceptive effects. *Anesthesiology* **70**, 780–6.

198. **Edwards, M., Serrao, J.M., Gent, J.P. and Goodchild, C.S.** 1990: On the mechanism by which midazolam causes spinally mediated analgesia. *Anesthesiology* **73**, 273–7.

199. **Rosland, J.H. and Hole, K.** 1990: 1,4-Benzodiazepines antagonise opiate-induced antinociception in mice. *Anesthesia and Analgesia* **71**, 242–8.

200. **Clavier, N., Lombard, M.C. and Besson, J.M.** 1992: Benzodiazepines and pain: effects of midazolam on the activities of nociceptive non-specific dorsal horn neurons in the rat spinal cord. *Pain* **48**, 61–71.

201. **Shipton, E.A., Minkowitz, H.S. and Becker, P.** 1993: Patient-controlled analgesia in burn injuries: the subcutaneous route. *Canadian Journal of Anaesthesia* **40**, 898.

202. **Shipton, E.A.** 1996: The relief of acute pain. *South African Journal of Surgery* **34**(1), 40–3.

203. **Shipton, E.A.** 1996: Modern use of neuraxial opioids in acute pain. *South African Journal of Surgery* **34**(4), 180–5.

204. **Irwing, G., Allwood, C.W., Levin, V. and Shipton, E.** 1996: Cancer pain: a South African perspective. In Parris, W. (ed.) *Cancer pain management: principles and practice.* Newton: Butterworth-Heinemann, 561–6.

205. **Shipton, E.A.** 1994: Technological advances in regional anaesthesia. *South African Medical Journal* **84**, 128–9.

206. **Shipton, E.A.** 1994: Management of intractable pain. *Medicine Today* **5**(4), 12–19.

207. **Shipton, E.A.** 1994: The management of intractable pain – treating cause the fundamental principle. *Medicine Today* **5**(3), 14–16.

208. **Alexander-Williams, J.M. and Rowbotham, D.J.** 1998: Novel routes of opioid administration. *British Journal of Anaesthesia* **81**, 3–7.

209. **Gutsche, B.B.** 1995: Spinal and epidural anaesthesia for obstetrics. *American Society of Anesthesiologists Annual Refresher Course Lectures* **236**, 1–7.

210. **Morgan, P.** 1995: Spinal anaesthesia in obstetrics. *Canadian Journal of Anaesthesia* **42**(12), 1145–63.

211. **Rubinow, A.** 1998: Pain of osteoarthritis and its management. Rheumatic pain. *Newsletter of the IASP Special Interest Group on Rheumatic Pain* (Jul), 1–5.

212. **Hirst, R.A., Lambert, D.G. and Notcutt, W.G.** 1998: Pharmacology and the potential therapeutic uses of cannabis. *British Journal of Anaesthesia* **81**, 77–84.

213. **Zeidman, S.M. and North, R.B.** 1994: General neurosurgical procedures for management of chronic pain. In Raj, P.P. (ed.) *Current review of pain.* Korea: Sung in Printing Company, 103–16.

214. **Breitbart, W., Rosenfeld, B. and Passik, S.D.** 1998: The Network Project: a multidisciplinary cancer education and training program in pain management, rehabilitation, and psychosocial issues. *Journal of Pain and Symptom Management* **16**(1), 18–26.

215. **Latimer, E.J., Crabb, M.R., Roberts, J.G., Ewen, M. and Roberts, J.** 1998: The patient care travelling record in palliative care: effectiveness and efficiency. *Journal of Pain and Symptom Management* **16**(1), 41–51.

216. **Papantonio, C.** 1998: Alternative medicine and wound healing. *Ostomy Wound Management* **44**(4), 44–6.

217. **Wainapel, S.F., Thomas, A.D. and Kahan, B.S.** 1998: Use of alternative therapies by rehabilitation outpatients. *Archives of Physical and Medical Rehabilitation* **79**(8), 1003–5.

218. **Drivdahl, C.E. and Miser, W.F.** 1998: The use of alternative health care by a family practice population. *Journal of the American Board of Family Practitioners* **11**(3), 193–9.

219. **Astin, J.A.** 1998: Why patients use alternative medicine: results of a national study. *Journal of the American Medical Association* **279**(19), 1548–53.

220. **Astin, J.A.** 1997: Stress reduction through mindfulness meditation. Effects on psychological symptomatology, sense of control, and spiritual experiences. *Psychotherapy and Psychosomatics* **66**(2), 97–106.

221. **Lindholm, L. and Eriksson, K.** 1993: To understand and alleviate suffering in a caring culture. *Journal of Advanced Nursing* **18**(9), 1354–61.

222. **Taylor, L.K., Kuttler, K.L., Parks, T.A. and Milton, D.** 1998: The effect of music in the postanesthesia care unit on pain levels in women who have had abdominal hysterectomies. *Journal of Perianesthetic Nursing* **13**(2), 84–88.

223. **Good, M. and Chin, C.C.** 1998: The effects of Western music on postoperative pain in Taiwan. *Kao Hsiung I Hsueh Ko Hsueh Tsa Chih* **14**(2), 94–103.

224. **Field, T., Peck, M., Krugman, S. *et al.*** 1998: Burn injuries benefit from massage therapy. *Journal of Burn Care and Rehabilitation* **19**(3), 241–4.

225. **Howdyshell, C.** 1998: Complementary therapy: aromatherapy with massage for geriatric and hospice care – a call for an holistic approach. *Hospice Journal* **13**(3), 69–75.

226. **Alden, P. and Heap, M.** 1998: Hypnotic pain control: some theoretical and practical issues. *International Journal of Clinical and Experimental Hypnosis* **46**(1), 62–76.

227. **Crawford, H.J., Knebel, T., Kaplan, L. *et al.*** 1998: Hypnotic analgesia: 1. Somatosensory event-related potential changes to noxious stimuli. 2. Transfer learning to reduce chronic low back pain. *International Journal of Clinical and Experimental Hypnosis* **46**(1), 92–132.

228. **Danziger, N., Fournier, E., Bouhassira, D. *et al.*** 1998: Different strategies of modulation can be operative during hypnotic analgesia: a neurophysiological study. *Pain* **75**(1), 85–92.

229. **Clark, A.J.M.** 1995: Chronic pain – anything new? *Canadian Journal of Anaesthesia* **42**(5), R55–R61.

230. **Loeser, J.D.** 1997: The future of pain management. In Jain, S. (ed.) *Current concepts in acute, chronic, and cancer pain management.* New York: World Foundation for Pain Relief and Research, 449–55.

231. **Macrae, W.A., Davies, H.T.O. and Crombie, I.K.** 1992: Pain: paradigms and treatments. *Pain* **49**, 289–91.

232. **Shipton, E.A.** 1992: The spinal route – quo vadis? *South African Medical Journal* **81**, 1–3.

233. **Orne, M.T.** 1992: Non pharmacological approaches to pain relief: hypnosis, biofeedback, placebo effects. In Aronoff, G.M. (ed.) *Evaluation and treatment of chronic pain.* Baltimore: Williams & Wilkins, 430–9.

INDEX

Numbers in **bold** refer to figures